Medical, Surgical and Anesthetic Nursing for Veterinary Technicians

(formerly *Medical Nursing for Animal Health Technicians*)

2nd Edition

Edited by
Paul W. Pratt, VMD

Production Manager: Elisabeth S. Stein
Production Assistant: Matthew B. Davidson
Cover Illustration: Michele McCrea Wallentin

American Veterinary Publications, Inc.
5782 Thornwood Drive
Goleta, CA 93117

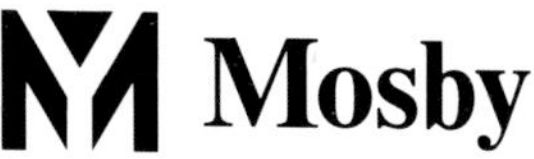

St. Louis Baltimore Boston Carlsbad Chicago Naples New York Philadelphia Portland
London Madrid Mexico City Singapore Sydney Tokyo Toronto Wiesbaden

97 98 99 00 01 02 / 9 8 7 6 5 4 3

ISBN 0-939674-49-1

Library of Congress Catalog Card Number: 94-70822

Printed and Bound in the United States of America

Authors

Wilbur A. Aanes, DVM, MS
Professor
College of Veterinary Medicine
Colorado State University
Fort Collins, CO 80523

Ahmad R. Abdullahi, DVM
Resident
College of Veterinary Medicine
North Carolina State University
Raleigh, NC 27606

R. Allen, Jr.
General Manager
Silver Creek Ranch
2500 East Valley Road
Montecito, CA 93108

G.J. Benson, DVM, MS, Dipl ACVA
Professor
Department of Veterinary Clinical Medicine
College of Veterinary Medicine
University of Illinois
Urbana, IL 61801

Colin C. Bullmore, DVM
Hamlin Pet Clinic
RR5, Box 5273
Moscow, PA 18444

Joann Colville, DVM
Department of Veterinary and Microbiological Sciences
North Dakota State University
Fargo, ND 58105

Thomas P. Colville, DVM, MSc
Director, Veterinary Technology
Department of Veterinary and Microbiological Sciences
North Dakota State University
Fargo, ND 58105

Laura A. Downey, DVM
Community Practice Clinician
School of Veterinary Medicine
Purdue University
West Lafayette, IN 47907

Karl Faler, MA
4411 Lacey Boulevard
Lacey, WA 98503

Kate Faler, DVM
4411 Lacey Boulevard
Lacey, WA 98503

Cynthia S. Intravartolo, RVT
Berwyn Animal Hospital
2845 South Harlem Avenue
Berwyn, IL 60402

Linda R. Krcatovich, LVT
Veterinary Technician
Food Animal Department
Veterinary Teaching Hospital
Michigan State University
East Lansing, MI 48823

Kristine A. Kazmierczak, RVT
Department of Small Animal Clinics
College of Veterinary Medicine
Purdue University
West Lafayette, IN 47907

Charles R. Kuhn, MS
2445 Sycamore Glen Drive
Sparks, NV 89431

Ann M. Lamar, LVT
Veterinary Technician
Veterinary Teaching Hospital
Michigan State University
East Lansing, MI 48823

Hui-Chu Lin, DVM, MS
Assistant Professor
Large Animal Surgery and Medicine
College of Veterinary Medicine
Auburn University, AL 36849

Pam Phegley, RVT
Department of Veterinary Clinical Sciences
School of Veterinary Medicine
Purdue University
West Lafayette, IN 47907

Mimi Porter, MS
Equine Therapist
4350 Harrodsburg Road
Lexington, KY 40513

J. Catharine Scott-Moncrieff, VMB, MA, MS, Dipl ACVIM
Department of Veterinary Clinical Sciences
School of Veterinary Medicine
Purdue University
West Lafayette, IN 47907

C.H. "Skip" Tangner, DVM, MS, Dipl ACVS
Animal Surgical Clinic
2915 NW 122
Oklahoma City, OK 73120

J.C. Thurmon, DVM, MS, Dipl ACVA
Professor
Department of Veterinary Clinical Medicine
College of Veterinary Medicine
University of Illinois
Urbana, IL 61801

Steven D. Van Camp, DVM, Dipl ACT
Associate Professor
College of Veterinary Medicine
North Carolina State University
Raleigh, NC 27606

John T. Vaughan, DVM
Dean
College of Veterinary Medicine
Auburn University, AL 36849

Carrie B. Waters, DVM
Department of Veterinary Biomedical Sciences
College of Veterinary Medicine
University of Missouri
Columbus, MO 65211

Preface

In the 9 years since publication of the first edition of this book, veterinary practice has changed dramatically, not only in technical advances, but also in the way veterinary technicians are employed. In years past, technicians were largely underused and sometimes considered merely an extra set of hands to be used in restraining animals during treatment. Today, veterinary technicians have become an indispensable part of the veterinary health care team. Their education encompasses the many complexities of veterinary care and includes most of the areas studied by veterinary students. In practice, technicians now perform many of the diagnostic and treatment procedures formerly done only by veterinarians.

This book describes many of the clinical procedures performed by technicians in veterinary practice. Its title has been revised in keeping with the trend toward standardization of the title *veterinary technician,* and also to reflect the book's greatly expanded content.

I am grateful to our group of highly qualified authors for sharing their expertise and clinical experience with our readers. Their contributions will help technicians provide superior care for their veterinary patients.

Paul W. Pratt, VMD
Editor

Contents

1

First Aid

J. Colville

First aid is the emergency care and treatment of a patient with an injury or sudden illness before definitive medical and surgical care is available. The primary objectives of first aid are to keep the animal alive until it can be seen by the veterinarian and to make the animal comfortable.

Legal and Ethical Considerations

Much can be done by a veterinary technician knowledgeable in first-aid techniques to help an animal in an emergency situation. Prompt first aid often means the difference between life and death for a badly injured or severely ill animal.

In providing first aid to an animal in the absence of a veterinarian, however, a technician must be careful not to overstep his or her legal and ethical limitations. What a veterinary technician is legally entitled to do varies with the laws of each state or province. In general, offering a diagnosis, prescribing medications and performing even what could loosely be described as surgery should be scrupulously avoided without the supervision and/or advice of a veterinarian. This prevents potential legal difficulties for the veterinary technician and veterinarian if an inappropriate or unsuccessful treatment is administered. Also, it maximizes the animal's chances of recovery by preventing the potentially disastrous effects of misdiagnosis under the pressure of an emergency situation. Finally, technicians will avoid undertaking procedures or administering medications for which they are not qualified by training or experience.

When a veterinary technician is confronted with a medical emergency and the veterinarian is not immediately available, it is better to apply basic first aid designed to improve the animal's chances of survival than to undertake drastic actions that could make the situation worse.

When emergencies occur with the veterinarian available, veterinary technicians may work as part of an emergency care team, with specific individual duties. In these cases a veterinarian is present to make critical decisions. This chapter is directed primarily to situations when a veterinarian is *not* immediately available and the veterinary technician must administer first aid until the veterinarian arrives.

Transporting Injured Animals

Veterinary technicians may be called upon to provide clients with information on how to transport injured animals. The goal in transporting an injured animal is to get it to a veterinary facility as quickly as possible without making its condition any worse or causing injuries to the people trying to help it. This is accomplished by taking a moment to think about how the injured animal can be transported most safely before attempting to move it.

Injured or severely ill animals are often in pain and may act out of instinct. Avoiding personal injury must be an important concern of anyone attempting to attend to such an animal. Taking such precautions as applying a gauze, rope or necktie muzzle to a dog, handling a small dog or cat through a towel or blanket, and avoiding the powerful hooves of an injured large animal indirectly benefits the animal while maintaining human safety.

Often an animal's condition can be stabilized somewhat before attempting transport. Controlling hemorrhage, applying a temporary splint to a fracture, or hosing down a victim of heatstroke are all procedures a veterinary technician or an owner can do. Talking over the telephone with a person who has an injured animal often allows a veterinary technician to advise on how to best handle the animal for transport to the clinic.

Large animals usually can be transported only in a trailer or truck. Some advance planning can often make a great deal of difference in the animal's condition on arrival at the veterinary clinic. The animal should be well bedded for cushioning if it is recumbent. Also, it should be adequately restrained with ropes and/or panels to prevent further injury during transport.

Small animals may be carefully carried in the arms or in a box or basket if their injuries and/or disposition allow it. Animals with suspected spinal injuries, with extensive trauma, or those that are unconscious are best transported on a blanket, or preferably on a rigid platform, such as a board or even a wooden or screen door. If necessary the animal can be secured to the makeshift stretcher with belts or ropes to ensure minimal movement during transport.

Initial Examination and Management

Usually there is no time to obtain a detailed history or perform a thorough physical examination when presented with an acutely injured or ill animal. Often the situation dictates that first-aid treatment for obvious life-threatening conditions be carried out as the animal is being examined for further, less obvious or urgent injuries.

In an emergency situation an animal must be examined quickly and decisions made logically on how best to carry out the basic objectives of first aid. The most serious, life-threatening conditions must be considered before attention is turned to other matters. Remember that emergency patients are not just a fractured leg or a large burn, but entire animals whose overall well-being must be the overriding concern in rendering first aid.

Priorities

Stay Calm: In an emergency situation there is a natural tendency for one to become excited and try to do everything at once. Also there is the tendency to panic and become incapable of doing anything useful. To aid a severely injured or ill animal, a veterinary technician must maintain a clear head and be able to think logically in assessing the situation and formulating a first-aid plan.

Notify the Veterinarian as Soon as Possible: First aid is of great benefit to the patient and may well save its life, but the patient should receive the more complete care that only a veterinarian can provide. Depending on the perceived severity of the situation, the veterinarian may be notified of a pending emergency while the veterinary technician is waiting for the patient to arrive.

Ensure Your Own Safety: Be certain that the animal is adequately restrained for your own protection and to prevent further injury to the animal.

Evaluate the Patient: Perform an orderly initial evaluation of the patient so that you are not distracted from unseen problems by obvious problems. If you follow a strict protocol with each animal you evaluate, you are less likely to overlook something important. The evaluation recommended below can be done in a minute or less.

View the animal from a distance to assess the level of consciousness, abnormal body or limb positioning, presence of blood anywhere on or near the animal, and breathing patterns.

Approach the animal from behind to assess its awareness of movement and any reaction to the movement.

Ensure Adequate Respiration: Note the color of the mucous membranes. Listen to the breathing sounds. If necessary, clear the airway of debris or fluid. This usually involves moving the tongue. You may have to use suction, if available, to remove fluid or mucus. Intubate the trachea if necessary. Check for blood in the nose or mouth. Capillary refill time can be assessed at the same time.

Stop Hemorrhage: Though minor bleeding can be temporarily ignored, major hemorrhage should be controlled with pressure or tourniquets. Clamping exposed major vessels with hemostats may be the only way to stop some major hemorrhages.

Treat for Shock if Necessary: (This will be discussed later.)

Proceed with Further Examination and First-Aid Treatment: After your initial assessment and treatment for altered vital signs, you can proceed in a less urgent manner.

Equipment and Supplies

The needs for first-aid equipment and supplies vary from clinic to clinic, but the following list includes items that typically are very useful. These items should be kept together in an emergency treatment "ready" area or on a "crash cart." Make sure the area/cart is fully stocked at all times, especially after it has been used. In some clinics the cart is checked daily to make sure all necessary drugs and equipment are present.

Baking soda
Bandaging materials (gauze pads, roll cotton, roll gauze, tape)
Blankets, towels
10% dextrose
Endotracheal tubes, various sizes
Examination gloves
Forceps for removing foreign bodies
Hemostats
Hydrogen peroxide
Ice
Lemon juice or vinegar
Oxygen
Sterile, isotonic saline
Stethoscope
Stomach tubes, various sizes

Table salt
Thermometer
Tourniquet
Towel clamps
Water-soluble lubricant (*eg,* K-Y Jelly)

Species Considerations

Because various animal species are cared for in veterinary hospitals, it is important to evaluate each animal in the context of what is normal and desirable for its species. For example, a healthy horse may lose a liter of blood without severe consequences, while loss of a relatively small amount of blood can be fatal for a parakeet.

The methods for handling animals, particularly in an emergency situation, must be appropriate for the species. Large animals, such as horses and cattle, usually cannot be restrained by strictly physical means because of their strength and size. Squeeze chutes and stocks are often needed, along with ropes and halters. Small animals, such as dogs and cats, can usually be restrained manually, though muzzles, towels, blankets and leashes are often needed.

The safety of the personnel working on an animal, as well as that of the animal itself, is an important consideration in any procedure undertaken. The steps necessary to ensure safety and to facilitate efficiency must be carefully planned and executed, and must be appropriate for the species being treated.

FIRST AID FOR SPECIFIC CONDITIONS

Shock

Signs

- Weakness and/or unconsciousness
- Pale mucous membranes
- Cool skin and extremities
- Rapid heart rate
- Weak pulse
- Shallow, rapid breathing
- Poor capillary refill

First Aid

- Maintain respiration
- Control bleeding
- Keep warm
- Position with the head lowered
- Monitor pulse and administer CPR if necessary

The term *shock* is used to describe a very complex and dangerous clinical syndrome. It is generally characterized by inadequate perfusion of blood to tissues by the cardiovascular system. This results in cellular hypoxia. If uncorrected, hypoxia can lead to cell death, which, on a massive scale, can have disastrous and frequently fatal consequences.

Cause

There are many potential causes of shock, including:

- *Decreased blood volume,* usually resulting from severe loss of blood or plasma, as seen with severe hemorrhage. Decreased blood volume can be from external hemorrhage that is readily apparent, internal hemorrhage, which is more difficult to ascertain, or severe loss of plasma from such serious external lesions as extensive burns.
- *Severe stress,* either physical or psychological. Such things as extensive traumatic injuries or severe pain can be inciting causes of shock.
- *Infection* with certain toxin-producing bacteria. Some of these bacterial toxins affect blood vessels, causing blood to "pool" in certain areas of the circulatory system. This in turn can cause a consequent precipitous drop in blood pressure.
- *Abnormal cardiac function.* Conditions that seriously interfere with the normal pumping action of the heart, such as severe heart failure, myocarditis, cardiopathy or severe arrhythmias, can cause shock.

Pathophysiology

When there is a considerable drop in blood pressure, the body attempts to compensate and maintain circulatory function. The heart rate and force of contraction increase. Peripheral arteries and veins constrict. Blood is redistributed in an attempt to maintain the blood supply to the brain and heart at the expense of the peripheral circulation. Blood flow to peripheral areas, such as the skin, muscles, intestines and kidneys, is decreased, with resulting hypoxia of these tissues. Anaerobic cellular metabolism, resulting from this hypoxia, produces increased amounts of lactic acid, upsetting the delicate acid-base balance of the body and resulting in acidosis. Damage to organs, such as the intestines and kidneys, can be severe.

If the blood supply to the brain is reduced, changes in the level of consciousness are seen. These changes range from excitement to unconsciousness.

Clinical Signs

The signs of shock are related to the body's attempts to maintain cardiovascular function through changes in cardiac function and redistribution of blood to the vital organs. Signs of shock include:

- *Pale mucous membranes.* This can best be evaluated at the gingivae, conjunctivae and the inner aspect of the vulva or prepuce.
- *Coolness of the skin and extremities*
- *Increased heart rate*
- *Weak pulse*
- *Shallow, rapid breathing*
- *Poor capillary refill.* To evaluate capillary refill, apply sufficient pressure to an unpigmented area of the gingivae with a finger to cause the area to turn white. Upon releasing the pressure, the normal pink color should return within 1-2 seconds. A refill time longer than 2 seconds indicates poor peripheral circulation.
- *Weakness and/or unconsciousness*

First Aid

Maintain respiration by keeping the respiratory passages clear, administering oxygen if possible, and giving artificial respiration if needed. Impaired respiration contributes to the hypoxia already present in the animal.

Control bleeding to help prevent a further decrease in the circulating blood volume and oxygen-carrying capacity.

Keep the animal warm with blankets, water recirculating blankets, towels and/or hot water bottles (wrapped in towels to prevent burning).

Evaluate peripheral perfusion by comparing the toe web temperature with the rectal temperature. Place a thermometer probe between any 2 hind limb toes. Stabilize it with a light dressing. Record the toe web and rectal temperatures simultaneously. Normally the toe web temperature is less than 7 F lower than the rectal temperature. If the difference is greater than 10 F, the animal is in shock. A difference of greater than 20 F indicates deep shock.

Position the animal with the head slightly lower than the rest of the body to help maintain blood supply to the brain.

Monitor the pulse. If cardiac arrest occurs, administer cardiopulmonary resuscitation (CPR).

Cardiac Arrest

Signs

- Unconsciousness
- Lack of respiration
- Lack of pulse
- Lack of heartbeat

First Aid

- Artificial respiration (15-20/minute)
- Cardiac massage (60/minute)

Cardiac arrest is the cessation of effective heart function. It usually occurs as either *ventricular fibrillation,* in which the heart "quivers" randomly, or as *asystole,* in which the heart becomes "limp" and stops all activity. In either case the circulation of blood stops, depriving the tissues, especially the brain, of needed oxygen. This hypoxic brain damage is generally reversible if circulation is restored within 3-4 minutes. After this period, irreversible brain damage is likely to have occurred. Even if circulation is eventually restored after 3-4 minutes, the animal's behavior and/or function will probably not return to normal.

It is vital to *act immediately* in a case of cardiac arrest if there is to be any chance of recovery.

Clinical Signs

Clinical signs of cardiac arrest include unconsciousness, lack of respiration, lack of pulse and lack of a detectable heartbeat.

Cardiopulmonary Resuscitation

Without special equipment, cardiopulmonary resuscitation (CPR) usually is not effective in large animals, such as horses and cattle, because of their size. This discussion, therefore, deals with animals small enough (dogs and cats primarily) for effective CPR to be carried out by 1 or 2 people without special equipment.

CPR consists of *artificial respiration* and *external cardiac massage.* The basic underlying cause of irreversible brain damage from cardiac arrest is cerebral hypoxia. Reestablishing circulation does little or no good if the blood being circulated is not adequately oxygenated. Also, without adequate ventilation, carbon dioxide levels in the blood rise rapidly and the animal becomes severely acidotic, compounding the problem. Establishing adequate ventilation through artificial respiration is vital to effective CPR.

Artificial Respiration: To perform artificial respiration, intubate the animal with an endotracheal tube, if possible. Inflate the cuff (if present), and artificially ventilate the animal at the rate of 15-20 breaths/minute by blowing into the end of the tube, using an Ambu resuscitation bag, or by connecting the tube to an inhalant anesthesia machine. Be sure the anesthetic vaporizer is turned off and the pop-off valve is closed. With pure oxygen flowing, compress the rebreathing bag. If endotracheal intubation is impossible, cup your hands tightly around the muzzle and ventilate by blowing into the nose 15-20 times/minute (Fig 1).

Regardless of what artificial respiration technique is applied, after inflating the lungs for each breath, release all pressure completely and allow the lungs to deflate passively before administering the next breath. This release of pressure is important for adequate respiratory gas exchange and to allow return of blood to the heart via the large veins in the thorax.

External Cardiac Massage: The valves of the heart allow one-way blood flow only. If the heart can be compressed rhythmically by applying pressure to the thorax over the heart, the valves open and blood flows in the appropriate direction. This is the principle of external cardiac massage.

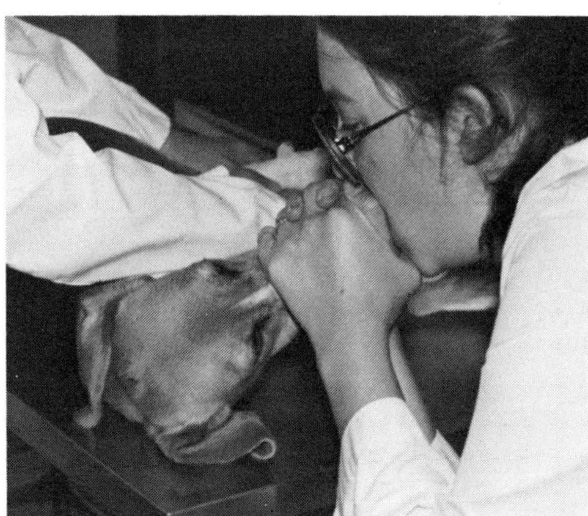

Figure 1. Artificial respiration is given by cupping the hands around the muzzle and blowing into the nares.

The heart is most efficiently massaged by compressing the thorax, as this is the narrowest dimension of the thorax in most dogs and cats. With the animal in lateral recumbency and the foreleg in a position as though the animal were standing, compression is applied to the area of the thorax underlying the elbow. In very small animals, the chest can be compressed between the fingers and thumb of one hand (Fig 2). In medium-sized animals, compression can be accomplished with one hand on each side of the thorax (Fig 3). In larger animals, compression is best applied from the top by compressing the chest between the hands and the tabletop or floor (Fig 4).

Compress for a count of 2 and release for a count of 1, at a rate of 60 compressions/minute. The effectiveness of cardiac massage

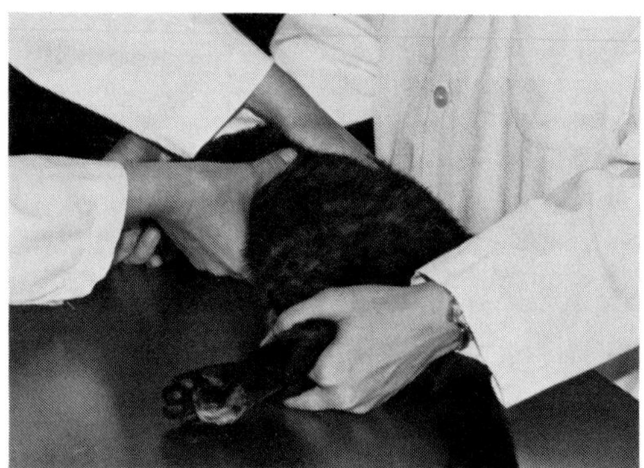

Figure 2. External cardiac massage is applied to cats or other small animals by compressing the chest between the fingers and thumb.

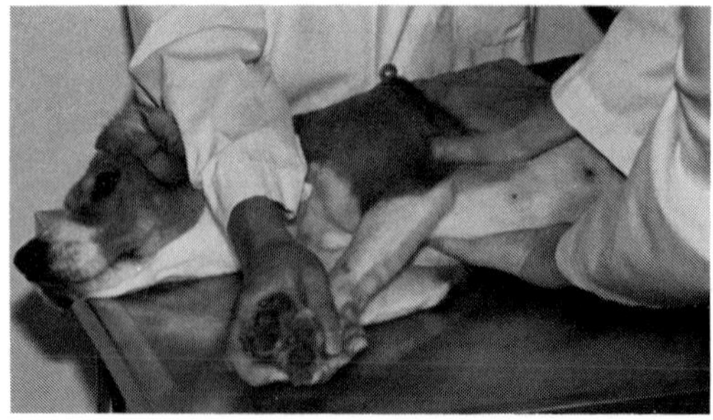

Figure 3. External cardiac massage is applied to a medium-sized dog by compressing the animal's chest between the hands.

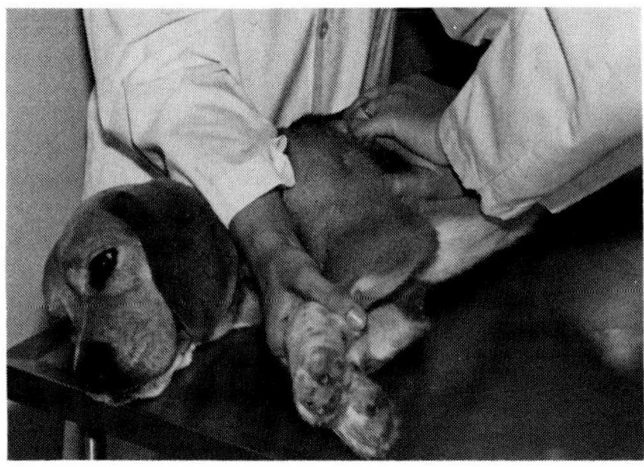

Figure 4. External cardiac massage is applied to larger animals by compressing the chest between the tabletop and hands.

can be evaluated by having someone else palpate for a pulse wave during each chest compression.

The ratio of respirations to chest compressions should be about 1 respiration to each 4 chest compressions. Check periodically to see if a spontaneous heartbeat and breathing have resumed. If they have not, continue CPR until a veterinarian can examine the animal.

Hemorrhage

Signs

- Arterial blood (bright red, spurts rhythmically)
- Venous blood (dark red, flows freely without spurting)
- Capillary blood (oozes into wound without much pressure)

First Aid

- Apply pressure
- Apply a tourniquet if necessary
- Treat for shock if necessary

Cause

Hemorrhage, the escape of blood from damaged blood vessels, can cause serious problems. Profuse hemorrhage can decrease the circulating blood volume sufficiently to cause shock. Hemorrhage that is not severe enough to cause shock may still cause tissue hypoxia, which can stress the animal and compound other concurrent problems. Even mild hemorrhage can delay wound healing and contribute to development of infection, as blood is an excellent medium for bacterial growth.

Hemorrhage can occur from individual blood vessels (arteries, veins or capillaries) or from groups of vessels. Hemorrhage from arteries generally is the most serious, while capillary hemorrhage generally is the least serious. Arterial bleeding is characterized by bright red blood that spurts under considerable pressure in time with the pulse. Blood escaping from veins is dark red and flows freely without spurting. Capillary blood oozes into a wound without much pressure.

First Aid

Hemostasis is the arrest of hemorrhage. In first aid, hemostasis is usually accomplished by applying pressure directly to the hemorrhaging area or by applying a tourniquet or pressure directly to the wound to slow the flow of blood through hemorrhaging vessels. Tourniquets are applied either above or below the wound depending on if it's arterial (above) or venous (below) blood.

Pressure can be applied by direct digital pressure or with a pressure bandage. Direct digital pressure is very effective and involves placing a clean cloth over the wound and applying pressure. If no cloth is available, effective pressure can be applied directly with the fingers.

A *pressure bandage* is a bandage firmly applied over a clean cloth on the wound. It must not, however, be applied so tightly as to cause damage from impaired circulation. Incorporating something bulky, such as a small gauze roll, rolled-up gauze sponges or crumbled pieces of cloth or paper, into the bandage over the wound helps apply direct pressure to the hemorrhaging area (Figs 5, 6).

A *tourniquet* can be a commercially available rubber or fabric one or made from roll gauze, a necktie or a belt. It can temporarily help reduce bleeding from an extremity while a pressure bandage is applied. It also can be helpful in combination with pressure for very serious bleeding. On a limb it should be applied proximal to the wound to help control arterial hemorrhage or distal to the wound to control venous hemorrhage.

Though a tourniquet can be a great aid in hemostasis if used properly, it also can cause serious damage if improperly applied. It should be applied tightly enough to slow or stop hemorrhage but loosely enough so that a finger can easily be slipped beneath it. Slowly release the tourniquet for 1 minute every 10 minutes and do not reapply it unless necessary.

Open Wounds

Signs

- Abrasion – surface scraped off
- Incision – clean cut
- Laceration – tissues torn
- Puncture – small opening on surface

First Aid

- Control hemorrhage
- Treat for shock if necessary
- Protect the wound

Cause

Open wounds are injuries that disrupt the surface of the skin or mucous membranes. The major types of open wounds include abrasions, incisions, lacerations and punctures.

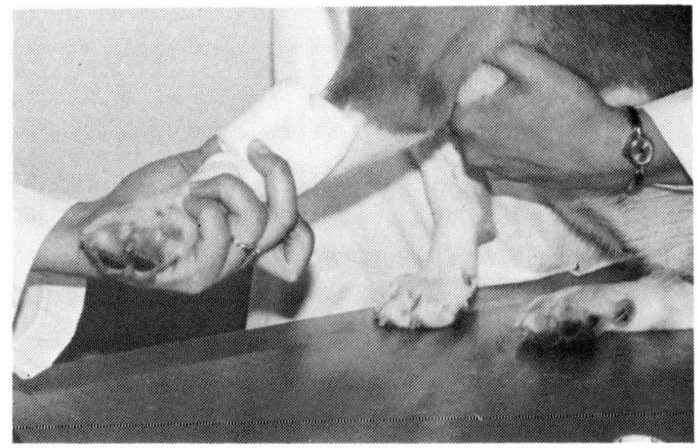

Figure 5. A pressure bandage can be applied by placing a small gauze roll over a gauze sponge.

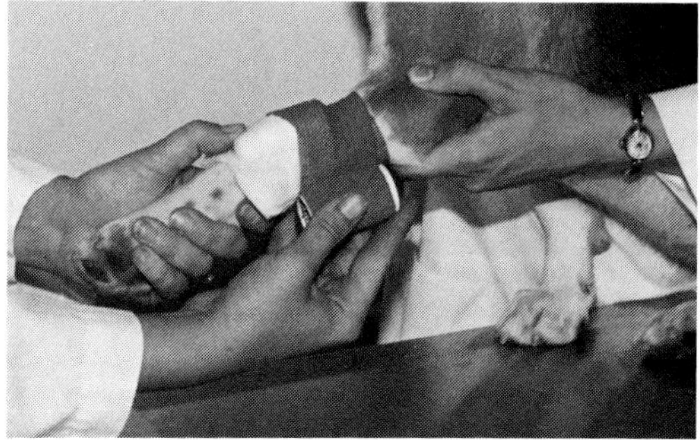

Figure 6. Elastic wrap is applied over the gauze roll to complete the pressure bandage.

Abrasions occur when the skin or mucous membrane is "scraped" off. Though they may be painful, abrasions usually are not very serious unless they are extensive, very deep or involve vital structures.

Incisions are clean cuts made by sharp objects, such as pieces of glass or metal. Depending on their size, depth and location, incisions can cause damage to underlying structures and/or allow infections to develop.

Lacerations have ragged, irregular edges and can be serious for the same reasons as incisions. The degree of tissue trauma can be greater with lacerations than with incisions.

Punctures are made by pointed objects, such as nails, teeth and projectiles. They usually appear as relatively small openings in the skin, but the damage beneath the surface can be quite extensive. Unless they are known to be shallow and small, punctures should be assumed to be deep and serious.

First Aid

First aid for wounds, in order of decreasing importance, involves control of hemorrhage, treatment for shock, if necessary, and prevention of further trauma and/or contamination of the wound. A cold compress applied to a fairly fresh wound can help control hemorrhage, prevent or reduce swelling, and help reduce pain. Self-trauma can be prevented with adequate restraint and use of such devices as muzzles and Elizabethan collars on small animals, and neck cradles or cross-ties on large animals. The wound can be protected with a sterile, or at least clean, dressing secured with gauze and/or tape.

Penetrating Foreign Bodies

Cause

Penetrating foreign bodies are objects that have penetrated the skin and are still present. They may include such objects as needles, fishhooks, porcupine quills and splinters. The damage caused by external foreign bodies may be superficial and limited to the skin, or may extend to deeper structures and tissues. For this reason, all penetrating foreign bodies should be considered potentially serious.

First Aid

The general principle of first aid for penetrating foreign bodies is to remove the object if it can be done *easily* without causing further trauma or pain, and to treat the wound appropriately. If, however, the object cannot be easily removed, or if removing it would cause further trauma (*eg,* barb on a fishhook), it is best to leave it in place and try to keep the animal as comfortable as possible until the veterinarian can examine it. Anesthesia and surgery may be necessary before the object can be safely removed.

Fractures

Signs

- Pain
- Swelling
- Diminished function
- Abnormal angulation or movement
- Crepitus

First Aid

- Handle gently
- Cover and protect wounds
- Control hemorrhage and treat for shock if necessary
- Apply a temporary splint if possible

Fractures, or broken bones, can be classified according to many criteria. The simplest classifications, from a first-aid standpoint, are according to the extent of the fracture and the integrity of the skin over the fracture site.

If the bone is not completely fractured, it is called an *incomplete (greenstick) fracture.* A *complete fracture* is one in which the bone is broken into 2 or more segments. A *comminuted fracture* is one in which the bone is broken or splintered into more than 2 segments. In *simple (closed) fractures,* the overlying skin is intact. In a *compound (open) fracture,* the bone protrudes through the overlying skin.

Clinical Signs

The signs of a fracture depend on the location and extent of the fracture, the temperament of the animal, and the presence and extent of other injuries. Common fracture signs include: pain at or near the injury site; swelling and bruising at or near the injury site; decreased or absent function of the affected part (*eg,* inability to bear weight on a fractured leg); abnormal angulation and/or movement of the affected part; and crepitus (grating when the broken ends of a bone rub together). *Do not deliberately test for crepitus* because it causes pain and may produce further injury.

First Aid

The main objectives of first aid for fractures are to prevent further injury and to make the animal more comfortable. An animal with a fracture is in severe pain, and the sharp ends of the fracture fragments can cause considerable damage to surrounding tissues. Handle the affected animal gently. Do not move it more than is absolutely necessary, and use proper restraint to prevent personal injury. Control any serious hemorrhage and treat for shock if necessary. Cover and protect any serious wounds, particularly in the case of a compound (open) fracture.

Many fractures, particularly those in the distal (lower) part of a limb, can be effectively stabilized with a temporary splint. This can decrease movement and prevent further trauma at the fracture site. An effective temporary splint can be made from virtually any reasonably stiff material, such as rolled up magazines or newspapers and pieces of wood or cardboard.

To apply a temporary splint, pad the leg with such material as cotton or cloth, place the splint material against or around the leg, and secure it with tape, strips of cloth, rope or string. Try to immobilize the joints proximal and distal to (above and below) the fracture site with the splint.

Another even more effective temporary splint is a modified Robert Jones bandage (Figs 7-12). This type of splint also helps reduce or prevent the swelling that often contributes to pain associated with a fracture. This swelling makes subsequent reduction of the fracture by the veterinarian more difficult. It is applied by wrapping many layers of roll cotton around the leg (large animals may

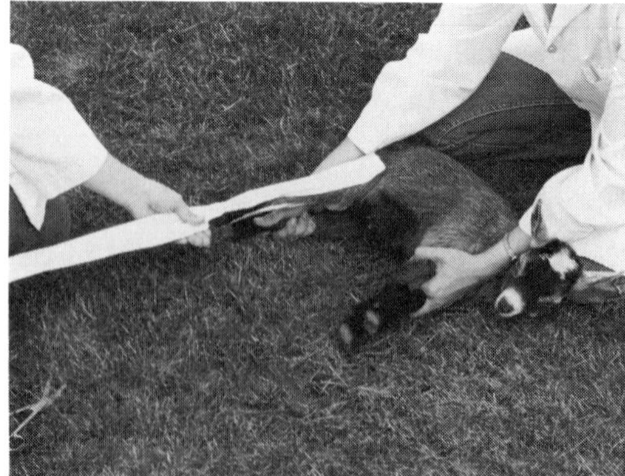

Figure 7. To apply a Robert Jones bandage, adhesive tape is put on the medial and lateral surfaces of the affected limb, with the pieces of tape joining distad at a distance about equal to the length of the leg.

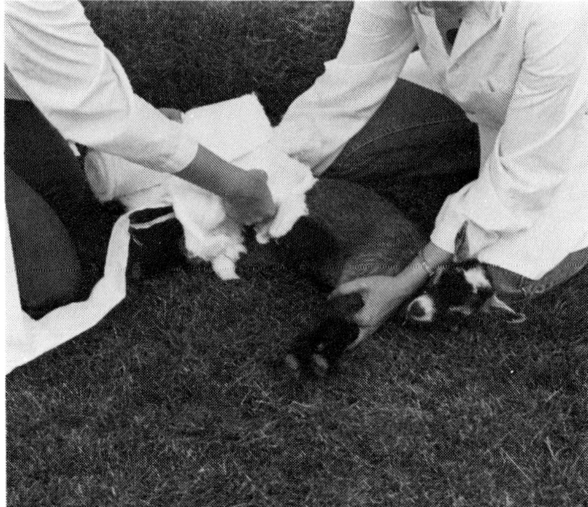

Figure 8. Roll cotton is unrolled and the paper removed. Then the taped leg is wrapped with the roll cotton.

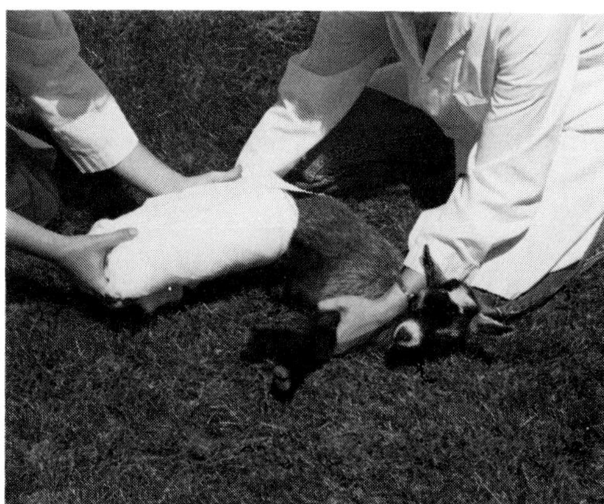

Figure 9. After the roll cotton is applied, the tape stirrup is reflected up over the cotton.

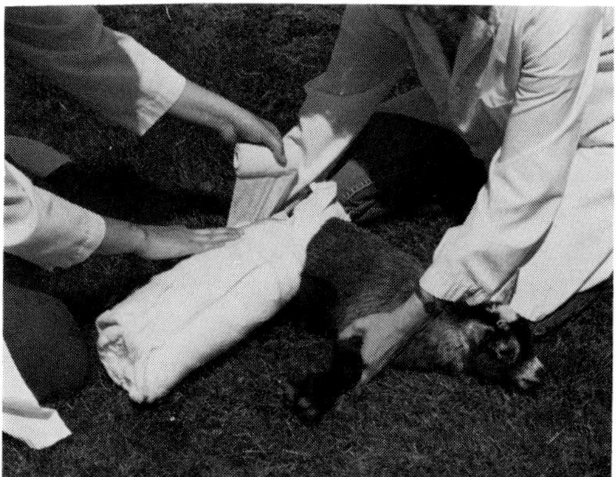

Figure 10. Elastic wrap is firmly applied over the roll cotton and reflected tape stirrup.

require several rolls) and then compressing the roll cotton with an elastic wrap.

Dislocations

Signs

- Pain
- Swelling
- Abnormal joint function
- Abnormal joint position or angulation
- Apparent shortening of limb

First Aid

- Control hemorrhage and treat for shock if necessary
- Avoid movement of joint

A dislocation is a displacement of a bone from its normal position in a joint, usually as a result of trauma.

Clinical Signs

The signs of a dislocation, like those of a fracture, can be quite variable but generally include pain, particularly when the joint is moved, swelling around the dislocated joint, abnormal or absent function of the affected joint, abnormal angulation of the leg at the affected joint, and apparent shortening of the limb. Abnormal angulation caused by a fracture occurs *between* the joints, not *at* the joint (assuming the fracture does not involve the joint).

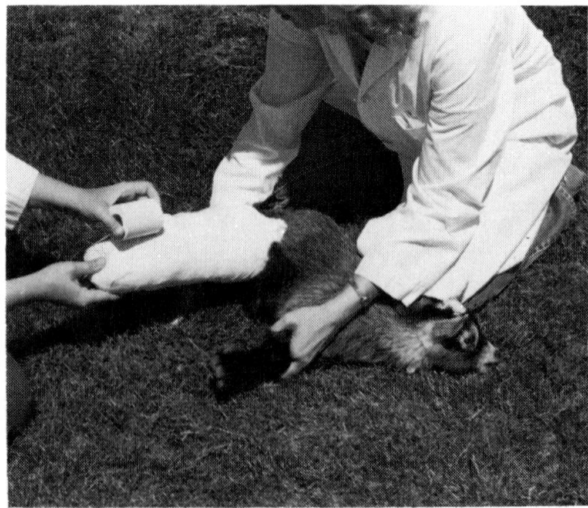

Figure 11. The elastic wrap is then covered with adhesive tape.

First Aid

First aid for dislocations is mainly symptomatic. Reduction usually requires general anesthesia because of the pain involved and the muscle spasms that must be overcome. An animal with a dislocated joint may be in severe pain and should be handled carefully and with adequate restraint to ensure personal safety. Control any serious hemorrhage and treat for shock if necessary. Avoid movement of the affected joint as much as possible, and keep the animal quiet and as comfortable as possible.

Head Injuries

Signs

- Altered level of consciousness
- Abnormal vision
- Abnormal pupil size and pupillary response
- Abnormal posture and movement
- Abnormal respiration
- Hemorrhage from the ear canals

First Aid

- Keep animal quiet and observe for changes in status
- Maintain respiration
- Control hemorrhage and treat for shock if necessary
- Treat any serious wounds
- Administer CPR if necessary

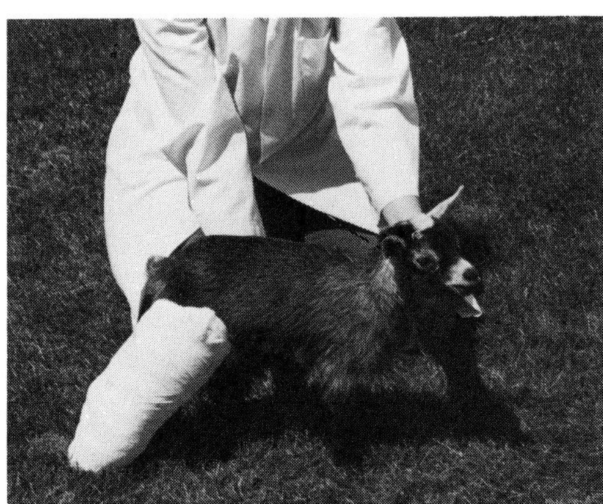

Figure 12. Completed Robert Jones bandage.

Cause

Because the head is a vital and vulnerable part of the body, cranial trauma frequently has more serious consequences than equivalent trauma to other parts of the body. Head injuries may include bruises, wounds, hemorrhage or fractures.

Clinical Signs

Signs of brain damage may be obvious or subtle. Severe brain damage can result in instant death, while very slight damage can cause slight functional and/or behavioral changes.

A variety of clinical signs may be observed in brain-damaged animals. The level of consciousness may range from normal alertness to coma. Initial consciousness followed by lapse into unconsciousness usually indicates severe injury. Brain damage may result in blindness or altered pupillary function and/or size.

Pupils that are abnormal on initial examination and become normal on subsequent examination indicate a favorable prognosis. Abnormal ocular findings include miosis (pupillary constriction), mydriasis (pupillary dilation), anisocoria (pupillary size different in the 2 eyes), lack of response to light or dark, nystagmus (horizontal, vertical or circular movement of the globes), and proptosis (globe prolapsed from the orbit).

Brain damage may also cause a head tilt, inability to stand or walk normally, partial or complete paralysis, altered muscle tone (flaccidity or rigidity) and convulsions. Abnormal respiration in the absence of respiratory tract lesions indicates possible damage to the respiratory control center in the brainstem. Hemorrhage from the external ear canals is another indication of severe cranial trauma.

First Aid

First aid for cranial injuries is directed toward preventing further damage and maintaining vital functions. The animal should be kept quiet and comfortable, and observed closely for changes. Respiration should be watched closely and the trachea intubated if necessary. Control serious hemorrhage, treat serious wounds, treat for shock if necessary, and be prepared to administer CPR if necessary.

With proptosis, protect the prolapsed globe against further injury. To prevent corneal drying, use gauze sponges soaked in a cool hypertonic solution (10% dextrose). The hypertonic solution also helps reduce ocular swelling.

Spinal Injuries

Signs

- Pain in neck or back
- Weakness of limbs
- Paralysis of limbs
- Anesthesia of limbs

First Aid

- Avoid movement of spine
- Maintain respiration
- Control serious hemorrhage and treat for shock if necessary

Cause

Most serious spinal injuries are caused by trauma or degeneration of intervertebral disks. Traumatic injuries usually involve vertebral fractures or dislocations, with associated damage to the spinal cord. Degenerated intervertebral disks can herniate dorsally to compress the spinal cord.

The severity of spinal injuries is often related to the type and severity of clinical signs exhibited. Pain and/or weakness generally indicate less serious damage than do anesthesia and/or paralysis.

Clinical Signs

Clinical signs seen with spinal injuries depend on the location, nature and severity of the damage. Typical signs of spinal trauma include pain, weakness, paralysis and loss of feeling in the limbs.

Spinal injuries can cause pain, usually in the neck and/or back region. If able, the animal walks gingerly, with its back and neck kept rigid. Weakness may be evident in the rear legs and perhaps also in the front legs. The animal may not be able to support itself.

Any paralysis usually affects the rear legs but may also affect the front legs, depending on the location of the injury. There is a complete absence of pain perception when a painful stimulus, such as pinching a toe, is applied to the foot. (However, even animals with a severed spinal cord show reflex withdrawal of a pinched toe.)

First Aid

First aid for spinal injuries is directed at preventing further trauma to the spinal cord. Animals with suspected spinal injuries should be kept quiet and moved as little as possible. A spinal injury is always serious, but as long as the spinal cord is maintained intact, the situation is not hopeless. The animal should be transported with minimal movement of the spine. If possible, it should be carried on a rigid platform, such as a board. General first-aid care should be given to other problems, such as hemorrhage, extensive wounds or shock.

Convulsions

Signs

- Muscle twitches
- Collapse
- Uncontrolled shivering, paddling and thrashing

First Aid

- Keep the environment quiet
- Prevent the animal from injuring itself

Cause

Convulsions, also called seizures, epileptic seizures and "fits," result from abnormal brain activity. This causes involuntary contractions (localized or generalized) of skeletal muscles.

Potential causes of convulsions include epilepsy, toxicities (lead, antifreeze, insecticides, rodenticides), infections (distemper, toxoplasmosis), CNS tumors, metabolic disturbances (diabetes mellitus), and developmental conditions (hydrocephalus).

Clinical Signs

The signs of convulsions depend on their type and severity. Some affected animals may show altered behavior that signals a convulsion is about to begin. This "aura" can take many forms, such as lip licking, twitching muscles and restlessness. The convulsion itself usually begins with involuntary muscle twitches and contractions. The animal may apparently lose consciousness, collapse, paddle, shiver, twitch and shake.

Convulsions usually last from a few seconds to a few minutes. The animal may appear dazed and disoriented for a time immediately following a convulsion. Prolonged, continuous convulsions are called *status epilepticus* and can be very dangerous for the animal.

Seizures cannot be shortened by first aid; they have to run their course. They can be prolonged, however, by continued stimulation from bright lights, loud noises or rough handling. It is important to remember that brief convulsions usually are not harmful to the animal; however, an animal can injure itself by falling or thrashing.

First Aid

First aid should be directed at 2 main areas. *Keep the environment as quiet as possible* to avoid prolonging an otherwise brief seizure. *Keep the animal from injuring itself.* Be sure it is on the floor or ground, and remove furniture and other objects it might knock over. After the seizure has run its course, quietly and calmly reassure the animal as it emerges from the postseizure period of disorientation.

Hypoglycemia Associated With Diabetes Mellitus

Signs

- Disorientation
- Weakness
- Hunger
- Convulsions
- Coma

First Aid

- Feed normal meal
- Rub Karo syrup or honey on the gums
- Check for unobstructed airway
- Treat for shock/hemorrhage

Cause

Hypoglycemia (low blood glucose level) is seen in diabetic animals following an overdose of insulin, excessive exercise, or a delayed or missed meal. If the blood glucose level falls slowly, the areas of the brain most metabolically active are affected first. This leads to early and milder clinical signs. If the blood glucose level drops rapidly, the less metabolically active areas of the brain become affected, leading to more severe clinical signs.

Clinical Signs

If the blood glucose level drops slowly, the patient may show a series of progressively more severe clinical signs (disorientation, weakness and hunger) leading to convulsions and/or coma. If the blood glucose level drops rapidly, the patient may develop convulsions or coma without displaying any other clinical signs.

First Aid

First aid is aimed at raising the blood glucose level. If clinical signs are mild, the patient should be fed a normal meal. Karo (corn) syrup (Best Foods) or honey can be rubbed on the tongue or gums. If clinical signs have progressed to convulsions or coma, apply small amounts of Karo syrup or honey to the tongue or gums until the animal revives. Comatose diabetic patients with a history of insulin overdose, strenuous exercise or a missed meal should receive the above first-aid therapy. In addition, make sure there is an unobstructed airway. Look for signs of hemorrhage and/or shock.

Epistaxis

Signs

- Hemorrhage from the nose

First Aid

- Keep animal calm
- Apply ice packs over nasal passages
- Elevate the nose
- Treat for shock if necessary

Cause

Epistaxis, or hemorrhage from the nose, can have many causes. Trauma, strenuous exercise (especially in horses), nasal tumors, blood clotting disorders, and violent sneezing can cause an episode of epistaxis.

Epistaxis of relatively short duration is not usually a serious problem. Prolonged epistaxis, however, can be serious. Severe blood loss can result in anemia, hypoxia and shock. Respiration can be impaired by partial obstruction of the respiratory passages and aspiration of blood into the lungs.

First Aid

First aid for epistaxis is aimed at getting blood to clot at the source of the hemorrhage. The animal should be kept as quiet as possible because rapid, excited breathing decreases the chances of a clot forming. Ice packs placed over the nasal passages can help hasten clot formation, as can elevation of the nose. Treat for shock if necessary.

Respiratory Obstruction

Signs

- Gagging or choking
- Difficult breathing
- Cyanosis
- Unconsciousness

First Aid

- Keep the animal calm
- Remove any pharyngeal foreign bodies
- If necessary, compress chest forcefully a few times
- Pass an endotracheal tube if possible and/or necessary
- Administer oxygen
- Give artificial respiration if necessary

Cause

The causes of respiratory obstruction vary and include: foreign bodies (bones, balls, toys, food); trauma to the nasal passages, pharynx, larynx or trachea; tumors; infection; allergic reactions; and inhaled irritants.

Clinical Signs

The signs of a respiratory obstruction are related to impairment of normal gaseous exchange and include gagging or choking, dyspnea (difficult breathing), cyanosis (mucous membranes turn dark purplish blue) and unconsciousness.

First Aid

First aid for respiratory obstruction is directed at reducing the body's need for oxygen and increasing the rate of gaseous exchange. The animal should be kept as cool, calm and quiet as possible to minimize its need for oxygen and heat elimination. Check for foreign bodies in the pharynx by carefully pulling the tongue forward and examining the throat visually or manually. If a foreign body cannot be removed manually or with forceps, compressing the chest forcefully a few times may expel it. Do this by placing the animal in lateral recumbency and compressing the thorax with the hands from above or with the hands on either side of the chest. Repeat as necessary.

Administration of oxygen to an animal with impaired respiration can be life saving. An inhalant anesthesia machine with the vaporizer turned off can be used with a face mask or endotracheal tube, if possible. Give artificial respiration, if necessary.

Rib Fractures

Signs

- Painful respiration
- Pain and crepitus at fracture site
- Flail chest

First Aid

- Keep the animal calm and quiet
- Administer oxygen
- Stabilize flail chest with a towel clamp

Clinical Signs

Clinical signs include painful respiration, pain and crepitus at the fracture site, and flail chest. The last occurs when multiple rib fractures produce a "floating" segment of the chest wall that moves paradoxically (in on inspiration, out on expiration) and interferes with proper expansion of the lung.

First Aid

First aid for rib fractures is aimed at increasing the efficiency of respiration. The animal should be kept as calm and quiet as possible. Administer oxygen if necessary and possible. If flail chest is present, stabilize the floating segment by grasping its central portion with a towel clamp and applying traction abaxially (outward).

Diaphragmatic Hernia

Signs

- Difficult breathing
- Muffled heart and lung sounds
- Peristaltic sounds in the chest

First Aid

- Keep the animal quiet and calm
- Elevate the cranial end of the animal
- Administer oxygen if necessary
- Give artificial respiration if necessary
- Treat for shock if necessary

Cause

A diaphragmatic hernia is a tear in the diaphragm that allows protrusion of abdominal viscera into the thorax. It may be congenital or, more commonly, traumatic.

Clinical Signs

The signs of diaphragmatic hernia are related to impingement of the herniated abdominal contents on the lungs, which prevents normal lung expansion. The severity of signs depends on the site and size of the diaphragmatic tear, amount of abdominal viscera in the chest, and activity of the animal. The condition of an affected animal can change very rapidly as abdominal organs move in or out of the thorax.

Typical signs include dyspnea (difficult breathing), and peristaltic sounds and muffled heart and lung sounds on thoracic auscultation. The degree of dyspnea depends on the extent of abdominal organ displacement into the thorax. Severe dyspnea may lead to cyanosis and collapse.

First Aid

First aid for diaphragmatic hernias is aimed at maintaining respiratory function and preventing more abdominal viscera from slipping into the thorax. Keep the animal as calm and quiet as possible. Elevate the cranial end of the animal to help prevent additional abdominal contents from slipping into the chest. Administer oxygen if the animal becomes cyanotic or loses consciousness. Give artificial respiration and treat for shock if necessary.

Bloat in Ruminants

Signs

- Abdominal distention
- Labored breathing
- Anorexia
- Decreased or no eructation
- Possible cyanosis
- Possible collapse

First Aid

- Keep the animal quiet
- Pass a large stomach tube if possible

Cause

Bloat in ruminants is an excessive accumulation of gas, free or trapped in a foamy froth, in the rumen. Mild bloat is not an emergency, but severe bloat causes a great deal of discomfort and interferes with respiration through pressure on the diaphragm. This interferes with normal expansion of the lungs. Severe bloat can be fatal.

Clinical Signs

Signs of bloat in ruminants include abdominal distention, labored breathing, anorexia, decreased or no eructation, cyanosis and collapse.

First Aid

First aid for bloat is aimed at diminishing the body's oxygen needs and attempting to remove the gas from the rumen. Keep the animal as calm and quiet as possible. Pass a large, well-lubricated stomach tube, if possible, to relieve the pressure. This, however, may not be effective in cases of frothy bloat.

Gastric Dilatation in Dogs

Signs

- Abdominal distention
- Difficult breathing
- Possible cyanosis
- Possible shock

First Aid

- Keep the animal quiet and calm
- Pass a stomach tube if possible
- Administer oxygen if possible
- Treat for shock if necessary

Cause

Gastric dilatation in dogs is the canine equivalent of bloat in ruminants. The stomach rapidly distends with gas and may undergo volvulus (torsion). The distended stomach compresses the caudal vena cava, decreasing venous return to the heart, impinging on the diaphragm and compromising respiration. The animal can rapidly become acidotic and hypoxic, with subsequent shock and possible death.

Clinical Signs

Signs of gastric dilatation in dogs are similar to those of bloat in ruminants and include abdominal distention, dyspnea (difficult breathing), cyanosis and shock. Nonproductive retching may be present in dogs with gastric volvulus.

First Aid

First aid for gastric dilatation is aimed primarily at minimizing the animal's oxygen needs and attempting to relieve gastric distention. Keep the animal as calm and quiet as possible. If possible, pass a well-lubricated stomach tube to relieve the pressure. If gastric torsion or volvulus is present, it may not be possible to pass the tube into the stomach, so do not force it. Administer oxygen if possible and treat for shock if necessary.

Colic in Horses

Signs

- Pawing at the ground
- Kicking at the abdomen
- Restlessness
- Rolling
- Flank-watching
- Abnormal posture

First Aid

- Keep the animal walking until the veterinarian arrives
- Look for signs of shock

Cause

Colic in horses is a syndrome related to abdominal pain. Causes include gastrointestinal tract disorders (impaction, bowel displacements, strangulation, infarcts, ulceration), urogenital tract abnormalities (uterine torsion, uterine rupture, urolithiasis, bladder rupture), ascarid impaction in weanling horses within a day of deworming, and foreign body obstruction in horses that habitually chew and ingest foreign material (wood, rope, nylon, etc).

Clinical Signs

Depending on the severity of the pain, a horse may exhibit discomfort by pawing, kicking at its abdomen, lying down and getting up (restlessness), rolling, flank-watching or adopting an abnormal posture. A horse in pain can thrash about and injure itself. Other signs of pain include sweating and panting.

First Aid

First aid is directed at keeping the horse from injuring itself. The horse should be walked continuously (as safely as possible) until the cause of the colic can be determined by the veterinarian. Check for signs of shock.

Gastrointestinal Foreign Bodies

Cause

Gastrointestinal foreign bodies consist of virtually anything other than food, water or medication swallowed by an animal. Metal, cloth, wood, bones or rubber may be ingested during normal feeding (large animals), play or chewing (horses, small animals).

The dangers of GI foreign bodies include gastrointestinal perforation, laceration, abrasion and partial or complete bowel obstruction. Many foreign bodies, even sharp ones such as needles, pass harmlessly through the GI tract without causing any difficulties. Ingestion of a foreign body without subsequent clinical signs (vomiting, abdominal pain) does not necessarily constitute an emergency situation.

A common foreign body in cats is string or thread that becomes looped around the base of the tongue and trails down the esophagus into the GI tract. The intestine attempts to move the firmly anchored string caudally, resulting in intestinal plication (accordion pleating) and possible intestinal laceration and/or necrosis.

First Aid

First aid for GI foreign bodies is primarily symptomatic. *Do not attempt to make an animal vomit a foreign body.* This may cause more damage and trauma than leaving the foreign body where it originally lodged. Some foreign bodies in the mouth or pharynx can be removed easily without causing further damage.

If a string or thread is found looped around the base of a cat's tongue, *do not attempt to pull it out.* This can severely damage the GI tract. Instead, carefully cut the string or thread, and observe the animal closely. After it is cut, the string may pass through the tract uneventfully. If the obstruction persists, surgery may be necessary.

Rectal Prolapse

Signs

- Reddish mass protruding from the anus
- Straining

First Aid

- Lubricate well and replace if possible
- Keep prolapsed tissue moist
- Apply hypertonic solution if possible

Cause

Rectal prolapse is an eversion of the rectum through the anus. It occurs most frequently in young animals from excessive straining in attempts to defecate.

Dangers with a rectal prolapse include drying and necrosis of the exposed, everted rectal mucosa, and swelling of the prolapsed mass from impaired venous return. Arteries continue to pump blood into the prolapsed mass, but pressure at the anus may partially occlude veins draining blood from the mass.

Clinical Signs

The prolapsed rectum appears as a reddish tubular or globular mass protruding from the anus. It is frequently accompanied by severe straining. The mass may be small and round or large and long, resembling a sausage.

First Aid

First aid for rectal prolapse is aimed at replacing the prolapsed mass or, if this is not possible, protecting the exposed mass from trauma and drying. Small, recent prolapses may be replaced without much difficulty. Gently clean the mass with warm water. Lubricate the mass well, and apply gentle constant pressure to replace it. If the mass cannot be easily replaced, keep it moist and protected by surrounding it with gauze sponges or cloth moistened with isotonic saline (or tap water if saline is not available). Use of a hypertonic solution, such as 10% dextrose, instead of saline not only prevents drying but also osmotically decreases the swelling.

External Hernias

Cause

A hernia is a protrusion of an organ or tissue through an abnormal opening. *Abdominal hernias* are most common. They consist of abdominal contents that protrude through an opening in the abdominal musculature and are covered by skin only. Hernias may be congenital or the result of trauma and/or weakened tissues. Most are visible externally.

The main danger with hernias is that the herniated tissues, especially if they include portions of the GI tract, may become strangulated at the hernial opening. Also, herniated tissues may be exposed if the skin over them is broken.

Incisional hernias occur at the site of a disrupted surgical incision. *Inguinal hernias* occur in the inguinal region (groin), usually through the inguinal ring. *Perineal hernias* occur in the perineal region, beside the anus. *Umbilical hernias* occur at the umbilicus, on the ventral midline.

A hernia usually appears as a soft, "doughy" swelling. It may be *reducible,* in which case the contents can be easily pushed back through the hernial opening, or *irreducible,* in which case the contents cannot easily be replaced.

First Aid

First aid for reducible hernias consists of replacing the contents and bandaging the area for support to prevent its immediate recurrence. In the case of irreducible hernias, keep the animal quiet and prevent it from traumatizing the hernia.

Paraphimosis

Signs

- An abnormally sustained penile erection

First Aid

- Gently clean if necessary
- Apply icepacks if severely swollen or traumatized
- Lubricate well and advance prepuce over penis
- If not reducible, protect and keep moist
- Apply hypertonic solution if possible

Cause

Paraphimosis is an inability of the engorged penis to retract back into the prepuce following erection. It usually occurs after coitus and is recognized as a sustained erection after the penis should have retracted back into the prepuce.

First Aid

First aid for paraphimosis is aimed at protecting the exposed penis and attempting to replace it into the prepuce. Gently clean the penis if necessary. If it is severely swollen (edematous) and/or traumatized, cold packs may help reduce swelling before replacement is attempted. Lubricate the penis and preputial opening well. Gently advance the prepuce over the penis. If the prepuce cannot be easily advanced over the well-lubricated penis, keep the penis moist by surrounding it with gauze sponges or cloth moistened with isotonic saline (or water, if saline is not available). Use of a hypertonic solution, such as 10% dextrose, can help reduce swelling osmotically.

Uterine Prolapse

Signs

- A reddish mass protruding from the vulva

First Aid

- If prolapse is small, attempt replacement by gently cleaning, lubricating and applying pressure
- If not replaceable, keep prolapsed tissue moist and protect
- Apply hypertonic solution if possible

Cause

Uterine prolapse is eversion of the uterus through the vaginal opening. It usually occurs shortly after parturition. Dangers with uterine prolapse include swelling of the prolapsed tissues from impaired venous return, and drying and necrosis of the exposed uterine mucosa.

Clinical Signs

A prolapsed uterus appears as a reddish mass protruding from the vulva. It can vary in size from small to large.

First Aid

First aid for uterine prolapse is aimed at replacing the uterus or, if that is not possible, protecting it. If the prolapse is small, replacement can be attempted by gently cleaning the exposed mucosa, if necessary, lubricating it well, and applying constant gentle pressure. If the prolapse is large or replacement is unsuccessful, keep the exposed tissues clean and moist (use isotonic saline, water or a hypertonic solution, such as 10% dextrose), and prevent self-trauma.

Dystocia

Parturition, or the birth process, can be divided into 3 normal stages (see Chapter 9).

The *first stage of labor* consists of uterine contractions and dilation of the cervix. The dam acts restless and uncomfortable.

The *second stage of labor* consists of the actual delivery of the fetus. The dam's intermittent, forceful abdominal contractions increase in frequency up to expulsion of the fetus.

The *third stage of labor* consists of delivery of the placenta. This usually occurs almost immediately after the birth of small animals but may take several hours in large animals.

Dystocia, or difficult labor, can be maternal or fetal in origin. Causes of *maternal dystocia* include abnormalities of the pelvis that narrow the birth canal, weak uterine contractions, uterine torsion or psychological disturbances. Causes of *fetal dystocia* include a large fetus, twinning or malpositioning.

In many cases, particularly in companion animals, more aid is given during parturition than is needed. This aid can actually produce dystocias through maternal distraction by unnecessary human participation. Most births occur with no problems or need for human intervention.

First Aid

It is beyond the scope of this discussion to describe all of the potential problems that can occur during parturition and the steps necessary to resolve them, but there are certain general procedures that can facilitate the birth process once the decision to intervene has been made.

Cleanliness: Anything that touches the neonate or is inserted into the dam's birth canal should be sterile or very clean. The environment in which the birth is taking place should be as clean as possible.

Lubrication: Use sterile water-soluble lubricant (*eg,* K-Y Jelly) liberally to aid extraction of the fetus and prevent injury to the dam's birth canal.

Traction: If traction is necessary to help with the delivery, it should be applied only to the fetus's legs and *not* to the head, if possible. The slippery fetus should be grasped with cloths, towels or gauze sponges and pulled gently and steadily. Work *with* the dam, not against her, by pulling when she has a contraction.

Care of Neonates

If placental membranes cover the face of the neonate and the dam does not quickly remove them, do so manually. Allow the dam to clean the neonate and stimulate respiration if she will. If she is not so inclined, it may be necessary to clear the neonate's nose and mouth of fluids and rub it gently but vigorously with a soft towel or cloth to stimulate respiration.

Burns

Signs

- Minor burns indicated by reddened skin and blisters
- Major burns indicated by edematous or charred skin

First Aid

- Keep animal quiet and prevent self-trauma
- Irrigate chemical burns
- Apply cold compresses
- Monitor vital signs and treat for shock if necessary

Cause

Burns can have many possible causes, including scalds from contact with hot liquids (water, grease, tar); flames or smoke inhalation; chemicals; radiation (sunburn); and electricity (chewing on electrical cords or lightning strike).

Burns can be classified several different ways. For the purposes of first aid, they can be conveniently divided into minor (superficial) burns and major (deep) burns.

Minor burns, though painful, are not generally life threatening. Recovery is usually rapid unless they are very extensive.

Major burns cause extensive tissue destruction that extends down into, and even through, the deepest layers of skin. In addition to the extensive tissue damage itself, with its attendant pain and healing problems, complications can result from loss of the protective skin covering and subsequent inflammation of exposed tissues. These include extensive fluid, electrolyte and protein loss, shock from fluid, electrolyte and protein imbalance, and infection that begins locally and can spread systemically.

Clinical Signs

Signs of the 2 main categories of burns differ mainly in the appearance of the affected skin. Minor burns are painful and the skin is reddened (this may be difficult to see if the haircoat is heavy and/or the skin is darkly pigmented). Blisters may be present, and the hair may be singed but still firmly attached. Major burns are also painful. The skin may be edematous, charred or entirely destroyed. Hair may fall out. If major burns are extensive, the animal is usually reluctant to move.

First Aid

First aid for burns is aimed at preventing further damage and reducing pain. Keep the animal quiet and prevent self-trauma. Apply cold compresses to help lessen pain and inflammation. If it will be some time before the animal can be seen by a veterinarian, apply either a sterile (or at least clean) dry dressing or one moistened with sterile isotonic saline. Do not apply oily dressings to burns. Monitor the vital signs and treat for shock if necessary.

If the burn is from a corrosive chemical, irrigate the wound well with sterile isotonic saline or plain tap water if saline is not available, so as to dilute and wash away the corrosive material.

Frostbite

Signs

- History of exposure to severe cold
- Affected tissues may be reddened, pale or scaly

First Aid

- Warm the affected area rapidly in lukewarm water, then dry it
- Prevent self-trauma

Cause

Frostbite is the freezing of tissues, usually in the extremities, such as the ears, tail and limbs.

Clinical Signs

The signs of frostbite can be quite variable, but usually the history of exposure to severe cold is helpful. Frostbitten tissues may be reddened or pale, and may be scaly.

First Aid

First aid for frostbite is aimed at warming the affected tissue and minimizing tissue trauma. Do not rub or massage the frozen tissues and do not apply snow or ice. Warm the affected area rapidly in lukewarm water. Immerse the area or use warm moist towels that are changed frequently, then gently dry the area after it is warmed. Finally, prevent self-trauma.

Heatstroke

Signs

- Elevated rectal temperature
- Weakness
- Collapse
- Rapid pulse
- Bright-red mucous membranes
- Shock

First Aid

- Cool the animal
- Monitor the rectal temperature and stop treatment as temperature approaches normal
- Treat for shock if necessary

Cause

Heatstroke, or hyperthermia, is an excessive elevation of the body temperature caused by high environmental temperatures. The condition frequently is accompanied by stress of some kind. Usually the animal has been confined in an area with a high ambient temperature, such as a dog in an automobile with the windows rolled up on a hot day, or an animal confined outdoors on a hot day with no access to shade and/or water.

Clinical Signs

Most of the signs of heatstroke are nonspecific. A history of exposure to high environmental temperatures is helpful in determining if an animal is affected. Typical signs include elevated rectal temperature (generally 105-110 F), panting, weakness, collapse, rapid pulse, bright-red mucous membranes (may turn pale as the animal goes into shock) and shock.

First Aid

First aid for heatstroke is aimed at quickly reducing the animal's core (internal) temperature. The first consideration is how best to cool the animal. It should be taken out of the sun and, if possible, immersed in or sprayed with cool water. Treat for shock, as needed. Measure the rectal temperature every 5 minutes and stop treatment as the temperature approaches normal. In very severe or unresponsive cases, cold-water enemas may be useful, but they prevent use of the rectal temperature to monitor progress. Once the rectal temperature is back to near normal, dry the animal off to prevent hypothermia.

Hypothermia

Signs

- Subnormal body temperature
- Shivering
- Decreased pulse rate
- Weakness
- Unconsciousness
- Shock

First Aid

- Warm the animal
- Monitor the rectal temperature and stop treatment as the temperature approaches normal
- Treat for shock if necessary

Cause

Hypothermia is an abnormal lowering of the body temperature, usually resulting from exposure to low environmental temperatures or drugs that interfere with normal body temperature regulation, such as anesthetics and some tranquilizers.

Clinical Signs

Many of the signs of hypothermia are nonspecific. A history of exposure to low environmental temperatures or to drugs that interfere with normal body temperature regulation is helpful in determining if an animal is affected. Typical signs include subnormal rectal temperature (<95 F), shivering (may be inhibited by some drugs), decreased pulse rate, weakness, unconsciousness and shock.

First Aid

First aid for hypothermia is aimed at elevating the animal's core temperature. This is accomplished with warm-water baths, blankets or towels, recirculating water blankets, hot-water bottles (wrapped in towels to prevent burning), or careful use of electric heaters. Be careful not to burn the animal. Monitor the rectal temperature and stop treating as soon as the rectal temperature approaches normal. Treat for shock if necessary.

Eye Injuries

General First-Aid Principles

Because the eyes are such delicate and vital structures, the aim of first aid for eye injuries is to prevent further damage to the area. This can be accomplished by adhering to some general first-aid principles.

Do not attempt to overtreat ocular injuries, as this may cause more damage. Do not force the eyelids open to examine the eye. Cold compresses, gently applied, may help relieve pain and reduce swelling and inflammation. If a bandage is to be applied to protect an injured eye, apply a bandage to the normal eye also, as movement of the uncovered normal eye causes unwanted movement of the injured eye. Finally, do not apply pressure to an injured eye. The eye can be easily ruptured if the sclera and/or cornea are weakened.

First Aid for Eyelid Injuries

The most common eyelid injuries are contusions and/or lacerations. The most effective first aid for these is to control hemorrhage with direct pressure or cold compresses. Bandage for protection, if necessary, and prevent self-trauma.

First Aid for Injuries to the Globe

Subconjunctival hemorrhage is a common result of head trauma. It looks serious but usually is not a problem in itself and seldom requires treatment. However, it should be a signal to look for other ocular lesions.

Chemical irritants can cause severe eye damage. Affected eyes should be irrigated with sterile isotonic saline or plain water, as soon as possible, for 10-15 minutes.

Abrasions, contusions and lacerations of the globe are among the most serious ocular injuries. First aid is aimed at stopping hemorrhage, preventing swelling, preventing further damage and relieving pain. Gentle application of cold compresses is helpful, but application of pressure to the damaged eye must be avoided. The eye can be irrigated to remove foreign material, if necessary, and bandaged for protection. Prevent self-trauma.

Ocular Foreign Bodies

Signs

- Grossly visible foreign bodies in the eye
- Eyelids clamped shut
- Rubbing at the eyes
- Swollen eyelids

First Aid

- Remove superficial foreign bodies if possible
- Do not remove foreign bodies protruding from the eyeball
- Control hemorrhage and swelling if necessary
- Protect the eye

Cause

Ocular foreign bodies may consist of virtually any foreign material, such as wood, metal, stone, dust and other debris. They may be the primary cause of an eye injury or may be secondary. They may lodge beneath the eyelids but external to the globe itself, partially penetrate the globe, or penetrate the globe to lodge entirely within the globe.

Clinical Signs

The signs of an ocular foreign body are largely nonspecific unless the foreign body is grossly visible. They include blepharospasm (eyelids clamped shut; do not force the eyelids open), rubbing or pawing at the eyes, and swollen eyelids.

First Aid

First aid for ocular foreign bodies depends mainly on their position. Foreign bodies external to the globe possibly may be removed by irrigating with sterile isotonic saline or by careful manipulation with a sterile cotton swab. If the foreign body cannot be easily removed, leave it alone and protect the eye from self-trauma (bandage and/or Elizabethan collar or cross-tying).

Foreign bodies protruding from the globe should *not* be removed, as this may result in collapse of the globe. Protect the eye from further damage and do not apply any pressure to the globe. Foreign bodies within the globe should not be disturbed. Protect the eye from further damage, control hemorrhage and swelling with cold compresses if necessary, and do not apply any pressure to the globe.

Proptosis

Signs

- Globe protruding from the socket

First Aid

- Do not try to force the globe back into the socket
- Keep the eye moist
- Protect the eye from further trauma

Cause

Proptosis is displacement or prolapse of the globe out of the socket. The eyelids close behind the displaced globe, preventing its return. This occurs most commonly in brachycephalic dogs, such as Pugs, Pekingese and Bulldogs, as a result of trauma. Proptosis is very serious because, unless promptly treated, the proptosed globe may swell and rapidly dry out, resulting in permanent damage and blindness.

Clinical Signs

A proptosed globe is very obvious as it protrudes prominently from the socket.

First Aid

First aid for a proptosed eye is aimed at keeping the globe moist and preventing further damage until it can be replaced in the socket. Do not attempt to force the globe back into the socket. The lids, which are closed behind it, usually prevent replacement; further damage to the eye may result from any applied pressure.

The globe should be kept moist by applying cold fluids directly, or soaking gauze sponges and gently applying them to the globe. Sterile isotonic saline or a hypertonic solution, such as 10% dextrose, which can help reduce swelling, should be used. If neither of these is available, tap water can be used. Keep the animal quiet and protect the globe from further trauma.

Suspected Poisoning

Cause

Animals can be poisoned by any of numerous potentially toxic substances. Sources include poisonous plants, toxic chemicals and medications. Toxicity can result from ingestion of or direct contact with the toxic substance.

Clinical Signs

Very few poisons produce distinctive signs. Most cause such nonspecific signs as excitability or depression, weakness, incoordination, salivation, vomiting, diarrhea, abdominal pain, convulsions and/or shock.

Poison Control Centers

A large number of government-sponsored Poison Control/Information Centers are located throughout the US and Canada. They can provide up-to-date information on poisons and appropriate treatment. The telephone number of the nearest center should be listed in the local telephone directory or can be obtained by contacting the nearest human hospital. Keep this number posted by the telephone so you can quickly locate it during an emergency.

First Aid

First aid for suspected poisoning is directed at maintaining vital functions and limiting the poison's effects by removing it from the animal's system, diluting it or neutralizing it with an appropriate antidote. Because very few toxins have specific antidotes, most animals are treated symptomatically. Timely supportive therapy may mean the difference between life and death.

It is important to identify the source of the poison, if possible. Toxic chemicals frequently have antidotes or first-aid procedures listed on their label. Obtain as much information from the owner as possible. If possible, have the owner bring the suspected poison, in the original package if it is a chemical, to the clinic with the patient.

If the animal is conscious and able to swallow, try to induce vomiting. *Do not induce vomiting if the poison is a corrosive or volatile substance,* such as a strong acid, strong alkali or petroleum product. Induce vomiting in small animals with a teaspoon or more of salt placed on the back of the tongue or a teaspoon (5 ml) of hydrogen peroxide given orally every 5 minutes. If acids have been swallowed, give bases, such as sodium bicarbonate (baking soda), and water orally. For ingested alkalis, give acids, such as lemon juice or vinegar and water orally. For petroleum products and other corrosive substances, give water or milk orally to dilute the poison in the GI tract.

If the animal is unconscious, convulsing or in shock, give symptomatic first aid as needed. Try to prevent an excited or convulsing animal from injuring itself.

Use large quantities of soap and water to cleanse body areas contaminated with a toxic or corrosive substance.

References

1. Colville, in Pratt: *Medical Nursing for Animal Health Technicians.* 1st ed. American Veterinary Publications, Goleta, CA, 1985.

2. Kirk *et al: Handbook of Veterinary Procedures and Emergency Treatment.* 5th ed. Saunders, Philadelphia, 1990.

3. Crowe, in: *Proc No Am Vet Conf,* 1993.

4. Nelson and Feldman, in Kirk: *Current Veterinary Therapy IX.* Saunders, Philadelphia, 1986.

5. Monroe: Management of diabetic dogs. *Vet Technician* 14:137-141, 1993.

Notes

Notes

2

General Patient Management

C.C. Bullmore and C.R. Kuhn

General patient management involves several related areas, including admissions, medical records, physical examination, patient handling and hospital care. The chapter is subdivided into small and large animal sections to make clear some fundamental differences between these 2 groups of animals from the standpoint of the technician. A small section on medical calculations is also included.

Admission of Small Animal Patients

Initial Client Contact

The telephone conversation is usually the client's first contact with the veterinary hospital. Good client-hospital relations are critical at this stage. The potential client can be won or lost before the patient has even seen the doctor.

Answering the telephone constitutes an overlap of duties between the receptionist and technician. It may be necessary for the technician to schedule appointments or to assist a client in determining if a veterinary examination is needed. Most clients do not realize that the veterinarian cannot talk to everyone who calls about their pet. Often they are equally ignorant of the training of the technician and that you are qualified to help answer their questions about animal health. Tactfully inform them that the doctor is with a patient, seeing a client or in surgery, and cannot be interrupted at this time. Avoid the phrase, "The doctor is busy." The assumption on the part of the client might be that if the doctor is too busy, he or she should call another veterinarian. Explain that as a well-trained technician you can assist them.

Scheduling appointments at first glance seems very routine. There are some major points that should be noted, however. Most veterinarians take about 15 minutes per office visit or about 4 calls per hour. The basic information needed to schedule a visit includes: client's full name; pet's name and breed; reason for the visit; telephone number where client can be reached during the daytime; and regular or new client? With this information the receptionist can have the medical record pulled before the client walks in the door. Being able to greet the pet by name is good public relations. Having the record ready is a time saver and helps project an image of efficiency.

The client's full name and animal's name are needed to avoid pulling the wrong record. Knowing the breed of the pet can have a bearing on the amount of time needed for the appointment. (Practitioners often need more time with birds and exotic pets and charge more for these office visits than for dogs or cats.)

The reason for the visit is important in using time most economically. A complicated (and more time consuming) case should be scheduled adjacent to a simple call, such as a vaccination. Thus, if the first appointment takes more than the allotted time, part of that time can be made up with a routine vaccination call scheduled next. If an infectious disease is suspected, it can be of benefit to schedule the pet when fewer other animals would be exposed, such as during the slowest part of the day or the last call before lunch. With coughing listed as the major reason for the visit, a technician can explain that it would be best for the pet to wait outside or in the car until the doctor is ready. Other clients appreciate not having their animal exposed to one that may have a contagious disease.

Being able to reach the client by telephone can be very helpful if an emergency arises. Prolonged surgery or an unexpected emergency case may require rescheduling of their appointment. A new client can be advised to come a few minutes early to fill out the information needed for a medical record. Realizing that this client has never previously been to your hospital can save much frustration in looking for a medical record that has not yet been made. Being prepared by having the record ready and knowing why the pet is scheduled for a visit can help the doctor greatly in budgeting valuable time.

There are always a few people who do not realize they need an appointment to see the doctor. Many of these clients would not dream of walking in unannounced to their hairstylist. But then, Fifi just needs a shot and her ears checked, not a facial, manicure, shampoo, wash and set. Grin and bear it. Try to fit these people in between scheduled appointments, but let them know that a wait is to be expected and that an appointment is required for future visits. Take clients with regularly scheduled appointments first if they are on time for their visits.

When genuine emergencies are involved, a rapid assessment is needed to determine the seriousness of the problem (see Chapter 1). Breathing difficulty, bleeding, poisonings, shock or convulsions should take priority, regardless of scheduling. The medical record can be pulled after the patient has been given an emergency examination to determine the need for immediate life-saving measures. Often the owner's level of concern for the pet's condition is not matched by the results of the examination. Some clients are overly concerned and can exaggerate or misread clinical signs. When a genuine emergency exists, prompt action on the part of the technician is required.

If the pet is to be admitted to the hospital for treatment or observation, some form of identification (ID) is needed. A cage card, including the date of admission, name of owner and patient, can be attached to the animal's cage or run. Some hospitals use an ID neck band that can be typed or marked with a waterproof marker to avoid possible confusion if the pet were moved without also moving the appropriate cage card.

History

A proper diagnosis can depend as much on a history as it does on the findings of the physical examination. On a routine visit, some history is volunteered by the client to the receptionist or technician. Important pieces of information often are not explained by the client because they were not recognized as relevant to the current problem. Eliciting a good history from a client is an art that can be learned by a technician to save time for the doctor and help avoid errors of omission that could be costly for both the client and patient by delaying proper diagnosis.

Questions should be asked without prejudice. A totally different answer can be obtained to a question, depending upon how that question is asked. Try not to put words in the client's mouth. If asked, "Has your cat been drinking a lot of water lately?" it is easiest for a client to say, "yes" or "no." But if asked, "Has your cat's water consumption increased, decreased or remained unchanged, or can you tell?", the owner may admit that 3 cats drink out of the same bowl and s/he cannot be sure what this cat's water consumption has been. Ask questions that offer alternatives, including "I don't know." It may be necessary to ask the same question more than once but in a different manner.

The history should begin with the basic complaint. What was it that caused the owner to be concerned enough to seek professional help? How long has the problem been present? In what order did the signs appear? (Which came first, the vomiting or the diarrhea?) Has the owner given any medication or tried to treat the problem? What effect did this have, if any? Has the pet had this problem before? If so, when? What was done for the problem at that time? What previous illnesses or accidents has this animal had? Some of these questions may not seem relevant to the client (or the technician), but the answers to these questions could supply the missing piece of data needed to determine a diagnosis.

More generalized questions should be asked after the initial complaint has been investigated. Where does this pet live: indoors, outdoors or both in and out? What part of the country is the animal from? Some diseases have a definite geographic distribution. What type of diet is fed: dry, canned, semimoist packets or table food? What brands are offered most often? Is the pet eating normally? Are bowel movements regular and normal in color and consistency? (Does the owner know what the bowel movement habits of this pet are?) Has the owner seen any evidence of vomiting? Are the urinary habits normal? When were the last vaccines given and for what diseases? Many owners reply, "The shots are up to date," but often they do not know what "up to date" really means. Get specific dates and types of vaccinations given or assume that they are overdue.

Are any other pets in the household healthy? Does this pet have any contact with other animals? Has the patient been boarded in a kennel or groomed by a professional groomer in the last 30 days? Contact with other animals may be a significant factor. Has this animal been exposed to any toxic substances? Remember to consider garden and household products, as well as garbage containers, plants, medication and foreign objects. All of this information can be useful in establishing a list of possible diagnoses.

When dealing with a genuine emergency, maintenance of life functions is primary. Some basic information is needed, but obtaining a detailed history must be postponed until emergency medical care has been rendered. More reliable responses to questions can be obtained after the owner has had time to calm down. The one major exception regards suspected poisoning cases. Exposure to any toxic substances must be discussed with the client immediately. Did the client observe the pet eating or drinking a poisonous substance? Has the owner used any snail bait, fertilizer, herbicides, insecticides, etc, that the pet could have contacted? If possible, the container of any suspected intoxicant should be brought to the hospital with the patient. First-aid instructions often can be found on the box or bottle, along with the chemical ingredients of the contents. With this information, the local poison control center can help by providing specific recommendations for treatment.

Small Animal Medical Records

Until recently, most veterinarians in private practice have kept medical records on a card index system filed alphabetically in a set of small drawers, each about the size of a shoe box. The cards may be 3 x 5 or 5 x 7 inches and contain all of the medical information on one or more pets over a several-year period. The disadvantages of this record system are obvious. Lack of space discourages proper recording of detailed information. Cramped wiring and numerous abbreviations become routine, making interpretation of the entries very difficult for another veterinarian treating the same animal. Ancillary information, such as lab results, may have to be filed separately. To obtain the complete record on a patient means going to 2 or more places, which is time consuming and increases the chance of a misfile. Changing addresses on the cards is inconvenient. Outdated files cannot be easily identified for removal to update the system. The only advantages to this system are that it is very inexpensive and records can be stored in a minimum amount of space.

Another type of record is the single sheet, with medical information on one side and the financial record for that client on the other. This style uses a sheet that is 11 x 6¾ inches, with the owner's last name placed in the top right-hand corner. The records are stored by rows in large bin, with the name visible by partially overlapping each sheet. When a sheet is removed, a gap appears in the sequence of files, thus helping to eliminate misfiling. On the reverse side of the page are several columns designed to classify the client charges by category (surgery, radiology, medication, etc), and indicate amount paid and balance due. This is superior to the card system because it offers more space and a record of all financial transactions. However, there are still space and filing limitations for adding laboratory data sheets and the need for more detailed record keeping, as would be required for lengthy hospitalization.

A good medical record system uses a file folder with the capacity to handle 8½ x 11-inch sheets. These files can be color coded, using bands on the edge of the folder to represent letters of the alphabet or a numeric code system that can be individualized to the size of the practice (Figs 1, 2). Misfiling is minimized by color coding, since an error stands our clearly. Each pet can have a separate section of the folder, divided by a card, to avoid confusion if the client has several animals. Year bands can be used to allow periodic culling of old files to keep the system updated. The record system should be scanned annually and any file with a 3-year-old band should be considered inactive and removed. The important advantage to this filing method is that more space is available for detailed record keeping on each patient. Laboratory results, radiology and surgical reports, previous medical records, and letters can all be placed in the folder for easy retrieval.

A medical record, regardless of the style employed, must contain the following information to meet legal standards and the requirements of the practice code:

1. Client's name, home address and telephone number.

2. Work address and telephone number (not required but very useful).

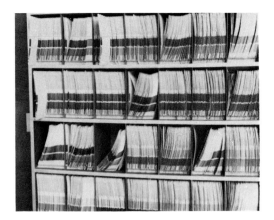

Figure 1. A color-coded file folder system.

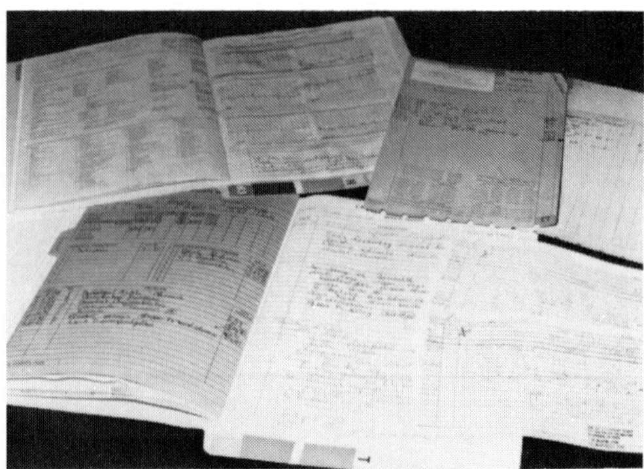

Figure 2. File folder records (upper and lower left) compared with the single-sheet record (upper right) and 5 x 7-inch card records (lower right).

3. Name and full description of the animal (species, breed, sex, neutering status, birthdate, color).

4. Medical information:

a) Dates of hospital visits or periods of custody of the animal.

b) History of the animal's condition, including reason for visit.

c) Physical examination findings and diagnosis.

d) Treatment and medication used (with complete directions).

e) Results of laboratory tests, radiographs, etc.

f) Progress and disposition of the case.

Medical record requirements vary among states. The above outline should be sufficient to meet most standards. In addition to these requirements, some states recommend keeping a separate surgical log, containing the date of surgery, client and patient name, type of surgery performed, and surgeon's name. This record can prevent confusion regarding the particulars of any surgery performed by that hospital. In some states, a radiology log is also required to record dates, exposure factors and patient information for every film made.

The file folder medical records system allows each hospital to design its own sheets. One simple alternative would use only 3 basic forms: registration, history and worksheet. The first page of the record would be a client registration form, filled out by every new client on the initial visit and updated when current information changed, such as a new address or telephone number (Fig 3). Credit information, including driver's license number and employment data, can also be included on this sheet. A more complex registration form includes basic questions about the pet as an aid in establishing a history (Fig 4).

Following the registration form is a medical-surgical summary sheet, with a complete description of the patient at the top (Figs 5, 6). Background information can be tabulated, including vaccination dates, heartworm tests, fecals, previous surgeries and radiographic studies, as well as long-term medical problems. This allows the doctor or technician to become familiar with a patient's previous history quickly, without need to leaf through many pages of written records.

The bulk of the medical record is the worksheet, which contains information on the current problem, answers to history questions, physical examination findings, laboratory test results, diagnoses, treatments, and daily progress notes. The worksheet is essentially a simple, lined page with space for the date, remarks, and charges in a column at the edge.

For hospitalized patients, some basic information is recorded in the medical record by the technician each day before the veterinarian examines the patient. Included should be the rectal temperature, pulse rate and respiratory rate. The temperature may be recorded in Fahrenheit or Celsius (Table 1). The pulse and respiratory rates should be recorded in beats and breaths per minute, respectively. Also of value is information on appetite, urination, bowel movements and any vomiting. A code system can be used for the last items and the information recorded on the patient's cage card by the person cleaning and feeding that patient each morning (Table 2). A cage card is large enough to record this data for several days if used properly (Fig 7).

Physical Examination of Small Animals

Vital Signs

Before a patient is examined by the doctor, a brief history should be obtained and the vital signs checked by the technician and recorded in the medical record, regardless of the reason for the visit. Many problems may be detected by performing these basic tasks on all patients, even apparently healthy ones. Normal rectal temper-

Figure 3. Registration form suitable for use in file folder record system.

REGISTRATION FORM

PLEASE PRINT

DATE ____________

NAME ____________ (LAST / FIRST / MIDDLE INITIAL) SPOUSE ____________

ADDRESS ____________ (STREET) CITY ____________ ZIP CODE ______ HOME PHONE ____________

OCCUPATION ____________ WORK PHONE ____________

EMPLOYER ____________ ADDRESS ____________ CITY ____________ ZIP ______

SPOUSE'S EMPLOYER ____________ ADDRESS ____________ CITY ____________ ZIP ______

REFERRED BY ____________

PROFESSIONAL FEES ARE TO BE PAID AT THE TIME THEY ARE RENDERED. PLEASE CIRCLE YOUR PREFERRED METHOD OF PAYMENT

CASH CHECK

SIGNATURE OF OWNER ____________

SIGNATURE OF PERSON PRESENTING THIS PET FOR TREATMENT IF OTHER THAN OWNER ____________

SPECIES ____________ BREED ____________ COLOR ____________

PET'S NAME ____________ SEX ______ ALTERED: YES[ ] NO [ ] BIRTH DATE ____________ (MONTH DAY YEAR)

DATE OF LAST VACCINATION ____________ TYPE ____________ WHERE ____________

____________ TYPE ____________ WHERE ____________

CREDIT REFERENCES ____________

DRIVER'S LICENSE NO. ____________

ature and pulse and respiratory rates (TPR) for dogs and cats are listed in Table 3. Be sure the thermometer has been shaken down and reads no higher than 96 F before rectal insertion. Using lubrication and a slight rotational movement, the thermometer is gently inserted about 2 inches and held in place for 2 minutes for a reliable reading. After the thermometer is removed and wiped off, the temperature obtained is recorded. Storing the thermometer in an antiseptic solution avoids cross-contamination between patients.

Figure 4. A detailed registration form includes some of the animal's history.

CARMICHAEL ANIMAL HOSPITAL
Registration

Client Information

Owner's Name and Address	Last	First		Middle
	Street	City	State	Zip
Referred By	Yellow Pages ☐	Relative or Friend ☐	Name ______	
Phone and Emergency Numbers	Home Phone	Husband Work Phone	Wife Work Phone	Emergency Phone
Method of Payment	Cash ☐ Check ☐	Mastercard ☐ Visa ☐	D.L. # ______	

Patient Information

Pet's Name ______ Breed ______

Sex ______ Date of Birth ______

Pet Obtained From? Breeder ☐ Pet Store ☐ Neighbor☐ Other☐

Has your pet been spayed (females) or neutered (males)?

Yes ☐ No ☐ If so, when? ______

Has your pet been vaccinated? Yes ☐ No ☐ If so, when? ______

For what? ______

What is your pets diet? Dry ☐ Canned ☐ Semi-moist ☐ Table food ☐

Are there other pets in the household? Yes ☐ No ☐

If so, what kind? ______

Is your pet currently taking medication? Yes ☐ No ☐

If so, what kind? ______

Does your pet suffer from any allergies? Yes ☐ No ☐

If so, what kind? ______

Do you have any problems with its behavior? If so, check below:

Housebreaking ☐ Biting ☐ Disobeying ☐ Running off☐

Fighting ☐ Disturbing neighbors ☐ Other ☐ ______

A DEPOSIT IS REQUIRED ON ALL HOSPITALIZED PATIENTS, BALANCE TO BE PAID UPON DISCHARGE. MASTERCARD, AND VISA SERVICE AVAILABLE.

Signature of owner or responsible party ______ *Date* ______

The pulse is taken at the femoral artery, inside the thigh, or by palpating the heart in smaller animals. A stethoscope can be helpful in recording heart rates in obese animals. Respiratory rates can be taken by observation, or by placing a hand on the thorax. Pulse and respiratory rates should be recorded as the number counted in one minute. With practice, counting for 10-15 seconds and then multiplying by 6 or 4, respectively, speeds up this procedure.

Figure 5. The medical/surgical summary sheet provides space for a detailed history of the animal's previous medical problems on one page.

CARMICHAEL ANIMAL HOSPITAL

CLIENT:			PATIENT:	
SPECIES:	BREED:	SEX M M/C F F/S	BIRTHDATE:	COLOR:

D.H.L.-P.											
RABIES											
PARVOVIRUS											
F.V.R.-C.-P.											
DENTISTRY											
FECALS											
WORMING											

SURGICAL PROCEDURES		DATE
1		
2		
3		
4		
5		
6		
7		
8		

RADIOGRAPHIC PROCEDURES		DATE
1		
2		
3		
4		
5		
6		
7		
8		

DATE ENTERED	PROBLEM NO.	PROBLEM	DATE RESOLVED

DRUG SENSITIVITIES	

General Assessment

When first looking at an animal from a distance, you should note its general condition and attitude. The animal may be of normal weight, underweight or obese. Its disposition may be friendly, nervous, placid or aggressive. Careful observation can alert a technician to possible danger in the handling of a patient. Take the time to look from a distance first. Get a feeling for the pet's overall ap-

Figure 6. Another style of medical/surgical summary sheet provides space for information on previous major and minor medical problems, radiographic results and any drug idiosyncrasies.

BRENTWOOD PET CLINIC

MEDICAL–SURGICAL SUMMARY

Client's name____ Animal's name____ Birth Date____

Sex____ Breed____ Color____ Referred by____

DHL-P											
Rabies											
FVR-C-P											
FECALS											
DENTISTRY											
WORMING											

ACUTE SELF-LIMITED (TEMPORARY) PROBLEMS

Prob. No.	PROBLEM	Dates of Occurance 1	2	3	4	5	6	7	8	9	10
A											
B											
C											
D											
E											
F											
G											
H											
I											
J											
K											
L											
M											
N											

MAJOR PROBLEM LIST

Prob. No.	PROBLEM–Active	Date Entered	Date Resolved
1			
2			
3			
4			
5			
6			
7			
8			
9			
10			

RADIOGRAPHIC PROCEDURES	Date
1.	
2.	
3.	
4.	
5.	
6.	
7.	
8.	
9.	

SURGICAL PROCEDURES	Date
A.	
B.	
C.	
D.	
E.	
F.	
G.	

DRUG SENSITIVITIES

1.
2.
3.
4.
5.

pearance and temperament before proceeding with the physical exam.

Physical Examination

Animals may be examined in several ways. I prefer the front-to-back system. Starting with the nose, I examine the animal anatomically, finishing with the rear feet and tail. For the purpose of teaching, however, an organ system approach is best. After mastering the basic technique, pick the method of examination that you feel confident in using.

Vital signs are checked initially, followed by obtaining an accurate body weight to the nearest pound if over 25-30 lb, or the nearest half-pound if under 25 lb. Though most of us are more comfortable using pounds and ounces, it is more appropriate to use the metric system of weights and measures (see following section on Medical Calculations). Accurate weights are essential in a medical record for calculating doses and to assess weight loss or gain in subsequent visits.

In a routine physical examination there are 9 areas to consider in the organ system approach. Use your senses to describe the findings. Sight, smell and touch (palpa-

Table 1. Centrigrade (celsius) and fahrenheit temperature equivalents.

Centrigrade (C)	Fahrenheit (F)
36.0	96.8
36.5	97.7
37.0	98.6
38.0	100.4
38.2	100.8
38.4	101.1
38.6	101.5
38.8	101.8
39.0	102.2
39.2	102.6
39.4	102.9
39.6	103.3
39.8	103.6
40.0	104.0
40.2	104.4
40.4	104.7
40.6	105.1
40.8	105.4
41.0	105.8
41.2	106.2
41.4	106.5
41.6	106.8
41.8	107.1
42.0	107.5

tion) are all important. Describe the location, appearance, and size of any abnormalities. Do not make diagnoses; simply record what you see. Avoid drawing conclusions as to why the problem exists.

1. *The Skin:* Is the haircoat shiny and glossy or dry and brittle? Are there areas of hair thinning or hair loss (alopecia)? Does the

Table 2. Common cage card abbreviations.

Appetite	**App**	**Urination**	**Urine**
none	0	none	0
ate small portion	⊝	normal	+
ate half meal	⊖	large volume	++
ate full meal	⊕	bloody urine	BU
Bowel Movements	**BM**	**Vomiting**	**Vomit**
none	0	none	0
normal stool	+	vomited once	+
soft stool	S	vomited twice	++
diarrhea	D	bloody vomitus	BV
bloody diarrhea	BD		

Figure 7. This cage card has columns in which information on an animal's appetite, bowel movements, urination and any vomiting is recorded daily.

Owner: Patient:

DATE	APP	BM	URINE	VOMIT	INSTRUCTIONS

dog or cat have a scratching or itching problem (pruritus)? Are there skin lesions? Are there red, inflamed areas (erythema)? Does the animal have fleas, ticks or lice? Do you detect an abnormal odor to the skin? If the patient tolerates handling, be sure to feel every part of its surface. A long coat can hide significant lesions.

2. *Eyes and Ears:* Can the patient see and hear? Owners sometimes state that the pet has a problem seeing or hearing; however, clients are often unaware of these problems until they are pointed out. Moving an object before an animal's eyes and noting if it tracks the object with its eyes is a good test of vision. Be careful not to create a current of air by moving a large object, such as the hand, too quickly and close to the face, as this air movement can be detected by the pet and misinterpreted by an examiner as visual perception. Tossing a cotton ball in the air usually elicits a response in a normal patient without causing any artifactual errors.

What do the eyes look like? Are they both open? Is there an ocular discharge or evidence of tearing (lacrimation)? Chronic overflow of tears (epiphora) is common in small breeds of dogs and leaves a reddish-brown discoloration of the hair in the corners of the eyes. Is the white of the eye (sclera) reddened or discolored? Are the pink mucous membranes that surround the eye (conjunctivae) pale, normal or irritated? Is the cornea clear and shiny? Are both pupils of equal size? Do they respond to light by constriction? Does the pupil appear black? Is there a grayish-blue haziness or white opacity (cataract) in the pupil? Is the third eyelid (nictitating membrane) partially protruding over the eye?

Do the ears have an odor? Are they clean or filled with exudate? Is any ear discharge wet, dry, dark, creamy, bloody, etc? Does the animal show any head-shaking behavior? Are the ears painful when handled? Does the ear flap (pinna) have any discolorations or swellings? Does the animal respond to sound?

3. *Musculoskeletal System:* Watch the animal walk to detect any lameness problem. Stand in front of the patient and, using one hand on each limb, gradually move from the shoulders down past

Table 3. Normal temperatures, pulse rates and respiratory rates for cats and dogs.

	Cats	Puppies	Adult Dogs	Toy Breeds
Rectal temperature				
F	100.5-102.5	100.5-102.5	100.5-102.5	100.5-102.5
C	38.0-39.1	38.0-39.1	38.0-39.1	38.0-39.1
Pulse rate (/min)	110-130	70-220	70-180	70-220

the elbows and wrist (carpus) to the digits. Asymmetry of the limbs can be detected more easily when comparing the left and right sides simultaneously. Do the same for the rear legs by standing behind the animal and palpating the limbs from the hips down past the stifles to the tarsus and toes. Palpate the thorax and trunk to check for lumps or pain. Gently flex and extend each joint of all 4 legs, checking for smoothness of motion, swelling, pain or muscle wasting (atrophy). It may be necessary to place the dog or cat on its side while examining the joints of the proximal limbs (Fig 13).

4. *Respiratory System:* Is there a nasal discharge from one or both nostrils? Is sneezing or coughing evident? Palpate the larynx and trachea gently. Does tracheal manipulation elicit an exaggerated cough response? Are the respirations shallow or deep in nature? Auscultate the lungs, beginning with the large airways (trachea and bronchi) in the cranial portion of the thorax and moving to the central thorax to listen to the intermediate airways. Finish with the smallest airways (bronchioles) in the caudal portion of the thorax. In normal animals, respiratory sounds are heard only during inspiration and the very first part of expiration. The majority of expiration is thus silent. To properly auscultate the chest, a quiet room is essential. Politely request that everyone stop talking for a few minutes. Hold the dog's mouth closed to prevent panting. Respiratory sounds are faint and require practice to discern.

5. *Cardiovascular System:* Initially check the color of the oral mucous membranes. Do not be misled by the presence of brown or black pigment, sometimes found in the gums (gingivae) of some animals. Look for a bright, healthy pink color that indicates good perfusion. Chow Chow dogs have dark blue-black pigment in the gums, lips and tongue. To the novice this may appear abnormal. Capillary refill time (CRT) is tested by pressing on the gum above the canine tooth with a finger, quickly releasing the pressure and timing how long it takes for reappearance of a pink color in the blanched area. Normal CRT is 1-2 seconds. A pale gum color or prolonged CRT indicates anemia or a circulatory disturbance. The femoral pulse rate has already been counted while checking vital signs. Its character should be described as strong, weak or irregular. Further descriptions of the pulse character may be made by the doctor.

The next step is auscultation of the heart. Begin in the pulmonic area, on the left side of the chest at the third intercostal space, ventrally toward the sternum. The aortic area is located in the fourth intercostal space at the costochondral junction (area where rib bone and cartilage join). The mitral area is located in the ventral fifth intercostal space, near the sternum. The last area of cardiac auscultation is in the tricuspid area, on the right side of the thorax at the fourth intercostal space, near the costochondral junction. At each of these points, the valve that corresponds to the name of the area can be heard most distinctly (Fig 8). The normal heart sound should consist of 2 separate beats, with a silent interval between them: LUB DUB, LUB DUB, LUB DUB, etc. Any additional sounds, or blurring together of the first and second sounds constitute a heart murmur. When evaluating the heart, it is important to check the heart rate and compare it with the pulse rate palpated at the femoral artery. The pulse rate can be lower than the heart rate (pulse deficit) in certain medical conditions.

6. *Gastrointestinal System:* Begin at the mouth by examining the teeth. A brownish discoloration of the teeth, known as calculus, may be seen in some middle-aged and older pets. This material can cause the gums to recede, resulting in premature loosening and loss of the teeth (periodontal disease). Inflammation of the gums (gingivitis) is indicated by a reddening along the gum line and usually is secondary to the presence of dental calculus.

Is the tongue symmetric? Can the animal swallow normally? Is there a problem with drooling or excessive salivation?

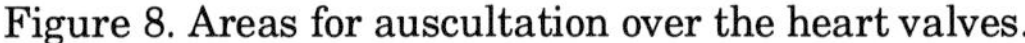
Figure 8. Areas for auscultation over the heart valves.

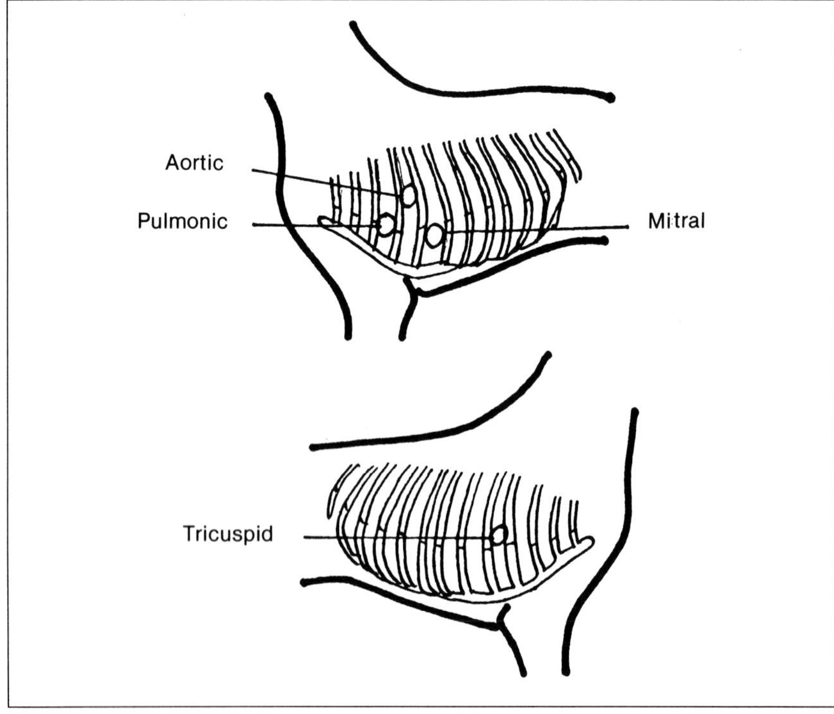

Palpation of the abdomen is useful in assessing the stomach, intestinal tract, liver and spleen. A distended stomach or painful loops of bowel may be evident; palpation can elicit a reaction from the patient. Some tenderness may be expected with any normal animal as a result of nervousness. Extreme tenderness or crying can indicate pain and a possible abdominal disturbance. Gas, fluid or normal stools can be palpated in the intestinal tract after some practice. The liver margin may be palpable in slender dogs and most cats, protruding just caudal to the rib cage. In large dogs or obese animals the liver may not be felt. The spleen, a flat, tongue-shaped organ in the mid-abdomen, is not usually palpable unless enlarged by disease or use of certain drugs. Any masses that cannot be identified should be noted. Tumors of the spleen, liver or intestinal tract may be detected early by skillful abdominal palpation. Be gentle when examining the abdomen, particularly if pregnancy is a possibility. If you encounter an animal that vigorously resists abdominal palpation, by tensing the abdominal muscles, it is better to skip that part of the examination and notify the doctor than to traumatize the animal by attempted palpation.

Examine the anus to determine if the anal sacs, on either side of the anus, are distended or if any irritation or abnormal lumps are present. A digital rectal examination, using a lubricated glove, can be used to detect prostatic enlargement or displacement in male animals. This type of examination may be helpful in assessing the character of the stool and can also be used to aid in expressing distended anal sacs.

7. *Reproductive and Urinary Systems:* Examination of the reproductive system of male animals should begin at the penis. In the dog, gently retract the prepuce and examine for irritation on the surface of the penis. A certain small amount of thick, greenish discharge is present in all normal male dogs. Excessive licking or irritation of the prepuce may be evidenced by redness or pain on examination. Next, examine the scrotum. Is the scrotal skin irritated, thickened or discolored? Palpate each testis individually. Are they symmetric and uniform in size and shape? Is there pain on examination of the scrotum or testes? Testicular asymmetry, a disparity in testicular size, may indicate a testicular tumor, atrophy or previous infection.

In female animals, begin the reproductive tract exam at the vulva. Is there a vulvar discharge? Describe the quantity and appearance of any discharge found. Is there swelling of the labia, indicative of estrus or infection? The internal reproductive tract of non-pregnant females is usually not palpable. Observing a scar or palpating steel sutures in the abdominal wall can indicate that the animal has been spayed. Lack of such a scar or palpable sutures does not rule out a previous spay operation. Careful palpation of the mammary glands is important, especially in older bitches. Examine each gland and nipple individually, progressing from the most cranial gland, caudad. Small cystic growths or nodules may not be visible but may be evident on careful, systematic palpation.

When palpating the caudal abdomen, the full or partially full urinary bladder may be evident as a smooth-surfaced, egg-shaped structure that slips easily between the fingers and thumb when felt. If urine has recently been voided or only a small amount is present, the bladder may not be palpable. Pain on palpation of the urinary bladder, especially in male cats, may indicate an infection or obstruction. Bladder stones (calculi) may be palpable with practice. Though in cats both kidneys are palpable behind the rib cage, ventral to the spine, only the left kidney may be felt in dogs. The cat's greater flexibility permits a more complete abdominal exam.

8. *Lymph Nodes:* The mandibular lymph nodes are palpable at the angle of the jaw as firm ovoid masses. The prescapular nodes are located cranial to the shoulder blades. Obesity may prevent palpation of these lymph nodes. The axillary lymph nodes, located in the "underarm" area, and the inguinal lymph nodes, located in the groin, are not palpable unless they are pathologically enlarged. The popliteal lymph nodes are palpable in normal animals caudal to the knee (Fig 9).

As all of the lymph nodes commonly examined are symmetric from one side of the animal to the other, an enlargement on one side can indicate inflammation or infection in the area drained by that node. Pain upon palpation of the nodes should be recorded.

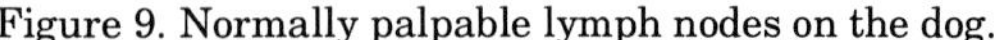

Figure 9. Normally palpable lymph nodes on the dog.

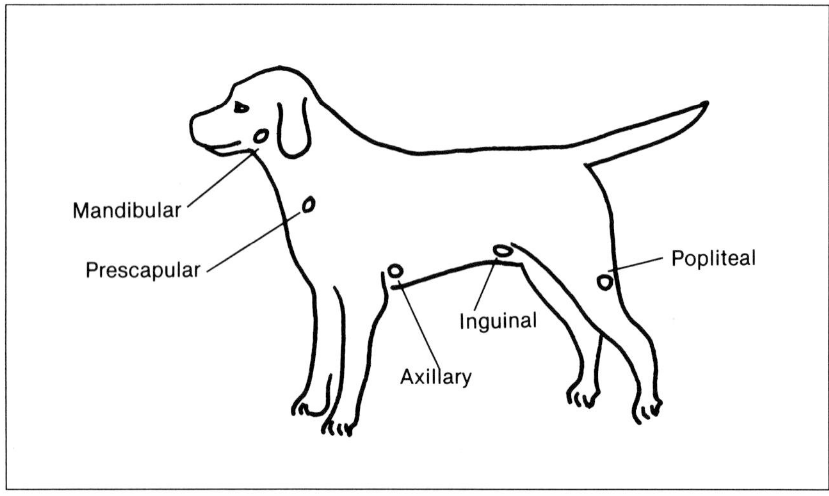

Generalized enlargement of all lymph nodes can occur in some infectious diseases and lymphosarcoma.

9. *Nervous System:* When first examining the animal, determine if the gait and mental attitude are normal. Is there lameness? Does the animal have a stumbling or uncoordinated gait (ataxia)? Is the animal bright and alert or is there evidence of mental depression, listlessness and lethargy? Injury to the brain or cranial nerves may manifest itself as a head tilt or nystagmus. Nystagmus is the involuntary, rapid horizontal or vertical movement of the eyeballs. Aimless wandering in circles or head pressing against a wall or other objects also indicates brain disease.

Pain, weakness or paralysis of the forelegs or rear legs may indicate spinal cord disease. These patients should be examined with extreme care to prevent injury to the examiner and further injury to the patient by manipulation. Pain sensation in each limb may be tested by pinching the toes with the fingers or small hemostats. The normal response is withdrawal of the limb and an indication that the patient felt the pinch by turning the head, curling the lip or crying. Simple withdrawal of the limb, without conscious recognition by the patient, can be a spinal reflex and, thus, not a true test of whether the animal has sensation or not.

Check the anus to determine the presence of normal tone. An open, flaccid anal sphincter indicates caudal spinal cord damage. Can the patient urinate? Is the urinary bladder overdistended and easily expressed upon palpation? Does urine flow just in response to gravity and not due to a conscious effort by the patient? Both of these situations could indicate neurologic bladder damage.

A peripheral nerve injury may be manifested as failure to respond when one limb is stimulated by a pinch or as lameness. The patellar tendon (kneejerk) reflex can be elicited in normal animals by sharply tapping the patellar tendon with the handle of a pair of scissors and watching the response. This reflex may be difficult to determine in a nervous or tense patient. An intact patellar reflex does not necessarily mean the spinal cord is intact, as the reflex remains intact even if the cord is severed completely anywhere cranial to the midlumbar cord.

Proper neurologic examination requires a veterinarian's training, but the above basic examination can alert the technician to the presence of gross neurologic deficits.

Handling and Restraint of Small Animals

Dogs

It is a good idea to require all clients to have their dogs on a leash upon admission to the veterinary hospital. Surprisingly, many owners fail to realize the importance of this simple safety precaution. Watching the animal enter the reception room and observing its responses enable you to assess the personality of the pet in advance of direct contact. Some dogs that are normal at home can become very nervous or even vicious in a veterinary hospital. The owner may volunteer the information that the dog has bitten a handler previously. Do not rely upon the client to give you advance warning that an animal is belligerent.

A small dog (under 40 lb) can be easily lifted by placing one arm around the animal's neck to control the head and using the second arm to scoop up the rear end (Fig 10). An alternative to scooping the animal around the rear legs is to place an arm under the abdomen, cranial to the rear legs, and lift the dog beneath the abdomen. If an abdominal injury or pregnancy is suspected, this second method of lifting should be avoided. For a larger dog, a 2-person lift allows better control and less strain for the technician (Fig 11).

Examination tables are smooth surfaced to prevent animals from attaining a good grip that may make holding a pet more difficult. The technician should be on the opposite side of the examining table from the veterinarian. The dog should be standing or in normal sternal recumbency, with the forelegs stretched out in front. The head must be controlled at all times. For nervous animals, a hugging grip, with the arm around the neck, allows the best control. The second arm can be placed around the abdomen and thorax, stabilizing the animal against the technician's body (Fig 12). Having the owner stand in front of the pet, where he or she can be clearly seen, is often an advantage, as frequently the animal attempts to turn and look at the owner. An easy-going,

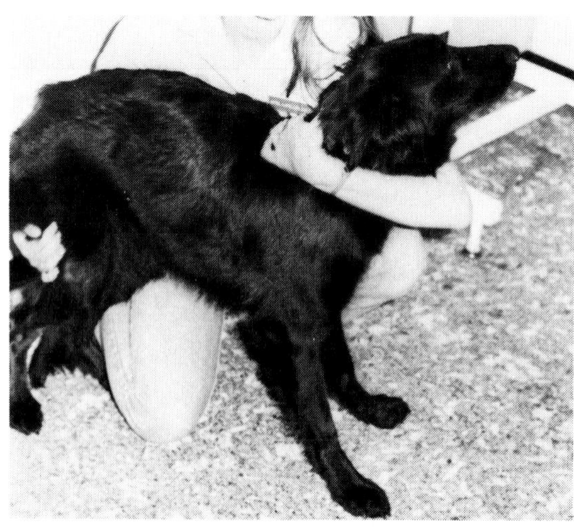

Figure 10. Dogs can be safely lifted with one arm around the neck and the other beneath the rear legs.

friendly animal can be examined with minimal restraint, as no painful procedures are anticipated in a routine physical exam.

To restrain a dog on its side, the forelegs are held in one hand with the middle finger separating the legs (Fig 13). The second hand holds the rear legs in a similar manner. The dog should be positioned with the legs held away from the handler and perpendicular to its body. Using one elbow to hold the dog's neck on the table prevents raising the head. The other elbow can be used to press down on the dog's rear quarters. For large dogs, only the lower limb of each pair (nearer the table surface) must be gripped, as it is the lower limb the dog uses to right itself from a prone position. This restraint position is useful when examining the joints, making an ECG and giving some types of injections.

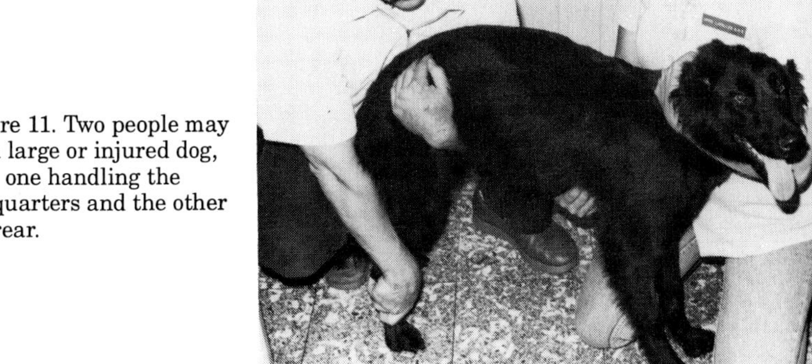

Figure 11. Two people may lift a large or injured dog, with one handling the forequarters and the other the rear.

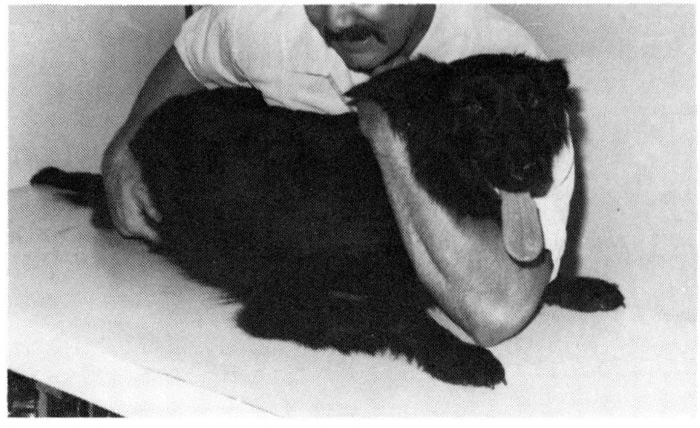

Figure 12. Standard restraint position for examination of a dog.

For an ear examination, one hand is placed on the muzzle and the second behind the skull, with the elbow holding the animal's chest and trunk into the technician's body (Fig 14). Such a position prevents gross movement of the head when the ear is being examined with an otoscope. With exceptionally painful ear conditions, sedation may be required to allow a full examination.

For administration of IM and SC injections, the normal restraint position is adequate, hugging the head with one arm and controlling the torso with the other (Fig 12). For IV injections, the animal handler must control the head with one arm while extending the foreleg with steady pressure and occluding the cephalic vein (Fig 15).

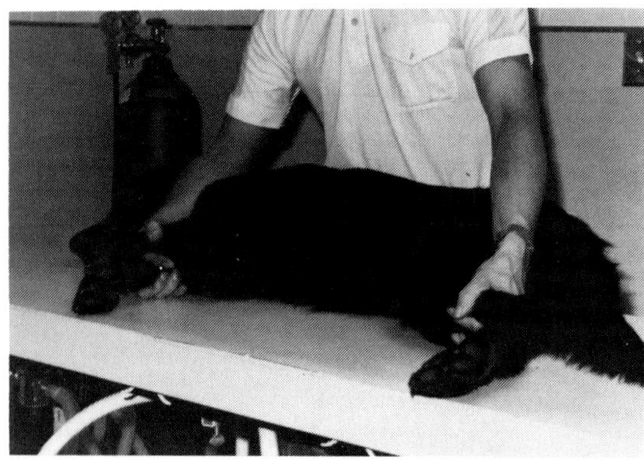

Figure 13. Dog kept in lateral recumbency for IM injection or electrocardiography.

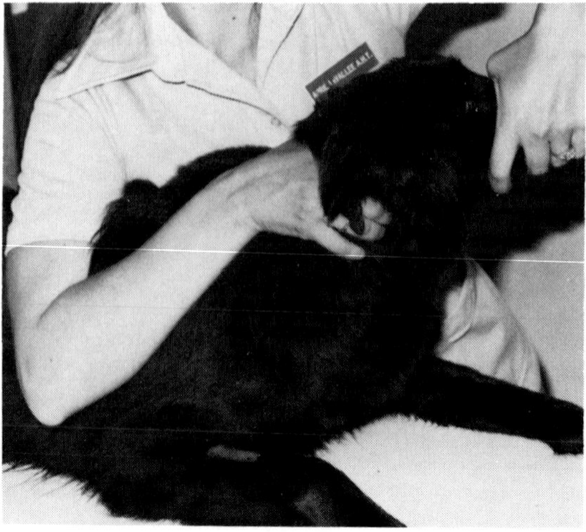

Figure 14. Restraint for ear examination limits head movement.

Animals that are excessively nervous, reluctant or downright belligerent may require a muzzle for the safety of the handler. A muzzle can be fashioned from nonstretch gauze tied over the nose, crossed beneath the chin and then tied in a bow behind the head (Figs 16, 17). It is important to explain to the pet owner that it is easy for the dog to breathe through the nose while the mouth is tied closed. This is not a painful or uncomfortable procedure for the dog, but it may be misinterpreted by the client as unnecessary or even cruel unless properly explained in advance.

For the patient that is totally unmanageable, a restraint pole or "come along" may be needed to allow injection of a sedative (Fig 18). This pole should not be used in the presence of the client. The adjustable loop of the pole should be maneuvered to include the head and one front leg of the small dog and then tightened down to prevent escape. Incorporation of one front leg in the noose prevents inadvertent strangulation of the patient due to struggling that may overtighten the loop. This device should be released as soon as possible after the injection is completed. The patient should be allowed to calm down and feel the full effect of the medication before the examination is begun.

For an IM injection, an alternative to the restraint pole is to thread the dog's leash through the cage bars. By pulling the head against the bars, a rear leg can be safely grasped and the injection made. If a dog is known to be difficult to handle, tranquilizers may be dispensed for the owner to administer before the animal is admitted to the hospital. Tranquilization may not be advisable if it jeopardizes the dog's health or masks signs of illness.

Figure 15. Restraint for IV injection of the cephalic vein in the dog (a) and cat (b).

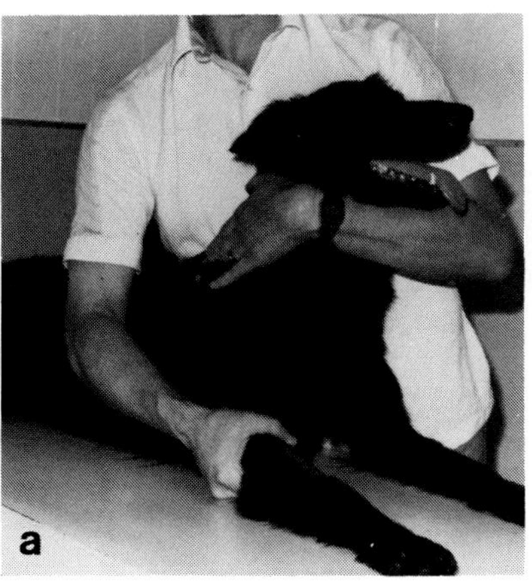

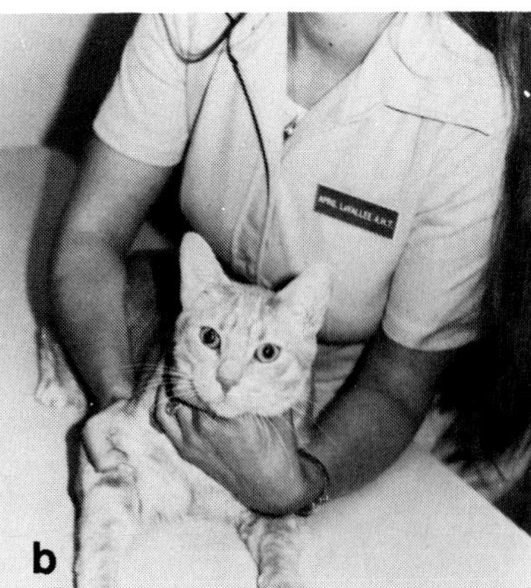

Moving slowly and calmly and avoiding unnecessary noise enable an animal handler and veterinarian to examine most animals. If a dog is reluctant to follow the handler on a leash when taken into the hospital, it helps to have the owner leave first. When the client is out of sight, most dogs follow the handler with little problem. Some animals do not respond to gentle handling and may require more physical restraint or use of tranquilizers. These animals may be strays that have had little human contact or may be excessively fearful, maladjusted pets that only do well with their owners, in familiar surroundings. Others may be genuinely in pain and only reacting instinctively when handled by strangers in an unfamiliar environment.

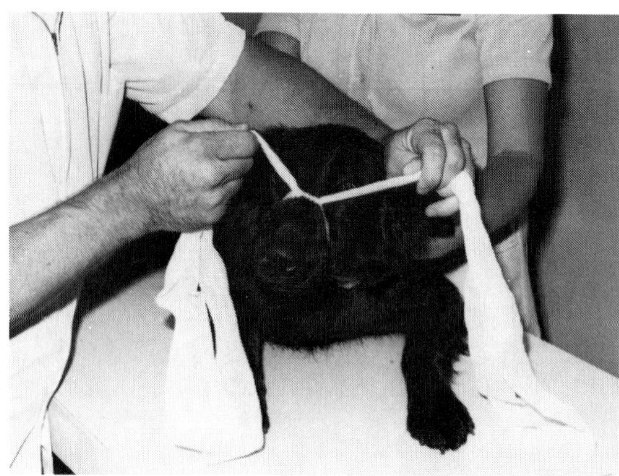

Figure 16. The first loop of a gauze muzzle is tied over the bridge of the nose, while the assistant steadies and points the dog's head toward the operator. The ends of the tie are looped under the chin and pulled behind the dog's head.

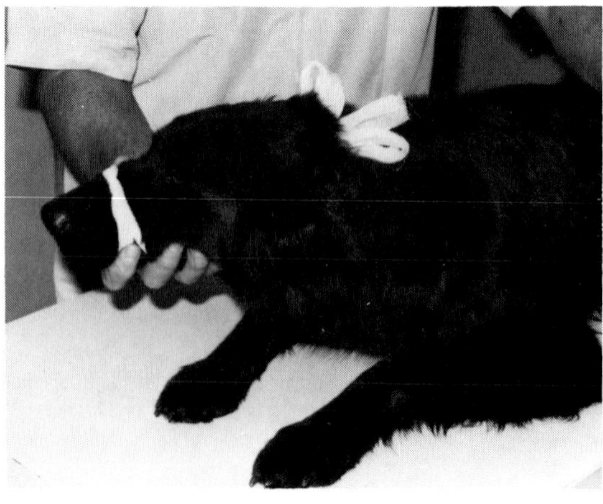

Figure 17. After the ends are looped under the chin and pulled behind the head, they are tied in a bow for easy removal, avoiding pinching the ears.

Cats

Bringing the cat to the veterinary hospital in a cardboard box or other suitable carrier is highly recommended, as this prevents altercations between pets in the waiting room, as well as preventing injury to the owner. Examining a cat that has already been made nervous by a dog in the waiting room can be difficult. Minimal restraint is the most successful way to examine most cats. Giving injections or taking blood samples is more challenging because of the smaller size, flexibility and agility of cats.

To examine the ears, the handler should use one hand under the chin and neck and the other to restrain the forelegs (Fig 19). Very nervous cats may be wrapped in a large, thick towel, with just the head exposed (Fig 20).

A towel can also be used to pick up a difficult cat by throwing it completely over the animal, then scooping it up. Particularly aggressive, biting cats can be handled with thick leather gloves that have a wide cuff to protect the lower forearm. It is far safer to se-

Figure 18. A well-constructed restraint pole or "come along."

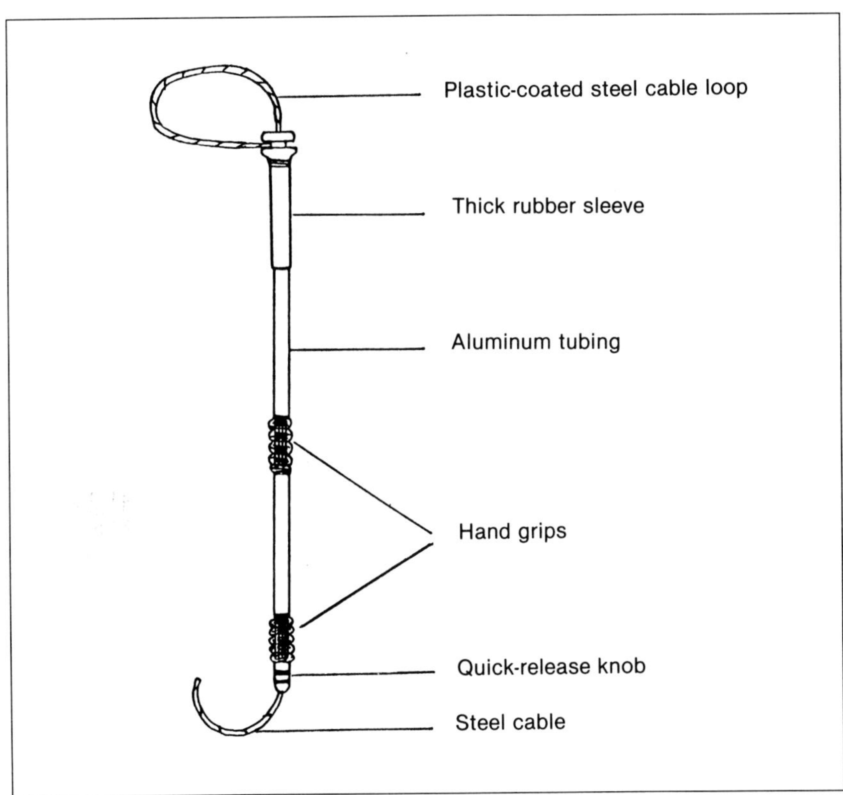

date these patients than to attempt to examine a frightened animal. Cats do not respond to physical restraint or a firm tone of voice as well as dogs. Struggling with a fractious cat can lead to injury that could be avoided with use of a sedative.

Cats are best carried under the arm, with the fingers separating and controlling the forelegs (Fig 21). The elbow is used to hold the cat's body against the waist and hips of the handler. The free hand can then be used for opening doors or controlling the head as necessary. Carriers should be used whenever possible when admitting or discharging patients from hospital wards.

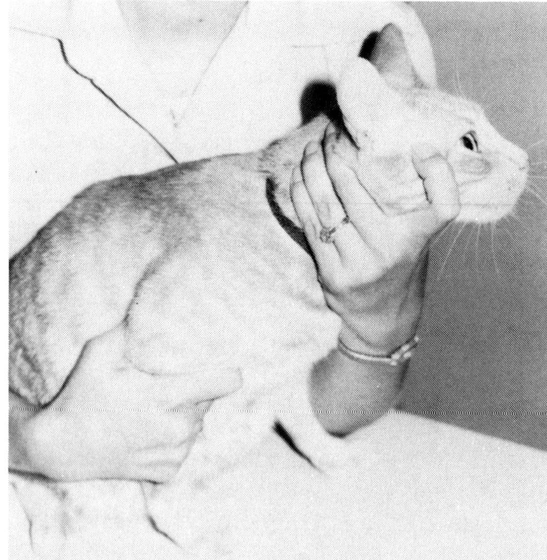

Figure 19. Restraint of a cat for ear examination or treatment.

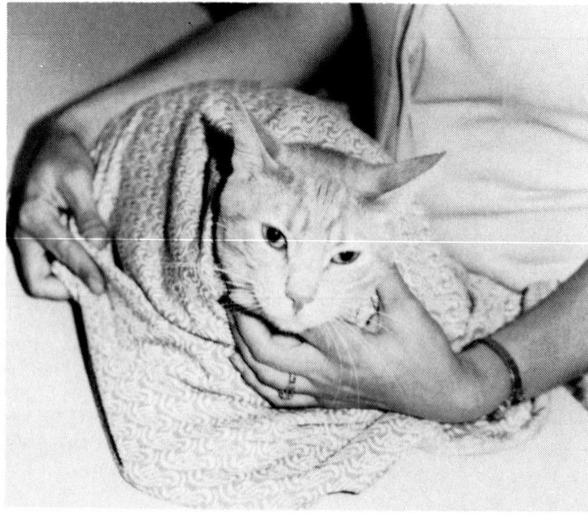

Figure 20. Wrapping the cat in a towel allows easy pill administration and manipulation of the head.

It is considered reasonable to hold a cat by the scruff of the neck, using the loose skin, only when no other means of restraint is possible. Holding the cat at arm's length prevents injury to the handler and does not harm the patient if done properly. It is preferable not to use this form of handling in view of the client, as it is commonly misinterpreted as cruel. Under no circumstances should a dog be picked up from the ground using the loose skin over the neck and back area, as such handling is unnecessarily painful for dogs.

Subcutaneous injections are usually not painful and require minimal restraint. The handler may simply distract the cat's attention by scratching or petting while the injection is made. More restraint is needed for an IM injection. With the cat in lateral recumbency, the head and forelegs are fully controlled using both hands. The rear legs are managed by the person giving the injection (Fig 22). After the injection, the cat should be released quickly to avoid unnecessary struggling.

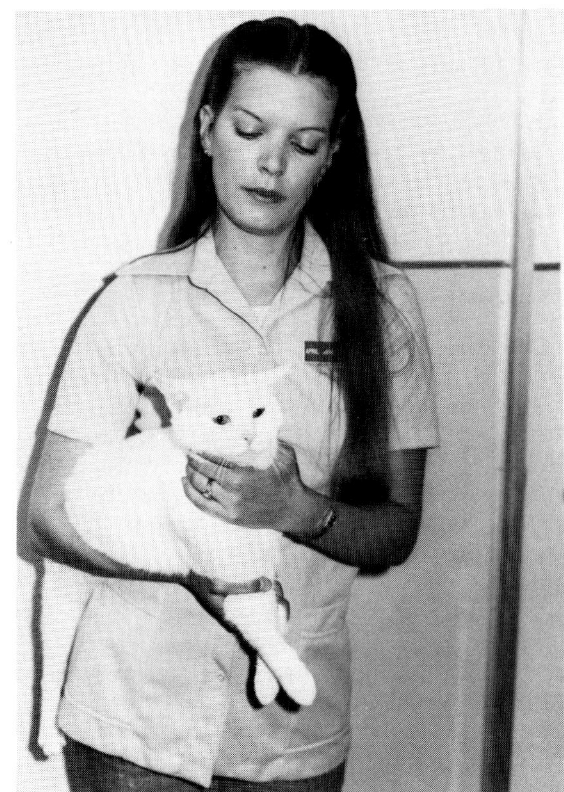

Figure 21. The forelegs of the cat are controlled and the body supported by one arm, while the other remains free to manipulate the head or open doors.

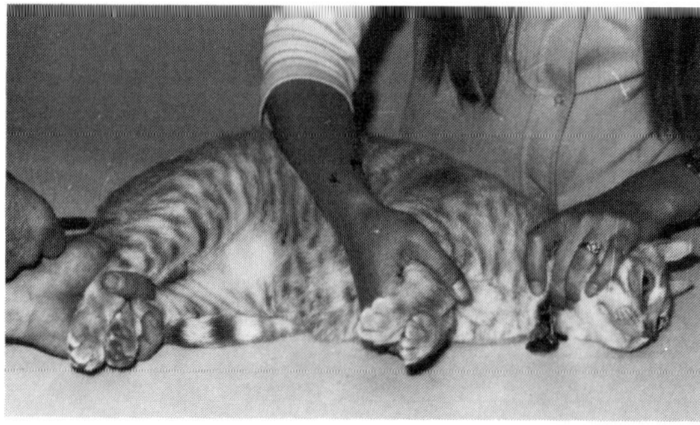

Figure 22. Cat held in lateral recumbency for IM injection.

Hospitalization of Small Animals

Observation

The veterinarian normally examines all hospitalized patients at least once daily to assess the progress of treatment. The technician may be responsible for the animal's cleanliness, feeding, watering and, most important, noting any changes in its condition. The technician is in a unique position to observe each patient because these other duties provide more contact time to notice behavioral changes. A good observer makes notes on significant events, such as passage of urine or feces, eating, drinking, vomiting, coughing and any change in attitude. Notations can be made on cage cards or in the medical record under daily progress notes.

Feeding and Watering

Feeding and watering the animals is a basic duty performed by the kennel person or technicians, depending on the hospital. Ideally, each cage should contain a metal ring to support a stainless-steel bowl so it cannot be tipped over by the animal. The bowl should be washed and properly disinfected daily. Fresh water should always be available for hospitalized pets unless specifically prohibited by the doctor in charge of the case. Some doctors use the abbreviation NPO, nothing per os or nothing by mouth, for those patients.

Feeding schedules vary for different types of patients. Normal puppies and kittens should be fed every 6-8 hours, while most adult animals are only fed once or twice daily. Typically, all patients allowed food are fed early in the morning to determine if their appetites are good before the morning examination and treatment. Paper disposable dishes are sometimes used because they are sanitary, light to carry and noiseless, and do not require washing. Animals scheduled for surgery or blood tests that day should not be fed. Patients undergoing general anesthesia should not be fed because of the danger of vomiting and subsequent inhalation of the vomitus. Aspiration pneumonia is a serious postanesthetic complication. Feeding may affect the results of blood tests and make proper interpretation difficult. Vomiting patients should not be fed until examined by the doctor.

Sanitation

After moving the animal and before cleaning the cage, check to see if any samples of stool, urine or vomitus have been requested in the medical record or on the cage card. Place the appropriate samples in sealed containers and refrigerate. Mark the cage card to indicate appetite, bowel movement, urine, etc, and then remove the cage papers and clean the cage. The best cages are stainless steel or fiberglass and do not have square corners or pitted surfaces. Spray all surfaces with a standard disinfectant solution, (*eg,* Roccal-D: Winthrop, Nolvasan: Fort Dodge) and wipe off, including the ceiling of the cage. Remove the water bowl and replace it with a clean one. Wash down the cage bars to remove feces, urine and saliva. Add new cage papers, if they are used, and move to the next patient. Remember when moving an animal to also move the cage card to avoid misidentification.

Temperature Control

Patients recovering from surgery or suffering from hypothermia may need an artificial source of heat. Warm water circulating pads provide a uniformly warm, but not overly hot, surface on which a sick animal can rest. With this type of pad, electrical shock is very unlikely, dangerous hot spots do not develop, and the animal will not become overheated. The disadvantages include the relatively high cost and vulnerability to damage by teeth and claws. Standard electrical heating pads must be wrapped in a towel and checked regularly for signs of wear or cord fraying. Overheating and burns are possible from improperly maintained electrical heating pads or improper use, such as allowing an animal to lie on a hot pad, unattended, for hours.

An incubator is ideal for puppies and kittens. Used human pediatric incubators are often available from medical equipment dealers. An oxygen tank and vaporizer may be added to the incubator to provide an intensive care unit for smaller patients (Fig 23). Hot-water bottles can be used to warm a puppy or kitten if care is taken to avoid burns.

Recumbent Patients

Decubital ulcers (bed sores) are uncommon in small animals because few of these patients are recumbent long enough to develop pressure sores. Most patients that do not show signs of recovery in a few days are euthanized. Human convalescent patients may develop such sores from prolonged bed rest. Proper padding of the cage floor is important to keep recumbent patients comfortable. (See section on large animals in this chapter.)

Any patient that is in lateral recumbency while recovering from anesthesia or immobilized by a splint should be gently rolled to its opposite side at least hourly to help prevent circulatory problems. When a patient is forced to remain on one side for a prolonged period, blood tends to pool in the dependent limbs and organs. The pulmonary air spaces (alveoli) tend to collapse from the effect of gravity in the dependent lung lobes. As a result, the lower lung has more blood but less open alveoli, while the upper lung has less blood and more open alveoli. This is known as a mismatching of perfusion and ventilation. By frequently turning the patient and encouraging deep breathing with an occasional vigorous rub, circulatory compromise can be prevented.

In recumbent patients with an indwelling urinary catheter, the catheter can be hooked up to a used IV infusion set taped into an empty IV bottle placed on the floor. This simple system allows continual urine flow by gravity, measures the amount produced, and keeps the patient dry. An alternative approach, if the volume of urine produced need not be recorded, is to place the patient on a grate elevated 1/2-1 inch off the cage floor. Grates are often used with feline patients being treated for urethral obstruction with an indwelling urinary catheter.

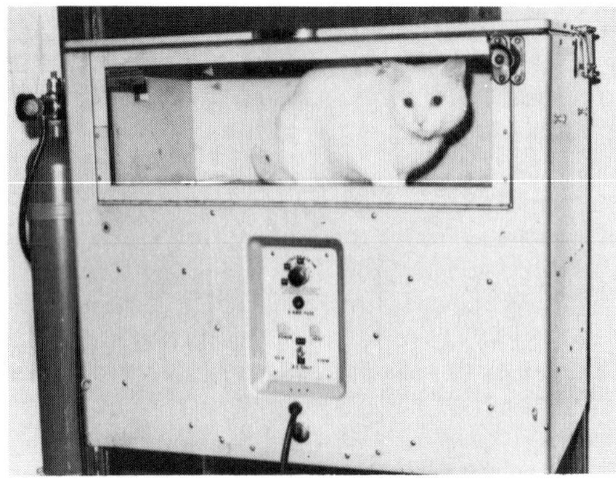

Figure 23. Pediatric incubator converted to a small intensive care unit by addition of an oxygen tank and vaporizer.

Preventing Self-Trauma

When urinary or IV catheters, splints, bandages or sutures are used, there is a danger of self-trauma or destruction of the device by chewing or licking. To prevent such occurrences, an Elizabethan collar can be used (Fig 24). Some felines are able to reach over such collars if they are not fitted properly. Plastic Elizabethan collars, fastened with snaps, may be purchased, or collars can be made from corrugated cardboard and taped around the animal's neck. These devices discourage dogs and cats from licking sutures, chewing bandages or splints, and pulling out catheters. Several brands of distasteful sprays and creams also are available to stop chewing or licking.

Intravenous catheters rarely are licked or chewed excessively by animals if they are properly inserted and are not painful. They must be checked frequently for the presence of tissue swelling or infection that may initiate self-trauma. The few animals that continually try to chew out a catheter, despite all restraint devices, should be tranquilized if their health permits.

Patient Discharge

While the primary purpose of a veterinary hospital does not involve grooming pets, appearances do count. Before any hospitalized patient is discharged, it should be brushed and checked to see if it is clean. Any pet confined to a cage is likely to develop an odor that is objectionable to the owner. If the animal's condition permits, the animal should be bathed, dried and combed out. Wipe the eyes free from any discharge, clip the nails as needed, remove any bandages from previous IV injection or catheter sites and use a

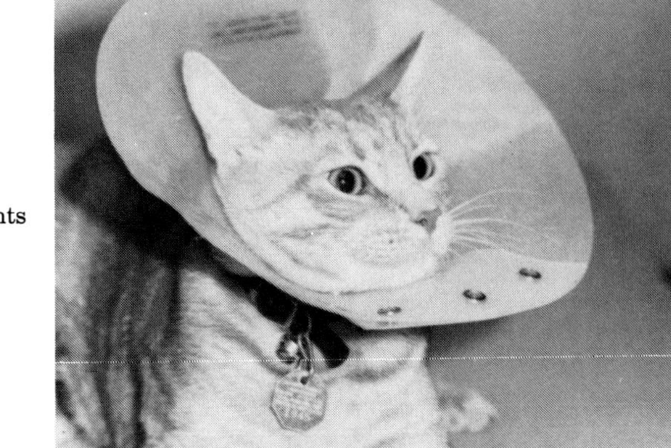

Figure 24. Plastic Elizabethan collar prevents self-mutilation.

scented spray to lightly touch up the coat when dry. Never send an animal home with fleas. These small steps are always appreciated by clients. Try to ensure that the pet looks healthier, is cleaner, and smells better than when it arrived.

Isolation

A well-designed isolation facility in a veterinary hospital has a separate entrance for pets with suspected contagious diseases. Patients admitted to the hospital for a possible infectious disease should be taken directly to isolation and assumed to be contagious until proven otherwise. The medical record should be marked to indicate the location of this patient. Hospitals not having a completely separate isolation area can help reduce the danger of contamination by keeping surrounding cages empty, moving the patient as little as possible, and disinfecting instruments and washing one's hands after handling the animal. Table 4 contains a list of common infectious diseases of cats and dogs.

The isolation facility must have an area for cages, runs, a sink, a treatment table and medical supplies. A separate ventilation system is desirable. A clean smock should be worn and left in the isolation unit when duties are completed. This simple procedure helps prevent exposure of other patients to contamination from clothing. Hands should always be washed between patients, especially those with an infectious disease. Using disposable gloves when handling animals with fungal skin diseases and scabies is recommended. A surgical mask is probably not routinely needed but is recommended in rabies suspects and in birds with psittacosis, both zoonoses that can be transmitted by inhalation of aerosolized organisms.

Table 4. Common infectious diseases of dogs and cats, necessitating isolation.

Dogs	Cats
Canine distemper	Feline panleukopenia
Canine infectious hepatitis	Toxoplasmosis
Leptospirosis	Feline leukemia virus infection
Parainfluenza	Upper respiratory infections
Canine parvovirus enteritis and other enteritis	Feline infectious peritonitis
Sarcoptic mange	Notoedric mange
Dermatomycosis (ringworm)	Dermatomycosis (ringworm)

Care should be taken in handling soiled cage papers, as saliva, blood, urine and feces may contain infectious organisms. All staff members working in the isolation unit must adhere to these basic sanitation procedures if they are to effectively prevent the spread of disease. Clients should be informed that a recovered pet may shed the infectious agent for several days or weeks. When discharged from the hospital, these pets should have limited contact with other animals for a reasonable period, according to the doctor's instructions.

Identification of Small Animals

Cage cards and ID bands have already been mentioned. It must be emphasized that if a hospitalized patient is moved within the hospital, the appropriate cage card must follow the animal. In large facilities, a more complete animal description may be required to avoid identification errors.

All pet owners should be encouraged to buy personalized name tags for their pet's collar that include name, address and telephone number. Collars may be removed and returned to the owner upon admission of the pet to the hospital as a safety precaution, as a collar buckle or tag can become entangled in the cage bars or kennel fencing, resulting in strangulation. Such an accident could result in a negligence suit against the veterinary hospital. Also, loss of a collar, lease, favorite toy or blanket in the kennel or hospital ward environment can upset the client. It is best not to take any such items into the hospital when a patient is admitted for any reason.

Dog licenses are another form of identification. The licensing of dogs is a method of ensuring proper vaccination against rabies. When a pet is vaccinated for rabies, the client usually is issued a rabies tag listing the hospital name, address and a serial number. A log is kept at the hospital to allow identification of any lost animal if the tag number is known. This extra service fosters good relations with clients, as many lost pets can be reunited with their owners with a simple telephone call.

Pet health insurance is now available and promises to become more widespread in future years. Proper identification of an insured animal is required to avoid insurance fraud. Some companies are issuing ID tags with a complex code of letters and numbers to avoid the problem of an owner switching tags from an insured animal to another that is not insured. The encoded data on the tag includes policy number, type of coverage, and a complete animal description.

Tattooing

Tattooing is becoming more popular as a method of identification in dogs and occasionally in cats. Its main advantage is that it is permanent. It is also slightly more costly than other identification methods and causes some minor discomfort for the animal during the procedure. Dogs may be tattooed inside the pinna (ear flap) or on the inner thigh. Veterinarians, dog clubs or breeders may provide this service, using a numbering system to identify the pet. Some owners require that their telephone number or driver's license number be used for identification purposes. Some national registry organizations use the owner's Social Security number for a more recognizable and uniformly identifiable code system. However, obtaining an owner's name from only the Social Security number can be very difficult.

There are 2 basic types of tattoo equipment: the vibrator tattooer and the tattoo clamp. The vibrator type uses 4-10 fine needles that vibrate at a high speed and implant the tattoo ink into the outer layer of skin with minimal discomfort. The area to be tattooed should be shaved and gently cleansed before the procedure. Tranquilization may be needed because of the noise produced by the vibrating unit.

The jaws of the tattoo clamp are designed to accommodate several inserts that consist of pins arranged in letters and numbers. These pins pierce the skin of the ear when clamped, leaving tiny holes that are then filled by gently massaging tattoo ink into the area. These tattoo markings are not easily removed and can last the lifetime of the pet. In young animals the markings expand as the pet grows. Black ink is used for most skin. Green ink is available for darkly pigmented skin that may obscure a black tattoo.

Implants

In recent years, encoded implants have begun to be used for identification of animals. A small, tubular implant is injected SC under the patient's skin, using a large-bore needle. The encoded implant contains a serial number specific for that animal. The encoded information can be detected by applying a special electronic instrument near the skin surface in the area of the implant.

This method of patient identification is advantageous in that it is permanent and cannot be altered or detached. A disadvantage is that a special instrument is required to obtain the information from the encoded implant.

Medical Calculations

Systems of Measurement

There are 3 general units of measurement: length, weight and volume. Various systems have been developed to express these measures in standard units, and each system has a unit for measuring length, weight and volume.

The systems of measurement include the metric, apothecary, avoirdupois, troy and imperial. The first 3 will be discussed briefly to provide a basic understanding of terms used commonly in medical calculations.

Metric System: The units of measurement in the metric (decimal) system are the meter (length), gram (weight) and liter (volume). These basic units are then subdivided to form new units, which are multiples of 10 of the original unit; thus the term decimal system. There is a trend to use this system exclusively and internationally for measurement.

The metric system is based on a system of prefixes added to the basic unit to form these new measures. Once the 3 basic units and the prefixes have been learned, the system is the same whether one is measuring length, weight or volume. Table 5 lists the prefixes used in the metric system, along with their corresponding numeric equivalents. Thus, the prefix *kilo-* in front of a basic unit, such as a meter, means 1000. A kilometer is then 1000 meters. Similarly, *centi-* means 1/100 and thus a centimeter is one-hundredth of a meter. The metric system was originally designed in terms of the meter; the units for weight (gram) and volume (liter) were derived from it.

After a value has been measured, the results must be recorded, making sure to include the unit of measurement. Knowing that a measurement is 10 has no value unless we know that it is 10 centimeters (cm), 10 liters (L), or 10 kilograms (kg).

To illustrate use of metric system terminology, the weighing of a dog might be used as an example. If the dog weighs 12,400 g, the weight can be expressed as 12.4 kg because 12,400 x 1 kg/1000 g = 12.4 kg. The general rule is to express the measurement in the largest appropriate unit, maintaining a whole number if possible. For example, if the object weighed only 950 g, the weight would not be recorded as 0.95 kg but as 950 g. In the same manner, it is generally preferable to report the length of an object

Table 5. Metric prefixes and their numeric equivalents.

Prefix	Numeric Equivalent
kilo-	1000 or 1×10^{3}
deci-	0.1 or 1×10^{-1}
centi-	0.01 or 1×10^{-2}
milli-	0.001 or 1×10^{-3}
micro-	0.000001 or 1×10^{-6}

as 17.2 cm rather than as 0.172 m, though both numbers indicate the same length.

In summary, the basic units of measurement in the metric system are the meter, liter and gram. The prefixes attached to each of these units indicate a part or multiple of that unit. Thus, 1 gram = 10 decigrams, 100 centigrams, 1000 milligrams, or 1,000,000 micrograms. By using these prefixes and their decimal equivalents, one can convert grams to kilograms by dividing by 1000 (1000 g = 1 kg), meters to centimeters by multiplying by 100 (1 m = 100 cm), or liters to milliliters by multiplying by 1000 (1000 ml = 1 L).

Avoirdupois System: This is the most commonly used measurement system in the United States. The units of measuring length are the inch, foot, yard and mile. Measurements of weight are the grain, ounce and pound. Fluid ounce, pint, quart and gallon are measurements of volume.

The principal advantage of the metric system over the avoirdupois system is the ease of conversion from one unit to another within a given measurement. That is the km, cm and mm are all multiples of 10 of the meter. As illustrated in Table 6, the conversion of avoirdupois units is not as convenient.

Apothecary System: Though the apothecary system is not commonly used today, the dosage of many drugs, such as morphine, aspirin, atropine, phenobarbital and nitroglycerine, is still expressed in apothecary units. With some modifications, the system is very similar to the avoirdupois system.

The apothecary system of weights consists of grains, scruples, drams, ounces and pounds (Table 7). The grain in the apothecary system is exactly the same value in the avoirdupois system.

Table 6. Avoirdupois units for length, weight and volume.

Length:	12 inches (in) = 1 foot (ft)
	3 ft = 1 yard (yd) = 36 in
	5280 ft = 1 mile (mi) = 1760 yd
Weight:	437.5 grains (gr) = 1 ounce (oz)
	16 oz = 1 pound (lb) = 7000 gr
Volume:	16 oz = 1 pint (pt)
	2 pt = 1 quart (qt) = 32 fluid ounces (fl oz)
	4 qt = 1 gallon (gal) = 8 pt

Volume in the apothecary system is measured in the same manner as in the avoirdupois system, with the addition of minims and drams. The units for length are the same as in the avoirdupois system.

The major difference between the apothecary and avoirdupois systems is the additional units in the apothecary system. It is important to keep in mind, however, the differences in the number of ounces that comprise a pound. Using the appropriate abbreviations for each system prevents confusion as to which system was used.

Conversion Between Systems

It may be necessary to convert values from one measuring system to another. The process of conversion is exactly the same as in converting between different units of measurement within the same system. The following is a general procedure for conversion:

Step 1: Find the appropriate conversion table and value.

Step 2: Multiply the original value by the appropriate conversion factor.

Step 3: Report the results in the new units.

Because the grain is an equivalent weight, the inch an equivalent length, and the fluid ounce an equivalent volume in the apothecary and avoirdupois systems, only one conversion is given: 15.4 gr = 1 g; 1 in = 2.54 cm; 1 fl oz = 29.6 ml.

An example is the conversion of 10 mg/kg to the appropriate mg/lb (avoir). As the conversion factor is grams, the dosage must first be converted from mg/kg to mg/g:

Step 1: 1000 g = 1 kg

Step 2: 10 mg/kg x 1 kg/1000 g = 10 mg/1000 g = 1 mg/100 g

Step 3: Dosage is 1 mg/100 g

The next conversion is from mg/g to mg/gr:

Step 1: 15.4 gr = 1 g

Step 2: 1 mg/100 g x 1 g/15.4 gr = 1 mg/1540 gr

Step 3: Dosage is 1 mg/1540 gr

Table 7. Apothecary units for weight and volume.

Weight:	20 grains (gr) = 1 scruple
	3 scruples = 1 dram = 60 gr
	8 drams = 1 oz = 24 scruples

Finally, to convert mg/gr to mg/lb:

Step 1: 7000 gr = 1 lb

Step 2: 1 mg/1540 gr x 7000 gr/lb = 7000 mg/1540 lb = 4.55 mg/lb

Step 3: Dosage is 4.55 mg/lb

An alternative to this long procedure involves applying the information that 2.2 lb = 1 kg. If this conversion had been used in the previous example, only 3 steps would be involved:

Step 1: 2.2 lb = 1 kg

Step 2: 10 mg/kg x 1 kg/2.2 lb = 4.55 mg/lb

Step 3: Dosage is 4.55 mg/lb

Prescriptions sometimes are written in what are referred to as household equivalents, such as the teaspoon, tablespoon and glassful. Their metric and avoirdupois (apothecary) equivalents are as follows:

1 teaspoon (tsp) = 5 ml

1 tablespoon (tbsp) = 15 ml = 1/2 fl oz

1 glassful = 240 ml = 8 fl oz

Table 8 contains the equivalents for the metric, apothecary and avoirdupois measurements of length, weight and volume.

Calculating Drug Dosages

Before medication is given by mouth or injection, 4 basic facts must be known: the patient's weight; the required dosage; the concentration of the medication; and the frequency of administration. The weight of the patient is already known from the physical examination and is in the medical record in pounds or kilograms. The dosage of most commonly used drugs and their frequency of administration are found in standard reference texts and in the drug's package insert. The dosage may differ from one species to another. The concentration of the drug is found on the container, in mg or gr for tablets and capsules and mg/ml for oral liquids and injectables.

To calculate the amount of drug to be given, multiply the patient's weight by the dosage from the reference source, *eg,* 15 lb x 10 mg/lb = 150 mg. If the medication comes in 100-, 200- and 500-mg tablets, the amount of drug, divided by the size of the tablet, equals the number of tablets to be given, *eg,* 150 mg/100-mg tablet = 1.5 tablets.

To calculate the amount of medication to be injected, multiply the patient's weight by the drug's dosage and divide by the drug's concentration, *eg,*

$$\frac{15\text{ lb} \times 10\ ^{\text{mg}}\!/_{\text{lb}}}{100\ ^{\text{mg}}\!/_{\text{ml}}} = 1.5\text{ ml}$$

It may be necessary to change the concentration of a liquid medication by diluting it with sterile water to enable more accurate dosing. A good example is ketamine HCl (Ketaset: Bristol), which comes in a concentration of 100 mg/ml. In anesthetizing small birds with ketamine HCl, it is important to dilute the drug to avoid overdosage.

Problem: Dilute a sample of ketamine HCl by a factor of 10.

Solution: Ketamine HCl is available in a concentration of 100 mg/ml. If diluted by a factor of 10, the final concentration would be 10 mg/ml. Take 1 ml of ketamine and add 9 ml water. The 100 mg of drug has been diluted to a total volume of 10 ml. The new concentration is then:

$$\frac{100 \text{ mg}}{10 \text{ ml}} = 10 \text{ mg/ml}$$

Table 8. Metric, apothecary and avoirdupois equivalents for weight, length and volume.

Weight:	1 mg = 1/60 gr
	15 mg = 1/4 gr
	30 mg = 1/2 gr
	60 mg = 1 gr
	1000 mg = 1 g
	2.2 lb = 1 kg
	1 oz = 28 g
	8 oz = 1/2 lb = 227 g
	16 oz = 1 lb = 454 g
Length:	1 mm = 0.04 in
	10 mm = 1 cm = 0.4 in
	1 in = 2. 54 cm
Volume:	1 ml = 1 cubic centimeter (cc)
	100 ml = 1 deciliter (dl)
	1000 ml = 10 dl = 1 liter (L)
	1 tsp = 5 ml
	1 tbsp = 15 ml
	1 fl oz = 30 ml
	8 fl oz = 250 ml = 1 cup
	16 fl oz = 500 ml = 2 cups = 1 pt
	32 fl oz = 1000 ml = 4 cups = 1 qt
	1 gal = 4000 ml = 4 qt = 8 pt

When dealing with percentage problems, remember that percent means parts per hundred, *eg,* 10% equals 10 parts per 100 parts. In the metric system, percent of solution equals grams of solute (substance dissolved) per 100 ml solvent (liquid base). For example, a 5% solution of drug A contains 5 g drug A in 100 ml water (or other vehicle).

Sodium thiamylal (Bio-Tal: Bio-Ceutic) is a short-acting barbiturate anesthetic for IV use that is stored in powder form and requires reconstitution in sterile water for use. To prepare this solution, 2 basic facts are required:

1. What amount of drug is in the bottle?
2. What percent concentration is desired for use?

The amount of drug in the bottle is recorded on the label. The percent concentration desired may be 5%, 4% or 2%, depending on the intended use. To mix a 5% solution, take 5 g of drug (solute) and add 100 ml of water (solvent), *ie,*

$$5\% = \frac{5 \text{ g drug}}{100 \text{ ml water}}$$

Problem: To mix a 4% solution in a bottle that contains 5 g of drug, how much water is required?

Solution: Remembering 4% = 4 g/100 ml, a simple proportion equation can be set up:

$$\frac{4 \text{ g}}{100 \text{ ml}} = \frac{5\text{g}}{\text{X}}$$

where X = number of ml of water needed for a 4% solution. Solving for X, X = 125 ml.

To mix a 2% solution in the same bottle containing 5 g of powder, 2% = 2 g/100 ml. Therefore:

$$\frac{2 \text{ g}}{100 \text{ ml}} = \frac{5\text{g}}{\text{X}}$$

Solving for X, X = 250 ml.

On occasion it is necessary to mix a more dilute solution from a concentrated mixture. An example is found in mixing a 5% or 10% solution of dextrose for IV administration.

Problem: How much 50% dextrose is required to make a liter of 10% dextrose?

Solution: 50% means 50 g/100 ml and 10% means 10 g/100 ml. In a liter of 10% dextrose there are 100 g of dextrose, *ie,* 10 g/100 ml x 1000 ml = 100 g. Therefore, 100 g of dextrose would equal 200 ml of 50% dextrose, *ie,*

$$\frac{50 \text{ g}}{100 \text{ ml}} = \frac{100\text{g}}{\text{X}}$$

Solving for X, X = 200 ml of 50% dextrose. To make this solution, add 200 ml of 50% dextrose to 800 ml of sterile water. The resulting liter contains 10% dextrose.

Sample Problems

Using the sample chart below, answer the following problems for these hypothetical medications. The answers follow the last problem.

	Dosage		
Drug	**Dog**	**Cat**	**How Supplied**
Avitrollin	5 mg/lb PO q12h	10 mg/lb PO q12h	50-, 100-, 200-mg tabs
Betamide	not used	20 mg/lb IM q8h	50 mg/ml
Chloraplex	50 mg/lb IV q6h	25 mg/lb IV q6h	100 mg/ml
Desoxythane	4 mg/10 lb PO q24h	not used	8-, 16-, 32-mg tabs
Episol	½ gr/5 lb IM q8h	½ gr/5 lb IM q8h	1 gr/ml

PO = per os (by mouth)
IM = intramuscular
IV = intravenous

q24h = once daily (every 24 hr)
q12h = every 12 hr
q8h = every 8 hr
q6h = every 6 hr

1. How much Chloraplex is required for one injection for a 10-lb Dachshund?
2. If asked to give Desoxythane to a 60-lb German Shepherd, how many tablets and what size would you use?
3. A 5-lb cat needs a 2-week supply of Avitrollin. How many tablets and of what size would you dispense?
4. The patient in question 3 also needs an injection of Betamide. In preparing the injection, how much medication would you withdraw from the vial into the syringe?
5. A 30-lb Corgi is hospitalized and requires Episol injections for 2 days. The doctor wants to know if one 10-ml vial of medication is enough to properly treat the dog for both days. If more medication is needed, how many more 10-ml vials must be purchased?

Answers to Problems

1. Patient's weight × dosage for dog = amount of medication:

$$10 \text{ lb} \times 50 \ {}^{\text{mg}}\!/\!_{\text{lb}} = 500 \text{ mg}$$

$$\frac{\text{amount of medication}}{\text{concentration}} = \text{volume of injection}$$

$$\frac{500 \text{ mg}}{100 \ {}^{\text{mg}}\!/\!_{\text{ml}}} = 5 \text{ ml}$$

2. Patient's weight × dosage for dog = amount of medication:

$$6 \text{ lb} \times \ 4 \text{ mg}/10 \text{ lb} = 240 \text{ mg}/10 \text{ lb} = 24 \text{ mg}$$

$$\frac{\text{amount of medication}}{\text{size of tablet}} = \text{number of tablets}$$

24 mg/8-mg tablet = 3 tablets
24 mg/16-mg tablet = 1½ tablets
24 mg/32-mg tablet = ¾ tablet

All 3 answers are correct. The choice of which size of tablet to administer rests with the technician and may be influenced by the number of each tablet size available.

3. Using same 2 formulas above with the values plugged in:

$$5 \text{ lb} \times \text{mg/lb} = 50 \text{ mg}$$

$$\frac{50 \text{ mg}}{50 \text{ mg per tablet}} = 1 \text{ tablet}$$

If other-sized tablets are used, it requires splitting the tablets into halves or quarters, which is not desirable. One 50-mg tablet given twice daily for 2 weeks:

$$1 \text{ tab} \times 2/\text{day} \times 14 \text{ days} = 28 \text{ tabs.}$$

4. Using 2 basic formulas:

$$5 \text{ lb} \times 20 \text{ mg/lb} = 100 \text{ mg}$$

$$\frac{100 \text{ mg}}{50 \ {}^{\text{mg}}\!/\!_{\text{ml}}} = 2 \text{ ml}$$

5. Using 2 basic formulas:

$$30 \text{ lb} \times \tfrac{1}{2} \text{ gr}/5 \text{ lb} = 15 \text{ gr}/5 = 3 \text{ gr}$$

$$\frac{3 \text{ gr}}{1 \ {}^{\text{gr}}\!/\!_{\text{ml}}} = 3 \text{ ml per dose given}$$

As this drug is given q8h, 3 injections are needed per day of hospitalization. Therefore, 3 ml/injection × 3 injections/day × 2 days = 18 ml.

Because one vial contains only 10 ml of drug, there is not enough medication to treat the dog both days. Another vial is required to have enough for both days of treatment.

Admission of Large Animal Patients

Initial Presentation

The introduction to a large animal patient almost always begins by telephone contact. The technician's job is to determine the immediate presenting complaint and the urgency with which the problem should be treated. Determining the reason for the call or the seriousness of the injury or current morbid state is the first objective. Many horse owners overstate the urgency with which their animal should be attended. Also, "poor doers" on a range may be on their last legs but can recover with immediate and proper care.

Admission of large animals to the hospital, or treatment in the field, requires owner registration and compiling of patient information. Owner registration entails collection of the owner's personal data, including place of residence and business, registered ranch or farm name, if any, source of referral, any insurance policy number for the animals and means of payment. Client records may be indexed by alphabet, zip code, date of last visit or whatever means the veterinarian and office staff find most effective (see Small Animal Medical Records).

Clients presenting large animals at the hospital or clinic should be handled with patience and courtesy. Horses should be quietly unloaded with the help of the owners to minimize the animal's anxiety. Untie the horse through the escape door first, toss the rope over its neck, open the back door and drop the backbar or chain. Have an assistant or the owner stand at the door to guide the horse down the ramp and grab the lead rope. Speak quietly and always approach the animal at an angle, never from behind. Once the horse is unloaded, circle the horse out of kicking range and lead it to a convenient spot for ease of examination. Tie the horse with a slip knot in the lead rope, never by the bridle reins, to a secure post, avoiding fence rails or gates. Be calm and confident. A nervous handler creates a nervous horse, resulting in more difficult examination and treatment.

Food animals (cattle, sheep, swine) should be unloaded with a minimum of shouting,arm waving or excitement. Lead or herd them calmly to a holding pen or enclosed alleyway. Most presentations of food animals at a hospital involve purebred or show animals that usually are accustomed to being handled and moved about. Move confidently, yet cautiously, as even the most apparently passive 4-H cow may turn cantankerous and cause serious injury if mishandled.

Unannounced arrivals at the hospital usually find the veterinarian on call in the field. It is best to politely inform those clients of the doctor's rigorous schedule and suggest an appointment another day. However, many clients travel a considerable distance with trailer in tow, making a return trip most unattractive. In these cases, and in emergency situations, it is best to refer the client to another practitioner in the area or contact the doctor by radio or telephone, if possible, for advice.

Large Animal Medical Records

History and Presenting Complaint

Horses: Before the horse is examined, either at the hospital or in the field, initial patient information must be obtained. Information on the age, sex, breed, color, registration (if applicable), and geographic location of stabling or pasture should be obtained. Specific information regarding previous illness or injury, diet, vaccination history, parasite control, type of housing, and animal contacts should be recorded. The presenting complaint should be noted, along with clinical signs, any abnormal behavior or recent changes in diet or location, vital signs, and location of injury or wound, if applicable. Copies of herd health records, if available, should be included with the record.

Any description of past illness or injury should include the date of illness, clinical signs, extent and location of any wound, treatment and length of illness. Any bad habits arising from the illness or manifesting themselves at other times should be recorded. These may include cribbing, head shaking or eating unusual objects (pica).

The immunization history is of critical importance in any medical record. An equine vaccination history should include the date of and age at vaccination and the type of vaccine used. There are many conflicting opinions regarding strangles vaccination. Current recommendations are to immunize the herd if one individual should contract the disease by placing the exudative pus from the infection in the feed of other horses. Venezuelan equine encephalomyelitis (VEE) has been largely eradicated, but vaccination may still be necessary in areas of outbreak.

Information on previous parasitic infections and results of treatment should be entered into the patient's file. Horses are affected by more than 75 internal parasites, with strongyles, ascarids, pinworms and bots being the most injurious. Prevention of internal parasites consists primarily of sanitary measures. An emaciated, unthrifty appearance generally indicates parasitism, but the diagnosis can only be confirmed by fecal examination.

External parasitisms include those by blowflies, mosquitos, lice, mites, screwworms, ticks and ringworm. Eradication programs involve sanitation, use of parasiticides and care of open wounds. Information on the animal's housing or any history of confinement should be recorded. The mental state of the horse should be considered when dealing with a horse accustomed to confinement. Stables should be properly insulated, drained and ventilated. Horses may injure themselves if stalls and the stable have not been surveyed for sharp projections, broken rails or poorly insulated wiring. Be aware of these potential dangers when recording the medical history.

Pastured horses have the advantage of free grazing exercise but run the risk of poisonous plants, broken fences and poor pasture. Become informed of the poisonous plants in your geographic location. Some common poisonous plants and shrubs are hemlock, green bracken, laurel, ragwort and monkswood. Broken or poorly constructed fences may cause horses to become entangled in barbed wire, wounded on splintered boards or nails, or tangled in rope or bailing wire. The time of entering information in the medical record is the ideal opportunity to alert both the veterinarian and client to potential hazards in housing by making an early note of it.

A notation in the medical record should be made regarding exposure to other animals. Respiratory infections are both very common and contagious among equidae. Joint pasturing also facilitates parasitism and spread of bacterial and viral diseases.

Food Animals: As with horses, specific information on cattle, sheep, goats and swine should be obtained regarding the individual, entire herd or flock when the initial complaint is discussed. When working with commercial operators, there are usually designated periods within the year when the entire herd is worked. Records should be updated at that time as to the current condition of the animals.

In commercial operations, herd records are updated when new calves are worked at 3-5 months of age. Separated calves are identified with ear tags, immunized, dehorned, castrated, weighed and branded. If older cows or bulls are worked at this time, the veterinarian may be involved in vaccinating, pregnancy and semen testing, deworming, recording weights and updating files.

Sheep are worked on a similar schedule, though that work is performed in shorter time because of the shorter gestation period and faster growth rate of sheep. Inquiry should be made into nutritional, reproductive and production programs for commercial flocks. The nutritional history should be compared with National Research Council nutrient and mineral requirements.

As for all patient records, questions should be asked regarding vaccination history, parasite control programs, parturition season and type of housing or shelter provided. Production records are critical tools for sheep and hog operations in monitoring drops in weaning percentages, birthing rates, and overall production levels. Such records are critical in commercial operations for superior returns and also enable the veterinarian to quickly and efficiently analyze the continuing needs of that operation.

Record systems for horses and food animals should include a treatment record and case summary. For entire herds this information may be incorporated into herd records. Records for purebred animals are handled somewhat differently because of the commercial value of the animals involved. In purebred beef operations, each animal should be assigned its own record, allowing close assessment of its performance and tracking of the medical record. This ensures a more individualized assessment of medical problems, subsequent treatment and production performance.

Case summary reports should be entered into each file after the animal is treated. Information regarding diagnosis, treatment procedures, dates of treatment and disposition of the animal should be included. When dealing with herd records, the number of swine farrowed, sheep docked or calves branded should be recorded. After creating each file, the summary report should be readily available for easy access of information.

Physical Examination of Large Animals

Horses

When a new patient is first examined, the vital signs and general appearance should be first evaluated. Table 9 summarizes the vital signs for horses and food animals. These values may be artificially elevated, depending on recent exercise, stress, general condition and stages of pregnancy or lactation. The technician should be adept at recording the vital signs to save time for the doctor.

When viewing a horse for the first time, stand back and inspect the animal from the side at 20-30 feet. Look for an alert attitude, with the horse standing squarely (resting one hind leg is normal, resting a foreleg indicates disease in that leg or elsewhere) and the ears erect and active. The eyes should be bright, the haircoat sleek and shiny in summer, but heavier in winter, and free of parasites or lesions. The hoof walls should be smooth and pliable, not misshapen or split. The frogs of the hoof should be well shaped and resilient, with no offensive odor or discharge from the cleft.

The animal in question should interact normally, if pastured with other horses. The appetite should be good, the droppings well formed and moist, with no parasites or mucus visible, and the urine thick and yellowish. Have the horse trotted and watch for soundness while observing the stride and gait. Watch for clumsy movement or a great deal of side movement. Make the visual appraisal while taking note of any abnormalities, and then begin a systematic examination of the organ systems.

Palpate and gently probe over the body of the horse. Take the extra time to calm the horse while searching for abnormalities or tender areas. The equine digestive system is unique because of its large cecum. Fluid contents forced from the cecum to the large intestine continues to be digested for several days, producing heat and gas. This process normally is accompanied by intestinal noises, or borborygmi, which are healthy, churning noises of the colon.

After the digestive tract, a horse's feet and legs create more medical problems than any other body system. The foot must be capable of absorbing tremendous shock during locomotion. The foot consists of a horny, somewhat elastic box enclosing the distal bones of the limb, which are cushioned by fibro-fatty pads. The most distal bone of the leg, the third phalanx, has elastic wings extending above the coronet, toward the heel. The more proximal second phalanx articulates with the third, forming the coffin joint. At the caudal aspect of this joint is the navicular bone, over which the flexor tendon courses. The sensitive sole covers the ventral aspect of the third phalanx, producing the overlying horny sole. The frog is formed on the ventral aspect of the plantar cushion.

A routine hoof-care program includes regular trimming and shoeing, daily use of a hoof pick, and painting with some type of hoof dressing to keep the hoof soft and free of cracks. Some hoof injuries can result in severe discomfort and lameness, sole bruises, corns, punctures, thrush, cracked hooves and heels, quittor, founder and laminitis.

Food Animals

As with horses, it is best to begin the physical examination by checking the vital signs and then moving to a visual appraisal for estimating general condition (Table 9). Food animals should be evaluated on the basis of their economically important anatomic systems.

Dairy cows are usually evaluated on the basis of their milk production and udder health. The udder should be structurally sound in all quarters, with no ligament breakdown, signified by a symmetric shape. Each teat should be examined for wounds, strictures, abnormal discharge or hardness, which may indicate mastitis. The feet and legs should also be observed for signs of lameness.

Dairy Herd Improvement Association (DHIA) records should be reviewed, noting any drops in milk production or butter fat content and increase in somatic cell counts. Be aware of the reproductive performance of each cow, noting abnormally long open (nonpregnant) periods and problems with dystocia. Keep in mind that production levels are critical in commercial herds. Good herd health programs ensure continued production at high levels. The technician should be able to review these records and find areas of poor performance for the veterinarian to explore.

As with dairy and beef records, sheep and swine production records should be closely scrutinized for problem areas in conception rates, weaning weights, feed conversion levels, mortality losses and areas of declining production levels. Attention should be directed to proper conditioning of both sheep and swine. Both these species produce valuable meat cuts from the rear legs and loin. Examine their legs and palpate over the lumbar area for excessive fat or leanness. Avoid rough handling and excitement before shipping, if possible. Swine are very susceptible to stress and can develop porcine stress syndrome, producing a soft, exudative cut of meat. Sheep should be closely examined for external parasites, such as mites, ticks and lice, that may damage the quality of the fleece. Special note should be made of the condition of the fleece, with reference to fiber quality and density. Poor fleece condition may indicate improper nutrition.

Restraint of Horses

J.T. Vaughan and R. Allen, Jr.

Despite use tranquilizers, sedatives, muscle relaxants and new anesthetic agents, restraint of horses remains an ability acquired

Table 9. Normal rectal temperature, heart rate and respiratory rate for horses, cattle, sheep and swine.

Species	Rectal Temp. (F)	Heart Rate (/min)	Resp. Rate (/min)
Horses	99.5-101.3	28-50	8-16
Cattle	100.5-103.0	40-70	10-30
Sheep	102.0-104.0	60-90	12-19
Swine	100.5-104.0	58-100	8-18

through experience. More than any other large domestic animal, horses must be handled as individuals. They must be protected from abusive restraint and from accidental injury when restraint is applied.

There are basically 4 psychological categories of horses: the well-mannered horse that has had good training and proper handling; the unbroken horse that has had little or no training or handling and is easily frightened; the ill-mannered horse that has had unfavorable exposure to people and has been poorly trained; and the rogue horse that may have had good training and proper training but still ferociously resists restraint for even the simplest procedures. Each of these types requires individual assessment as to the method and degree of restraint required. The ability to recognize individual differences and to take into account an animal's idiosyncrasies as reported by the owner or stable manager is necessary if minimal restraint is to be applied.

The method of restraint depends on many factors, including the animal's temperament, age, size, physical condition, procedure to be performed, and the equipment, help and drugs available. The duration of the procedure and the amount of pain or anxiety likely to be produced should be considered. The use of humane techniques is imperative. A professional responsibility is acquired when a patient is accepted for treatment. It is assumed that the practitioner and technician will protect the patient's well-being and prevent injury, especially that resulting from unwise application of restraint.

Because individual horses may react differently in a given situation, the method and degree of restraint required are often a matter of experimentation. In general, one should apply the least restraint possible initially while judging the animal's reaction as a procedure progresses. The general methods of physical restraint, in increasing order of severity, include halter and lead, skin twitch, ear hold, and nose or lip twitch. Other methods, such as raising a limb, the tail hold, and use of stocks and breeding hobbles, are useful in certain situations.

Halters and Leads

The most important assistant is the one restraining the horse's head. Use the halter and lead to exert control just as a rider uses reins and bits. Never try to restrain a horse by the halter alone because a lead attached to it provides much more control. Always be alert to divert the horse's attention from work being done by the operator, who may be at the opposite end of the animal. The assistant should usually stand on the same side of the horse as the operator, as this is the best position to prevent the animal from wheeling into or kicking the operator.

A horse should be led from the left or near side, the same side on which it is usually caught, bridled, saddled and mounted. When leading a horse during an examination, the assistant should walk or jog alongside the horse's head, facing the direction of travel and never looking back. If the horse does not follow willingly, it should be urged from behind by another person and not pulled by the halter. If there is only one assistant, a loop or rope can be dropped over the horse's hindquarters, crossed over the back and the ends passed up through the halter, to be pulled along with the lead to encourage the horse to advance. If this fails, the horse can be blindfolded and led or backed for short distances.

Halters are typically constructed of leather or braided rope (nylon or cotton). The latter are cheaper and stronger, and can be tied. They can be used with a chain shank for special restraint of spirited horses. The chain can be used over the muzzle, under the jaw, through the mouth, and over the gingivae (Figs 25-28). The last method has somewhat the effect of a war bridle and can be very effective in restraining horses that cannot be twitched or do not respond to a twitch. Chain shanks (leads) should not be used abusively, nor should they be used to tie a horse. When not used in the ways described, a chain shank is simply snapped in the halter ring at the bottom of the caveson (nose band) or doubled through the ring and snapped back on itself.

Special halters include heavy reinforced table halters for confining the animal to an operating table, and the dental halter, with a rigid loop of steel incorporated into the nose band. Both have D-

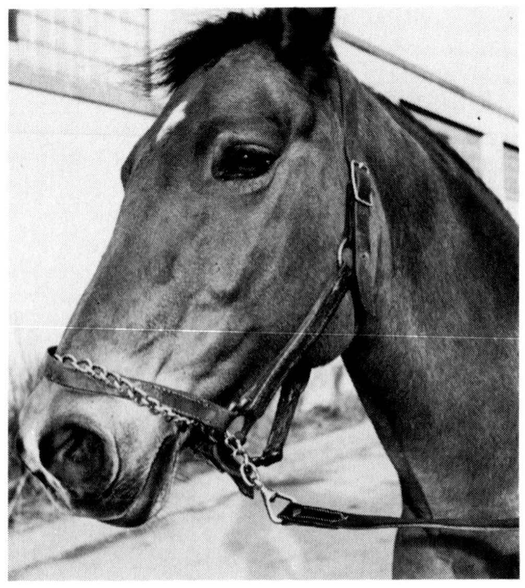

Figure 25. Use of a chain shank over the muzzle.

rings at the 4 quadrants of the nose band as well as the crown piece behind the poll, which make it possible to secure the head from any direction. The rigid nose band in the dental halter provides space to open the mouth for dental surgery without encroaching on the cheeks. The list of halter types also includes the stallion bridle, lunging caveson, Tennessee grass halters, and stable and track halters.

A word of caution is important at this point, however, concerning the use of cattle halters and temporary rope halters on horses. Both are "draw" halters, *ie,* they constrict around the head or muz-

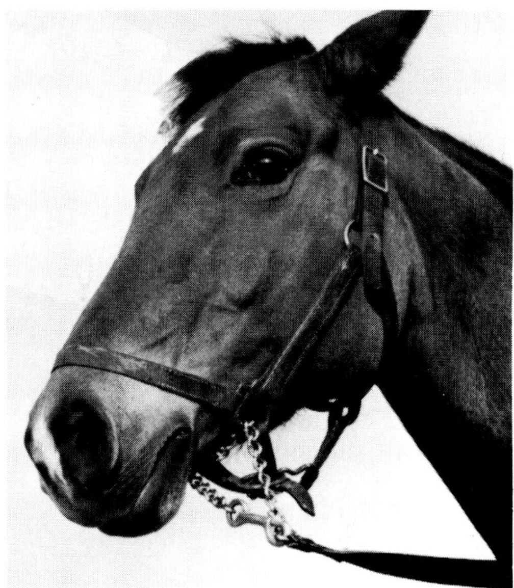

Figure 26. Use of a chain shank below the mandible.

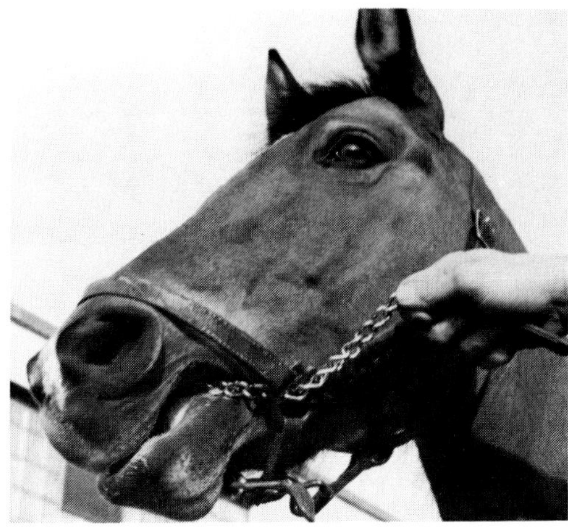

Figure 27. Use of a chain shank through the mouth.

zle when tightened. This can cause serious injury, especially if the horse is tied and attempts to escape. Trauma to the nasal bones and passages, hemorrhage and asphyxia have resulted from use of such halters. If it is necessary to improvise, one should make a knot in the lead rope to prevent halter constriction.

A horse of unknown temperament should never be left unattended when tied because it may become excited and struggle to free itself. This is hazardous, as the horse is likely to be injured or to injure persons nearby. One should never attempt to do anything to a tied horse, even such seemingly minor operations as examining the incisor teeth, inspecting an eye or taking the pulse. Many horses use the slightest excuse to sit back on their halters, invariably breaking a piece of tack. These "halter breakers" frequently cannot be tied at all.

Skin Twitch

Another method of restraint, especially useful on horses prone to strike with the front feet, is the skin twitch. The skin twitch is applied by grasping a roll of skin over the shoulders with both hands (Fig 29). As with any other method of restraint, the skin twitch works well on some animals but not on others.

Ear Hold

Horses that do not respond to halter or skin twitch restraint may respond to the ear hold. The left ear is firmly grasped with the

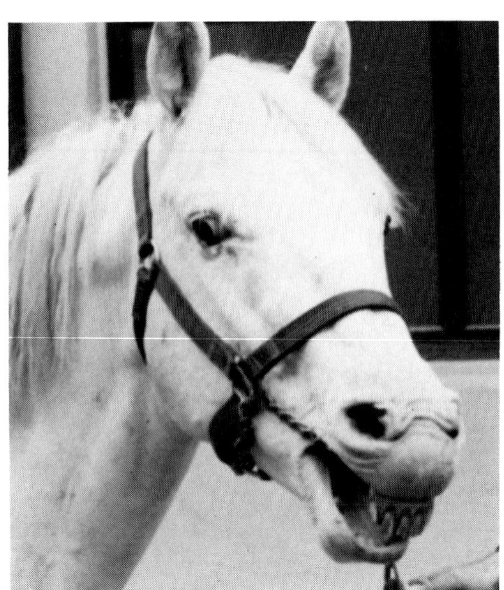

Figure 28. Use of a chain shank over the upper gingivae.

right hand, with the heel of the hand against the animal's scalp (Fig 30). The ear is squeezed and slight pressure is applied ventrad. The right forearm and elbow should be held firmly against the vertical ramus of the animal's left mandible, so the assistant is pushed away rather than hit in the face if the animal rears.

The ear hold can be very effective if correctly applied. However, it can result in a fallen ear or head-shy horse if applied abusively.

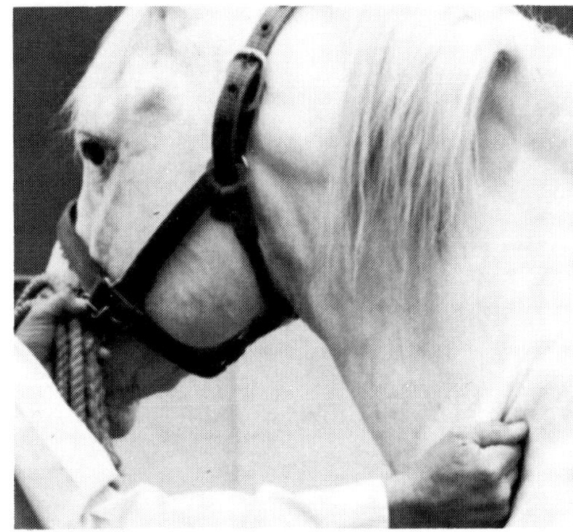

Figure 29. Application of the skin twitch to discourage a horse from striking.

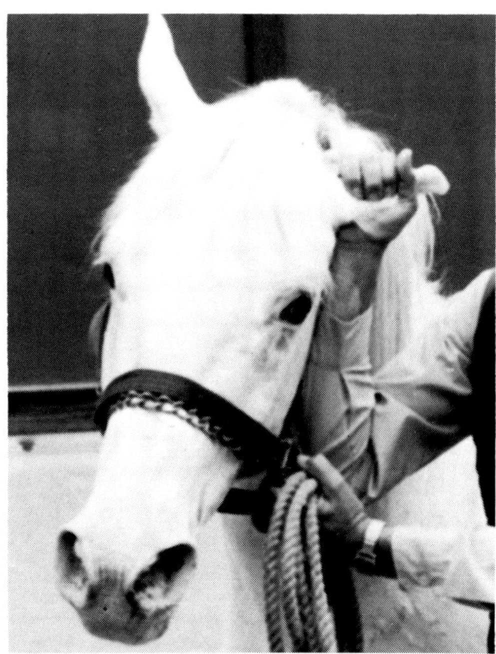

Figure 30. Grasping an ear to restrain the head.

Application of a rope or chain twitch to the ear is inhumane and usually results in permanent ear injury.

The ear hold should not be applied to show horses, such as the American Saddlebred, Tennessee Walking Horse, Hackney, Arabian, Morgan and others.

Lip Twitch

The twitch is one of the oldest and most widely used (and misused) restraint devices. Its exact effect on a horse has been argued, but nevertheless it effectively distracts the animal's attention and provides restraint. Twitching is most simply accomplished by firmly grasping the lip (usually upper) between the tips of the thumb and fingers. This often is necessary to hold the horse's head still long enough to apply the twitch to the lip. The conventional twitch consists of a loop of small chain or rope fixed to the end of a wooden handle about 36 inches long. The loop is applied over the lip, which is folded so that the mucosal surface is not exposed, and the loop is tightened by twisting the handle (Fig 31).

At this point some horses may strike or paw with one or both front feet. Therefore, the person holding the horse should be stand-

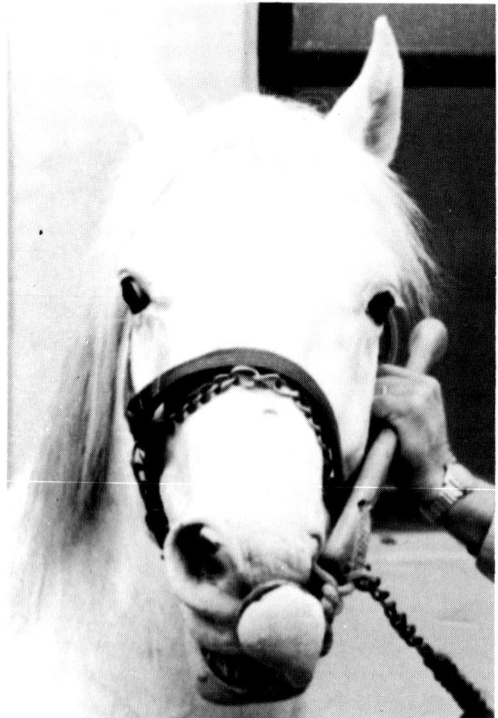

Figure 31. A rope twitch applied to the upper lip.

ing beside the left shoulder and the one twitching the horse should be beside or just in front of the first, so both are in a safe position. As the twitch handle is turned the last time, it should be held at its end so the handler will not lose control of the twitch if the horse pulls back or strikes. This is important because if the twitch is pulled from an assistant's grasp, the horse may use it as a flail and seriously injure anyone in the area. After the twitch has been applied, an assistant can hold the halter lead and twitch. This is the customary restraint for routine procedures, such as passing a stomach tube.

Some horses should never be twitched. Because of past abuse, they greatly resent the twitch and fight it, even after it is applied. These animals should be restrained in some other way. A twitch is most effective when used as needed. Its effect is greatest when first applied and is lost if the lip becomes numb. Therefore, one should alternate the pressure of the loop around the lip so that maximum pressure is applied when needed. The pressure is then reduced enough to allow sensitivity and circulation to return. When the upper lip becomes numb or if there is some reason not to use it, the lower lip can be twitched with almost as good effect (Fig 32).

The nose clamp has been used for many years (Fig 33). The modern version has a nylon cord and snap so it can be fixed to the halter, freeing one hand of the assistant.

War Bridle

This is a rope gag used to restrain a horse that tends to rear or resist a twitch. There are several variations, including Magner's modified war bridle (Fig 34). It should always be used in conjunc-

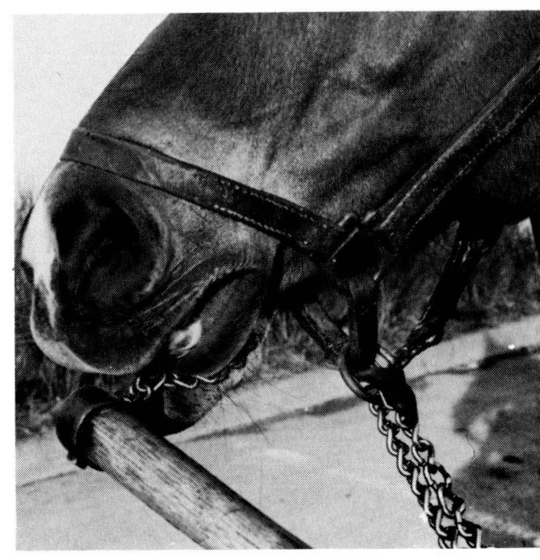

Figure 32. A chain twitch applied to the lower lip.

tion with a halter and lead, and never used to tie a horse. A war bridle can injure the horse if not used properly.

Another method of restraining the head involves holding the muzzle with the left hand and the nape of the neck with the right. The left thumb can be inserted under the noseband to prevent the horse from ducking its head. The right hand can grasp the mane or an ear for added restraint. This method is very useful for such procedures as floating teeth (Fig 35). Do not compress the nostrils and restrict breathing.

Restraint of the Feet

The manner in which the feet are restrained depends on how the horse has been handled. An animal that has been groomed daily and is accustomed to having its feet handled cooperates by picking up its feet. When the horse's feet have never been handled, some training may be required. Sedatives or tranquilizers are helpful.

Regardless of the horse, the approach is the same. The assistant stands at the animal's head and the horse is encouraged to stand with its weight on all 4 legs so its weight can easily be shifted to 3

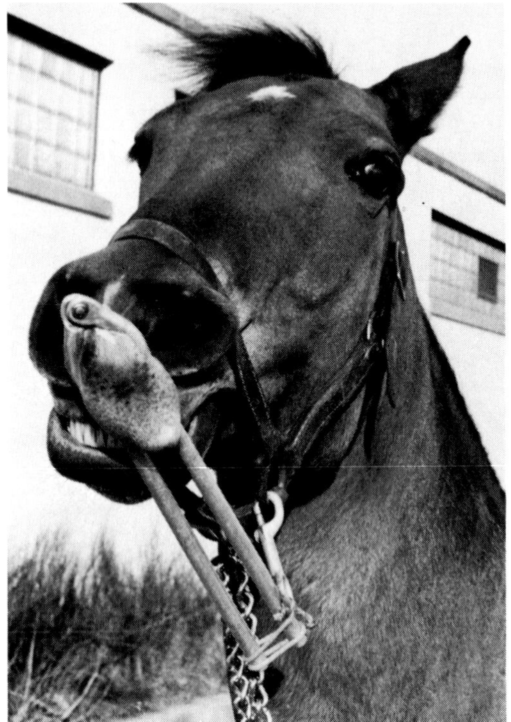

Figure 33. A clamp twitch applied to the upper lip is snapped on the halter.

legs. The operator should make his presence and intentions known to the horse. If a front leg is to be raised, a hand is moved down the leg to the fetlock and the volar digital nerves are pinched or the hair below the fetlock is pulled. This usually prompts the horse to pick up the foot. Some horses require more force, such as pushing the animal onto the opposite leg while flexing the one being raised.

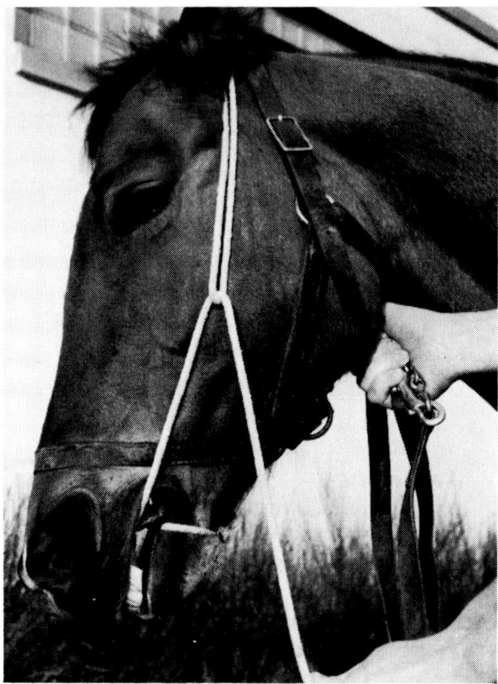

Figure 34. The war bridle.

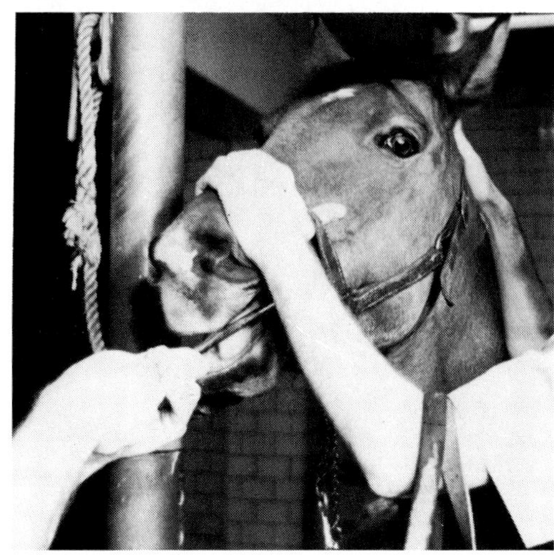

Figure 35. A method of head restraint for floating teeth.

If the horse's foot is held between the operator's knees to free his hands, the operator should crouch with his knees together and his toes pointed mediad. One should avoid pulling the horse's foot or leg laterad because it is uncomfortable for the animal.

Raising and holding a hind foot can be more difficult. A horse that cannot be approached safely from behind usually gives warning by moving away, feinting with the hindleg that is being grasped, or merely taking weight off the leg so it can kick at any time. The operator's hand nearer the horse is kept on the animal's tuber coxae, while the other is moved down the cannon bone to draw the leg craniad. The hock and toe are held in a flexed position when the leg is raised, partially restricting voluntary movement of that leg. As the leg is cradled between the operator's arm and leg nearer the horse, the cannon is propped on the inside of the thigh. The operator can then use his hands to clean the foot and perform the required procedure (Fig 36). The operator should position himself firmly so that he is not thrown off balance by the horse's struggling. When releasing the leg, the procedure is reversed: the operator's near hand is placed on the horse's tuber coxae and used to push himself to the front of the animal.

Many horses are accustomed to having all 4 feet examined and cleaned daily from the left side, with the operator reaching under and across when raising the feet on the right side. A front foot can be raised and held to prevent a horse from kicking with a hind foot (Fig 37). The front foot on the same side as the operator should be lifted because the horse is then unable to kick with the rear leg on

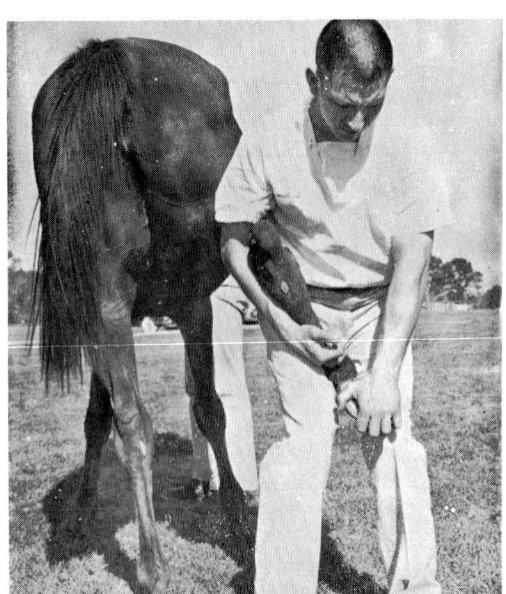

Figure 36. Position for examination or treatment of a hind foot.

that side. When holding a front leg,, one should avoid supporting the horse. A front leg is occasionally tied for restraint of a mare during breeding or for rectal examination (Fig 38). The rope or strap should be tied in such a manner that it can be released quickly to prevent the animal from casting itself. Tying a hind leg involves use of a single-rope sideline. This does not permit careful examination of the foot but may discourage kicking. For animals that resist these restraint methods, use of tranquilizers or sedatives is indicated. Rope burns can be avoided by using hobbles or bandages (Fig 39).

Tail Displacement

The tail is displaced for rectal or urogenital examinations, to discourage kicking, and to provide some support of the hindquarters during certain procedures, such as a standing castration and putting a horse on a surgery table. This can be done manually or with a rope tied in the end of the tail (Figs 40, 41). A tail rope is held and must never be tied to a stationary object if the horse is standing. When the animal is lying on a surgery table and secured by a halter and body belts, the tail can be tied. As a horse is getting on its feet, it can be assisted by lifting the tail.

The tail can be used to subdue unmanageable ponies and weanlings. One person can often restrain such an animal by grasping the halter with one hand and the tail with the other. The tail is held firmly over the animal's back by grasping it near the base and

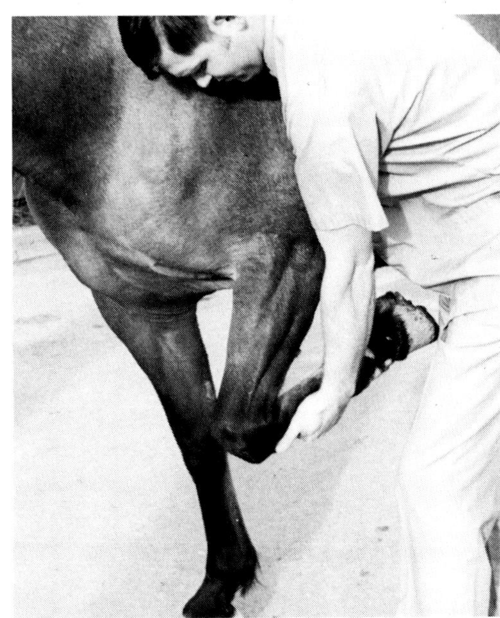

Figure 37. Manual restraint of a foreleg.

pulling it craniad. If the horse is not haltered and is small enough, the base of the neck is cradled in the other arm. To restrain a larger weanling, it is helpful to push the animal beside a smooth wall and lean into it while holding its head and tail. It is even better to back to back the animal into a corner of a stall. This provides safe restraint for stomach intubation, injections and other short procedures.

Young horses often react to head restraint by rearing and may fall over backward, strike the head, and suffer concussion and fractures. The restraint methods just described are safer for young horses that may be unbroken or only partially halter-broken. Abu-

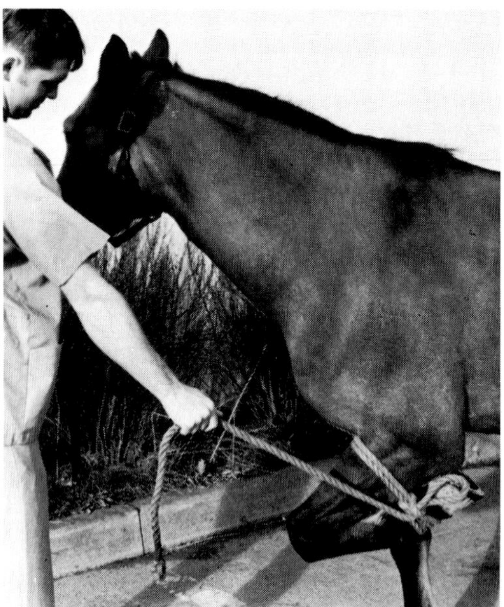

Figure 38. Restraint of a foreleg by tying.

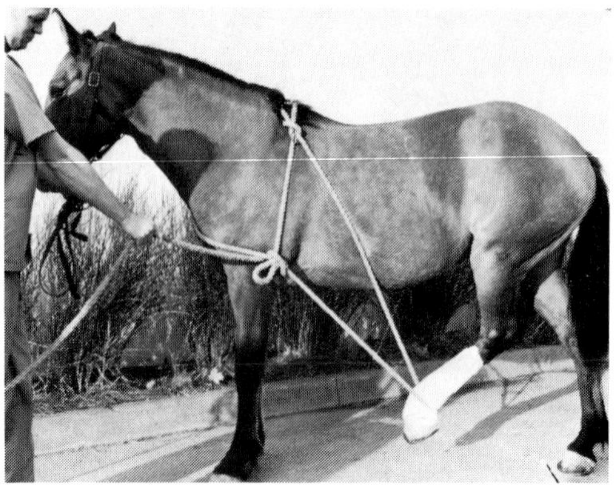

Figure 39. Use of a sideline to immobilize a hind limb. The bandage on the immobilized leg prevents rope burns.

sive application of tail restraint may cause fractures, especially in young animals. Coccygeal fractures can result in abnormal tail carriage caused by pain, paralysis or bone distortion.

Restraint of Foals

Suckling foals require special handling and foals should never be separated from the dam unless kept in a safe place, preferably with a "baby-sitter." Foals can become very excited when left alone and may hurt themselves.

When restraining young foals or weanlings that have not been halter-broken (even though they may be wearing one), one should not grasp the halter or apply one and attempt to hold the animal with it. The foal's reaction usually is to rear back and fall. Instead,

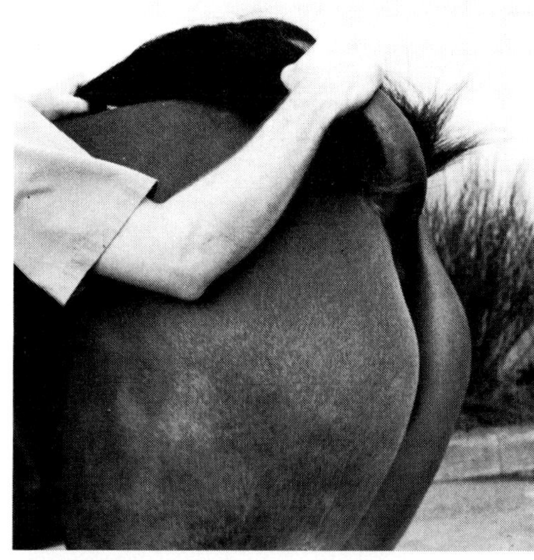

Figure 40. Manual displacement of the tail.

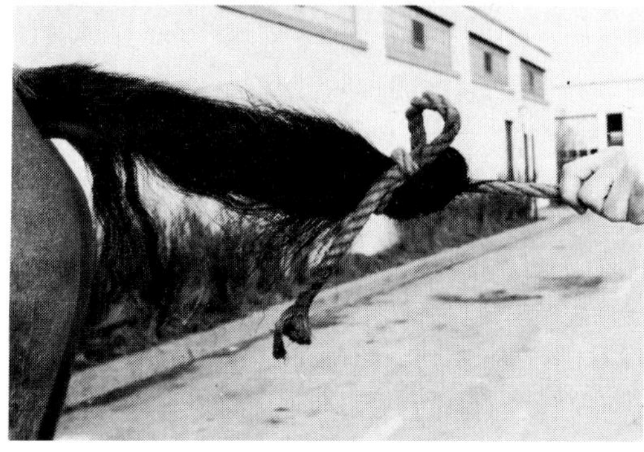

Figure 41. Use of a tail rope for restraint.

the foal should be cornered in a smooth-walled box stall free of buckets, tubs, sharp edges or other hazards, with the mare nearby, restrained by an assistant. The foal can then be cradled in the arms, one around the neck and the other around the rump (Fig 42).

Restraint in Stalls

Certain procedures are often more easily accomplished if performed in surroundings familiar to the animal. Passing a stomach tube, treating teeth, examining the eyes and medicating a wound are usually more easily accomplished in the animal's stall. Usually the best position for the assistant and operator is the center of the stall, with the horse led beside a wall. A fractious horse is restrained more easily this way. The operator keeps to the inside (normally the left) shoulder of the horse. By taking a short hold on the lead shank and placing the elbow of the same arm squarely against the side of the horse's neck, it is possible to keep the horse's head turned toward the handler and its hindquarters away.

Slings

As a rule, use of slings is indicated when the animal, once raised to a standing position, can and will support or partially support its own weight at least part of the time. If a horse will not support its weight at least partially, it is better off lying in a deep bed of clean, dry straw and turned or lifted at regular intervals. A sling may be used temporarily to raise a weakened animal to its feet. Horses have tolerated a sling well for many weeks (fracture cases), but the animal was able to bear its own weight and stand for long periods

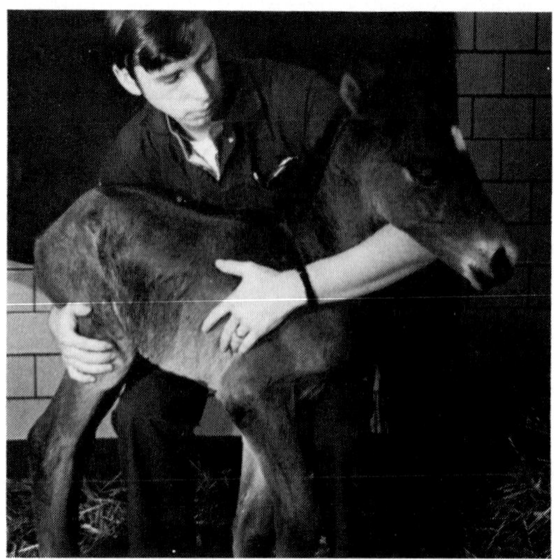

Figure 42. Restraint of a foal.

without the sling's support. When an animal hangs in a sling constantly, its death is certain.

There are many poor slings and a few good ones. The former are poorly constructed with inferior materials. A good sturdy, easily adjusted sling is a valuable possession. Though there are relatively few occasions for its use, nothing else will suffice when a sling is needed. The components of a sling are a wide belly band (the wider the better), a breast collar, breeching, a crupper, a single-tree, and a chain hoist (Fig 43). The breeching keeps the horse from falling out of the sling backward and must have the necessary straps to keep it from slipping up or down. The breast collar prevents the horse from slipping forward. All bands and straps should be buckled together in one unit and adjusted to fit the individual horse. The single-tree is the point of suspension above the horse and keeps the straps separated over the animal's back. The chain hoist is firmly anchored in the ceiling of the stall. It should be raised until the horse is lifted to a standing position and then lowered just enough to allow a hand to be slipped between the belly band and the horse when it is standing. This amount of clearance is necessary to remove constant pressure on the chest and abdomen. Otherwise, respiration and circulation are impaired.

The patient usually is tied loosely to one wall by the halter to prevent its turning in circles in the sling. This may not be necessary if the hoist has a swivel. Feed and water must be placed in easy access, and a hay net hung nearby is an added convenience. When first placed in a sling, the horse should be fully conscious. It is very difficult to put a partially anesthetized animal in a sling, especially if it is unable to use one or more legs. Tranquilization may help horses that rear and otherwise resist being placed in the sling. Time and patience are necessary until the patient adjusts to confinement.

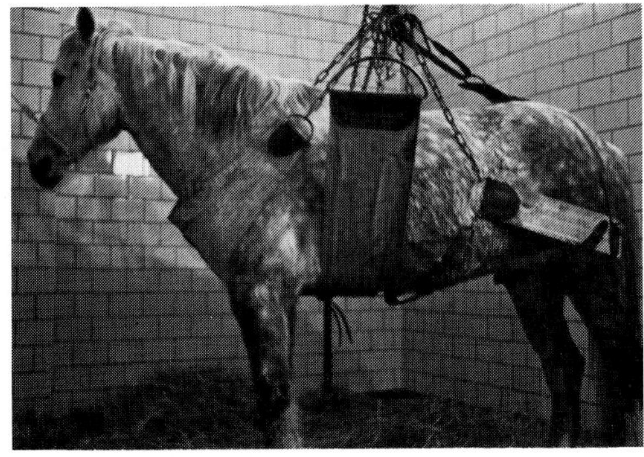

Figure 43. A satisfactory sling.

Stocks

Stocks are very useful to simplify examination and treatment, and are especially suitable for dental procedures and surgery on standing horses (Fig 44). Animals unfamiliar with restraint in stocks should be introduced gradually before the need for such restraint arises.

The use of a kickboard in conjunction with stocks enables one to work with relative safety around the rear of a standing horse. This is a heavy half-door constructed of either oak boards or heavy marine plywood with a reinforced backing. It can be hinged to swing open like half a Dutch door or can be slipped into the stocks behind the horse. It should be 40 inches high and wide enough to be braced against the uprights of the stocks. The side facing the horse should be smooth or padded, especially the top edge. The door should be fixed to the stocks with ropes or latches to keep it from falling forward against the horse. After the door is fixed in place, the horse should be backed against it. If allowed to move forward, the animal might be able to kick over the top of the door.

Casting Harnesses

Though casting harnesses are still used, such equipment is no longer required to restrain horses, and risks their injury. If casting harnesses are used, they should be employed in conjunction with tranquilizers, sedatives, general anesthetics and/or muscle relaxants to minimize the risk of injury. Most horses are cast with the use of drugs alone. They can be held by a halter or snubbed to a ring in the wall or some other stationary object to prevent falling backward and possibly striking the head on the wall or floor. Once anesthesia has been induced, the analgesia and muscle relaxation achieved render restraining ropes and harness unnecessary except to maintain the position of the limbs. Tight ropes and strained po-

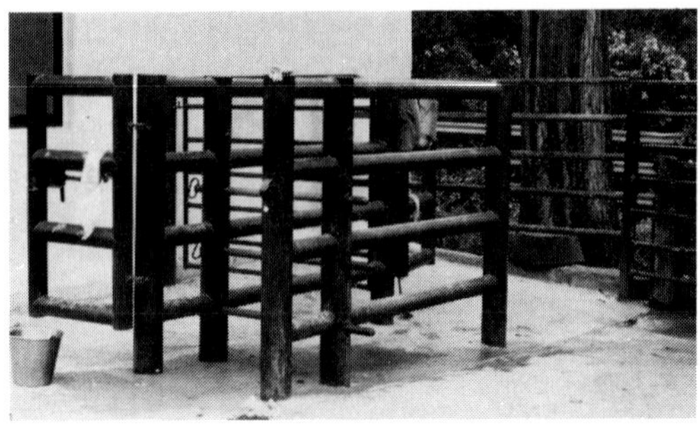

Figure 44. A well-constructed set of outdoor stocks. The hinged rear door is at the left and a padded neck cradle on the hinged front door is on the right.

sitions are contraindicated because they often result in peripheral nerve injuries, especially of the hind legs.

Breeding Hobbles

Breeding hobbles are used to prevent the mare from kicking during breeding. The restraining ropes extend from a breast collar, between the forelegs, and to the hocks or pasterns of the hind legs (Fig 45). They also can be used for restraint during rectal examination or any operation around the hindquarters. One should adjust the hobbles properly to prevent any slack and also provide for quick release in case of such emergencies as the stallion's catching a leg in one of the ropes or casting of the mare.

Restraint of Cattle

W.A. Aanes

Cattle may be restrained by many methods. The choice of a single method or combination of restraint methods depends on many factors. Careful consideration of these factors in selection of restraint should result in minimal stress to the animal and handler.

The response of most cattle to handling depends mostly on previous experiences. Beef cattle usually require more restraint than dairy cattle because they are handled less frequently and are commonly subjected to pain or discomfort when restrained. Dairy cows usually do not associate handling with pain, and their restraint should be minimal to avoid loss of milk production.

Bulls should never be trusted! Even a bull that appears to be gentle may suddenly change, especially during or after a painful

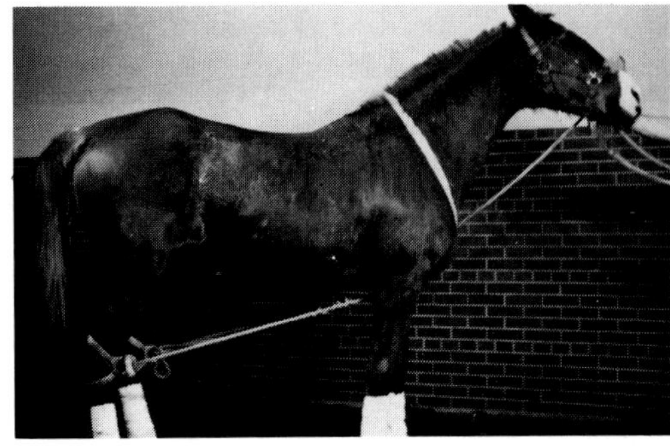

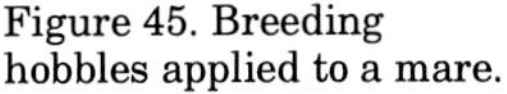

Figure 45. Breeding hobbles applied to a mare.

procedure associated with restraint. A beef bull is usually less dangerous than a dairy bull, but there are enough exceptions to heed the statement "The only safe bull is a dead bull."

Factors that determine the methods of restraint to be applied include size, age, strength and disposition of the animal, and the availability of mechanical restraint equipment. The examination or treatment procedure(s), their duration, and the amount of pain to be inflicted also influence the extent of restraint. Because cattle have very sensitive skin, few procedures can be accomplished without causing some pain. Judicious use of tranquilizers, local anesthetics and general anesthetics is indicated, in conjunction with physical restraint, to handle cattle effectively. The general principle of "the least restraint necessary to satisfactorily accomplish the task at hand" should be followed at all times.

Restraining the Head

Ordinary adjustable rope halters may be used to catch cattle in small pens. The halter should be adjusted so the crown of the halter can be dropped over the animal's head and the halter shank tightened under the jaw (Fig 46). The nose piece of the halter should be sufficiently long to keep the halter from damaging an eye or interfering with respiration. A common error in applying the rope halter is reversing the crown position so the pull on the halter shank is across the poll of the animal; this reduces the effectiveness of the restraint. In larger pens a lariat may be used to catch the animal and then a halter applied to prevent choking. A halter

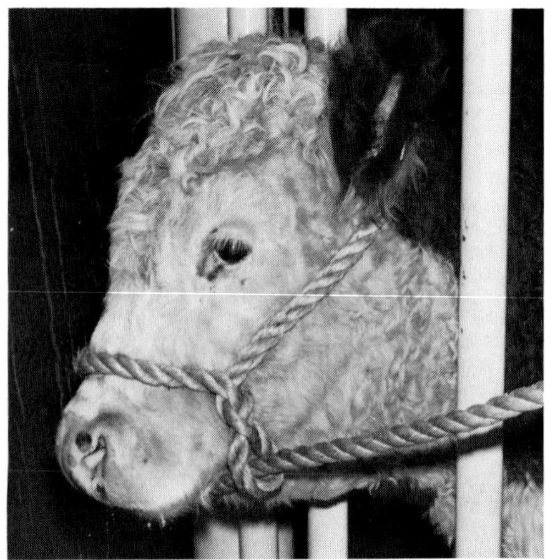

Figure 46. Properly applied rope halter.

can be used to effectively restrain the head of a "downer" cow during medication by tying the halter shank above the cow's hock (Fig 47).

If an ordinary rope halter is not available, an effective temporary halter can be made by putting the loop of a lariat around the animal's neck. A bight (loop) is formed in the standing part of the rope distal to the honda (eye at end of lariat). This bight is passed back to front through the lariat loop and adjusted over the nose. When properly adjusted, this temporary halter does not choke the animal. Any danger of choking can be avoided by tying the initial loop around the neck with a bowline (Figs 48, 49).

Another type of halter, called a "Wyoming slip halter," may be formed by splicing a metal ring into one end of a rope. A bight is formed in the standing part of the rope and is passed through the metal ring, forming 2 loops (Fig 50). The loop from the spliced end of the rope forms the crown of the halter and the bight through the ring forms the loop for the nose (Fig 51). Tension on the standing part of the rope shank tightens the loop around the nose. This halter is easily released by pulling the loop from the nose.

A nose lead (bull leader) used in conjunction with a halter is an excellent device for restraining cattle (Fig 52). The nose lead causes temporary pain and thus diverts the animal's attention. Pressure on the lead should be in a dorsal direction, against the alar cartilages, to avoid tearing the nose. There should be sufficient tension on the halter shank to prevent the entire weight of the an-

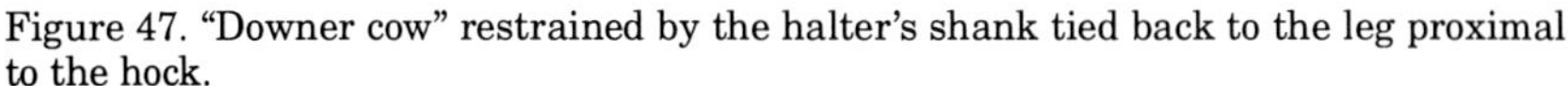
Figure 47. "Downer cow" restrained by the halter's shank tied back to the leg proximal to the hock.

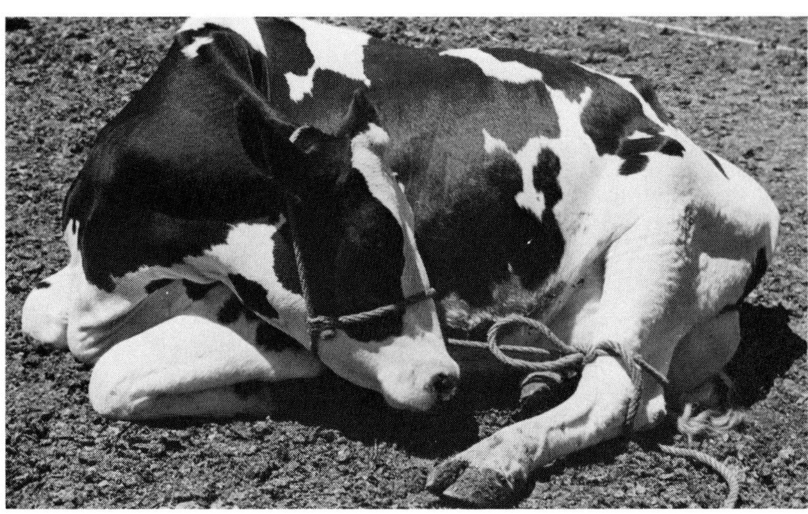

imal from pulling on the nose lead. If a nose lead is not available, the same type of restraint can be applied by grasping the nasal septum with the thumb and forefinger of one hand and supporting the animal's head with the other hand (Fig 53). The effectiveness of this restraint is limited by the strength of the individual applying it; it is a poor substitute for a nose lead.

The head of a gentle young animal may be held for simple examination and minor treatments by grasping the base of an ear with one hand, applying pressure against the head, and stabilizing the head with the other hand placed beneath the jaw. The head of an animal confined in a chute or stanchion may be examined by facing in the same direction as the animal, grasping its head, and holding it securely against the hip (Fig 54). Additional restraint can be applied by firmly grasping the animal's upper lip between the thumb

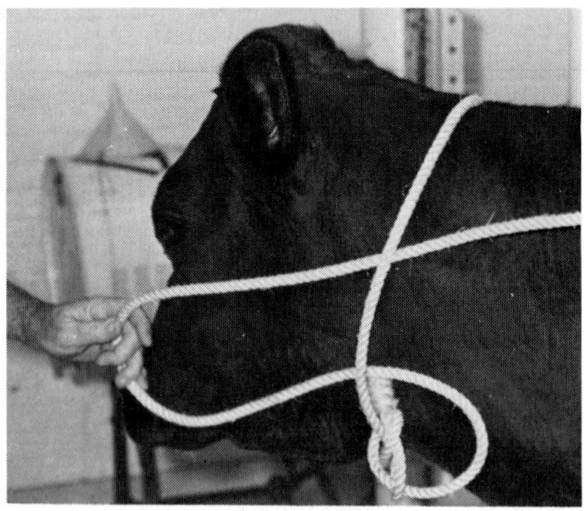

Figure 48. A temporary halter can be made by looping a lariat around the neck and pulling a bight through the loop toward the muzzle.

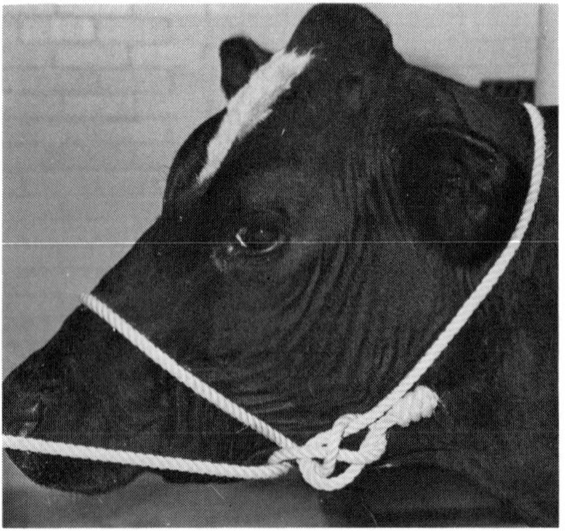

Figure 49. The bight is pulled over the bridge of the nose and adjusted.

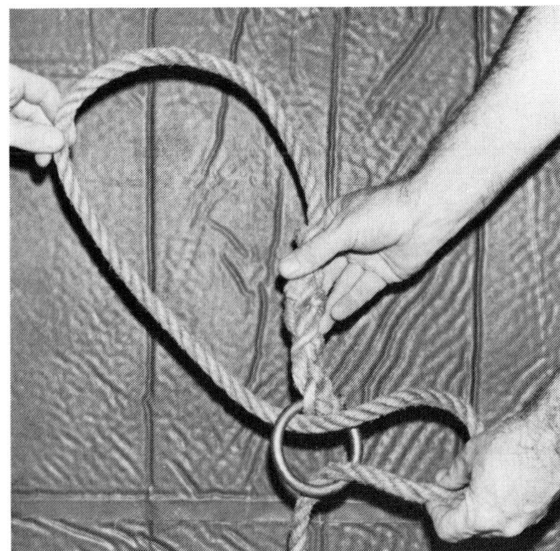

Figure 50. A Wyoming slip halter is made from a rope with an attached metal ring in one end.

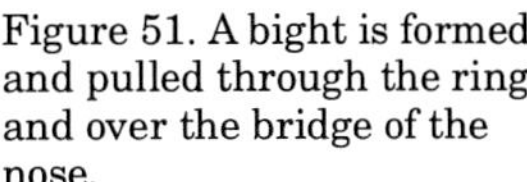

Figure 51. A bight is formed and pulled through the ring and over the bridge of the nose.

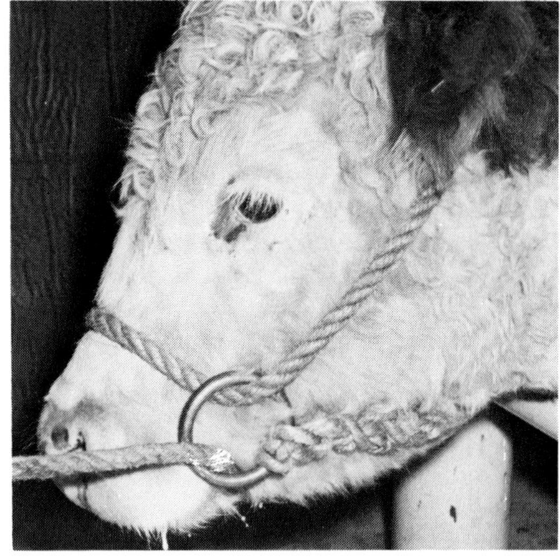

and fingers of a hand passed across the nose of the animal (Fig 55). This restraint is effective for oral examination and medication.

To restrain the neck of an animal during dehorning when a chute or head stanchion is unavailable, a bight can be formed in the loop of a lariat. This bight is then placed over a fence post and the collapsed loop is passed under and around the animal's neck. A second bight is formed in the loop and placed over the first bight on the post. The honda is drawn tightly to secure the animal's neck to the post (Fig 56). A nose lead can then be used to control the position of the animal's head for examination or dehorning.

Restraint of a Bull's Head

Use of a hood that completely blindfolds or allows the bull to see only in a ventral direction may aid in handling and moving bad-tempered individuals. A hood can also be used to protect the animal's eyes when it is being cast.

A nose ring is one of the most effective devices for restraint of a bull's head. Nose rings are commonly used on dairy bulls and

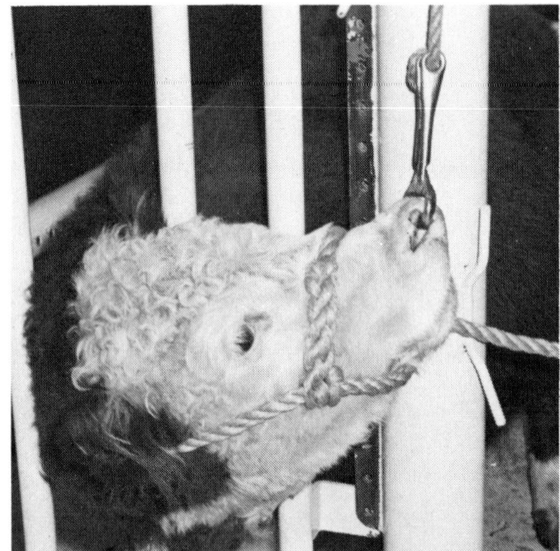

Figure 52. A nose lead should only be used with a halter.

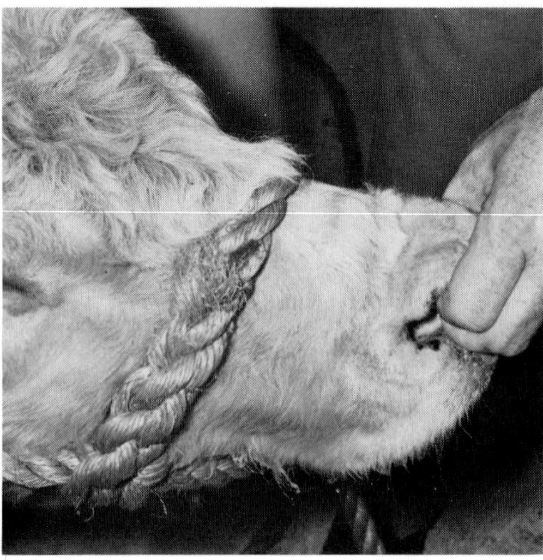

Figure 53. Cattle can be temporarily restrained by grasping the nasal septum with the thumb and forefinger.

should also be used on beef bulls that have bad temperaments or are handled frequently. The nose ring restrains by causing pain, thus diverting the animal's attention from the handler. A nose ring should not be used as the primary method of head restraint because the nose may be torn, resulting in loss of this important method of restraint. A bull lead and halter should be used for primary restraint of the head for examination and treatment.

When moving bulls, a commercial bull staff may be snapped into the ring to aid control of the head (Fig 57). It is safer to use 2 long lead shanks snapped into the ring; each shank is held by a separate handler on each side of the bull (Fig 58).

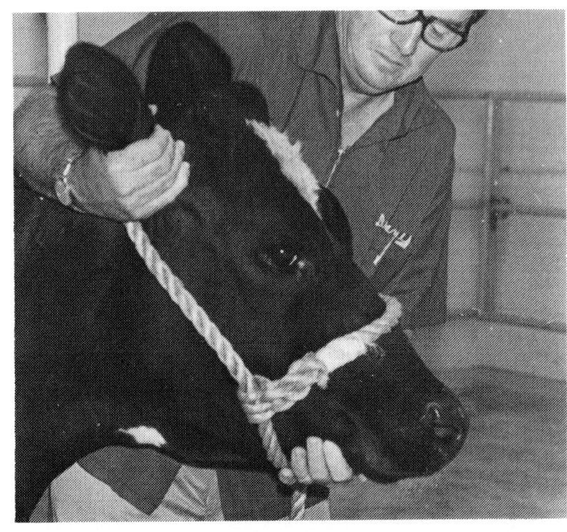

Figure 54. A cow in a stanchion can be restrained by holding the head against your hip.

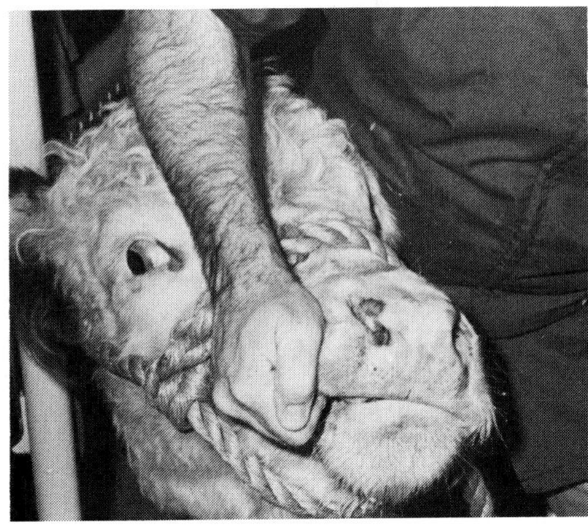

Figure 55. Grasping the upper lip facilitates oral examination and administration of medication.

When moving "unbroken" cattle where adequate corrals or chute systems are not available, the animal should be "double haltered" with a shank held to each side of the animal for control. An alternative method is to apply a single halter and lariat to a foreleg to reduce forward speed, thus throwing the animal off balance should it attempt to escape.

Restraint of the Body and Limbs

If a chute or stock is not available, uncooperative animals may be examined by securing the head to a strong fence post and applying a nonslip loop around the animal's neck. The standing part of the rope is then brought along the animal's side and tied to another fence post behind the rear legs. After pulling the animal snugly

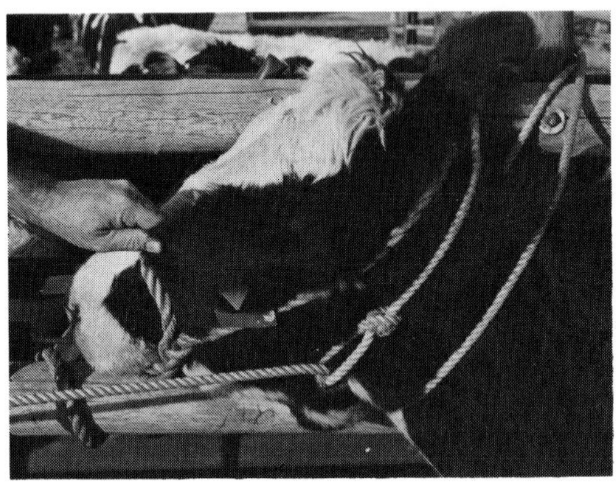

Figure 56. The head is secured to a fence in preparation for dehorning.

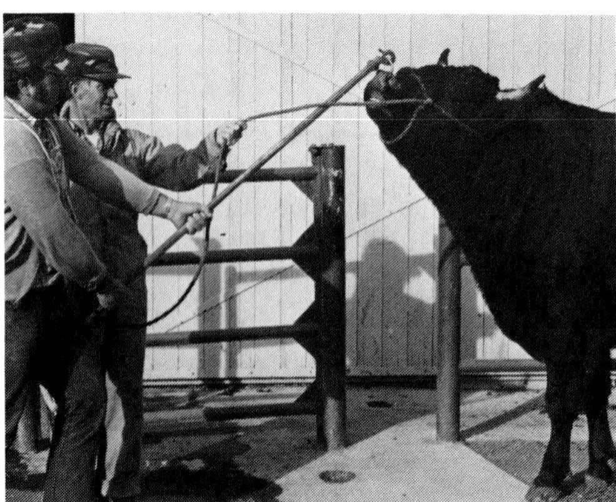

Figure 57. A bull staff is inserted through a bull's nose ring to control the animal.

against the fence, the handlers can approach and examine it (Fig 59).

Several methods of restraint may be employed to reduce or prevent kicking:

Tail restraint is applied by grasping the base of the tail firmly with both hands and bending it sharply in a dorsal direction (Fig 60). This causes pain and diverts the animal's attention when its legs, udder or external genitalia are examined and when performing minor operations. Care must be taken to bend the tail at the base because lateral movement may cause pain and fractures of the vertebrae without producing the desired restraint. Tail re-

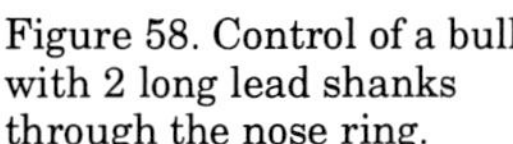

Figure 58. Control of a bull with 2 long lead shanks through the nose ring.

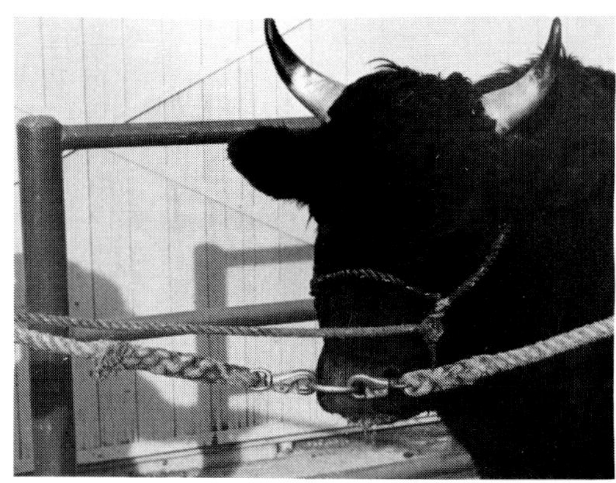

Figure 59. A halter secures the cow's head and a side line keeps the animal against the wall.

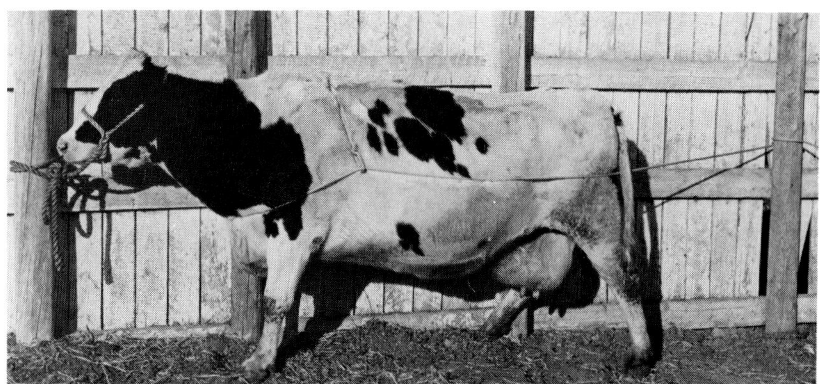

straint is often used in conjunction with a bull leader for minor procedures.

Milking hobbles may be applied to the hind limbs to prevent kicking (Fig 61). This restraint device is used most commonly on dairy cattle to prevent kicking. It is applied over the Achilles tendons, proximal to the hocks, and pulled sufficiently tight to prevent kicking. The device works well when cows are accustomed to its use. The hobbles should be applied cautiously because the hind legs may easily be injured when animals are not accustomed to this restraint.

A *flank rope* is effective for reducing kicking (Fig 62). This involves placing a lariat around the flank area, just cranial to the tuber coxae. The rope is tightened to reduce kicking. Excessive pressure may cause the animal to fall.

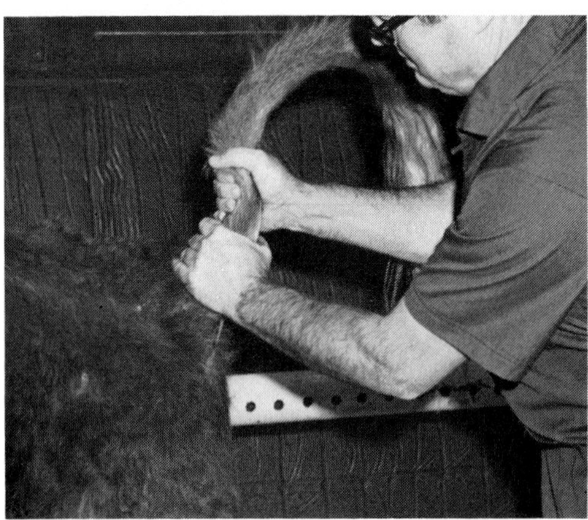

Figure 60. Restraining a beef cow by bending the tail dorsad.

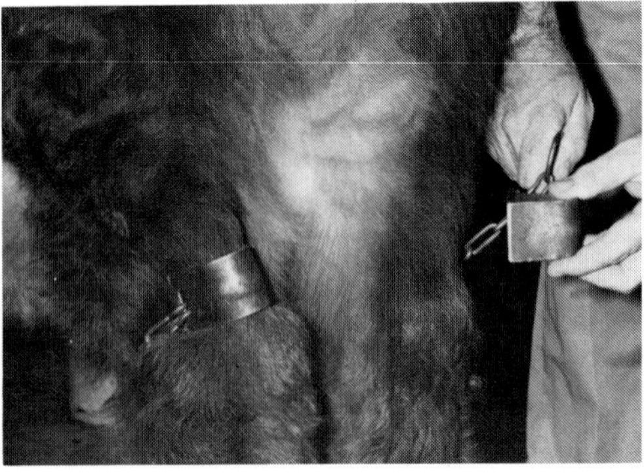

Figure 61. Milking hobbles applied to the rear legs to prevent kicking.

For minor examinations of the hindquarters of smaller animals, the *tail* can be *pulled* between the hindquarters and flank (Fig 63).

A *hock twitch* may be applied to a hind limb just proximal to the point of the hock (Figs 64-66). This restraint device consists of a piece of cotton rope about 20 inches long, with a loop braided in each end. A stick about 12 inches long is threaded through the loops of the rope and twisted until the rope binds the limb tightly.

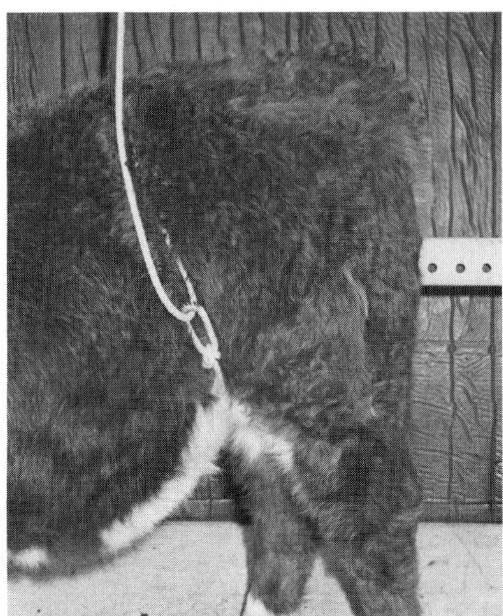

Figure 62. Flank rope used to prevent kicking.

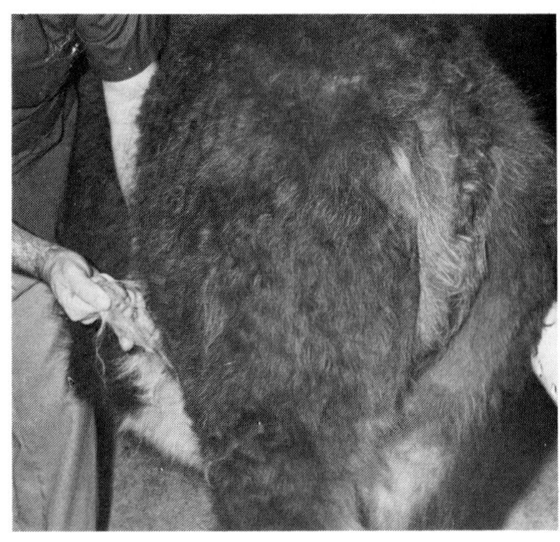

Figure 63. The tail is pulled between the rear legs to restrain the legs.

Pressure on the Achilles tendon tends to prevent flexion of the limb and aids in examination of the hind leg.

A *tail rope* effectively controls tail movements and is essential for reduction of contamination during surgical procedures (Fig 67). The switch of the tail is tied to a small (1/4 inch diameter) cotton rope with a quick-release knot (Weaver's). The opposite end of the rope is then secured to the neck, horns or opposite foreleg of the animal. The rope should *never* be tied to a fixed object because the tail may be torn off if the animal escapes the restraint when the tail is still secured.

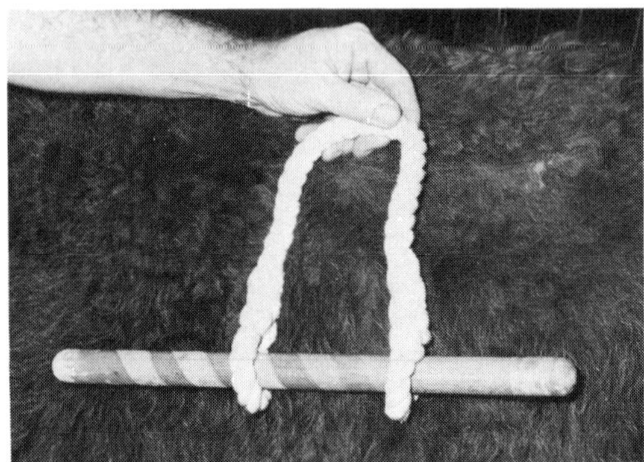

Figure 64. A hock twitch consists of 20 inches of rope with a foot-long stick inserted through the end loops.

Figures 65, 66. The hock twitch is applied by looping the rope around the hock and inserting the stick through the rope's end loops. The stick is twisted until the rope constricts the hock, allowing examination of the foot.

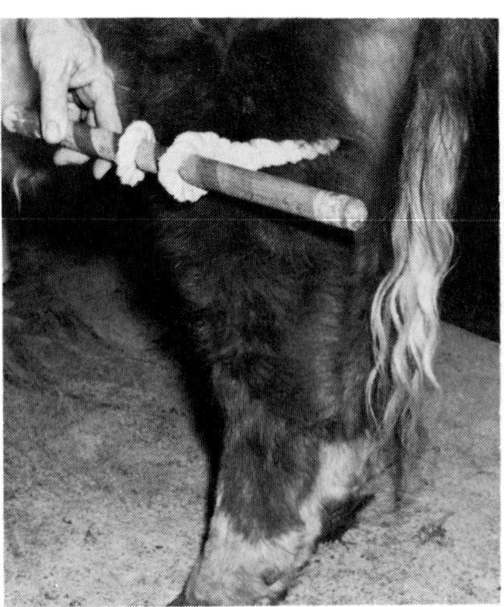

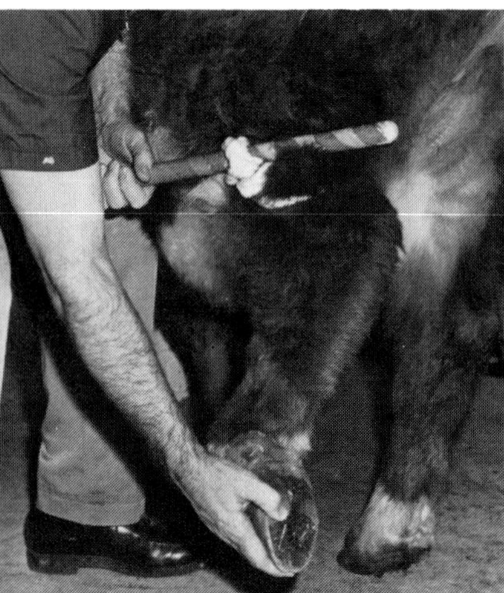

An *electroejaculator* can be used effectively to restrain the hindquarters for minor procedures. Excessive stimulation may cause the animal to "go down" or damage the muscles of the hindquarters.

A *front foot* is properly *picked up* by manually flexing the carpus and pulling the limb into a flexed position (Fig 68). Most cattle have a tendency to lie down when a front foot is flexed, however, making this manipulation difficult. A rope can be used to assist examination of a front foot by placing a loop around the pastern (Fig 69). The standing part of the rope is then passed over the withers and in front of the neck and a bight is formed across the vertical part of the rope. An alternative is to place a loop around the forelimb, proximal to the elbow and secure the loop to a beam above the animal. This supports the animal's weight while the operator examines the foot.

The hind foot of a gentle cow can be raised for examination by grasping the limb at the fetlock, slightly flexing the limb, and supporting the animal's weight with a hand or knee (Fig 70). The limb should be retained in a slightly flexed position because extending it results in kicking and loss of control of the limb. A nose lead can be used to pull the animal's head to the opposite side to facilitate this procedure. Most cattle do not cooperate sufficiently for satisfactory examination of a hindlimb without further restraint.

The *beam hook method* can be used when cows are stanchioned in a barn (Fig 71). For such restraint the animal must be positioned

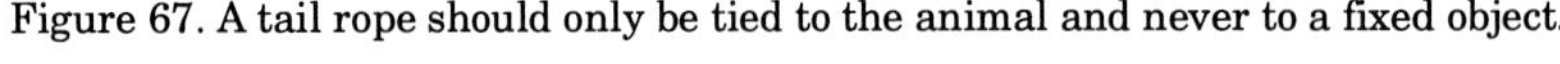

Figure 67. A tail rope should only be tied to the animal and never to a fixed object.

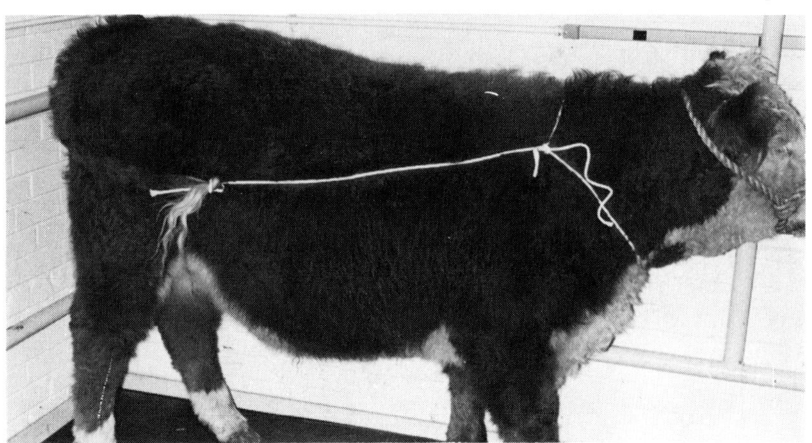

so that lateral movement can be prevented. The cow's head is restrained with a nose lead, pulled to the side opposite the leg to be examined, and a beam hook is fastened above and behind the cow. A loop of rope is then placed around the pastern of the hind leg to be lifted. The opposite end is passed through the ring of the beam

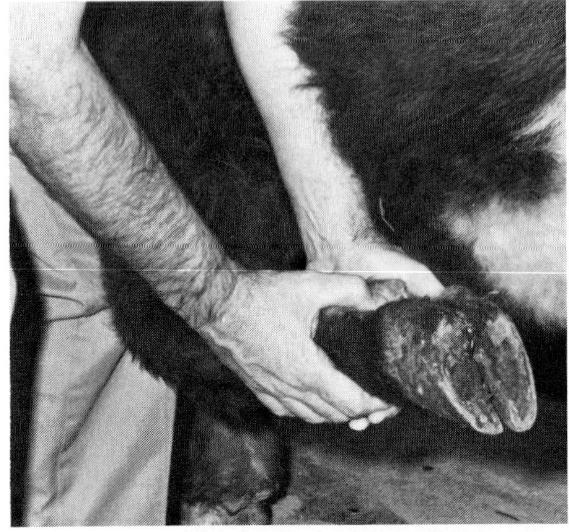

Figure 68. Raising a front foot for examination.

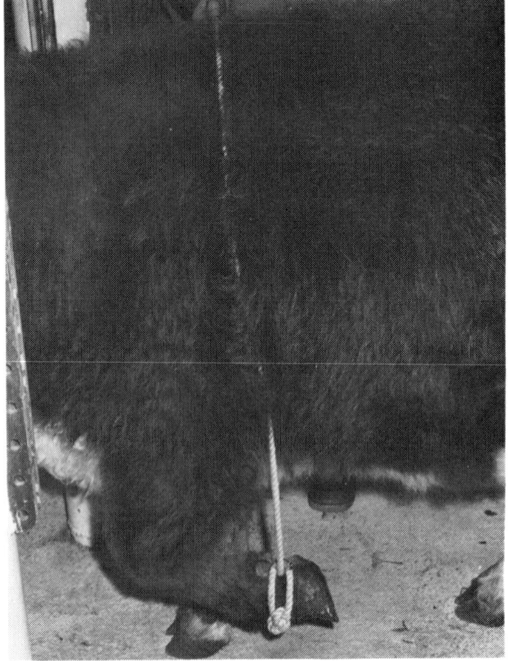

Figure 69. Rope looped over the pastern and led up over the back aids examination of a front foot.

hook so that the free end goes toward the head of the cow. The standing part of the rope is passed medial to the limb to be raised, brought around the limb craniodorsal to the hock, and a bight is formed around the standing part of the rope. The end of the rope is then carried forward and wrapped around a fixed object (stanchion). The foot to be examined is lifted off the ground and the

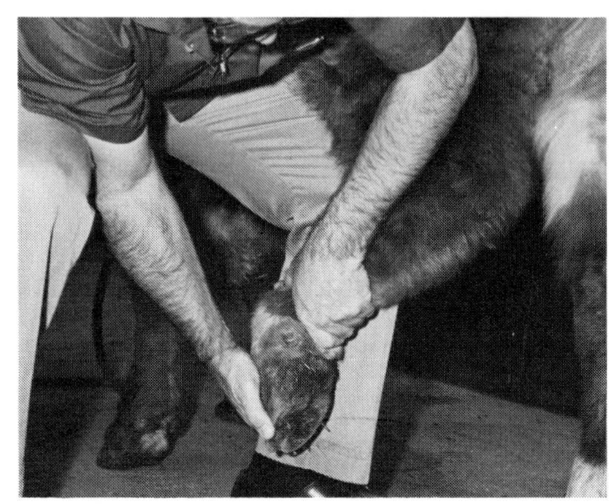

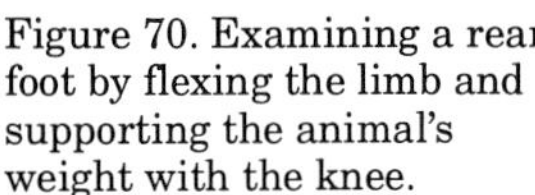

Figure 70. Examining a rear foot by flexing the limb and supporting the animal's weight with the knee.

Figure 71. Rope is looped around the pastern and led up over a beam hook and back down to the hock for examination of a rear foot.

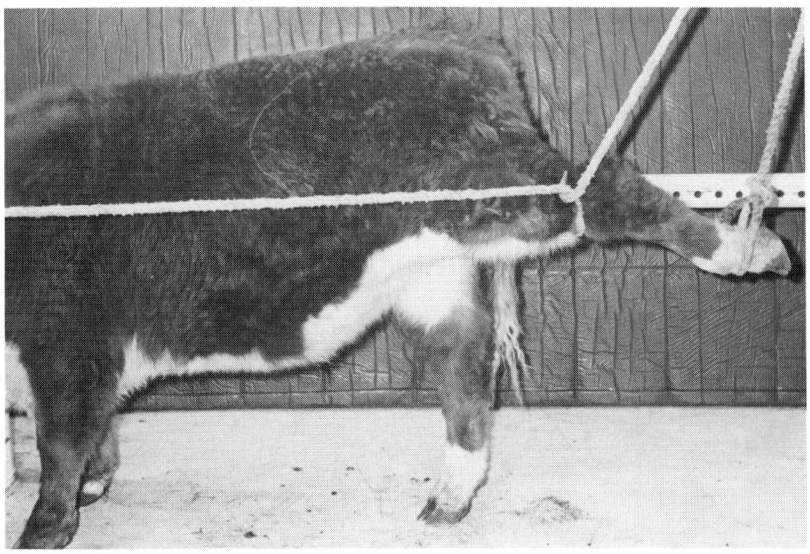

slack in the rope is removed. The animal will struggle when the foot is lifted and care must be taken to prevent its being injured.

Another method of examining a hind foot of a standing animal involves placing a fixed loop of rope around the limb (Fig 72). The loop is attached to a beam above the animal with a block and tackle to support the animal's weight so that the fetlock can be flexed to examine the foot.

The methods described so far are adequate for examination and treatment of many animals. Others, because of their temperament or the procedure, do not allow adequate examination and/or treatment. Other types of restraint are thus necessary.

There are several methods of casting cattle, each with its advantages and disadvantages. The animal's rumen should be empty when casting to avoid discomfort and possibly death from bloating. Though cattle are relatively easy to cast, care should be taken to select a place on which bruising will be minimal.

The "double half-hitch" method of *casting* is used commonly to restrain cattle (Figs 73, 74). It involves tying the animal's head in a fixed position with a halter. A loop of cotton rope is placed around

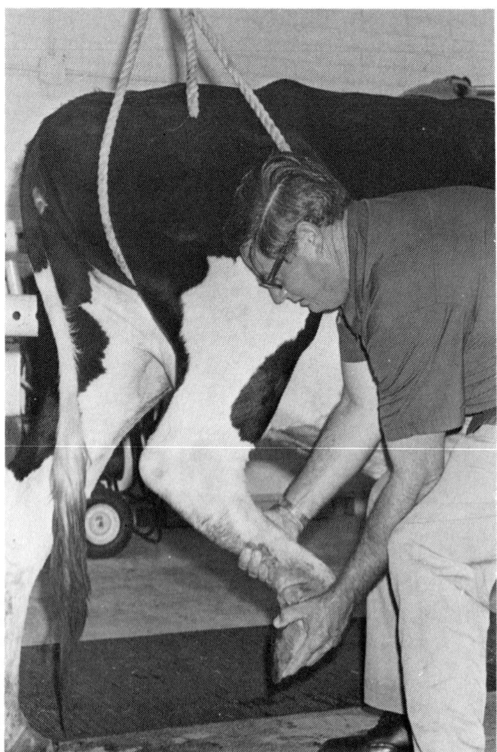

Figure 72. Placing a fixed loop around the proximal rear leg helps support the animal's weight during examination of the foot.

the neck and secured with a nonslip knot, such as a bowline. The loop is made large enough to prevent excessive pressure on the trachea during casting. The standing part of the rope is then used to form a half-hitch around the thorax, just caudal to the forelegs. A second half-hitch is made in the flank area, cranial to the tuber coxae. The half-hitches are tightened; tension applied to the standing part of the rope causes the animal to lie down. Most cattle are cast relatively easily in this manner. Constant tension must be kept on the casting rope to keep the animal down; otherwise ropes are applied to the forelimbs and hind limbs and secured to fixed ob-

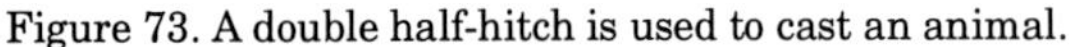
Figure 73. A double half-hitch is used to cast an animal.

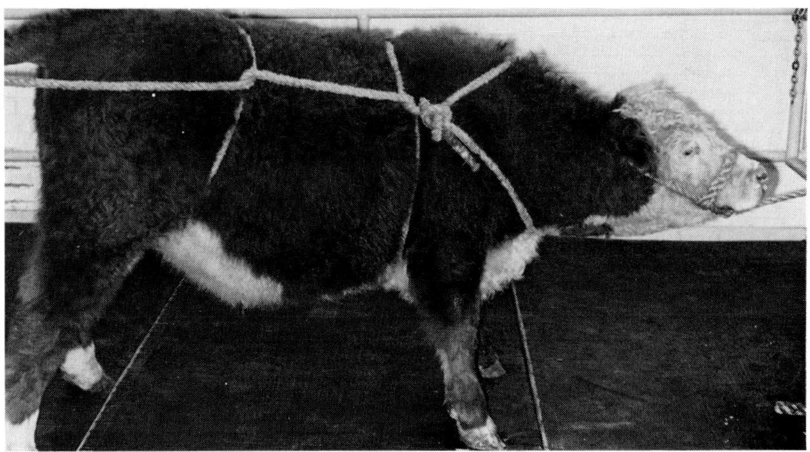

Figure 74. Tightening the half-hitches by pulling caudad causes the animal to lie down.

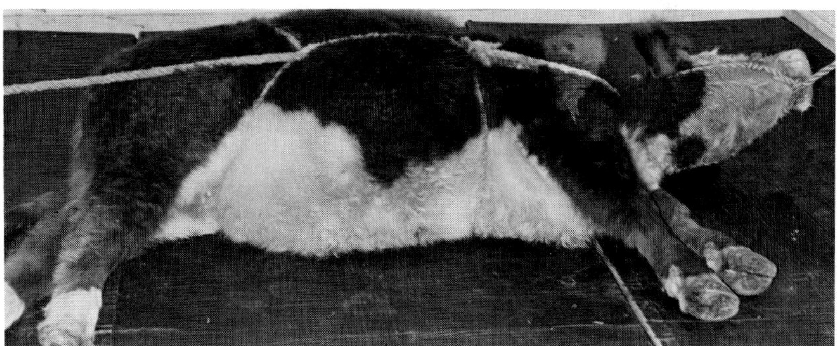

jects. This method of casting places pressure on the thorax and mammary vessels of a cow or external genitalia of a bull.

The "Burley method" of casting cattle involves using a 40-foot cotton rope (Figs 75-77). The cow's head is secured by a halter rope to a fixed object. The middle of the rope is placed over the neck of the cow cranial to the withers. The ends of the rope are carried between the front legs and crossed at the sternum. One end is carried up each side of the animal's thorax and the 2 ends are crossed again over the back. Each end is then passed down to the flank and caudad on the medial aspect of the hind limb. When the ends of the ropes are pulled backward simultaneously, the animal falls. The di-

Figure 75. The rope in position for casting an animal using the Burley method.

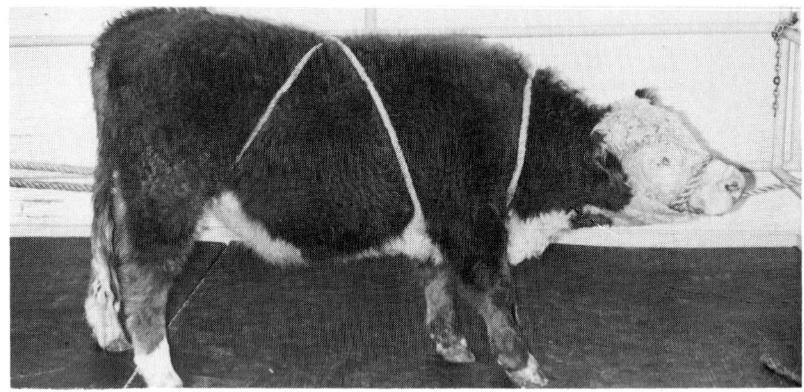

Figure 76. Pulling the ropes caudad causes the animal to fall.

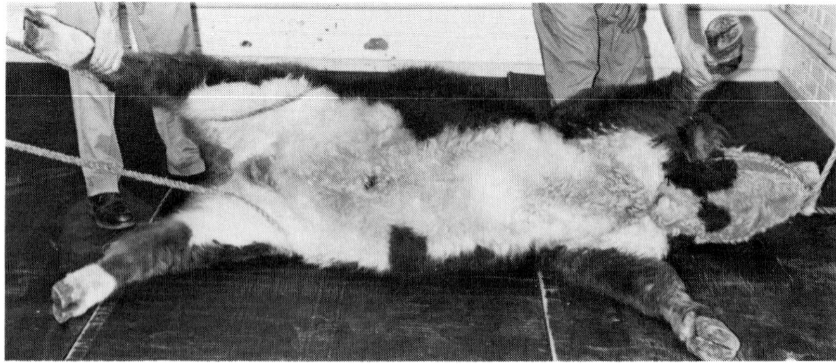

rection of the fall may be controlled by applying pressure to one side with both ends of the casting rope. The proximal hind limb can be tied while flexed by sliding the upper rope along the medial surface of the leg to the pastern, where a loop is formed. The limb is then flexed and tied with one or more "figure 8s" and secured with a half-hitch. The proximal forelimb can then be secured to the casting rope by flexing the limb and wrapping a cord around it several times. The cord is attached to the casting rope cranial to the sternum. The animal is turned and the opposite limbs are tied similarly.

The Burley casting method requires application of more pressure on the ropes to cast most animals than the double half-hitch. It has the advantages, however, of exerting less pressure on the thorax and avoiding any pressure on the mammary vessels of cows or the external genitalia of bulls.

A modified half-hitch method of casting and completely restraining cattle is especially effective in an open area where only one fixed object is available to restrain the animal (Figs 78-80). It involves tying the animal to a fixed object with a halter shank. A loop of cotton rope is placed around the animal's neck and secured with a nonslip knot (bowline). A half-hitch is then formed around the thorax caudal to the forelegs. The half-hitch is positioned at the level of the left elbow if the animal is to be cast on its right side. The standing part of the rope is passed over the back and medial to the right hind limb. The end of the rope is brought forward on the lateral side of the right hind limb and passed beneath the rope around the thorax. The bight formed by the rope around the hind limb is then dropped to the pastern distal to the dewclaws. At this point all slack is removed from the entire rope and the right hind foot is pulled craniad to the thorax. The standing part of the rope is pulled caudad and the animal is cast on its right side. After readjusting the rope to remove all slack, the standing part of the rope is brought to the left (upper side of the animal) and an overhand knot

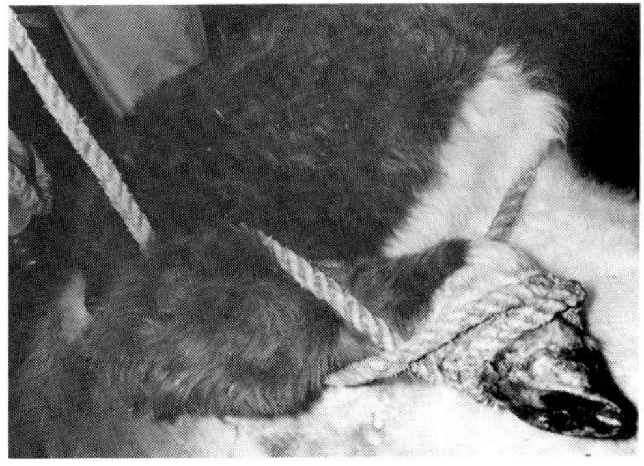

Figure 77. A loop is tied around the pastern of the flexed rear limb, followed by a figure 8 and a half-hitch.

is placed around the rope on the thorax. The standing part of the rope is then passed around the left hind pastern (from medial to lateral). The left hind limb is pulled craniad to the thorax and secured with 2 half-hitches on the left hind pastern. The forelimbs are restrained by tying a Tom Fool's knot near the honda of a lariat, placing the knot over the pasterns of both forefeet, and pulling the

Figure 78. Rope in position for the modified half-hitch method of casting.

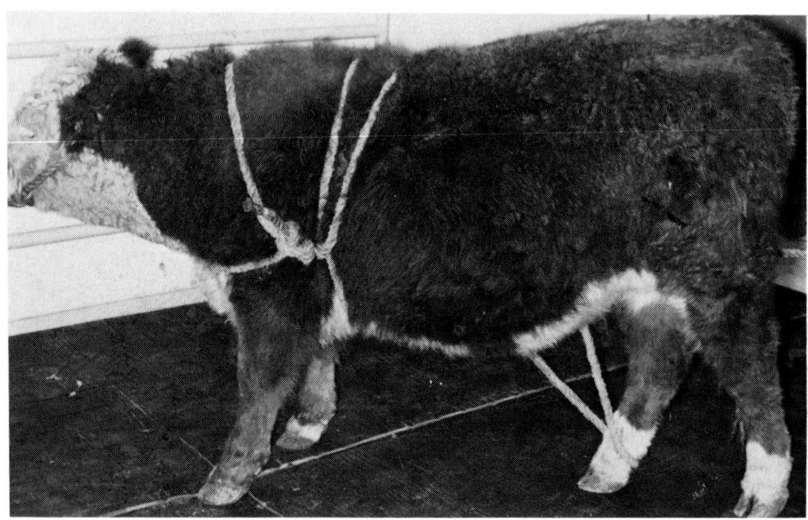

Figure 79. View from the opposite side in the modified half-hitch method of casting.

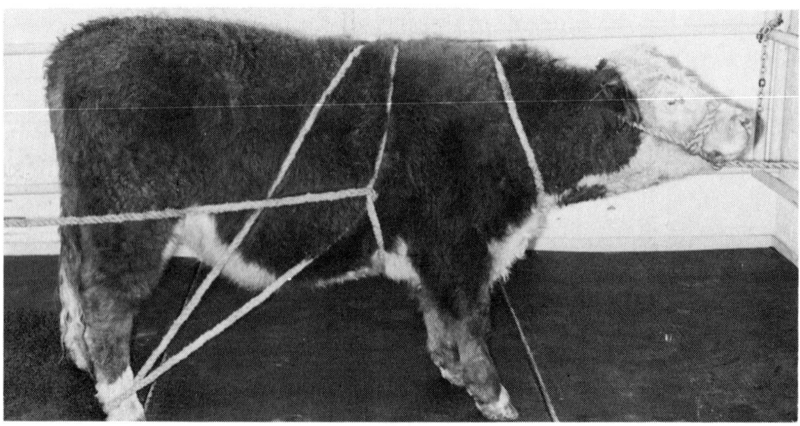

feet up to the sternum with the standing part of the rope over the withers secured to the honda with a halter tie. When the animal attempts to extend the hind limbs, the pressure of the standing part of the rope tightens the half-hitch around the thorax, tending to recast the animal. The animal can be cast on the left side by reversing the method of application.

If properly applied, this restraint affords complete control of the animal. It is essential that no slack develop in the rope during its application. If the half-hitch around the thorax slips back to the abdomen, there will be slack in the rope and the restraint will fail. Veterinarians and handlers have been reluctant to use this excellent method of restraint because of failures resulting from inadequate attention to keeping the rope taut at all times. I have developed a modification of this method that involves using the principle of the modified half-hitch method, together with a casting harness that eliminates this problem (Figs 81-88). This harness (Lane Manufacturing Co, Denver, CO) includes 2 metal plates; plate A has 4 metal loops and 2 metal pegs and plate B has 5 metal loops and a metal hook. The plates are joined with 3 adjustable leather straps designed so that animals of different sizes can be cast on the right or left side. The leather straps attach to the plates with tackleberry buckles; the length of the straps can be adjusted by "D" buckles. Adjustable hobbles are used to restrain the forelegs after the animal is cast and the hind legs are tied in the restrained position. Two ropes, one with a loop braided in one end, complete the harness.

The harness is placed on the animal and adjusted so that the plates (A and B) are located over the opposite sides of the thorax at the level of the shoulders. The adjustable leather straps are used to join the metal plates, one over the back caudal to the withers (back strap), one cranial to the forelegs (breast strap), and a third caudal to the forelegs under the sternum (belly strap).

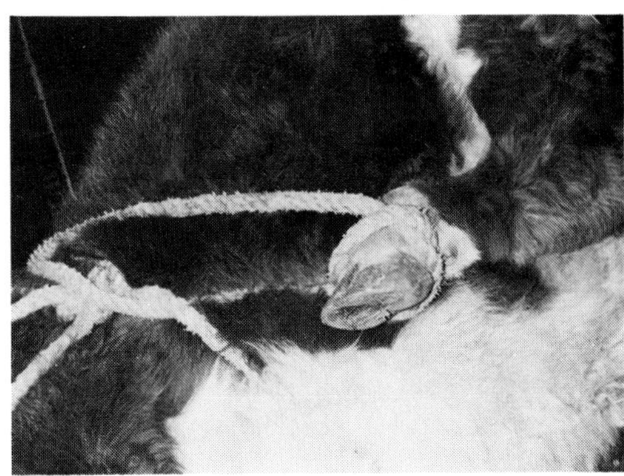

Figure 80. After the ropes are pulled and the animal falls, the rear leg is tied forward.

The braided loop of rope is secured over the upper peg of plate A and passed over the withers, cranial to the hook in plate B. The rope is then guided under the sternum, behind the forelegs and over the lower peg on plate A, passing from the front toward the back. It is then passed around the pastern of the hind leg on the side of plate A from the inside (medial) outward (lateral). The end of the rope is passed through a single metal loop on the back (caudal) side of plate A. The rope is now in position to cast the animal. A second rope is tied (bowline) to 1 of 2 loops on the caudal edge of plate B. This rope is passed from the inside outward, around the pastern of the hind leg on the same side as plate B and through the second loop on the caudal edge of plate B.

Figure 81. Bovine casting harness consisting of 2 metal plates (A, B), 3 adjustable leather straps, 2 ropes (1 with a loop braided in), and adjustable hobbles for the front legs.

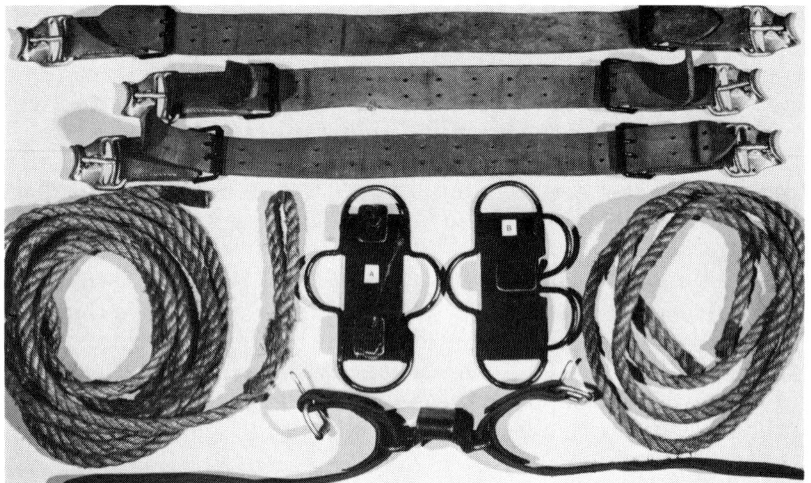

Figure 82. Closeup view of metal plate A.

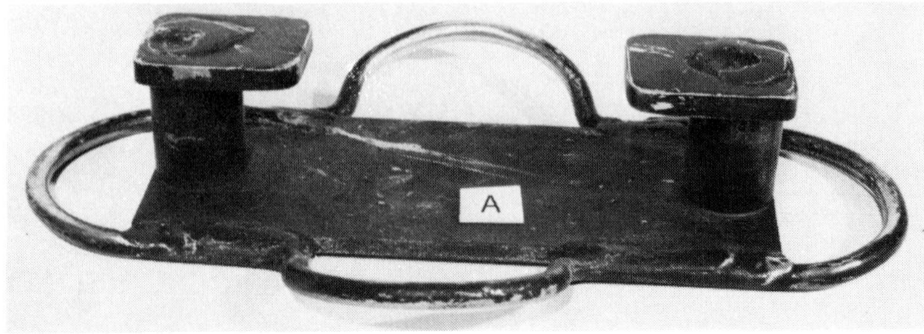

After the animal's head is secured to a fixed object, the rope on the side of plate A is pulled caudad to cast the animal (a sleeve is provided on each peg of plate A to facilitate proper tightening of the rope around the thorax). The hind leg is pulled craniad, toward the casting harness, and the animal usually goes down on this side (plate A). Tension is maintained on the rope while it is secured to itself by a halter tie behind plate A. An alternative and usually simpler procedure is to maintain tension on the rope at plate A after the animal is cast and tie the proximal hind limb to plate B

Figure 83. Closeup view of metal plate B.

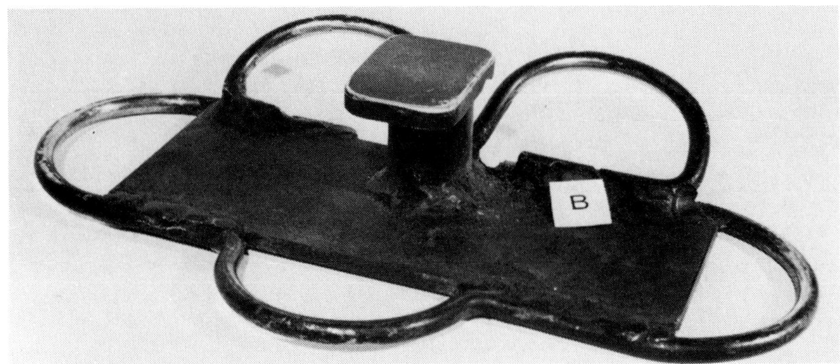

Figure 84. Casting harness in position, with metal plate A on the animal's left side.

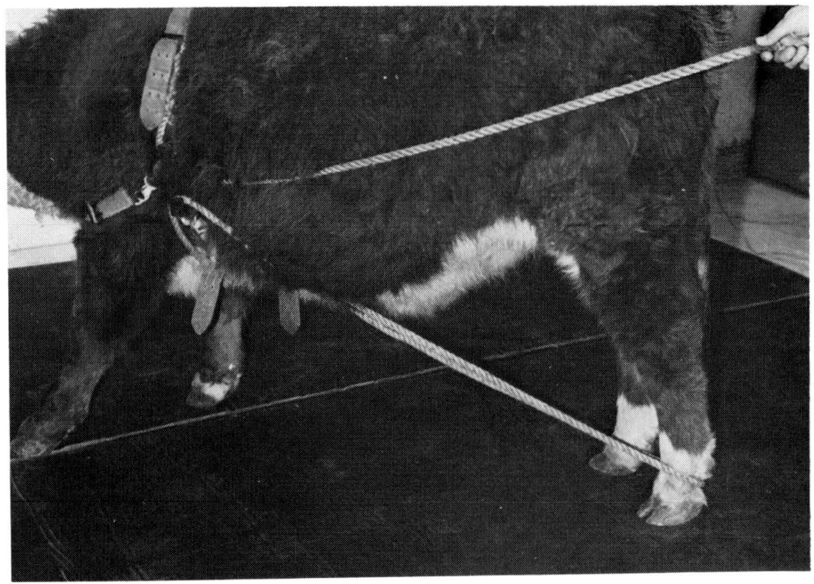

Figure 85. Casting harness in position, with metal plate B on the animal's right side.

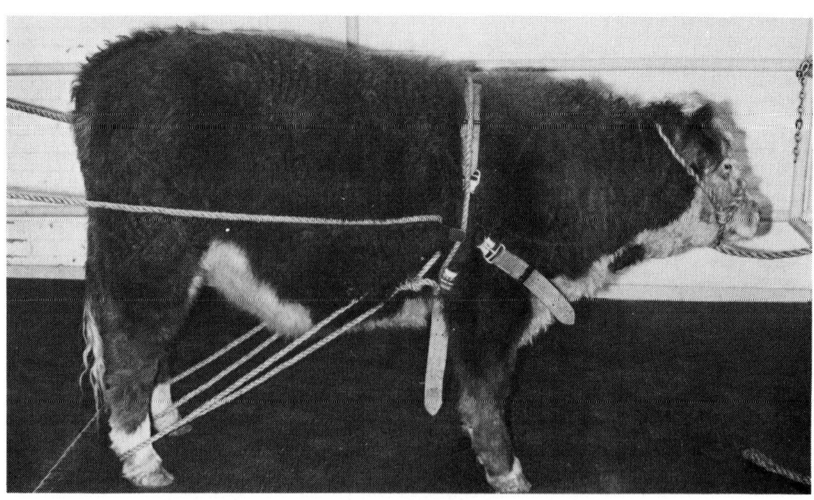

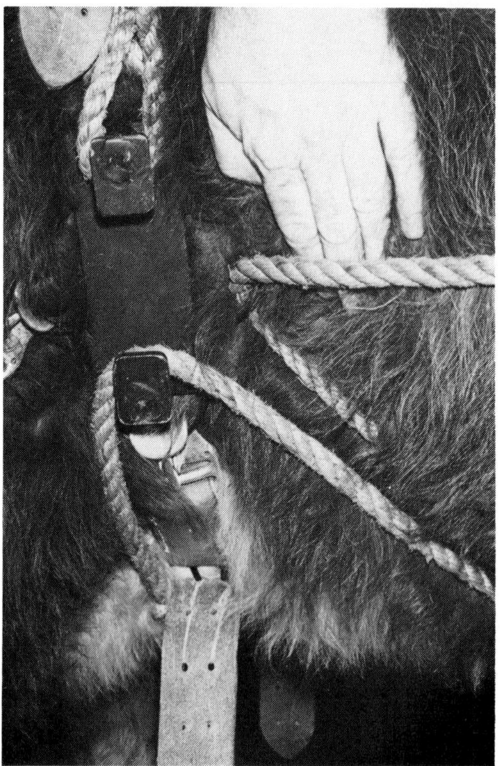

Figure 86. Closeup view of ropes coursing around metal plate A.

after pulling the hind limb close to the plate and securing the rope with a hitch. The animal is then rolled to the opposite side and the rope is tied at plate A as described previously. The forelegs are se-

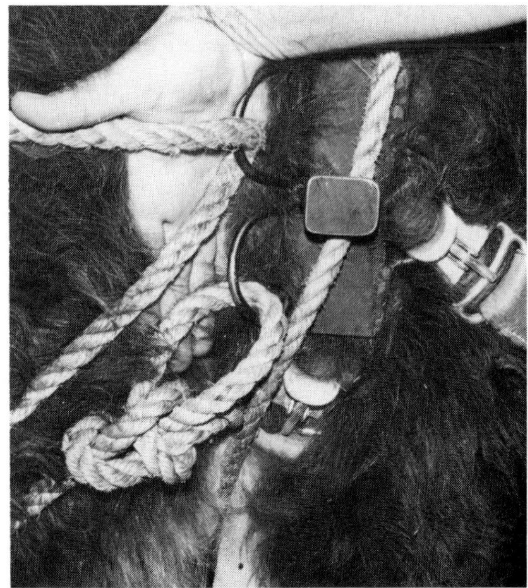

Figure 87. Closeup view of ropes coursing around metal plate B.

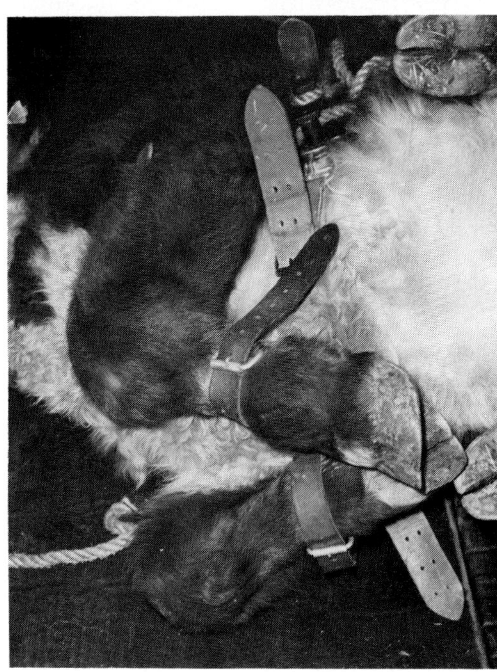

Figure 88. Forelegs restrained with hobbles.

cured to leather hobbles attached to the belly strap after the animal is cast and the hind legs are secured. At this time the animal is completely restrained and can be positioned as the handler desires.

This harness can be used to cast animals of all sizes. In mature cattle a sedative or tranquilizer should be given before applying it. With this harness, cattle can be cast on either the left or right side or placed on their back. After the animal is cast and properly tied, the harness keeps the animal in the cast position until it is released.

Restraint of Calves

Small calves can be efficiently restrained by hand by adequately trained handlers. The method is rapid and effective for such procedures as branding, vaccinating and castrating. In "flanking" a calf to lateral recumbency, the handler grasps the animal and stands at its side while facing the calf, reaches over its back, and holds the loose skin at the flank with one hand and places the other one under the forelimb (Figs 89-91). With a knee pressed against the calf's side, the calf is lifted off its feet so it falls to the ground in lateral recumbency. The proximal foreleg is held in complete flexion and the operator's knee is placed across the calf's neck to keep it restrained. If another assistant is available, this person can aid in restraining the calf by sitting on the ground behind the animal and holding the proximal hind leg and extending the distal hind leg forward by placing a foot on the Achilles tendon proximal to the hock and applying enough pressure to prevent kicking (Fig 92).

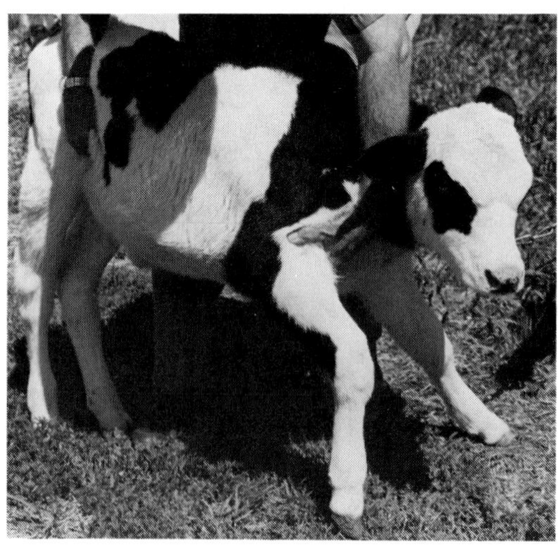

Figure 89. To "flank" a calf to lateral recumbency, the foreleg and skin of the flank are grasped.

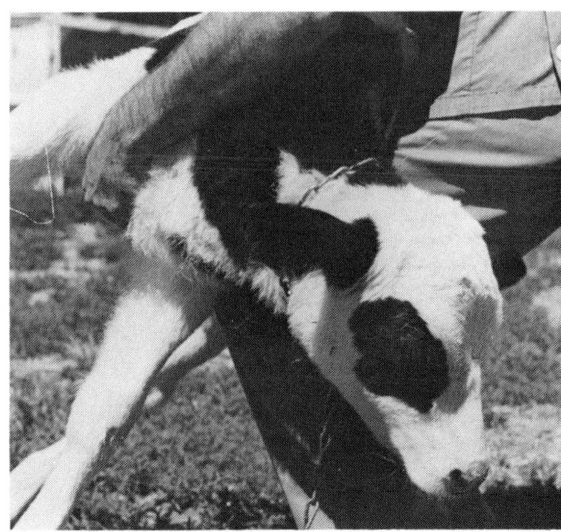

Figure 90. The operator's knees are used to raise the animal as it is flopped onto its side.

Figure 91. The operator's knee is placed on the calf's neck as the foreleg is held.

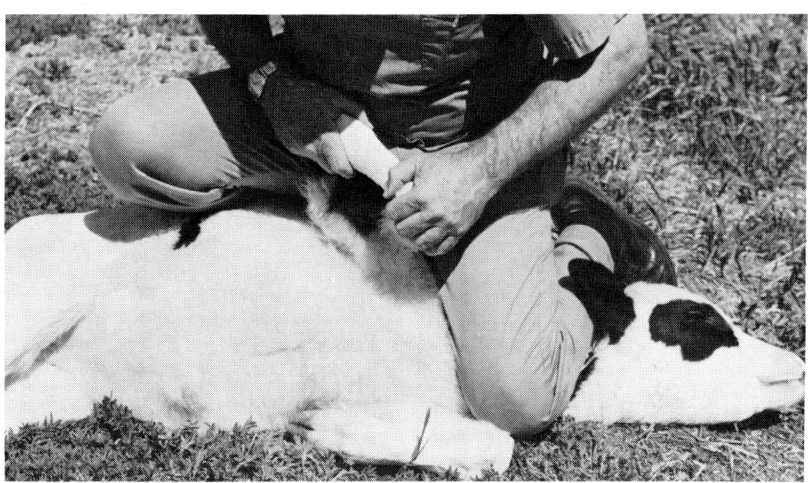

Another method of casting a calf is to grasp its flank and foreleg nearest the handler. By a rapid, coordinated movement, the calf is lifted so it falls on the opposite side. The operator then steps across the calf, placing his knee over the calf's neck, and maintains the upper forelimb in a flexed position (Figs 93-96).

In a third method of laying a calf on its side, the halter shank is passed around the hind limb from inside out, proximal to the hock. The end of the shank is then passed around the standing part of the rope and the hind limb is pulled craniad. This pulls the head to the same side, causing the calf to lose its balance (Figs 97, 98). After a calf is cast, it can be "hog tied" by placing a loop of rope around a forelimb proximal to the fetlock and pulling the hind limbs craniad to the forelimb. One or 2 loops are then passed

Figure 92. A second assistant grasps a rear leg to stretch the calf out for treatment.

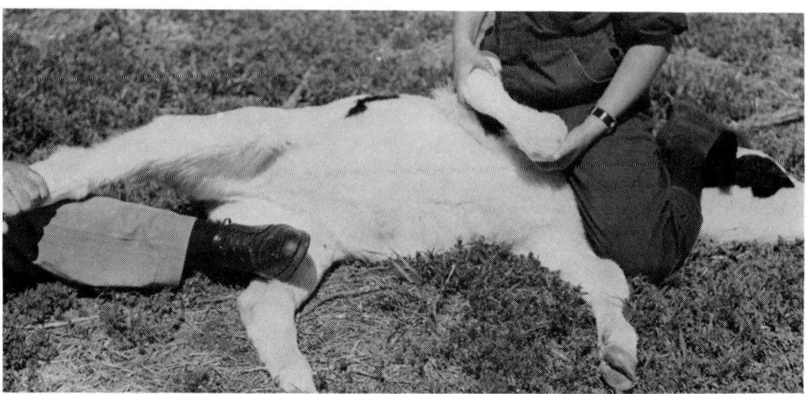

Figures 93, 94. Position to "flank" a calf from the near side is similar to that for flanking on the far side. The operator steps forward as the calf is lifted.

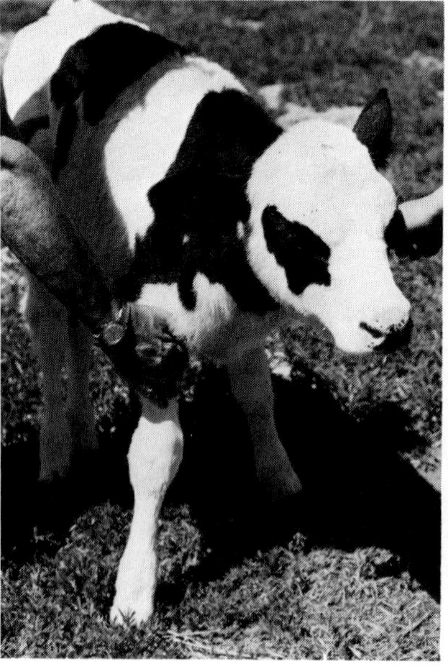

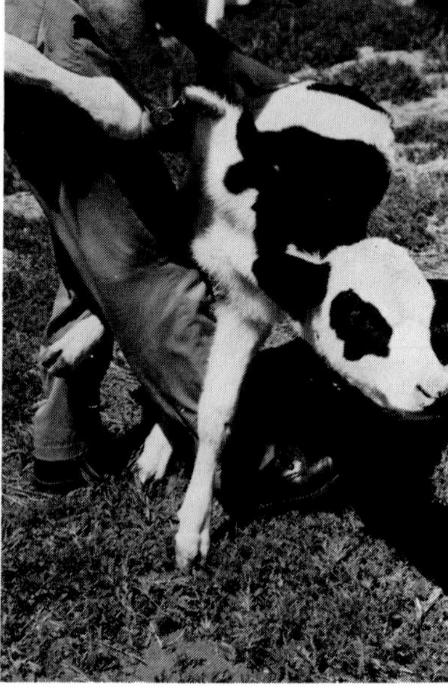

around the forelimb and both hind limbs to proximal to the fetlocks, followed by 1 or 2 half-hitches (Figs 99-101). "Hog tying" adult animals may cause injuries.

Restraint of Sheep

K. Faler and K. Faler

Sheep do not bite, strike or kick. Their only method of defense is running away or butting. Handlers must be steady, calm and patient, as excited sheep may exhaust themselves running, suffer from hyperthermia (especially if they are heavily wooled and it is a hot day), or injure themselves. They have strong social instincts (form a flock); a single sheep in a pen is harder to catch than if left with several others. Sheep become tame with gentle handling, and feeding grain from a bucket. They develop consistent daily patterns of feeding and confinement.

Catching and Moving Sheep

Drive a group of sheep into a pen, narrow alleyway or chute before attempting to single one out. Most domestic sheep will not

Fig 95. The operator's left leg is thrown over the calf as it falls and the foreleg is held.

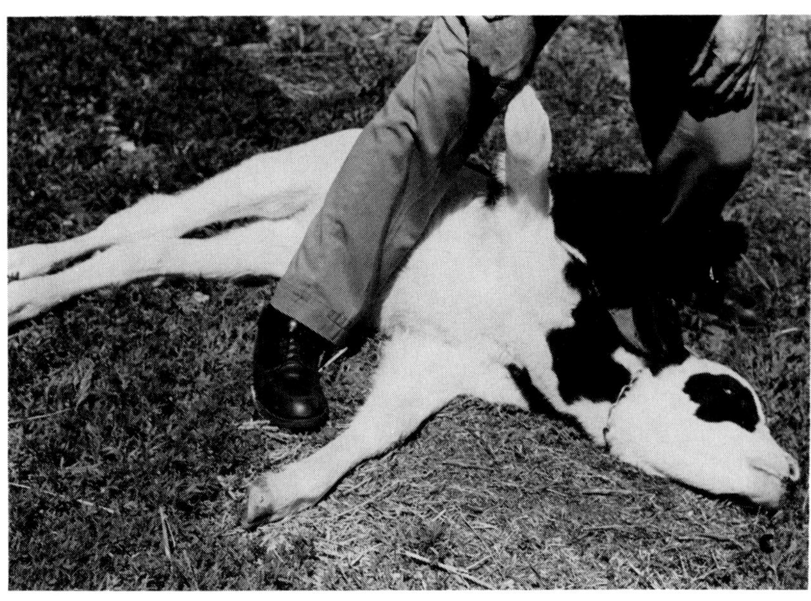

Figure 96. The knee is placed on the calf's neck while the foreleg is held.

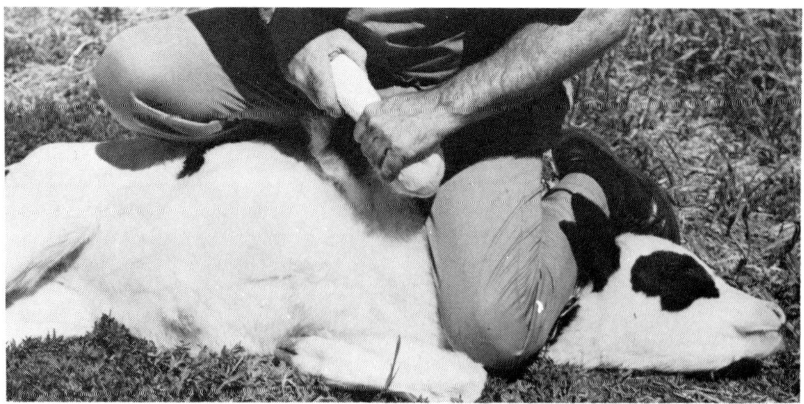

Figure 97. A halter shank is looped around the hind limb to pull it forward.

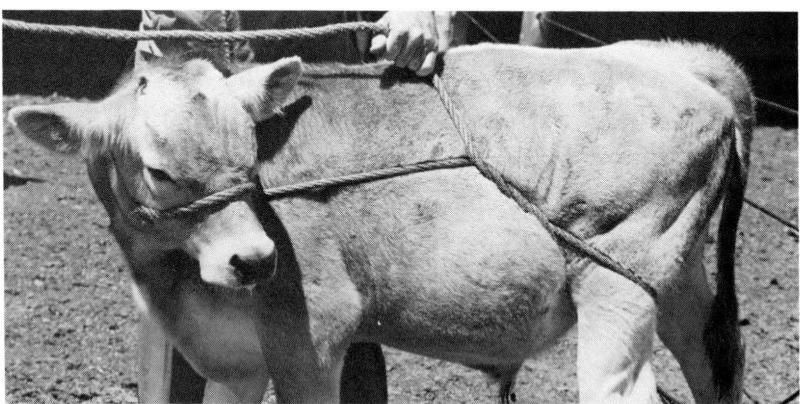

Figure 98. Tightening the rope pulls the head toward the rear, causing the calf to fall.

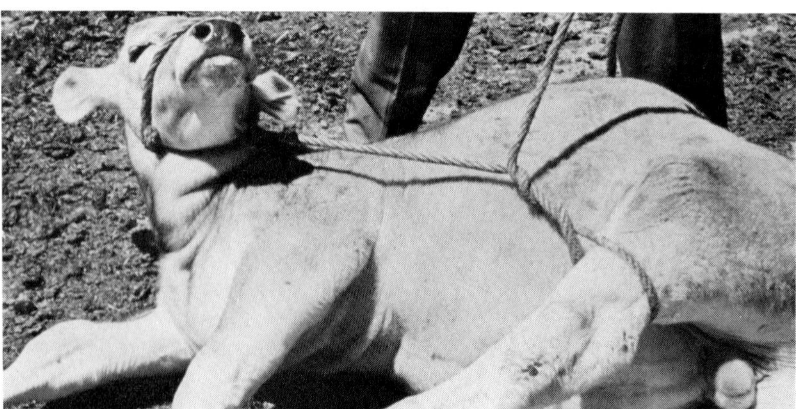

jump a barrier over 1.2 m (4 ft) high. Once the sheep are in the pen, an individual can be singled out by guiding it into a corner with a wooden or wire panel, or by calmly entering the group and catching the selected one as it flees past, with an arm under the chin or around the breast or horns (Fig 102). A shepherd's crook can be used to pull an individual from a group by snaring it proximal to the hock. Never grab a sheep by its wool or skin, as the wool may

Figures 99-101. Hog tying. First, a loop is made proximal to the front fetlock. The front leg is then brought back to the rear legs and all are secured with loops around them. A half-hitch secures the hog-tied calf.

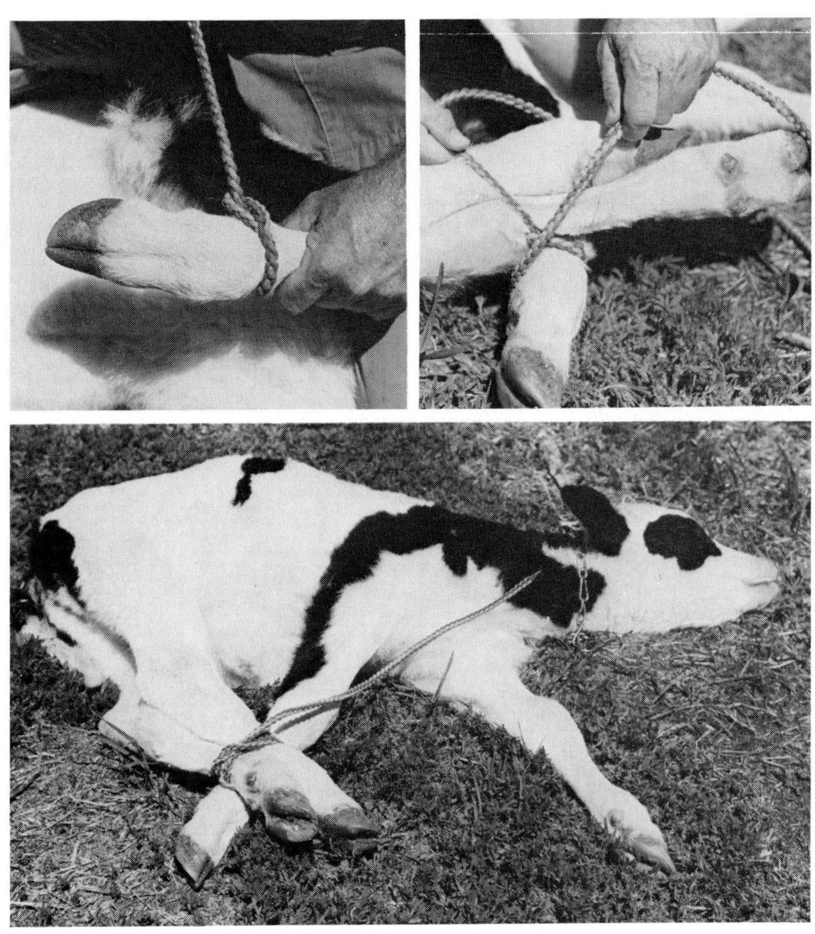

pull out, the skin may tear, or the underlying tissue may be bruised.

Sheep may be led by grasping under the chin and around the tail and guiding the animal in the desired direction. Sheep can be taught to lead, using a halter or collar.

Restraint of Adult Sheep

Two basic methods of restraint are used for adult sheep. The animal can be straddled at the shoulder, between the handler's legs, and the chin restrained in one hand for medication with a balling gun or drench (Fig 103). The mouth can be opened by pressing a thumb in the interdental space (caudal to the incisors, where the bit would rest in a horse's mouth). To limit motion, back the sheep into a corner before straddling it.

For examination of the oral cavity, udder, prepuce and testes or to trim the hooves, the sheep is set up on its rump, with all 4 feet in the air, by unbalancing it and rolling it over the handler's knee. It is not lifted off the ground. The object is to unbalance the animal, rather than to "muscle" it into position. To "set up" the sheep, stand at the animal's side, grasping the web of the flank in one hand and the muzzle with the other (Fig 104). Bend the sheep's head backward, beside the neck, while pulling up and toward yourself with the flank. A bent knee can be used as a lever to help roll heavy sheep over (Fig 105). The most important thing is to bend the head back as far as you can, rather than lifting it up and over the back. Improper technique results in the struggling sheep pivoting around the handler. Rather than bending its neck, a small sheep

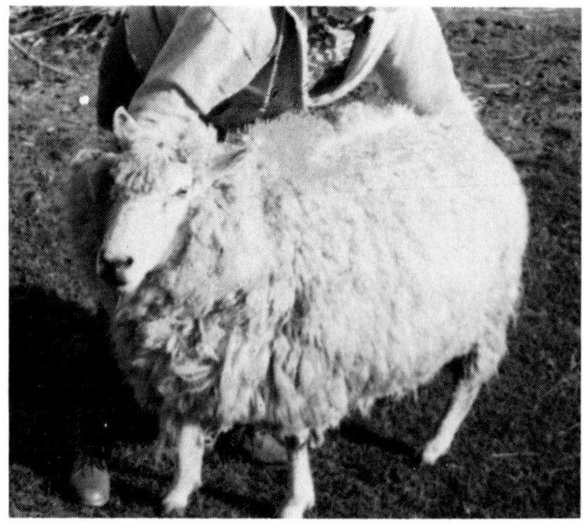

Figure 102. Sheep can be restrained with one arm placed under the chin and the other behind the animal's rump.

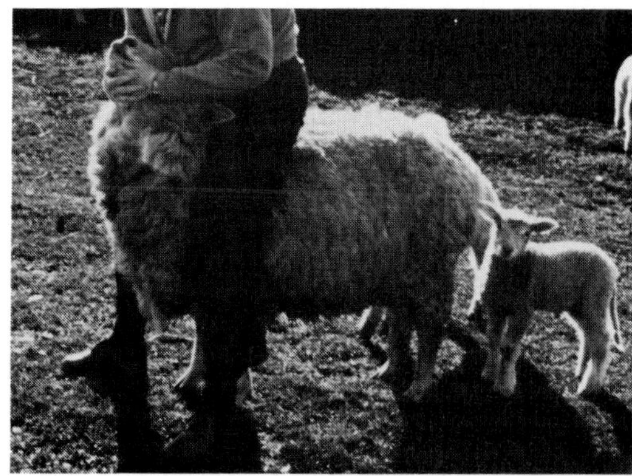

Figure 103. Sheep restrained for administration of oral medication.

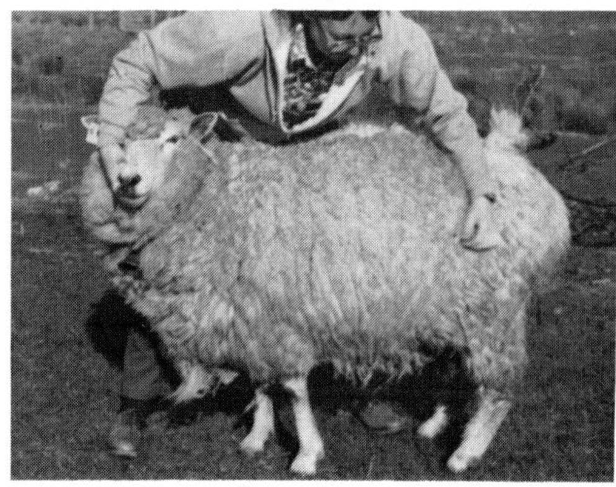

Figure 104. In the first step in setting up a sheep, the animal is pulled toward the operator by its muzzle and flank.

can be set up by reaching over the back and under the animal's chest to grasp the front leg nearer the handler. The leg is used as a handle (holding it above the knee) to rotate the sheep up onto its rump.

Once the sheep is set up, it is held between the handler's slightly spread knees (sheep's withers) and feet (sheep's rump) and slumped to one side. The front legs are held to stabilize the position and prevent flailing. The sheep's head may be tucked under one of the handler's arms for jugular venipuncture (Fig 106). Most sheep are extremely docile and quiet once they are "set up."

Tying 3 feet together with a thong or string after the sheep is set up allows immobilization in recumbency for most short procedures.

Head-locking systems, ranging from a pole set in the ground with a strap around the top to tabletop stanchions, are useful when help is limited.

Restraint of Lambs

Lambs are carried cradled next to the handler's chest, with one arm around the animal's breast and another around its tail (Fig 107). Lambs are presented for tail docking and/or castration by placing them on their back and grasping one front leg and one rear leg in each hand (Fig 108). This can be done over the handler's extended knee or while sitting.

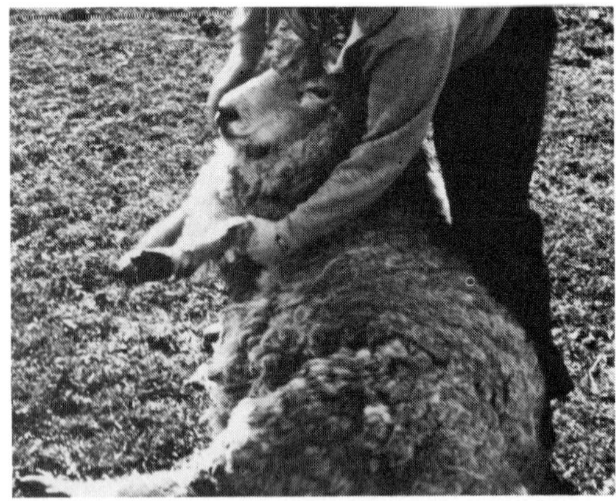

Figure 105. The sheep is rolled onto its side and set up, using the knee as a lever.

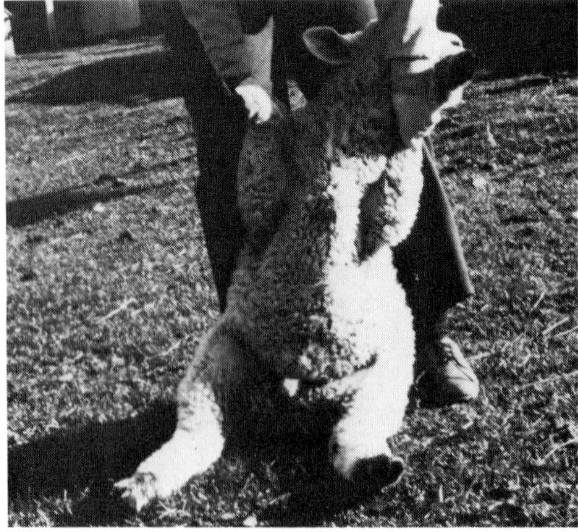

Figure 106. The sheep's head can be tucked under an arm for jugular venipuncture.

Restraint of Swine

K. Faler and K. Faler

The main danger of swine is their bite. Even baby pigs have sharp, pointed teeth that can inflict damage. Adult boars have tusks formed from elongated canine teeth. Because of their poor vision, pigs try to force their way through any small opening, even if

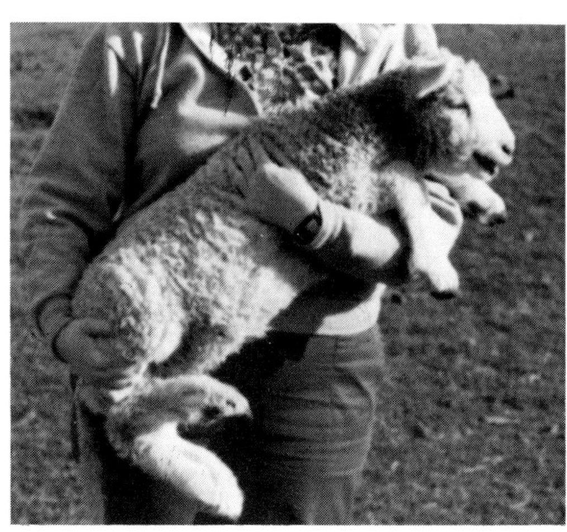

Figure 107. A lamb is supported by an arm under the rump and another under the chest.

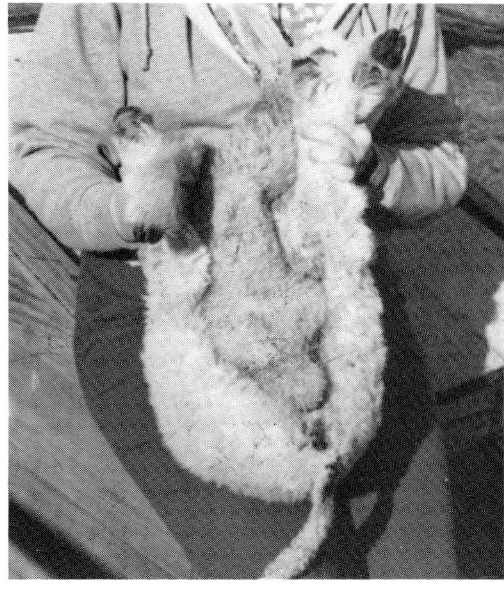

Figure 108. Lamb properly restrained for castration or tail docking.

it is between the handler's legs. Some tame pigs can be handled with a minimum of restraint, soft talk and gentle scratching of the skin. However, swine can move swiftly and the animal's head should always be watched, as they can turn and bite suddenly.

Individual behavior varies, but swine generally are unpredictable. It is best not to enter a pen without a readily accessible escape route. Sows with baby pigs and boars are especially aggressive. The streamlined body and tightly adhered skin of swine offer no handholds for grasping, except the legs. They are especially slippery when wet.

Swine can become stressed or hyperthermic (especially on a hot day) if chased or excited or if they struggle excessively when restrained. A calm, purposeful approach should be used during capture and the rectal temperature monitored on a restrained animal for signs of hyperthermia.

A hog that is rushing toward a handler may be discouraged by slapping it on the nose with a board or cane (pain can, however, cause further aggression); do not use a hand or foot, as the pig may bite it.

Most pigs squeal loudly in protest when they are restrained, even when they are not in discomfort. Squealing may excite other pigs, especially sows, but there is no physical way to stop it.

Never mix pigs of various sizes or add anesthetized or bleeding pigs to pens with normal animals, as they may be attacked by their penmates.

Moving Pigs

Pigs are very stubborn and cannot be led, as they usually move in the direction opposite from that desired by the handler. Swine should be handled in small pens or chutes. Trained pigs can be

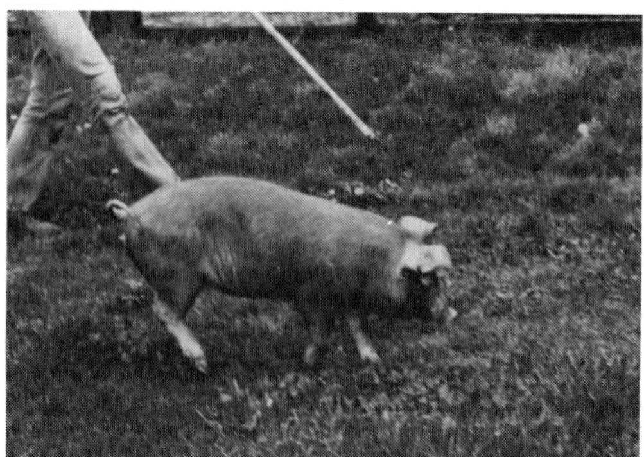

Figure 109. Pig being driven with a cane.

moved by using a wooden cane to tap them on the side of the head, turning them away from the cane (Fig 109).

A wood or wire panel is a good way to guide pigs or to pin them in a corner for closer examination. Keep the shield close to the floor or ground and tilt the bottom toward the pig so it cannot get its snout under the bottom and toss the barrier aside (Fig 110).

A pig will back away from a bucket or blindfold placed over its head. This behavior can be used to guide the pig backward in the desired direction. One hand or a second person pulling on the tail is an additional help while backing the animal (Fig 111).

Stationary Restraint

Small to medium-sized pigs (under 100 lb) are often restrained by holding them up by their front or rear legs by the standing han-

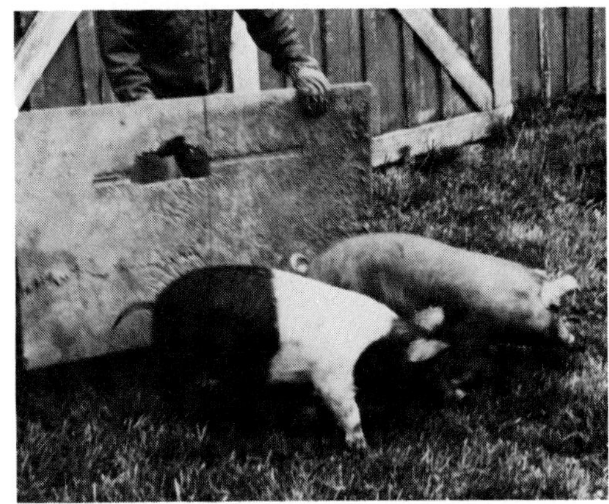

Figure 110. Wooden panel being used to drive swine.

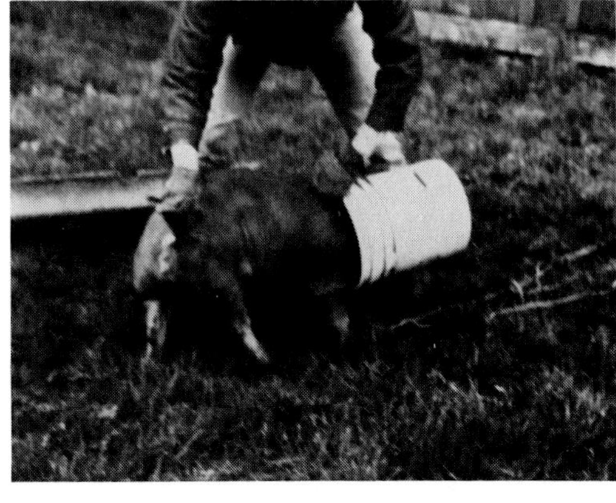

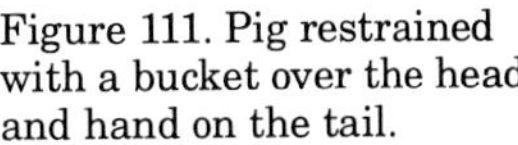

Figure 111. Pig restrained with a bucket over the head and hand on the tail.

dler. For additional control, the pig's back or head can be held between the handler's knees, depending on the amount of struggling (Fig 112). The pig can be held facing either direction, but keep in mind that it may be able to bite. If the pig is held so that its feet touch the ground, it will struggle less and it is not so tiring for the handler, as the pig's legs support some of its weight. The rear legs should be held proximal to the hocks and care taken not to twist the pig's legs.

Swine cannot be held by a single rope around their neck, as their response to such restraint is to back up and evade the noose. However, a loop over the head or snout can be combined with a half-hitch behind the front legs to form a harness that can be used to tie up or hold a pig (Fig 113). The first loop is applied over the neck without tightening it (or the pig will back up). The half-hitch is threaded around the pig or it is preformed and the pig encouraged to step through it. The handler should stand behind and to the side of the pig to cause it to move forward.

The snout rope or snare is used for pigs as the halter is for horses. It consists of a loop of 1/8- to 1/2-inch rope or cable placed caudal to the canine teeth and around the maxilla (snout). The pig automatically pulls back as the rope tightens and can be held or tied up for examination or treatment (Fig 114). Once the noose is tightened around the snout, constant tension must be maintained on the rope to prevent it from slipping out from behind the canine

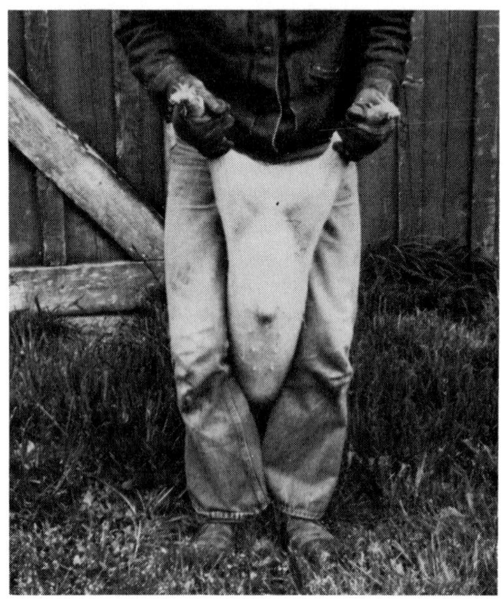

Figure 112. Pig held upside down and between the operator's knees.

teeth. The handler stands directly in front of the pig. This technique does not usually work for baby pigs. Snout ropes should not be left on for longer than 15 minutes, as they act as a tourniquet, cutting off the blood supply to the snout. Watch carefully that the animal does not chew through the rope while it is being restrained or that the rope does not slacken.

To place a rope around the snout, form a loop (through a honda or permanent eye on the end of the rope) and hold it in both hands. Approach from the side and rear of a quiet or confined animal. In many cases, the pig will open its mouth to chew on the rope, which is then tightened over the snout. However, pigs that have previously been restrained by this method may need to have the snare forced into the mouth by holding each side of the loop and "sawing" it back and forth while pulling toward the tail. If the pig moves during this process, the handler must move with it.

"Hog tongs," a large, blunted, pincer-like instrument, can be applied behind the ears to temporarily immobilize the head and snare the snout of a resisting pig by causing it to squeal and open its mouth. The tongs are removed once the snare is in place. Tongs

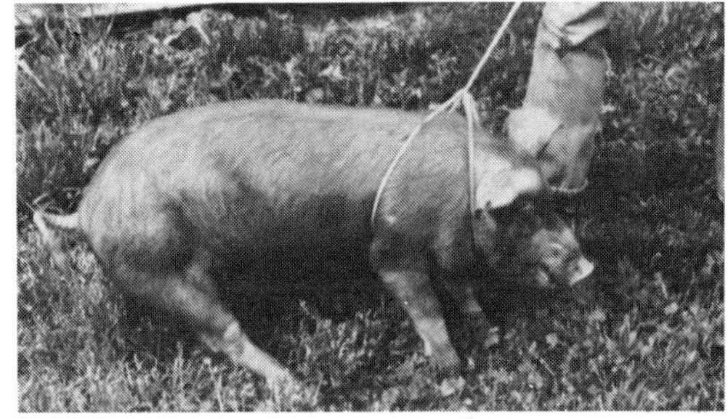

Figure 113. A half-hitch is combined with a loop around the pig's neck to form a harness.

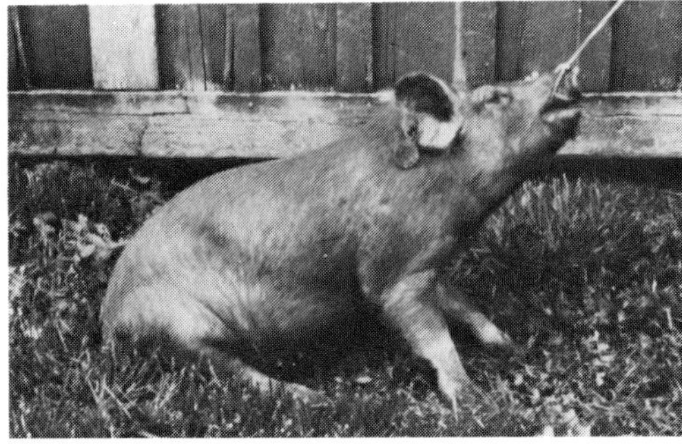

Figure 114. Pigs reflexively back up when a rope is thrown over their snout.

cannot be used effectively on pigs over 100 lb because of their thick neck.

A variety of snares with handles is available to make catching pigs easier and to lessen the danger by allowing distance between the handler and the pig. These snares consist of a loop, with the tail of the rope threaded through a tube. Once the loop is around the snout, it is tightened against the end of the tube (some types have a locking mechanism).

Casting Swine

A small pig may be laid on its side by reaching under its abdomen and pulling the legs farther from the handler out from under the animal. This can also be done with ropes around one rear and one front leg; the free ends are passed across the abdomen and over the back (Fig 115). The legs should be tied together once the pig is on its side.

A pig restrained with a snout snare may be stretched out by tying another rope proximal to both the hocks and pulling the rear feet back, fixing the pig between the 2 ropes on its side or back. A "bar hobble" or "hog shackle" works well for this and spreads the rear legs for castration or other procedures. It consists of 2 loops of chain on each end of a bar. Each loop is placed proximal to a hock and tightened with a common rope. Most pigs do not object to having their feet lifted to apply the chains.

A common method of casting pigs is to take the snout rope back along the animal's side, keeping constant tension on it, and make a half-hitch proximal to a hock. Pulling on the end of the rope causes the pig to lie down on its side, with the half-hitch up (Fig 116). This is a good position for castration.

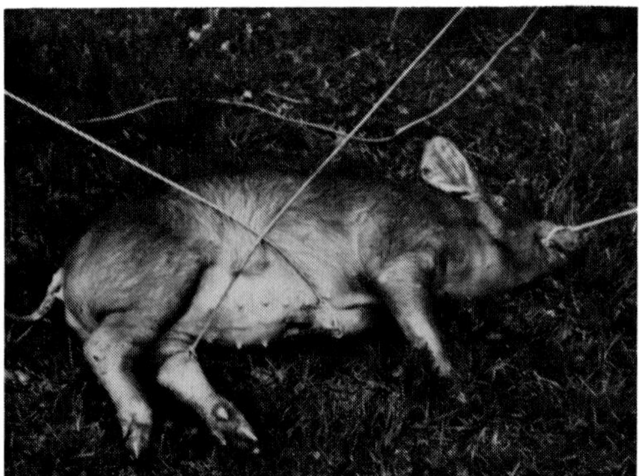

Figure 115. Pig restrained in lateral recumbency with a rope on the snout and ropes on the front and rear legs next to the ground.

For further restraint once the pig is cast, the legs may be trussed together or a person may kneel on the pig's neck and back.

Various types of troughs or cradles are used to hold small pigs on their back for surgery, examination and venipuncture (Fig 117). A bar or rope over the snout is used to hold the head down and the legs are tied or strapped down. Squeeze chutes or cages are used for bigger swine.

Restraint of Baby Pigs

Baby pigs should be captured with a minimum of chasing. They should be seized from behind by gripping them over the shoulder or by one or both rear legs. They are lifted up by both hind legs or scooped up with a hand under the animal's chest and over its back. Never lift them by a tail or ear only. They can be restrained between the knees of a sitting handler (Fig 118). Always restrain the sow before handling its babies because their squeals can make the sow very aggressive. Holding baby pigs with their head down may quiet them.

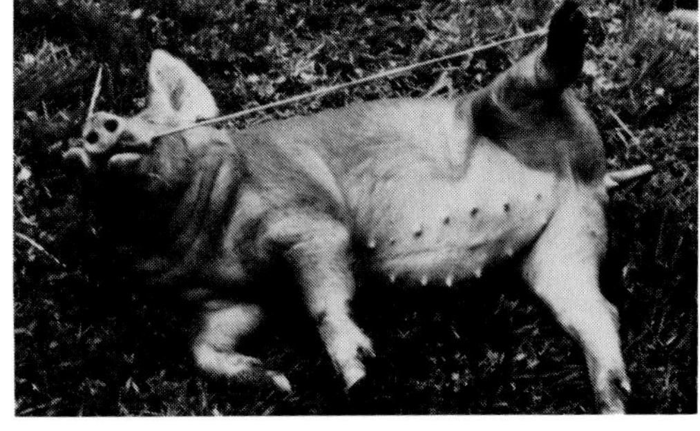

Figure 116. A heavy pig restrained for castration with a snout rope led back to a half-hitch around the rear leg.

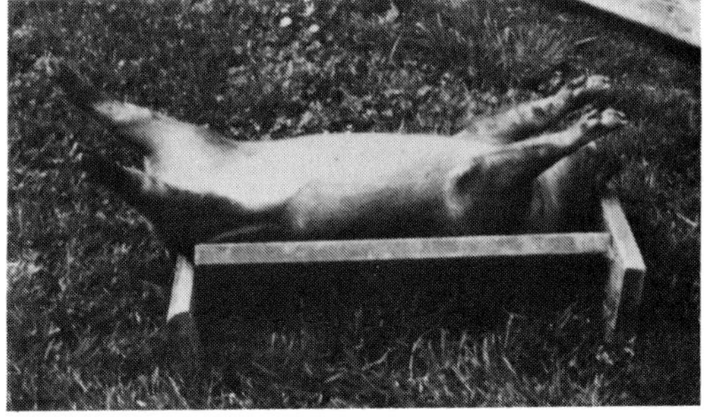

Figure 117. Pig restrained in dorsal recumbency in a trough.

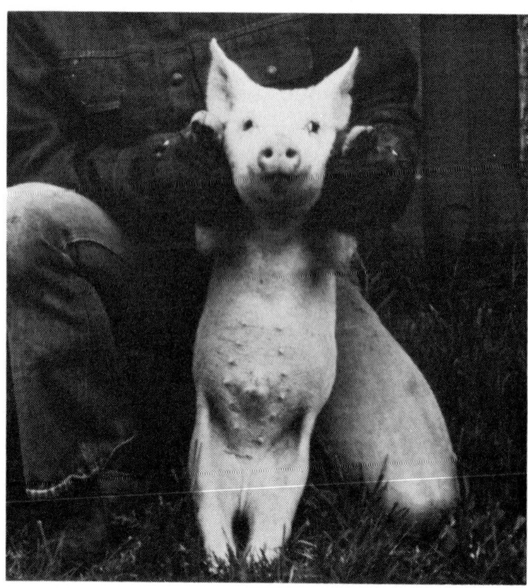

Figure 118. Baby pig restrained between the operator's knees.

Recommended Reading

Fowler: *Restraint and Handling of Wild and Domestic Animals.* Iowa State Univ Press, Ames, 1978.

Leahy and Burrow: *Restraint of Animals.* Cornell Campus Stores, Ithaca, NY, 1953.

Sonsthagen: *Restraint of Domestic Animals.* American Veterinary Publications, Goleta, CA, 1992.

Notes

3

Supportive Care

K. Faler and K. Faler

FLUID THERAPY

The body of animals contain 55-67% water by weight. The water is held within cells, between cells and in body cavities, and circulates in the blood, lymph and cerebrospinal fluid. Water is a solvent for chemicals, enters into chemical reactions, is involved in temperature regulation, acts as a lubricant and is a transport medium for nutrients and waste products. When more water is lost from the body than is taken in, the animal becomes dehydrated and many necessary functions are interrupted. If enough water is lost, the animal dies. Therefore, replacing lost fluid, maintaining hydration and monitoring fluid balance are all important aspects of health care.

Determining Degree of Dehydration

There are several methods to estimate how much fluid an animal has lost, and often more than one is used in the final assessment.

History

When the patient's history is taken, the frequency of urination, vomiting and/or diarrhea should be noted and the amount estimated. Ambient temperature, fever, stress, severe sneezing or coughing, neglect of stall-fed livestock or drought conditions can all contribute to dehydration and should be noted on the medical record. Frozen or contaminated water supply, spilled dishes, obstructed sipper bottle tips and too many animals drinking from a single water supply can also be contributing factors. Very weak or physically compromised animals may not be able to reach water easily. Several sources of water should be available to groups of animals.

Skin Fold Pinch

During physical examination, the percent dehydration can be estimated by the "4-6-8" rule. Loss of 4% of the body water is not evident clinically but is assumed if the animal has not taken in food or water for 24-60 hours, or if there has been water loss by any means (vomiting, diarrhea, excessive urination, blood loss, serum leakage from burns, etc). A 6% loss (moderate) is indicated when a pinched fold of skin slowly returns to its normal position, rather than quickly springing back. In addition, the eyes may be dull because of dryness and the animal may be depressed. At 8% dehydration (severe), the animal's skin stays in a tented position when pinched and feels coarse and leathery. The eyes are sunken into their sockets and the animal only sluggishly responds to any stimulus. When an animal is 12-15% dehydrated, death is imminent. The animal may be in shock and may twitch from muscle tremors.

Packed Cell Volume

A third way to assess hydration is with the packed cell volume (PCV), also called the hematocrit, and with the total plasma protein level. Fluid loss elevates the PCV and plasma protein level.

Dehydration in large animals and exotics is more difficult to assess than in small animals. Loss of skin elasticity, sunken eyes, a rapid weak pulse, weight loss, dry mucous membranes, cold extremities and low urine volume are all indications of deficient fluid volume. The severity of signs varies with the degree of dehydration. An improvement in the patient's condition with fluid therapy may be the only sign that dehydration was present.

Smaller animals dehydrate more rapidly than large animals because of their greater surface area in proportion to their smaller total fluid volume. Young animals may quickly reach a critical level of dehydration with only mild vomiting or diarrhea when they are not consuming liquids. These animals require fluid therapy.

Hydration

Volume

To hydrate an animal, lost fluids must be replaced, maintenance fluid needs met and any continuing losses offset. If the patient is consuming liquids, the amount can be subtracted from the volume given to hydrate the animal.

The amount of maintenance fluids required each day is estimated by multiplying the animal's body weight by 45 ml/kg (20 ml/lb). Percentage of dehydration is multiplied by the body weight to determine the percentage of body weight reduction because of fluid loss. For example, a 15-kg dog that is 6% dehydrated has lost 0.06 x 15 = 0.9 kg in fluid. Because 1 L (1000 ml) = 1 kg, the loss in body weight can be converted to volume (*eg,* 0.9 x 1000 ml = 900 ml lost). Continuing losses are estimated by observing the volume of vomit, diarrhea, etc. Adding maintenance needs to the amount of dehydration and any continuing fluid losses gives the approximate volume of fluids to be replaced.

If too large a volume of fluid is given IV, it passes out of the blood and into the air spaces in the lungs, "drowning" the animal. This occurs because the small blood vessels in the lungs are thinly separated from the air for effective exchange of O_2 and CO_2. When giving fluids IV, no more than one-quarter of the total volume needed should be infused in the first hour and one-quarter the second hour. The remaining half should be distributed over the rest of the day. Following this guide when giving large volumes of fluids IV prevents additional stress on an already compromised animal.

The amount of fluid given to an animal varies with kidney function, lung status, cardiovascular integrity and other factors. Therefore, the technician should always consult with the veterinarian regarding the volume of fluid to be replaced, during a given time, before starting therapy.

Routes of Administration

Fluids can be introduced into the body in several ways. They can be added directly to the blood stream (intravenous, IV), injected under the skin (subcutaneous, SC), deposited in the abdominal cavity (intraperitoneal, IP), or given by mouth or tube directly into the stomach (oral, per os, PO). Each method has advantages and disadvantages. The type of fluid necessary may influence the route of administration.

Fluid should be administered at room temperature or warmed to body temperature (floating the container in a sink of warm water works well) for severely debilitated or very small animals and for animals with an elevated body temperature.

IV Administration: Adding fluids directly to the blood stream is the quickest way to hydrate the animal. Because the solution is diluted by the blood, many substances that are irritating when given IM or SC can be safely administered by this route. However, fluids that contain potassium (K), calcium (Ca) or glucose should be given slowly, with careful monitoring.

To give fluids IV, a needle or catheter is inserted into a large vein, usually the cephalic or jugular (see Chapter 4), a piece of tubing is connected to it, and the tubing is attached to a bottle or bag of fluids. The tubing allows the fluid container to be held above body level so the solution can flow in by gravity. Alternatively, air can be injected into the fluid container to force the fluid out into the animal's vein. Small amounts of fluids can also be given directly using a needle or butterfly and a syringe. The fluid bottle is attached to the IV unit by puncturing the bottle's rubber stopper with a large needle or prong on the end of the tubing opposite that which is connected to the needle or catheter in the animal's vein. The tubing end nearer the fluid container usually has a clear, bubble-like chamber so drip speed can be visualized. For large animals, the IV unit may simply consist of a rubber tube with a flared end, which is slipped over the neck of the fluid bottle.

An air vent allows pressures to equalize as fluid leaves the bottle. The air vent may be built into the IV unit or created by puncturing the tubing with a needle inserted into the air space near the neck of the fluid container. Fluid flow is regulated by compressing the tubing or bag and by using needles with different diameters (gauge) in the animal's veins. The IV unit should be sterile, as the fluid moving through it is introduced into the blood and any microorganisms or chemical residues present may be harmful. Contaminated lines should be discarded, autoclaved if made from hard plastic or rubber, gas sterilized if made of thin plastic, or cold sterilized with a disinfectant and thoroughly washed with sterile water before reuse.

Most IV drip lines deliver 15 large drops/ml, but microdrip units deliver 60 small drops/ml and are used for long-term, slow infusion. IV pumps are also available to deliver a precise amount of fluid over a given time, such as 1 ml/minute. Some have an alarm to indicate when the fluid is not flowing and adjust to a lower rate to keep the vein open. Other safety features are available, such as shut down when air is present, depending on the model.

The speed of fluid administration varies with the percent dehydration, condition of the animal and the vein used. Giving fluids rapidly stresses the cardiovascular system but may be necessary in an emergency if hypovolemic shock occurs. Because of the great fluid capacity of large animals, solutions are often administered as fast as they can flow; in emergencies, a pump (pressure cuff around the container) or more than one line may be used. The optimal rate of fluid administration in drops/minute can be estimated, based on the volume to be administered in an hour and the delivery rate of the line (*eg,* 15 drops/ml x 250 ml fluid = 3750 drops ÷ 60 minutes/hour = 60-65 drops/minute or about 1 drop/second). It is best to consult with the veterinarian regarding the speed of fluid administration for each patient, then take care not to exceed it.

Check the patient frequently while IV fluids are being administered. Lung sounds should be normal (no wheezing or "wet" fluid sounds) and the pulse regular. If the catheter or needle has been dislodged from the vein, fluid flow into the patient stops or a SC swelling forms around the vein because of fluid accumulating outside the vessel. If either of these situations occurs, rethread the needle in the vein or replace the catheter. Before rethreading the needle, run a small amount of fluid through it to make sure it is free of blood clots. Do not try to unplug a needle or catheter while it is in the vein or the clot will enter the circulation and may occlude a small vessel (such as the coronary artery, which may cause a heart attack).

The drip may also stop if the air vent is obstructed, the line is kinked, the vein is blocked (*eg,* by flexing the limb or with a pressure bandage), or if the bottle is not held above the level of the vein.

Shut off the fluid flow before the bottle is completely empty to prevent air from entering the blood stream. Air emboli (circulating bubbles) are thought to be an infrequent cause of death, but they should be avoided. If air enters the line, close the tubing below the bubble and inject enough additional fluid into the line with a syringe to push the air back into the bottle, withdraw the air bubble with a syringe, or detach the line from the vein and run fluid through the tubing to push the air out.

After the fluid flow is stopped, the bottle can be changed or the therapy ended. A cap can be applied to the end of the catheter and taped in place for later use. If the catheter is not removed, a small amount of heparin (about 0.1 ml of 1000 units/ml) is injected through the catheter to prevent blood from clotting in the tube. The IV line can be reused only if sterile fluids have contacted the inside surface.

SC Administration: In dogs and cats, the skin is loosely attached to the underlying tissue, creating a large potential space for fluid to be deposited. It is then slowly absorbed as the body needs it. Horses and cattle generally have skin too tightly attached for SC fluid therapy, though this route is sometimes used for small volumes of fluid.

Fluid for SC injection should be similar to plasma in composition of dissolved particles (isotonic); 10-200 ml can be deposited in one area, depending on the size of the patient. More than one site can be used in an individual at the same time. In small animals, the back, from shoulders to tail, is used, but in swine the flank area (where the rear legs join the body at the abdomen) is the best site to use. The fluid is delivered from a syringe or IV line (see Chapter 4). In birds, fluid may be given in the skin folds of the wings.

The more dehydrated the animal is, the faster fluid is absorbed. Periodically checking the fluid deposit under the skin indicates how often to repeat the therapy. Pinching the needle hole in the skin after the needle has been withdrawn helps prevent leakage from the site. Fluids given SC take less time to administer than those given IV, but the return to normal hydration is slower. Also, SC administration is less likely to overhydrate a patient from IV infusion and is better tolerated in most patients.

IP Administration: The space around the abdominal organs (peritoneal cavity) offers a potential depot for fluids. They are absorbed more rapidly from this space than if given SC, but not as quickly as the IV route. Large volumes can be given, 100 ml to several liters, depending on the size of the animal, but the fluids should be of a plasma-like composition (isotonic). The method has a potential hazard of puncturing an organ but is still relatively safe (see Chapter 4). It is used in both small and large animal medicine for fluid therapy.

Because the peritoneum (membrane lining the abdominal cavity) has a good blood supply and is semipermeable, fluids deposited in the abdominal cavity equilibrate with the blood stream. Thus, the blood can be gradually cleared of many toxins by adding fluids to the abdominal cavity, letting diffusion take place and removing the fluid and accumulated material. The technique is called *peritoneal dialysis* and is used in treating kidney failure and poisoning. Using a needle or dialysis catheter, 200 ml to 2 L of fluid are injected into the abdomen and withdrawn after about an hour. In severe cases, dialysis is repeated 3-5 times a day. The volume of fluid collected after each treatment should be recorded and the entire procedure done as aseptically as possible because peritonitis (inflammation of the peritoneum) is a constant danger.

Oral Administration: Giving fluids by stomach tube, forced feeding or pharyngostomy tube (see Chapter 4) is the ideal way to hydrate an animal (Fig 1). Fluid volume and composition are of lesser importance than for other routes, as the animal's body selectively absorbs what is needed. The method is less traumatic to tissues and more natural than other techniques. In addition, it is the most practical way to administer adequate nutrients to an anorectic animal. Oral fluids need not be sterile and can be mixed in the veterinary clinic, and so are less expensive than purchased fluids.

The oral route is not used when vomiting, diarrhea, enteritis (intestinal inflammation) or GI obstruction is present, so as to avoid additional stress to the digestive system.

Intramedullary Administration: Whole blood and other fluids can be given rapidly in small animals through a large-bore needle

Figure 1. Tube feeding an orphan kitten. 1. The formula is placed in a large syringe attached to a plastic urinary catheter or rubber feeding tube. 2. The feeding tube is held next to the kitten to measure the distance from the tip of the nose to the last rib to determine how far the feeding tube must be inserted. 3. The syringe plunger is depressed to fill the tube with formula and expel the air before the tube is inserted into the kitten's mouth. With the kitten held firmly, the mouth is pried open with the thumb and forefinger while the tube is inserted with the other hand. 4. The tube is inserted to the predetermined length and an assistant slowly dispenses the formula from the syringe. (Courtesy of TFH Publications)

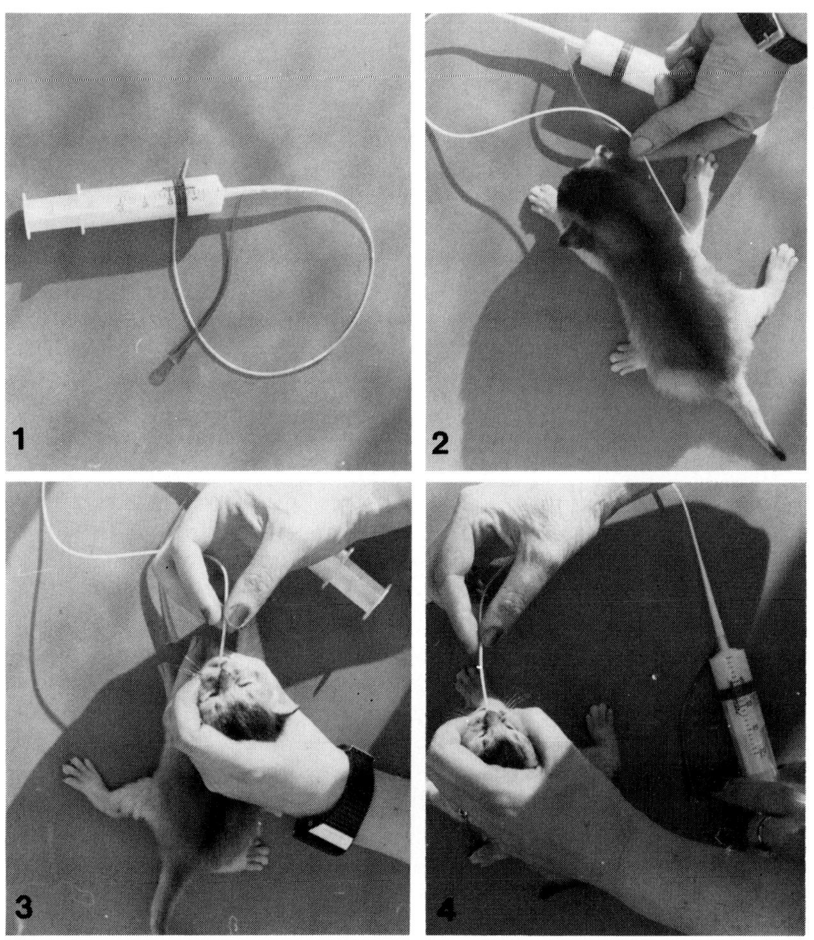

inserted into a long bone. A 20-ga needle in the proximal femur can be used for small kittens, ferrets, etc.

Fluid Types

Fluids for therapy consist of water and solutions of various electrolytes, amino acids, carbohydrates and vitamins. Electrolytes are ionic particles that can conduct electricity when in solution. Ionic particles are atoms charged by losing or gaining electrons. Common ions are K^+ (potassium), Ca^{++} (Calcium), Na^+ (sodium), Mg^{++} (magnesium), Cl^- (chloride) and HCO_3^- (bicarbonate). Electrolytes are necessary for the many chemical reactions in the body's normal function. When fluids are lost, so are electrolytes.

Different diseases cause different ion imbalances, so the fluid type for therapy depends on the animal's condition. For example, vomiting causes loss of HCl (hydrochloric acid) from the stomach. The Cl in HCl is normally recycled by the body during digestion, so Cl lost by vomiting should be replaced by administering a fluid rich in Cl. If a solution low in Cl is given, the patient's condition would worsen rather than improve as a result of the therapy. For this reason, always consult with the veterinarian regarding the type of fluid to give each patient.

In addition to the type of electrolyte present, the overall balance of all electrolytes in a solution is important. If the balance is similar to that of plasma, the fluid is called *isotonic.* If there are more electrolytes than in plasma, it is called *hypertonic* and if less than in plasma it is *hypotonic.*

Body fluids can move through the tissues, so the concentration of electrolytes remains the same throughout the animal (with a few exceptions). If, for example, hypertonic solution is given SC, fluid moves out of the animal's body into the SC space to dilute the solution until it is isotonic and the overall fluid composition of the animal is balanced. The patient is now more dehydrated, except for the SC space, than before therapy. Isotonic fluids can be given by any route, but hypertonic or hypotonic solutions are given IV or PO. Hypertonic or hypotonic fluids should be given IV slowly and with constant monitoring.

Isotonic solutions include whole blood, plasma, 0.9% sodium chloride (physiologic saline), 5% dextrose (glucose) in water, 2.5% dextrose in half-strength lactate, or lactated Ringer's solution (a balanced electrolyte solution, with lactate for energy). A plasma substitute (Dextran) is also isotonic and contains large molecules to help hold fluids in the blood stream.

Hypertonic solutions include 50% dextrose, 3% sodium chloride (table salt or saline), 10% calcium gluconate or 5% amino acid solution. Lactated Ringer's with 2% glucose, Peridial 1.5% or Inpersol 1.5% are hypertonic solutions used for peritoneal dialysis.

Hypotonic solutions are plain water or 2.5% dextrose.

Storage and Handling of Fluids

Fluids should be stored at room temperature and protected from excessive heat or cold. Expiration dates should be observed and supplies rotated to prevent outdating of solutions. Inspect the seals on any new container before using it to make sure it is sterile. Discard any solution that appears cloudy or contains a precipitate (visible solid material).

Determining the amount, route, rate and type of fluid therapy should be left to the veterinarian, as it requires a detailed knowledge of medicine and the patient's condition. However, giving fluids and monitoring hydration are valuable services the technician can contribute to patient care.

Fluid therapy has saved the lives of many patients, but it is a supportive or symptomatic treatment. The underlying cause of the fluid loss must be corrected and the animal must maintain its own fluid balance before the prognosis (predicted outcome of the case) becomes more favorable.

OXYGEN THERAPY

Oxygen (O_2) therapy is indicated when respiration is impaired. Oxygen deprivation (hypoxia) requires immediate attention, as it may be rapidly fatal. Administration of O_2 is a temporary measure until the condition that caused the poor oxygenation can be corrected. Typical uses of O_2 include supporting the newborn animal that is weak from a difficult or prolonged delivery (dystocia), aiding the patient with a blocked trachea (windpipe), or assisting a patient in respiratory distress caused by heatstroke, etc. If the hypoxia is caused by airway obstruction, removal of the blockage may be adequate to restore normal breathing without O_2 therapy. When hypoxia is caused by decreased numbers or function of circulating RBCs, a transfusion may be necessary before O_2 therapy is effective. Shock, reduced cardiac output, circulatory failure or anesthetic overdoses all cause hypoxia because blood is not adequately circulated to the tissues to deliver O_2.

A significant stimulus for respiration is high blood carbon dioxide (CO_2) levels. When the brain's respiratory center is depressed by drugs, trauma, chronic respiratory disease or anesthetic overdose, the body's sensitivity to CO_2 may be reduced and the animal depends on low blood levels of O_2 to trigger respiration. If O_2 is given to such an animal, the elevation in O_2 lowers the "hypoxic drive," resulting in a depressed respiratory rate and an increased O_2 deficit. For this reason, animals with chronic O_2 deprivation should be watched carefully for respiratory depression when pure O_2 is administered (the patient must breathe for O_2 to enter the lungs).

The nervous system is very sensitive to hypoxia and is the tissue damaged first when blood O_2 levels fall below normal. The interval between O_2 deprivation and tissue damage depends on a number of factors, including the animal's age, condition, activity and temperature. As a rule of thumb, 4 minutes of hypoxia causes irreversible brain damage in a normal animal, but neonates (newborn animals) may tolerate up to 10 minutes without harm. Resuscitative efforts may continue for longer than 10 minutes when O_2 therapy has been given or when the animal is colder than normal (hypothermia caused by immersion in cold water or exposure to cold temperatures).

If O_2 therapy is necessary for more than 2-3 days on a continuous basis, it may be prohibitively expensive.

Equipment for O_2 Therapy

Pure O_2 gas is compressed to 1900-2500 lb/square inch (psi) of pressure (at 70 F) and stored in green metal cylinders. Large tanks (G tanks) hold about 6000-7000 L and small tanks (E tanks) hold 500-600 L. Tanks are usually rented from and filled by commercial suppliers.

The cylinder is fitted with a gauge on the top (threaded onto the tank top) that indicates the amount of pressure in the tank, which is a direct reflection of the volume of O_2 in the tank, as gases expand to fill all space available. Tanks should be changed before they are completely empty to avoid running out of O_2 while treating a patient. Most tanks have a tag with perforations that is marked "Full," "In Use" and "Empty," and sections of the tag are torn off as the tank is used so that its status is clear to everyone. Some clinics have O_2 piped into surgery and treatment areas from tanks in storage areas.

In addition to the gauge, a regulator is attached to the top of the tank. It reduces the pressure of the O_2 leaving the tank to ≤60 psi, as the immense, unregulated pressure in the cylinder would otherwise damage lung tissue. The gauge and regulator are often combined into one device. A handle or wrench on top of the cylinder opens or closes the tank.

Because the tank is under pressure, opening it without a regulator attached (or with a poor one) or puncturing the cylinder may cause it to be propelled like a rocket by escaping gas. This can be very dangerous, depending on the volume of O_2 in the tank. For this reason, tanks should be handled gently, opened gradually and fixed firmly in position by chaining them to a wall when not in use. Tanks in use should be well attached to the anesthetic machine or a solid surface to prevent knocking the regulator off if the cylinder falls.

Oxygen itself is not flammable, but it supports fire (like "fanning the flames"). It should be kept away from cigarettes, open flames and electrical connections, such as electrocautery equipment. It is explosive in combination with other substances, such as cyclopropane, grease and oil. Valves and fittings should not be lubricated with oil or grease if they are used with O_2. Only equipment designed for O_2 use at the pressure delivered should be used.

Administration of O_2

The tank can be hooked up to a variety of devices to deliver O_2 to the patient. A simple tube can be attached and held to the patient's nose, inserted through an incision in the trachea, passed into the pharynx (back of the throat) or run into an oxygen chamber (aquarium, closed cage, etc) (Figs 2, 3). Oxygen can also be delivered through an endotracheal tube (tube in the windpipe) or nose cone. It can also be forced into the lungs using a rebreathing bag, Ambu bag or positive-pressure ventilation system (Fig 4). The rebreathing bag fills with O_2 by flow from the tank. The Ambu bag automatically refills when the pressure applied to it is released. The positive-pressure system uses a machine that takes over or assists respiration (see Chapter 1). In any case, the air is delivered to the lungs by a squeezing action of the O_2-filled chamber.

To administer pure O_2, the delivery system must be sealed so that no air mixes with gas from the cylinder. The flow of O_2 from the tank is regulated by a flow meter (often attached to the anesthetic machine), which delivers gas at 5 ml to 15 L/minute at room temperature under normal atmospheric conditions. The flow meter serves as another regulator to reduce the pressure of the gas leaving the tank, preventing damage to the lungs.

The correct level of O_2 flow for the patient is determined by the minute volume of the animal's breathing and gas leakage of the delivery system. Minute volume is the amount of air breathed per minute and is calculated by multiplying the tidal volume (amount of air exchanged in a resting breath) by the number of breaths per minute. Tidal volume can be estimated by assuming that 10 ml of air/kg of body weight are exchanged in one breath (5 ml/lb). (This figure is not valid for very large or very small animals). For example, a 10-kg animal taking 10 breaths per minute would require an O_2 flow of 1 L/minute (10 kg x 10 ml/kg = 100 ml x 10 breaths/minute = 1000 ml/minute).

The greater the number of leaks in the delivery system (*eg,* semi-open anesthetic machine), the higher the flow must be to deliver the necessary amount of O_2. A loose-fitting mask or vented O_2 cage may require 10-20 times the O_2 flow as that given by endotracheal tube.

The percentage of O_2 (50-100%) given to a patient varies with the cause of the respiratory distress and the length of therapy needed. Most of the O_2 is carried by hemoglobin in RBCs and only a small fraction is dissolved in the plasma. Once RBCs are saturated by O_2, increasing the percentage of O_2 administered has little effect on the animal. On the other hand, if the hemoglobin is not saturated, increasing the percentage of O_2 above that in normal room air (about 16%) aids hypoxic patients. Poor oxygenation of RBCs occurs when the respiratory rate is depressed, cardiac function is poor, alveolar (air sacs in the lungs) walls are too thick for good gas exchange, RBCs are damaged, etc.

Pure (100%) O_2 can be administered in emergencies, but severe toxicity occurs within 10 hours (at 2 atmospheres of pressure) in warm-blooded animals. The eyes of neonates are especially susceptible. Concentrations of less than 35% do not affect the retina (visual layer at the back of the eye), and in dogs the first 21 days after birth is considered the most critical period for eye damage from 100% O_2. Cold-blooded animals are not damaged by long-term pure O_2 therapy and also survive O_2 deprivation better than mammals and birds.

Under normal conditions, it is difficult to obtain 100% O_2 concentrations unless an endotracheal tube is used for administration. The typical concentration in an O_2 cage is 30-50%. When using an O_2 cage for small animals, initial flows of up to 10 L/minute are needed to wash out residual nitrogen in the cage; levels are then decreased for maintenance. Oxygen cages are the best way to administer O_2 to a conscious animal without constant supervision. Using a mask may cause the animal to struggle, compounding the respiratory distress by using up more O_2 in muscular activity. In sealed O_2 cages and anesthetic delivery systems, CO_2 levels should be maintained at less than 1.5% using an absorber containing soda lime.

The most efficient temperature for giving O_2 is 65-70 F, as the concentration of gas particles varies with temperature changes.

Pure O_2 decreases blood flow through the lungs. This reduces the volume of secretions by the respiratory tract and increases the thickness of mucus. The respiratory system is constantly exposed to foreign material and microorganisms from inhaled air. Mucus and other secretions trap inhaled particles and are swept out of the lungs and up the airways, clearing them of potentially harmful materials. Interference with this process increases an animal's sus-

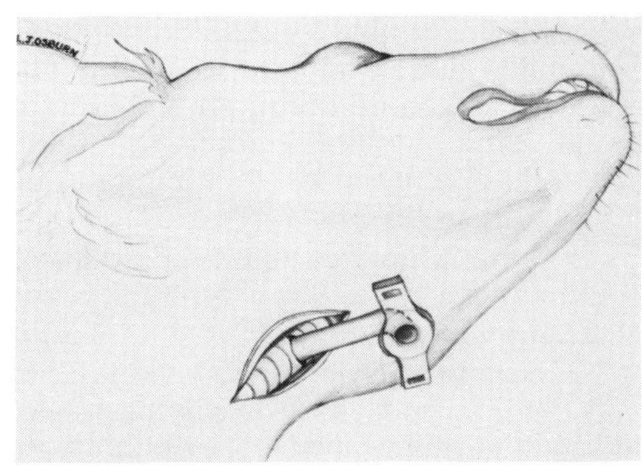

Figure 2. After incising the skin on the ventral midline of the neck and the ligament between 2 tracheal rings, a tracheostomy tube is inserted.

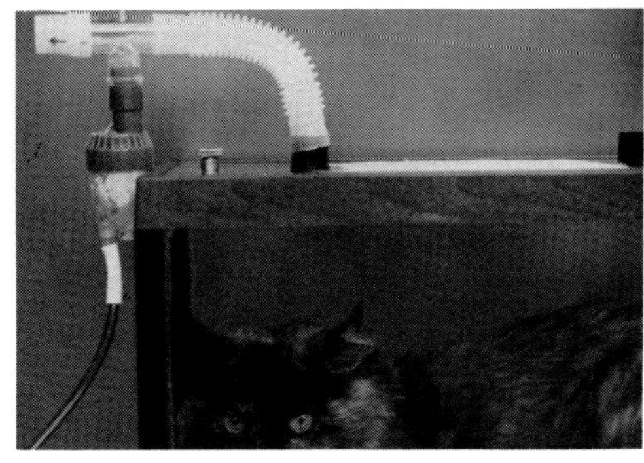

Figure 3. Anesthetic induction chamber used as a nebulization chamber for small animals.

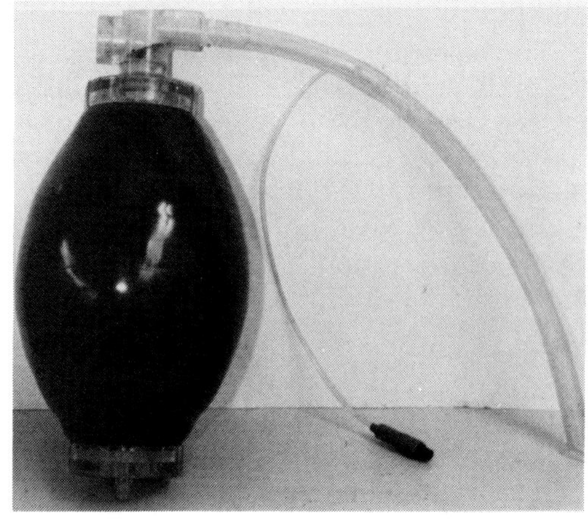

Figure 4. Ambu bag attached to an endotracheal tube, used for positive-pressure ventilation.

ceptibility to respiratory tract disease. Clearance of respiratory secretions is greatly delayed in dogs given 100% O_2 because of thickened mucus. In addition, pure O_2 further narrows airways in patients with severe pulmonary (lung) disease. Evidence of inflammation of the airways occurs in dogs after breathing pure O_2 for 6 hours or 75% for 12 hours.

As there is no treatment for oxygen toxicity, do not administer 100% O_2 for more than 5 hours without consulting the veterinarian.

In most instances, 30-60% O_2 is adequate for hypoxic patients and there is no risk of toxicity. Increasing the humidity of the O_2 (40-60% humidity is ideal) by bubbling it through ice water before it enters the O_2 cage helps prevent respiratory irritation due to high concentrations of O_2.

For cattle, an adaptation of the "Venti-Mask," designed for people, delivers an O_2 flow of 12 L/minute at 28% (because of the air vents). Oxygen is usually administered to large animals by face mask, endotracheal tube or nasal catheter (through the nose by tube).

In summary, to administer O_2 to a conscious patient, use an O_2 cage for small animals or a nasal catheter for large animals. If the patient is unconscious, use an endotracheal tube or face mask. Animals that are not breathing spontaneously must be assisted with an Ambu bag, rebreathing bag, positive-pressure ventilation machine (respirator), closed-chest massage, etc. The oxygen flow is turned on by twisting the handle on top of the tank and the flow is regulated by setting the meter. Pure O_2 can be safely given for up to 5 hours. Closely monitor the patient's pulse rate, mucous membrane color, and respiratory rate and depth.

ARTIFICIAL ALIMENTATION

The best diet is useless unless it is eaten, and many hospitalized animals refuse to eat. This is especially a problem with cats, young horses and small dogs. Often the animal can be supported with forced feedings until its appetite returns with its health and it adjusts to the clinic environment.

The process of supplying nutrients to animals that cannot (because of face, mouth or throat injury or surgery) or will not eat is called *artificial alimentation.*

Oral Alimentation

Forcing nutrients into an animal orally is less time consuming, less expensive and less risky than IV feedings. It allows the body to digest the food naturally and is the best way to supply a complete diet artificially. A functional digestive system (not inflamed or blocked) is necessary and the animal should not have vomiting or diarrhea.

Solid chunks of food, gruel and liquids can be administered as if they were medication, by "pilling" or "drenching" the animal (see Chapter 4). This method requires a docile patient with a pain-free, uninjured mouth, tongue, throat and esophagus (tube leading from the throat to the stomach).

Slurries of food can be deposited directly into the stomach with a tube passed through the mouth for small animals or nose for large animals (see Chapter 4). For small animals, a nutritionally balanced, canned food mixed with water (using a blender) is ideal. Mix one-quarter of a 1-lb can with 175 ml of water and divide it into 3-4 feedings/day for a 5-lb animal. Giving fluid by SC injection and feeding concentrated food sources (*eg,* egg yolk, baby food) reduce the volume and number of feedings/day.

For horses, a mixture of electrolytes, dextrose, dehydrated cottage cheese and 6-7 L of water can be used.[3] In cattle, use of a blend of vitamins, minerals, dextrose, dried skim milk, soybean meal and water is recommended.[4] Exact recipes, volumes and number of feedings should be determined by the veterinarian. Make sure all food particles are small enough to pass easily through the tube.

For long-term artificial alimentation, a pharyngostomy tube may be surgically implanted by the veterinarian (Fig 5). One end of the tube extends out of the esophagus, through the skin of the neck near the jaw, and the other rests in the stomach. Gastrotomy tubes may also be used. They are placed through the body wall, into the stomach. Food is given through the tube, which eliminates the need for repeated oral passage of a stomach tube. Pharyngostomy tubes are well tolerated by most animals and may remain in place for weeks. The skin around the tube and the incision (tube is sutured in place) should be washed daily with a mild antiseptic (*eg,*

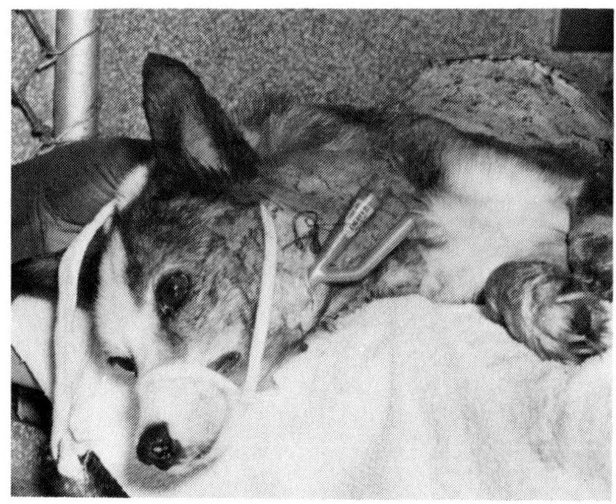

Figure 5. Pharyngostomy tube implanted in the esophagus of a dog, for artificial alimentation.

povidone-iodine) and water. The tube should be capped when not in use to prevent air from entering the stomach.

Concentrated nutrients are available in liquid or gel form (*eg*, Pet Kalorie, Sustagen) and can supplement the patient temporarily, but they are expensive and may cause diarrhea if given in large amounts or over an extended period. Complete liquid diets are available from several companies.

Forced feedings should not be continued longer than necessary. The patient should be encouraged to eat on its own by offering highly palatable food frequently (Hill's a/d is designed for this use).

Parenteral Hyperalimentation

An animal that is severely malnourished may not have adequate energy to digest its food. In addition, patients with serious digestive tract disease, chronic vomiting and/or diarrhea, acute kidney failure, inflammation of the pancreas, or GI surgery may (before or after) benefit from nutrients given IV. As with all artificial alimentation, the goal is to assist the animal while the condition preventing normal eating is resolved.

Parenteral hyperalimentation involves continuous IV administration of a hypertonic solution containing calories, proteins, vitamins, electrolytes and water. Calories are provided by fat (lipids) and sugars. Solutions typically contain 10% dextrose, crystalline amino acids, K, phosphate, Na, Mg, Cl, and vitamins B and C. Copper, zinc and multiple vitamins are added if therapy continues for more than a week. Some B vitamins and vitamin K must be given IM, as they are destroyed (oxidized) if placed in a high-glucose solution. Adding HCO_3 (bicarbonate) to the solution causes precipitation of Ca and Mg. The veterinarian may rotate the solutions to be used.

If a solution with more than 10% glucose is used, it should be administered through a large central vein, such as the jugular vein. Lipids are added (10-20%) by allowing a second, high-fat solution to mix with other infused fluids just before they flow into the vein. This method prevents the lipid from separating out from the rest of the solution (as happens with oil and water in salad dressings). If a high-fat solution is used to provide calories, the fluids may be given in a smaller vein in a limb, such as the cephalic.

The solution is best administered with an infusion pump, but any conventional unit (including microdrip) may be used. When administration of hyperalimentation solution is stopped, IV administration of 5% dextrose should be continued for a short time to gradually taper off the blood glucose level. As the patient begins to eat food, hyperalimentation is gradually discontinued.

Patients treated by hyperalimentation should be monitored carefully. Laboratory tests to determine the patient's response to therapy should be done regularly on blood, plasma and urine. Hydration status, body temperature, weight, and pulse and respiratory rates should be checked frequently. The IV catheter should be kept clean and dressings to hold it in place changed frequently. Any sign of localized or generalized infection should be reported to the veterinarian immediately.

CRITICAL CARE MONITORING

Ideally, every patient in critical condition should be observed 24 hours a day by a veterinarian. However, this is physically and financially impractical, so the technician must aid the veterinarian by reporting anything important to the doctor.

A significant part of any technician's job is *observation.* Consider clients who did not know their animal was sick until the signs were so advanced it seemed impossible anyone could be unaware of the problem. These clients were not good observers and their animals may have suffered because of it.

Careful observation is a learned skill that develops with practice. It involves comparing normal behavior or appearance against abnormal signs, and drawing conclusions. The more time spent observing normal and sick animals, both as individuals and as members of a species, the better judgment a technician has when monitoring critically ill patients. Time spent observing, touching, hearing or smelling hospitalized animals is never wasted, as it is gathering data for decision making. Part of the reason animals are hospitalized is so they can be observed frequently by someone capable of recognizing minute changes that could herald a problem.

Pulse, respiratory and heart rates all vary significantly in normal animals, due to exercise, excitement, environmental temperature, etc. However, an increase or decrease can also indicate a metabolic problem or other disease. The Appendix contains a table of normal physiologic values for several species. Any variation from them should be brought to the veterinarian's attention.

Consult with the veterinarian regarding how often to check vital signs and monitor the patient. As a rule of thumb for non-life-threatening cases, check the patient every 15 minutes for the first hour after hospitalization, every 30 minutes until the animal is stabilized, and every hour thereafter. Animals near death may have to be watched almost continuously. It is difficult to over-monitor a patient and usually the animal's condition indicates how often observation is necessary. Experience adds confidence in making this judgment.

Monitoring Body Temperature

Most mammals and birds can regulate their body temperature within a very narrow range. The range varies with the species and allows for internal conditions optimal for chemical reactions (homeostasis).

Monitoring body temperature is not useful in cold-blooded animals, such as snakes, lizards and other reptiles, because they equilibrate with the environmental temperature. However, they also have an optimal temperature for body functions and should be kept in that range by using an artificial heat source.

Warm-blooded patients sometimes lose control of their ability to regulate temperature. Elevated temperatures occur with heatstroke (see Chapter 1), infections, tight bandages, some poisonings, etc. Heatstroke causes the temperature to rise high and fast, and because of loss of temperature-regulating ability, the animal may easily be over-cooled during treatment. Infection with bacteria or viruses elevates normal temperatures, similar to turning up a thermostat. The way the temperature fluctuates varies with the disease. Some infections cause chronic low-grade fevers, others a sharp fever spike, and sometimes the temperature oscillates up and down. Close monitoring may provide clues to the source of the fever. Temperatures that rise rapidly usually indicate a worse prognosis than slowly rising fevers.

Temperatures may be measured rectally (see Chapter 2). However, the animal's behavior may also indicate that internal temperatures are not optimal. Animals with a fever may be depressed, have a dry nose, huddle in a corner or with other animals, feel warm to the touch and/or drink excessive amounts of water. Animals with a subnormal temperature may seek a source of warmth, be depressed and/or have cold extremities. In both cases, the patient often is anorectic (inappetent) and usually quiet and withdrawn.

A rectal temperature elevated 3 F (2 C) above normal is considered a fever. Excitement or extremely hot weather may increase the body temperature by 2 F (1 C), but only in unusual circumstances will it go higher. Allowing the animal time to adjust, then retaking the temperature, and considering other clinical signs, usually eliminate excitement as a cause of a fever.

The higher the rectal temperature goes, the more concerned a technician should be. Most thermometers do not measure beyond 106 F (42 C) and at 105 F (41 C), except for birds, the fever becomes harmful. The nervous system is especially susceptible to damage by fever. Fevers of 103-105 F (39-41 C) should be closely monitored and brought to the veterinarian's attention. The animal should be kept warm and quiet, and encouraged to drink liquids, and any other clinical signs treated. Animals with a fever above 105 F (41

C) should be treated by applications of ice packs or immersion in cold water and/or by drug administration. Any fever this high should be treated as an emergency.

The rectal temperature may be low when an animal is in shock, severely debilitated, suffering from cold exposure (hypothermia) or recovering from anesthesia. Conserve body heat by covering the animal and insulating it from cold surfaces, especially stainless steel. If the temperature drops to about 98 F (37 C), warm the patient with hot-water bottles, a heat lamp or heating pad. Be very careful that the patient does not get overheated by checking the temperature of the skin nearest the heat source frequently. Severely depressed animals may suffer burns as they cannot move away from an overly hot heat source. If the temperature drops below about 94 F (34.4 C), the animal may be near death and emergency measures must be taken to warm it. Immersion in lukewarm water is a quick way to increase temperature. The water may be gradually warmed to normal body temperature. Be sure to thoroughly dry the coat afterward to prevent chilling. Animals have survived with a body temperature as low as 75 F (24 C) when cooled in cold water or during open-heart surgery, but these are exceptional circumstances.

Young or old animals are less able to regulate their body temperature and should be watched carefully for chilling or overheating.

Because of their greater body mass, adult horses and cattle typically have slower temperature changes in disease and therapy than small animals.

Electronic probe systems for monitoring temperature are made by several companies. A very fast response time and "on-line" monitoring are advantages to these devices.

Monitoring Cardiovascular Function

Pulse

A pulse is created in arteries by expansion and contraction of the vessel walls with each heart beat. The pulse wave propagates like a limp rope that is whipped up and down. This wave moves much faster than the blood flows. A pulse is not normally observed in veins, as their anatomic structure tends to moderate pressure changes in these vessels.

A change in pulse rate or character indicates a difference in heart function or blood flow volume. However, the rate varies widely in normal animals because of excitement, anxiety or even normal respiration. An intermittent pulse (occasional pause between regular pulses) may be present in normal animals. Thus, judgment must be exercised when evaluating the pulse.

The character of the pulse normally is firm and regular. However, its rate and character may vary as the heart beat does, becoming harder or softer, larger or shorter, depending on the amount of blood flowing through the vessel.

If the pulse abnormality is caused by a heart defect, the veterinarian has usually detected it and the technician's main concern is a change in pulse, especially if it is gradually deteriorating in strength and/or rate.

A slow, soft pulse (thready) that is barely perceptible can occur with shock, diminished heart contraction strength or constriction of the heart by fluid in the pericardial sac (membrane around the heart). A fast pulse may occur when the tissues are not getting enough oxygen and the heart compensates by increasing its speed and subsequent blood flow.

A pulse deficit occurs when there are more heart beats than pulses present in a given time span (both must be monitored at the same time). The heart pumps blood inefficiently on abnormal beats, so no pulse may be felt then.

Pulse frequency (rate in beats/minute) is easy to evaluate, but character (soft, hard, long, short, etc) is much more difficult to assess. The strength of the pulse (amplitude) can be estimated by determining the amount of pressure needed to close off the vessel. Spending time feeling pulses gradually increases digital sensitivity and the value of this in critical care monitoring.

Electronic monitors are available to produce audible or visual indications of pulse rate.

Mucous Membranes

Color: The protective, keratinized layer of the skin's surface is absent in areas of the body that are moist and protected from injury and invasion by other means. These areas are called *mucous membranes* (mucosae) and line the body orifices. Because mucous membranes are hairless and thin, the blood within small vessels colors the tissue (unless the skin is naturally pigmented). This color serves as an important indicator of body condition.

The best areas to examine for mucous membrane color are the inside surface of the lip, gums (gingivae), tongue, inner eyelid, surface of the eye (sclera), and inner vulva or sheath. Most people find the lips and gums easiest to examine but the surface should not have any dark pigment that obscures the normal pink color. Good lighting is necessary to evaluate the color. Studies have shown that viewers may disagree on the depth of color of the mucous membrane.

If the mucosa appears blue-purple (cyanosis), the blood is low in O_2 content or blood flow to the tissue is decreased, so more O_2 is being extracted from the blood. Unoxygenated blood is dark red, but combined with skin pigment appears blue. Cyanosis is cause for concern and usually must be attended to immediately, though some heart conditions cause chronic, low-grade cyanosis. The deeper the shade of blue-purple, the more severe the condition, as the proportion of unoxygenated to oxygenated blood is greater.

Anemic patients may be low in blood O_2, but not cyanotic, because of low levels of functioning hemoglobin. This must always be kept in mind when monitoring such animals. If the cyanosis is caused by low blood O_2, then O_2 therapy is of benefit. On the other hand, if it is caused by poor blood flow to a tissue, O_2 therapy is less beneficial to the patient.

If an animal is cyanotic, check cardiac and respiratory function first. If neither is apparent, initiate cardiopulmonary resuscitation (CPR). If the heart is beating but the animal is not breathing, pass an endotracheal tube if possible and assist respiration with an Ambu bag, artificial respiration, manual compression of the lungs, etc (see Chapter 1). Oxygen therapy during this time may also be helpful. If the animal is breathing but the heart is not beating, electric shock, compression or injection of a stimulant may start it. If a cyanotic animal is breathing and the heart is beating, administer O_2. If O_2 does not improve the color, therapy to increase blood flow, volume or quality may be needed. In any of these situations, notify the veterinarian as soon as possible.

When the amount of blood flowing through the vessels in a mucous membrane is low, the tissue becomes pale or white (pallor). This could be caused by shock (as the blood is pooled elsewhere), loss of blood, or anemia. Whole blood transfusions may be necessary if the number of circulating RBCs is very low.

Mucous membranes may also be bright red, as in carbon monoxide poisoning, or muddy brown, as in nitrate toxicity.

Develop the habit of checking the mucous membrane color of any animal you examine.

Capillary Refill Time: The smallest blood vessels in the body are the capillaries. They join the arteries and veins to make a continuous vascular circuit. Not all capillaries are filled with blood at one time or there would not be enough blood left in the large vessels to circulate (this is an indication of the vast number of capillaries in the body). However, enough are normally filled in an area to color the mucosae pink.

A good measure of cardiovascular function is to determine how rapidly capillaries refill with blood after their supply has been shut off with pressure. To determine capillary refill time, gently press on the mucous membrane (usually the gum) with the tip of a finger (not the fingernail) until it blanches white. Then quickly remove the finger and note the time it takes for the color to return, which normally is in less than 1 second. Diseases that reduce cardiac output (the amount of blood leaving the heart), impair circulation or delay capillary refill time include shock, heart valve abnormalities and fluid in the pericardial sac.

Heart Rate

Interpretation of the various heart sounds is complex and usually requires a veterinarian to recognize any heart defect. Thus, patient monitoring involves primarily checking the rate of the beats. This can be done by palpation (feeling), auscultation (listening with a stethoscope), electronically (heart monitors) or indirectly by counting the pulse rate (see Chapter 2).

Report any of the following to the veterinarian: a progressively decreasing or increasing rate, a highly irregular beat, long pauses between beats, or a continuously rapid rate.

Monitoring Respiration

Interference with respiration can occur in the upper respiratory tract (nose, mouth, throat) or the lower respiratory tract (trachea, bronchi, lungs). It can involve a simple physical blockage of air conduction or a subtle thickening of alveolar walls, preventing gas exchange. Structures associated with the respiratory tract can affect breathing, such as the pleura (membrane covering the lungs) or ribs. Even diseases not associated with the respiratory tract, such as heart disease, anemia or gastric (stomach) dilatation, can influence breathing. Regardless of the cause of respiratory difficulty, it should be viewed as an emergency as adequate O_2 intake and CO_2 removal are essential for life. When establishing priorities in an emergency, adequate respiration should be the first concern, as apnea (no breathing) and subsequent asphyxia (O_2 starvation) are the quickest cause of death.

The respiratory and cardiovascular systems are closely linked, so a change in one is usually reflected in the other. Pulse rate and character, mucous membrane color and respiration all change as blood gas levels become abnormal.

Changes in respiratory rate, depth or pattern can be detected by observation, palpation or auscultation (see Chapter 2). Certain individuals or breeds may have variations in breathing that are considered normal. Respiratory sounds are usually harsher in young and/or small dogs and cats than in older or larger animals.

Respiratory Rate

The respiratory rate may be elevated with exercise, excitement, obesity, environmental heat, pain, structural changes in the lungs, low O_2 availability or change in the body's pH balance (measure of acidity or alkalinity). Animals acclimated to cold may show a rate increase of 6-8 times normal when brought indoors. Hyperventilation (prolonged, rapid, deep breathing) can cause loss of consciousness. Panting is normal in most animals but it does not elevate the body's O_2 level because the breaths are too shallow to exchange much air. The cause of rapid breathing must be determined before it can be corrected. Excited animals may be calmed by moving them to a quieter location, blocking their view of other animals or using tranquilizers. Fever, pain and abnormal blood pH (acidosis, alkalosis) may be treated with drugs or specific treatment (cold-water baths, etc). Oxygen can be given if rapid breathing is caused by hypoxia, but do not administer O_2 if the animal is already hyperventilating.

Low respiratory rates can occur with poisoning, overly deep general anesthesia or alkalosis (high blood pH). As therapy for hypoventilation (reduced breathing), the effects of some anesthetics may be reversed with antagonists, respiration may be stimulated with drugs or the pH can be adjusted with certain IV fluids. Oxygen should be given if the animal is cyanotic.

Depth of Respiration

The lungs are inflated by expansion of the thorax (chest), contraction of the diaphragm (drum-like muscle that separates the thoracic and abdominal cavities) and outward rotation of the ribs. Normally both the chest (thoracic breathing) and the abdomen (abdominal breathing) move with each breath. Pressure on the diaphragm from an enlarged structure (*eg,* the liver) or fluid in the abdominal cavity (ascites), and paralysis of the diaphragm may result in thoracic breathing only. Thoracic pain, as from pleuritis or broken ribs, can result in abdominal breathing only.

Deeper breaths cause greater expansion of the lungs. If chest expansion is not possible or is painful, the animal breathes shallowly. Several shallow breaths are required for the same amount of gas exchange as one deep breath. Thus, the rate of respiration is elevated with shallow breathing. Shallow breaths without an increase in respiratory rate rapidly lead to hypoxia and cyanosis. Shallow breathing occurs with pain, nerve damage or pressure increases in the thoracic or abdominal cavity.

The depth of respiration is evaluated by observing the degree of chest expansion or rebreathing bag (on the gas anesthetic machine) expansion. Some animals naturally have a greater lung capacity than others and the amount of expansion varies with exercise, so judgment must be based on experience. Panting represents shallow breathing and deep breathing is seen after exercise, so keep this range in mind when making observations of depth of respiration.

The term *Cheyne-Stokes breathing* refers to breathing with a gradual increase then decrease in the depth of respiration in a cyclic pattern.

Pattern of Respiration

The pattern or rhythm of respiration can be varied voluntarily or involuntarily. The length of time for inspiration and expiration should be equal and any variation is an abnormality of rhythm (a slight pause occurs between them). Dyspnea (difficult, laborious breathing) can occur with lung and/or airway disease. On expiration, the normal lung collapses and airways narrow, so small obstructions can easily trap air. Inspiratory dyspnea (forced inspiration), with flaring nostrils and gasping can occur with loss of lung elasticity, fluid buildup in the lungs (pulmonary edema), upper airway obstruction, exercise or excitement. Dyspneic animals should be monitored carefully and the veterinarian notified regarding their condition. An animal with dyspnea extends its head and neck, dilates the nostrils, rotates its elbows away from the chest, may breathe through the mouth, and has exaggerated movements of the chest and abdomen, and pronounced respiratory sounds, especially grunting.

Respiratory Sounds

A variety of respiratory sounds may be heard in disease. Most fall into 2 groups: rales (moist, bubbly sounds) and rhonchi (dry, whistling sounds). Normal respiration is almost silent, though air flow may be heard in airways, so any especially obvious respiratory sound should be reported to the veterinarian. Coughing and sneezing are other signs of respiratory disease that should be monitored and their frequency noted.

Controlling Pain

Dorland's Medical Dictionary defines pain as a localized discomfort, distress or agony caused by stimulation of nerve endings. In people, pain can be difficult to localize and may even be felt in a part of the body distant from an injury (referred pain). It can occur without a lesion (tissue defect), as pain in a "phantom" limb after amputation. Individual people can feel pain differently; the cause and prevention of pain are an area of intense medical study.

The fact that animals feel pain is well established, though this was not always believed. Observing an animal react to the prick of a needle or a fractured limb has convinced most people the pain that animals feel is analogous to that in people.

The discomfort of pain can cause behavior abnormalities, delay recovery from injury or disease, lead to further self-inflicted trauma or cause disuse of a body part. For these reasons, as well as for reasons of compassion for any suffering animal, the recognition and alleviation of pain should be an important goal of all technicians.

Animals in pain may express it with a whimper, yipe or growl when an area is touched or moved. Causing this reaction may be necessary so the veterinarian can make decisions regarding the severity, type, treatment, etc, of an injury or disease. Because the animal's vocal response to stimulation may distress the client and further trauma to the injured area must be avoided, handling of an animal in pain should be minimized.

Often the expression of pain is nonvocal. Animals may refuse to eat or become withdrawn, anxious (alert and looks around constantly), irritable or restless. Large animals may struggle to get away or become aggressive when handled. Some animals endure pain stoically or seek human companionship. Limping on a painful limb, tilting an infected ear downward, holding an inflamed eye closed, lying on only one side, reluctance to stand, arching the back, abnormal tail carriage (especially in swine), etc, are all signs of pain. Knowledge of normal behavior and the ability to predict how an animal may react to pain are important. Use caution when handling potentially dangerous animals in pain by using restraint devices (*eg,* muzzle, kick bar, etc).

Relieving pain is a task involving nursing skill. Check casts and bandages to make sure they fit properly and are dry. Offer highly palatable food if the patient is not eating or thin it to a gruel if the painful lesion is oral. If the animal is withdrawn, a kind word or touch may help. If the animal is restless and cannot find a comfortable position in which to rest, bedding a stall deeper or adding padding to a cage may induce relaxation. Watch for self-mutilation or excessive licking of an injured area. There are a wide variety of analgesic (pain relieving) and antiinflammatory drugs available if needed. Surgical correction of a defect may give the animal relief from pain. In general, use common sense to meet patient needs on an individual basis.

Monitoring Food and Water Intake

Any hospitalized animal should be monitored for food and water intake. A complete history should include the type, time and amount of food an animal is accustomed to eating. The change in environment when an animal is hospitalized may temporarily affect eating; if the patient has not consumed food and/or water for 24 hours, it should be brought to the veterinarian's attention. The amount of time an animal can go without eating depends on its activity level, size and body condition. A working, trim animal shows the effects of starvation more rapidly than a sluggish, overweight one. Refusal to drink liquids is of greater concern than loss of appetite (anorexia), as dehydration occurs more quickly than starvation.

Daily food and water intake should be recorded on the patient's chart. A standardized amount should be offered to each animal so the amount consumed can be estimated from the amount remaining.

Food

Canned food for dogs and cats and concentrate feeds for farm animals are usually more palatable than dry foods because of their higher nutritional and moisture content. Semi-moist foods fall in between them in palatability. Some animals, especially cats or small-breed dogs, eat only what they are accustomed to consuming, so a wide variety of foods should be stocked in the clinic. Mixing water or canned food with dry food and handling cat food with the fingers sometimes increases its acceptability to patients. Adding bottled baby food in meat flavors, cottage cheese, shrimp, meat broth or eggs may encourage animals to eat. For a docile animal, offering food by hand may start it eating. Dogs may want privacy when eating and typically consume their food in "meals." Cats are "snack" eaters; if dry food is left in the cage, they may consume it at night when the clinic is quiet. Farm animals eat most readily at dawn and dusk. Uneaten food should be removed in several hours. If the animal still refuses to eat, forced feeding may be necessary.

Herbivorous animals (ruminants, horses) find sweet feeds and grains most palatable. Mixing these in with forage may encourage eating. Use of high-quality hay and a variety of feeds is desirable. Because of the larger capacity of the equine and bovine stomach, they can go for longer periods without eating than dogs or cats. Two days of inappetence for an active horse or beef or dairy cow (where production is important) should be cause for concern, but up to a week without eating for a quiet pleasure horse in good condition is not dangerous to its health. Forced feeding by intubation may be required.

Correction of the underlying cause of anorexia is essential for its resolution. Drugs, including vitamins and corticosteroids, may help stimulate the appetite.

Excessive consumption of food may also be a problem. A change in diet, especially from a dry to canned food, may stimulate an animal's appetite. The stimulus of seeing and hearing other animals eat may also encourage an animal to bolt down its food. Large volumes of food may upset the digestive system, causing vomiting and diarrhea. They may make the patient lethargic and obese. This is especially a problem if the animal's activity is limited by confinement and if "treats" are given by hospital employees.

Water

As the section on dehydration indicates, animals must consume water to maintain a normal physiologic environment. Typically, animals consume water at 45 ml/kg (20 ml/lb) daily, but the exact amount varies with environmental temperature, activity level, individual metabolism and the moisture content of feeds.

Water consumption can be encouraged by lightly salting the food, adding broth, or frequently setting out a fresh supply Sometimes warming or chilling the water may increase intake. Adding water or broth to food or feeding succulent forage are other ways to increase liquid consumption.

A sudden switch in water source or adding medication to the water may have discouraged drinking and can be corrected. Most animals readily accept distilled water.

Using a wax pencil to mark the fluid level in the water bowl or bucket helps monitor intake. Only one person in the clinic should be responsible for filling water bowls or buckets and a standardized amount used. Spilled or evaporated water must be subtracted from the amount considered consumed and the daily intake noted on the patient's record.

If the animal refuses to drink, giving fluids by stomach tube or injection may be necessary.

Excessive fluid intake is also cause for concern. If an animal is using water internally, as for lowering body temperature or for metabolic processes, dilute urine is not produced. However, if the patient is drinking excessively (polydipsia) and urinating large volumes (polyuria), it is a sign of disease and should be reported to the veterinarian. Excited or bored animals may drink excessively, but if it happens continually, laboratory tests should be run to eliminate disease as a cause. Using ice cubes instead of liquid water slows water consumption of an excited patient.

Automatic watering systems should be checked on a regular basis for proper function. If an animal's intake must be monitored, water should be offered in a measured volume, or a flow meter should be installed in the line of an automatic watering system. Cats, rodents, ferrets and other animals can be taught to drink from a sipper bottle, but a bowl of water is usually preferred.

Monitoring Urinary and Fecal Output

The waste products of an animal are a direct reflection of its internal conditions. Each species has a normal range of volume, content and consistency, and deviations from normal can be a sign of disease.

Feces

The digestive tract is actually a tube within the animal, in which food is digested and nutrients absorbed. This system protects the delicate internal environment from the foreign, nonsterile and possibly toxic substances the animal consumes as raw material for body functions. Because the digestive system contacts substances from the environment, it is often a site of disease, and such signs as vomiting and diarrhea are common. When describing feces, any abnormal color, odor, consistency, content or volume should be noted.

Color: Feces are normally brown to green, depending on the species, but they may range from white to black abnormally. Bacterial breakdown of yellow bile pigments (from worn-out RBCs processed by the liver and excreted into the proximal small intestine) produces the normal brown color of small animal feces. If more RBCs are broken down than normal, as from a blood parasite, the feces are yellowish, as more bile is present than the bacteria can process. This can also occur if bacteria are not present (*eg,* with antibiotic therapy) to break the bile pigment into the brown color.

Black, tarry stools indicate bleeding into the proximal digestive tract (esophagus, stomach, mouth, small intestine). The blood is partially digested a it passes down the tract, resulting in the black color. Fresh blood, mixed throughout the feces or present in flecks, results from bleeding in the distal digestive tract (distal small intestine, colon, rectum), as it has not been decomposed. Blood may not be visible (occult blood) and a laboratory test is required to detect it.

The color of feces depends on the diet of the animal. White stools may indicate the patient has consumed large numbers of bones (small animals) or excessive milk (calves). Consumption of plant material turns feces green because of chlorophyll and is normal for large animals.

Consistency and Content: Normal consistency of feces varies among species and before and after weaning. Become familiar with the normal consistency of feces for each species. If a patient is producing stools more liquid or dryer than is typical, note it on the animal's record. The degree the stool varies from normal and the duration of the abnormality are important.

Canine and feline stools should be firm enough to be picked up with a paper towel and leave only a small spot on the original surface. They should not be hard and dry. In cattle, normal feces are pudding-like and retain a flat shape with ridges after striking the ground. Normal equine feces are dry enough to break apart when disturbed.

Foreign material in feces, such as aluminum foil, plastic, cloth or bone chips, should be reported to the veterinarian. Excessive amounts of mucus give a jelly-like, transparent look to the stool. Small amounts of undigested food are no cause for concern, but significant quantities on a regular basis indicate the digestive tract is not functioning efficiently. Horses with teeth that need floating (filing down to a smoother surface) or that consume large amounts of water at meal time sometimes pass whole grain in their feces.

Odor: The odor of fresh feces also varies with the species. A putrid odor occurs when animal protein (meat) is digested and accounts for the difference in smell between the feces of carnivores (meat eaters) and herbivores (grain and forage eaters). A fetid odor, reminiscent of decaying flesh, may indicate the surface of the digestive tract is diseased and sloughing, as in a parvovirus infection of dogs.

Volatile toxic materials, such as motor oil and gasoline, may impart their odor to feces.

Volume: Excessive volumes of feces are linked to large food intake, as one is not possible without the other. Inefficient digestion may force an animal to overeat to maintain itself. Poor digestion can result from a lack of the necessary enzymes or other substances to break down food (normally produced by the liver, pancreas, stomach and intestines).

Feces that contain excessive liquids also occupy greater volumes than normal. Ingesta (consumed food) is usually liquid when moving through the proximal digestive tract, but in the distal regions the liquid is absorbed and the feces compacted to their normal consistency. Liquid feces result when this function is lost, when food material is moving too fast for liquid to be absorbed or when nutrients are not absorbed into the body and they osmotically draw liquid from the tissues into the intestine.

Defecation: The way an animal defecates is determined by behavior and fecal consistency. Excessive straining or lack of straining when defecating is cause for concern.

Straining to defecate (tenesmus) may indicate constipation, a foreign body, inflammation or blockage of the distal intestine (in the proximal intestine this causes pain rather than straining, and in the stomach it usually causes vomiting). Radiographs, ultrasonography, palpation and/or rectal examination may be necessary for diagnosis. Laxatives, enemas or surgery are possible treatments.

Straining or not straining when passing liquid stools is an important diagnostic clue and should be noted on the record. Different diseases can produce different signs; for example, cattle with Johne's disease often do not lift their tails when defecating. Some animals with nerve damage or neurologic defects (such as some Manx cats) may not be aware of defecation.

Urine

Urine is plasma (the liquid fraction of blood, or blood without proteins and cells) filtered by the kidneys and changed by adding and removing substances. Because urine originates as plasma, its composition is a reflection of internal conditions and its production is an indication of kidney function.

Volume: Loss of the ability to concentrate urine leads rapidly to dehydration. Dilute urine is normally produced when water intake is high or when the kidneys have lost the ability to concentrate urine by resorption of water. A water-deprivation test may be necessary to test an animal's ability to concentrate its urine. Familiarity with the volume of urine normally produced by different species is essential for detection of polyuria (see Appendix).

Damage to the kidneys, shock, low blood volume, cardiovascular abnormalities and obstruction of the excretory ducts (ureters, urethra) can all cause low or no urine production. This rapidly leads to accumulation of toxic waste products in the blood (uremia). A cat with a urethral obstruction (urinary duct leading out of the body) can become dangerously uremic in 24 hours. Thus, male cats that strain to urinate, visit the litter box frequently, or have an excessively full bladder should be treated as an emergency. Urinary tract obstruction can lead to permanent kidney damage from pressure buildup.

The rate at which urine is produced is an indication of blood flow and kidney function (glomerular filtration rate). The bladder can be catheterized and urine production monitored by watching the drops/minute produced. Most animals produce urine at 20-50 ml/kg (10-20 ml/lb) in a day, which averages to about 1.5-2 drops/minute in a medium-sized dog. More urine production than this is not a problem, but less or no urine formation should be called to the veterinarian's attention, as it can indicate renal failure. Desert animals, such as gerbils, have highly concentrated urine for water conservation.

Physical Characteristics: The odor, color and consistency of urine vary with the animal's diet, species and metabolism. For example, horses and rabbits typically produce thick, opaque urine, and male cat and goat urine has a pungent smell.

Normal urine color ranges from pale to dark yellow, depending on its concentration. Red, cloudy urine indicates the presence of blood (hematuria), whereas clear, red urine (port wine colored) indicates the RBCs in the urine have lysed (broken open) and released their hemoglobin (hemoglobinuria). Some drugs excreted in urine may discolor it. Bright orange urine may be caused by poor liver function or excessive RBC breakdown.

Urea (from breakdown of protein in the body) in urine is degraded by bacteria into ammonia when urine is left standing after it has been excreted or if there is a bacterial infection in the bladder (cystitis). A ketone smell (like nail polish remover) indicates an energy imbalance in the body (excessive fats being degraded). Some toxins produce a "chemical" odor in urine.

Urine can appear cloudy because of the presence of yeast, crystals, molds, pus, mucus or contaminants from cage surfaces and fecal material. Crystals normally thicken horse, rabbit and rodent urine. The cause of increased urine turbidity can be determined by microscopic examination and other laboratory tests.

Vomiting

Vomiting may be caused by pain, toxins, infections, mechanical irritation, parasites, grass or hairballs, GI malfunction, tumors, drugs, distasteful odors, digestive tract blockage, foul tastes, metabolic disorders, throat irritations, neurologic problems and motion sickness. It may be preceded by restlessness, salivation, swallowing, nausea and retching in dogs, cats and swine. The time between eating and vomiting or regurgitation may help indicate the cause. If it occurs immediately after eating, it is termed *regurgitation* and the esophagus is implicated; if 30-60 minutes after eating, the stomach may be involved; and if 3-4 hours have passed since eating, the lesion may be in the small intestine. Problems in the large intestine do not usually cause vomiting. Vomiting related to specific foods may be caused by changes in diet, spoiled food, meals consumed too hot or cold, gulping food or food allergies. Typically, food allergies relate to the protein source of the food, such as a reaction to beef, chicken or eggs, but can also be a sensitivity to a preservative or another additive.

Vomiting not related to food intake may be caused by systemic (generalized) or localized infection, poisons and metabolic or neurologic abnormalities. Chronic digestive problems may cause periodic vomiting. Intermittent vomiting can be caused by a partial obstruction or other interference with digestive function. Obstructions closer to the mouth than the small intestine produce regurgitation of recognizable food material.

Cats vomit hair that accumulates in the stomach during grooming. The vomited hair may have a tubular shape or may be loose hair mixed with food or mucus. Cats with skin problems or ectoparasites may groom themselves more frequently and tend to have a bigger problem with hairballs. Cats with hairballs often cough or choke, along with the vomiting. Dogs and cats also may vomit after consuming grass, spoiled food or prey animals.

The volume of vomit decreases with the number of times the animal has vomited after a particular meal. If retching is severe, bile from the small intestine and liver stain the vomitus yellow to green. Protracted vomiting can lead to dehydration and electrolyte imbalances that can be fatal. Nerve receptors that send impulses to the vomiting center in the brain are found throughout the abdominal organs and may be activated by pain, infection, etc.

Projectile vomiting occurs when the stomach contents are ejected with force and is not preceded by retching and nausea. It can be seen with cranial (head) trauma or obstructions of the stomach or esophagus.

Fresh blood in the vomit is associated with bleeding from the mouth, pharynx or esophagus. Partially digested blood from the stomach appears as brown flakes resembling coffee grounds.

Horses and cows do not vomit unless they are very ill, due to the anatomy of their digestive tract. Horses vomit through their nose, rather than the mouth, inhale the vomit and usually die of aspiration pneumonia caused by the inhaled particles.

Regurgitation occurs when undigested food is brought up without retching. It happens normally in cattle, sheep, deer and other ruminants when they ruminate (chew their cud). It may be caused by overeating, or disorders of the stomach and/or esophagus.

The frequency, character (color, consistency, odor, content) and volume of vomit, and severity of retching should all be communicated to the veterinarian as they may provide clues regarding the origin of the disorder.

Monitoring Nervous System Injuries

Head and spinal cord injuries can result in coma, spasm, convulsion, paralysis, incoordination, and changes in pupil size and response to light. Progressive worsening of these signs indicates increasing pressure on the brain, a low brain O_2 level or other defects.

The animal's state of consciousness is evaluated by response to its name, painful stimuli (such as pricking its rump with a needle), change in position, etc. The patient may be alert, depressed, confused (animal is aware of its surroundings but does not react normally to stimuli), delirious (animal moves and may make sounds but is not aware of its surroundings), semicomatose (animal is unconscious but reacts to pain) or comatose (animal is unconscious, cannot be aroused and does not react to a painful stimulus).

Pupils that are dilated in bright light, constricted in low light or asymmetric (one dilated and one constricted) indicate a brainstem injury. Pupillary response to light is usually evaluated by shining a light in the eyes and observing the response of the pupil and comparing the response of one pupil against that of the other. Nystagmus (eyes rhythmically move back and forth horizontally or vertically) may indicate a skull fracture, bruising of the brain, damage to the middle ear or high intracranial pressure (inside the skull).

Any abnormal posture (head tilt, leaning), paralysis, rigid limbs, incoordination, etc, should be reported to the veterinarian.

Convulsions should be brought to the doctor's attention immediately as they can be fatal if protracted or if they affect the heart, certain blood vessels or the respiratory system (see Chapter 1).

Miscellaneous

Blood or pus exiting the anus, mouth, mammary gland, eyes, nose, ears or wounds may be significant and the veterinarian should be alerted. Excessive matter in the eyes, ears or nose may indicate disease. Lymph nodes are easiest to palpate (feel) when enlarged. Typically the easiest places to palpate them are below the ear, at the angle of the jaw, behind the knee, and where the neck joins the shoulder. Fluid accumulations in body tissues or cavities are also important. Breath that smells like spoiled fruit may indicate diabetes mellitus. Ammonia breath occurs with uremia. A musty smell on the breath of a comatose animal can indicate liver disease.

Conclusion

Recognition of when an animal is in difficulty is the first step in monitoring a critically ill animal. This may not be easy, particularly in birds, and seemingly inconsequential findings may precede disaster. Changes may be subtle even though one or more body systems are near collapse. An abnormal finding may easily be dismissed as unimportant, but such thinking can lead to deterioration in a patient's condition before the signs are taken seriously.

All clinical signs are interrelated. Any disturbance in the natural harmony of the body is often reflected in several abnormal signs. Thus, it is essential that all body systems be checked each time an animal is examined.

ELECTROCARDIOGRAPHY

Muscles contract in response to electrical stimulation. The pacemaker of the heart is the sinoatrial node (SA node), located in the top quarter (end opposite the pointed apex) of the right side of the heart. Other areas of the heart can produce impulses, but the SA node sets the pace for the heart beat. The electrical impulse it generates is conducted through the heart by specialized fibers. This allows contraction in a specific sequence, so blood is "milked" from the heart rather than with a uniform, simultaneous contraction, which is not efficient in pumping blood.

The heart is responsive to hormonal (*eg,* epinephrine) and nervous stimulation. It normally pumps all of the blood delivered to it by the veins and, like any other muscle, enlarges in response to increased work loads. Contraction rate and/or strength can increase or decrease as tissue needs change.

The electrocardiogram (ECG) measures electrical activity on the surface of the body, resulting from impulse flow through the heart. The electricity travels in all directions away from the heart but is measured in a standardized way.

The pattern of electrical flow through the heart is irregular with cardiac arrhythmias (irregular heart beats), is prolonged with heart enlargement due to a greater muscle mass to stimulate, and is abnormal when the heart muscle is diseased or affected by metabolic problems. The ECG is useful in diagnosing any of these conditions, detecting electrolyte imbalances, determining response to therapy for heart disease, monitoring a patient's condition during anesthesia and establishing a prognosis for cardiac abnormalities.

Making an ECG

The ECG machine consists of leads (wires) that attach to the animal, a terminal that interprets the electrical impulses and a device that displays the impulses on paper or a screen.

The leads are color coded. The black lead attaches to the left front leg, the white to the right front leg, the green to the right rear leg and the red to the left rear leg. The leads are composed of plastic-coated wires with alligator clips, plugs, needles or sticky pads on the free ends. The clips are clamped to the skin over the elbows and stifles of the patient. Good electrical contact between the animal's skin and the clips is essential so that the electrical impulse can be transmitted to the machine. Contact is enhanced by wetting the skin with alcohol, water or electrode jelly where the clips attach. Some machines have an extra lead (chest lead) that is attached to different sites on the animal. Sticky pads are used for long-term monitoring of the heart and must be used directly on the skin (hair is shaved off).

Contraction of muscles other than the heart also generates small electrical impulses, so the patient must remain immobile for a good ECG reading. Tranquilization and anesthesia affect the rate and rhythm of the tracing (pattern of the impulse on the ECG paper). Most animals are quiet enough for a good reading if patience and mild restraint are used.

In large animals, an ECG is performed with the patient standing, but small animal patients are usually held recumbent on their right side, with the legs parallel to each other and perpendicular to the body (Fig 6). Cats, severely ill patients or animals that resist being held in lateral recumbency may be allowed to rest in sternal recumbency (on their breast bone), but this position is not as desirable as lateral recumbency. The technique should be standardized for all patients. A wooden, Formica-topped or rubber-insulated table should be used to prevent impulse conduction to the table surface.

The machine traces the electrical flow on a piece of graph paper (electrocardiographic paper) and/or a screen. Paper speed is 25 mm/second or 50 mm/second. The faster paper speed (50 mm/second) spreads out the tracings so they are easier to read. Some anesthetic monitors show an ECG tracing but do not print it on paper; however, some models can record the tracing for later analysis.

Leads detect electrical activity in different planes through the animal's body and are called I, II, III, aVR, aVL and aVF (Fig 7). Lead I records electrical activity from the left front leg to the right front leg, lead II from the left rear leg to the right front leg, III from the left rear leg to the left front leg, aVR (augmented vector right) from the right front leg to the left limbs, aVL (augmented vector left) from the left front leg to the right front leg and left rear leg, and aVF (augmented vector foot) from the left rear leg to the front legs. As previously mentioned, some machines have a movable chest lead and recordings are made at 4 standard locations (over the 7th thoracic vertebra, at the 5th and 6th intercostal spaces near the edge of the sternum and at the 6th costochondral junction). By recording the electrical flow between each of these locations, a composite picture can be formulated of the heart's activity.

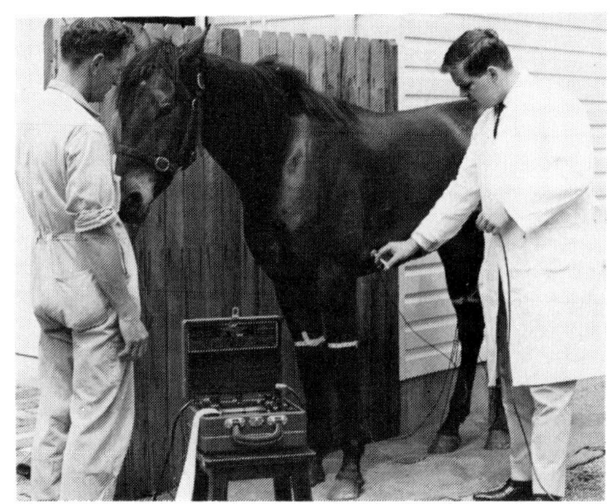

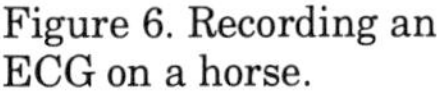
Figure 6. Recording an ECG on a horse.

Recording the ECG is simple. After the paper speed is set (usually 50 mm/second for small animals and 25 mm/second for large animals), about 6-12 beats of the heart are recorded at each lead setting. In addition, 20-60 beats on lead II are recorded to evaluate the heart's rhythm.

If the tracing is too high for the paper width (pen moves higher or lower than the paper width), the sensitivity of the machine may be reduced. If the tracing is too small to be easily read, the sensitivity can be increased. Machines with the capacity to change the sensitivity have a control marked "1/2, 1, 2" to double the height of the reading (2) or half it (1/2). The center of the tracing (baseline) should be in the middle of the paper and maintained there by adjusting the pen (stylus) position throughout the recording. The baseline changes with respiration and other muscular movements.

Machines that convert the signal to sound or digits can be used to send the tracing over telephone lines. This allows remote consultations.

Interpreting the ECG

The mammalian heart is composed of 4 chambers: 2 atria and 2 ventricles. The first small peak on the ECG tracing is formed as the electrical impulse travels through the atria and is called the P wave (Fig 7). The stylus moves up or down and returns to the baseline to record the impulse. The QRS complex is the second and highest peak and is formed by passage of the impulse through the ventricles. The R fraction of the complex is a large spiked wave. The final deflection is the T wave and results when the ventricles "recharge" (return to resting after depolarization). Tracings may contain additional landmarks but these are the major waves of diagnostic interest.

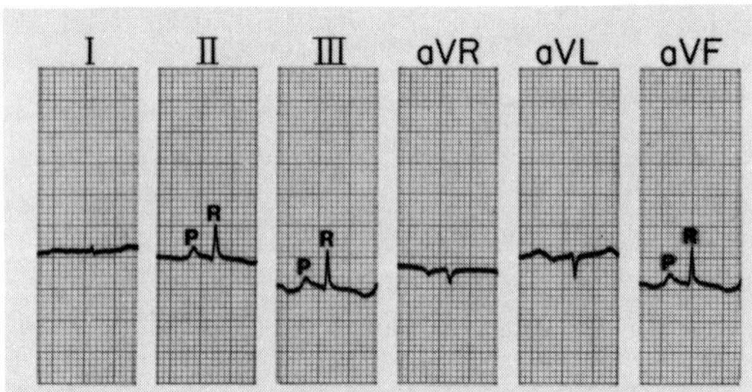

Figure 7. Normal ECG tracings from a cat, using the various leads.

The P, R and T waves should be clear on tracings from each lead for a useful ECG. Additional beats should be recorded if patient movements and other artifacts obscure the tracings.

Many technicians read tracings to free the veterinarian's time for other tasks. Reading the ECG involves measuring wave height and width, intervals between waves, and the heart rate.

At a paper speed of 50 mm/second, the large grids on the calibrated ECG paper are 0.1 seconds wide and 0.5 millivolt high (Fig 8). The small grids are 0.02 seconds wide and 0.1 millivolt wide. There are small lines (hash marks) on the top of the paper every 1.5 seconds at a paper speed of 50 mm/second and every 3 seconds at 25 mm/second (the lines are 7.5 cm apart). Counting the number of beats (P, QRS and T waves combined) between several lines and multiplying by the time in which the beats occurred determine the heart rate.

Measurements of wave heights and widths, and intervals between waves is done on the long lead II strip (Fig 8). Upward (positive) deflections are measured from the upper edge of the baseline to the peak of the wave and downward (negative) deflections are measured from the lower edge of the baseline to the lowest wave point. The width of the wave and intervals between waves are mea-

Figure 8. A normal lead-II ECG tracing. (Courtesy of Mosby-Year Book)

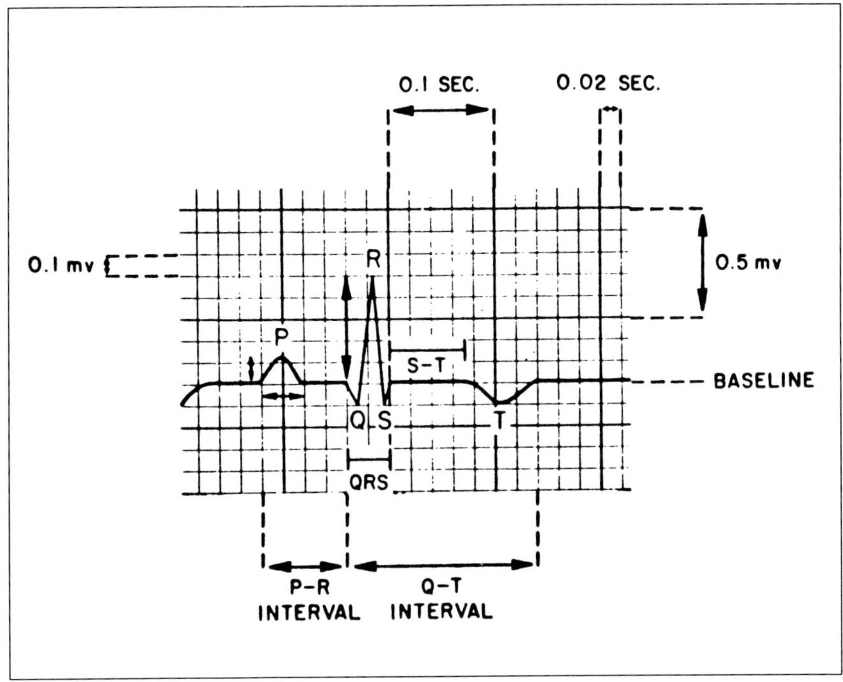

sured from the beginning to the end of the deflection. Measurements usually include the width and height of the P wave, QRS complex, T wave and ST segment. The lengths of the PR and QT intervals are also measured. Calipers and special ECG rulers are useful in measuring the tracing. Results are recorded in seconds or millivolts. It is a good idea to check all measurements twice.

Interpreting the ECG is a complex skill involving knowledge of cardiac structure and function, familiarity with species and breed variations, and an idea of how a given disease can affect the heart. The technician's function is to provide the doctor with readable tracings and measurements for medical analysis, not to interpret the tracings. Some veterinarians may refer tracings to specialists or use a system where the ECG is telephonically transmitted to an expert for interpretation.

Abnormal Tracings

Though interpreting ECGs is complex and should be left to the veterinarian, there are some potentially fatal conditions the technician should be able to recognize, so the veterinarian can be notified immediately. The following questions should be considered in a quick inspection of the tracing: Is there a P wave for every QRS complex? Is there a QRS complex for every P wave? Is the distance between P and R waves consistent? Are all of the QRS complexes alike and normal in shape? Do the beats occur regularly and at a normal rate?

If the answer to any of these questions is "no," the tracing may be abnormal. The more negative answers there are, the more serious the patient's condition and the quicker the veterinarian should be alerted.

Atrial fibrillation occurs when multiple ares in the atria generate electrical impulses (rather than just the SA node). The resulting irregular beat causes inefficient pumping of blood. The ECG shows a fast, irregular heart rate, with the P wave replaced by multiple waves of various sizes (they may be very short), and a normal or wide and bizarre QRS complex (Fig 9). A normal QRS usually follows a group of ripples that represent the P wave.

Ventricular fibrillation is similar to atrial fibrillation but is fatal in a very short time, as the heart pumps almost no blood. The tracing appears as waves of varying heights and widths (large and coarse or small and fine). Individual P, QRS and T waves cannot be recognized (Fig 10). The abnormal waves progress to a wavy or straight line as cardiac arrest occurs.

Ventricular premature contractions (VPC) occur when the ventricles beat separately from the pacemaker (SA node) impulse. It is a common arrhythmia of dogs. With VPC, the P waves are normal but may be bizarre, wide and deflected in a positive and/or negative direction (Fig 11). The typical VPC appears as 2 wide, tall waves close together and pointed in opposite directions. A succession of 3 or more VPC in a row is called ventricular tachycardia (fast heart beat).

ECG Artifacts

Artifacts in the ECG are distortions that are not related to cardiac abnormalities and that interfere with ECG interpretation.

Figure 9. ECG tracing from a cat with atrial fibrillation. (Courtesy of Mosby-Year Book)

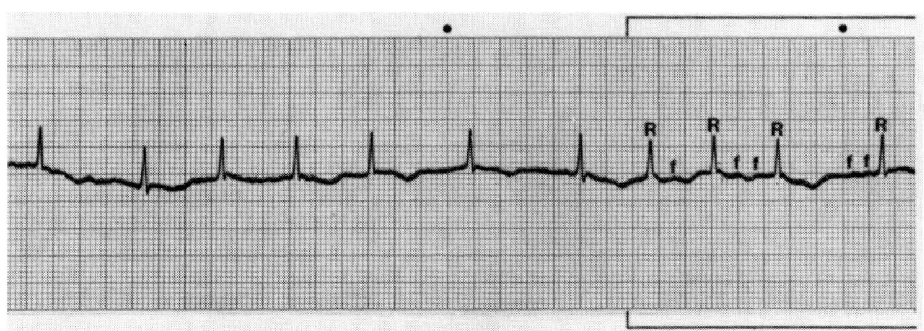

Figure 10. ECG tracing from a dog with ventricular fibrillation.

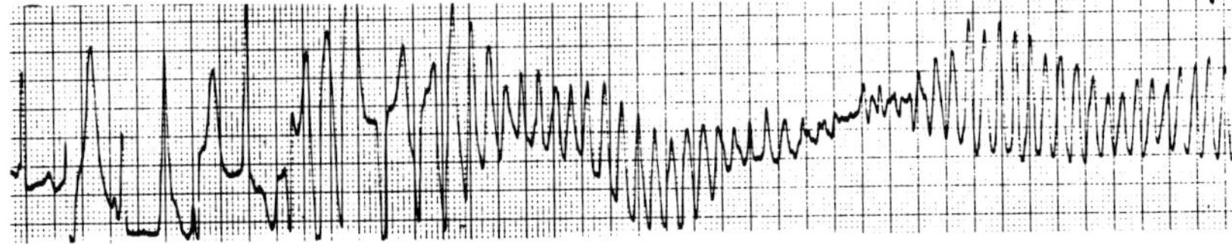

Figure 11. ECG tracing from a cat with premature ventricular contractions. (Courtesy of Mosby-Year Book)

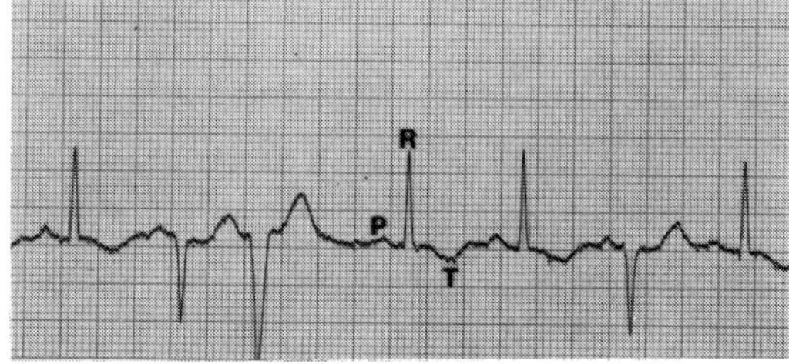

Electrical interference occurs as 60 sharp waves/second. If it is present, check to see that the machine is plugged into a properly grounded (3-prong) outlet, that the leads are all attached to a fleshy part of the limb (not a large fold of skin), that the leads are clean and not saturated with alcohol, that the leads are not touching each other and the clips well fixed to them, that all other electrical equipment in the room is unplugged (*eg,* x-ray machine), that fluorescent lights are turned off, that the table is moved away from the walls with electrical writing in them, that nothing is touching the clips (other than the patient), and that the table is properly grounded. Many ECG machines have a ground wire affixed to a cold water pipe in the clinic.

Body movements or respiration can produce ECG interference. To minimize it, discourage purring in cats, make sure the animal is comfortable, apply moderate pressure with a hand on the chest to reduce muscular tremor (nervous or cold shivering), or lower the sensitivity of the ECG machine. Televisions and other electronic equipment may also produce artifacts in the tracing.

POSTOPERATIVE CARE

Surgery, by its invasive nature, unavoidably injures and stresses the patient. During recovery from anesthesia, the patient's normal response to environmental stimuli and ability to protect itself from harm are depressed. The technician must assume responsibility for the patient's well-being in this helpless state and be especially diligent in monitoring body functions.

Immediately after the end of surgery, determine the rectal temperature, pulse and respiration rates and mucous membrane color, and inspect the incision site. If the animal's temperature is below 100 F (38 C), cover it with a blanket, towel or newspapers. Insulation beneath the patient is especially useful in conserving body heat. If the temperature is below 98 F (37 C), some external heat supply should be used, such as a heating pad, hot water bottle or infrared light. An unconscious animal cannot move if the heat source is too hot, so do not place heating devices in direct contact with the animal's skin; check the skin temperature frequently. Pale mucous membranes can indicate blood loss or shock, and cyanosis an inadequate oxygen supply. Administering pure O_2 for about 10 minutes after gas anesthesia has been discontinued speeds elimination of the anesthetics and the animal's recovery.

If the incision site is bleeding, direct digital pressure (with fingers and a gauze pad) or application of a cold, dry compress can be used to stop it. A small amount of seepage for a short time is normal. The veterinarian should be notified immediately of excessive incisional bleeding. Remove dried blood from the skin around the wound with 1-3% hydrogen peroxide. In some cases, a bandage to support the incision, prevent contamination or reduce joint motion may be useful.

Always deflate the cuff of the endotracheal tube before it is removed. Most veterinarians prefer to untie the tube from the animal's jaw for quick removal when the swallowing reflex returns; however, the tube may slide down the trachea and block an airway, so this practice is not recommended. Tying the tube with a quick-release knot is a safer method.

Once the animal's vital signs (pulse, temperature, respiration) are in the normal range, it can be moved to a recovery area with a cart, stretcher or small tractor (for large animals). When transporting the patient, do not stretch the incision site, and protect appendages and the head from banging against objects. Room temperature in the recovery room would be 68-72 F (20-21 C). The area should be dark and quiet but easily accessible for observation.

Small animals are usually placed in an empty cage, with adequate insulation from the cold cage bottom and the surgical site up or not in contact with the cage bottom. The animal's neck should be extended and the tongue should be drawn out of the animal's mouth so it does not lodge in the back of the throat and obstruct respiration. The exposed tongue is also a convenient monitor for cyanosis. Urinary catheters, chest tubes, IV drip lines and so forth should be firmly affixed to the animal to prevent dislodging during recovery from anesthesia.

Large animals may be placed in a padded stall or an open field during recovery from anesthesia. They are watched from a safe distance and kept as quiet as possible. An alternative method involves kneeling at the animal's head (with one knee on its neck) and holding the muzzle flexed slightly back along its neck. As the patient begins to recover consciousness and struggle, one person holds onto the animal's halter (while standing directly in front of the patient) to stabilize the head, and another holds onto the tail to stabilize the rear end. They assist the patient in standing and balance it until recovery is complete. Never approach the legs and feet of an anesthetized large animal.

Check the patient's vital signs at least every 15 minutes. Irregular heart beat, difficult breathing, cyanosis, signs of shock, and/or a very low temperature are cause for concern, and require appropriate therapy (see Chapter 1) and notification of the veterinarian.

The time required for recovery from anesthesia depends on the type and duration of anesthesia used and the patient's metabolism. An unconscious animal cannot respond to most stimuli and is unable to swallow or blink its eyes. Do not yell or try to arouse the patient quickly, as a true recovery from anesthesia requires elimination of the drug by the body and cannot be speeded in this way.

Turn (roll over) the patient every 30 minutes to prevent pooling of blood in the lungs of the dependent (down) side; the larger the animal is, the more important this is. Support the incision site carefully while turning the animal. Inspect dressings, bandages and bedding for signs of bleeding. Fresh blood is bright red, while old blood is dark red to brown. Palpate the toes, ear tips, etc, extending from bandages and casts for coolness or swelling, which may be evidence of improper application or constriction of blood vessels. A tight bandage interferes with blood circulation, causing cold, swollen and/or cyanotic toes or ear tips.

When the animal begins coughing and swallowing, remove the endotracheal tube by gently pulling rostroventrally (forward and slightly down). The cuff on the tube must be deflated before the tube is removed. The endotracheal tube should never be removed before the animal can swallow, as vomiting may lead to aspiration of vomitus and subsequent pneumonia. In addition, the unconscious animal may need O_2 therapy, using the endotracheal tube.

A semiconscious animal can respond to pain, has reflexes and can move somewhat but does not respond to verbal commands. If the patient is thrashing and may injure itself, pad the recovery area. Howling, whining and other noises do not necessarily indicate the animal is in pain; however, if they continue for more than 30 minutes, call it to the doctor's attention. Many animals have a dry mouth after surgery and rinsing it with a small amount of water may have a quieting effect. Keep the head below the level of the chest while rinsing so any excess water runs out of the mouth, not back into the lungs.

Soiling of the recovery area with urine, feces or vomit should be cleaned immediately, as the animal can easily roll in it. Shivering and uncontrolled movements are not uncommon, but persistent coma, convulsions, widely dilated, fixed pupils (do not respond to light), pupils of unequal size or rigid limbs are indications of a problem.

Semiconscious large animals should be approached with extreme caution. They should be provided with secure footing when attempting to rise so they do not injure themselves by slipping. A dimly lit, quiet recovery area may help make recovery from anesthesia more smooth.

The final stage in recovering from anesthesia is disorientation. Here, the patient responds to stimuli but is confused about where it is. Slow walking of horses during this stage may steady them.

A fully conscious animal is alert and able to appropriately respond to all stimuli. Chapter 8 contains a detailed discussion of anesthesia and anesthetic procedures.

Recovery from Surgery

A rectal temperature elevation of 1-2 degrees often occurs for up to 48 hours after surgery. A persistent or higher fever could be a sign of infection, especially if respiratory distress, vomiting or other signs accompany it. Postoperative inflammation can also slightly elevate the rectal temperature. Animals that have had catheters inserted, those that are debilitated, those that have lain on one side for long periods, or those that have had GI contents spilled into their peritoneal cavity are particularly prone to infection.

Check the incision site at least twice a day for inflammation (redness, heat, swelling, pain and/or a serous or purulent exudate) around a suture or line of sutures. Soreness and inflammation associated with incisions normally decrease daily.

Dehiscence (opening of the incision) can occur in debilitated animals, regardless of the surgeon's skill. Coughing, vomiting, strenuous exercise, infection, licking at the incision, and an inadequate diet all predispose wounds to dehiscence. Evisceration (spilling of bowels or other internal organs through a broken incision line) is frightening but seldom fatal if organs are protected from soiling and damage, and the wound is closed again in a short time. A watery, pink discharge from the wound indicates imminent dehiscence (separation of the suture line). If this is seen, bandage the wound firmly and alert the veterinarian. Most incision separations occur 6-8 days postoperatively.

Patients wearing an orthopedic device (cast, splint) may require 2-3 days to learn to rise and walk with it.

Because animals heal at different rates, suture materials are absorbed at different rates and the trauma produced by surgery varies, suture removal times may differ. The key to recuperation is rest and a proper diet. For large animal patients, drug administration, stall cleaning and patient examination should all be done at the same time so the patient can have long periods of uninterrupted rest. Overexertion and exposure to harsh environmental conditions should be avoided during the postoperative period.

Early ambulation (patient walking) usually is desirable to prevent joint stiffness, improve circulation and exercise muscles. It also encourages patients to urinate and defecate.

Licking and biting at incision sites and bandages should be strongly discouraged by using bitter-tasting compounds, Elizabethan collars, etc (see Chapter 2).

Flies can be a problem in the spring and summer. Wound exudates attract them and they may bite, lay eggs (which hatch into maggots that burrow into and liquefy tissues) and irritate the patient. Bandages, repellents and/or insecticides should be applied if flies have access to the patient.

Patients that cannot walk or that require long-term postoperative care should be treated as debilitated animals.

MANAGEMENT OF SHOCK

Shock is a state of circulatory collapse that can be fatal if untreated. It is precipitated by blood loss, pooling of blood in body vessels or cavities, or cardiac dysfunction. Causes of shock include endotoxins (from bacteria), CNS trauma, acute allergies (anaphylaxis), poisoning and severe injury.

Supportive care is aimed at maintaining the circulating blood volume with fluid therapy (except in neurogenic shock, where fluid therapy may increase intracranial pressure dangerously). Various types of fluid are given IV, including whole blood, plasma, saline or Ringer's solution, and blood volume is monitored with the PCV.

Blood or plasma pooling in body cavities may be removed and reintroduced into the cardiovascular system (autotransfusion) (Fig 12). Oxygen therapy may be useful in cyanotic animals. If kidney function is impaired and the blood volume is normal, diuretics are given to encourage urine production. Heart function may be monitored with an ECG.

Figure 12. Autotransfusion. In this dog with severe abdominal bleeding, a dialysis catheter (A) is used to transfer blood, via IV tubing (B), to a 4-way stopcock (C) attached to a 3-ml syringe (D) and a 60-ml syringe (E). The large syringe is used to aspirate blood from the abdomen and then to force it through a filter (F) and into the jugular vein.

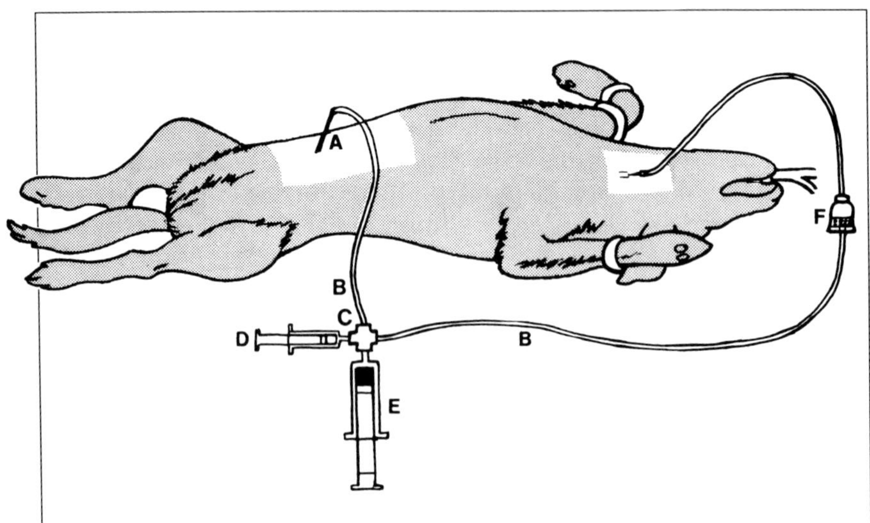

SUPPORTIVE CARE IN SPECIFIC DISEASES

Respiratory Disease

There are 3 phases of normal respiration. The lungs must fill with air and empty, the blood must flow through the lungs, and tissues must pick up and discard gases. A common sign of respiratory disease is dyspnea (difficult breathing). Exaggerated respiration is normal after heavy exercise, but not at rest. Dyspnea is commonly associated with hypoxia (low O_2), hypercapnia (high CO_2) and acidosis (low blood pH).

In all respiratory diseases, the patient should be kept quiet and at a comfortable temperature to minimize respiratory stress.

Nosebleed

Epistaxis (nosebleed) is caused by trauma to the nose, nasal infections, nasal tumors, coagulation (blood clotting) disorders, poisoning (warfarin or sweet clover poisoning), and racing in some hores. Bleeding can originate in any part of the respiratory system, not necessarily the nasal passages. Pulmonary bleeding is often indicated by frothy foam.

Supportive care can involve decreasing the blood volume (and blood pressure) with diuretics and use of agents that encourage clotting, such as vitamin K. Bleeding originating in the nasal blood vessels is treated by direct pressure using a tampon or packing the nose with gauze, decreasing blood flow to the area with cold packs, elevating the head, or use of epinephrine or cocaine.

Free blood in the lungs may interfere with breathing, lead to pneumonia, and cause shock from blood loss.

Exudates

Respiratory exudates can be serous (clear and watery), mucoid, mucopurulent (mucus mixed with pus), purulent (pus), serosanguineous (watery blood) or hemorrhagic (bloody). Exudates can be caused by viral, bacterial or fungal infections, foreign bodies (*eg,* grass awns), tumors, irritants (gasoline or ammonia) and allergies (pollen, dust, etc).

Nasal discharges may exit one or both nostrils, depending on the area involved.

Supportive care may involve use of hot packs (to break up mucous obstructions and stimulate circulation), antibiotics, nose drops, vaporizers (humidifiers), nebulizers (see Chapter 4), O_2 therapy or bronchodilators.

Exudates may also accumulate around the lungs (in the pleural space), between the lung lobes (in the medastinal space) or in the alveoli of the lungs themselves. Accumulation of exudate around the lungs can interfere with lung inflation. Exudates in the lungs can compromise gas exchange. Fluids around the lungs can be drained periodically using a needle and syringe or indwelling chest tube, or continuously with a suction device. Withdrawal of large amounts of fluid can be harmful and can dehydrate the animal. The source of the fluid must be determined by cytologic examination, radiography or ultrasonography to formulate a prognosis (eventual outcome). Aveolar fluid can only be removed through use of diuretics or by correcting the underlying cause of the problem.

Inspiratory Noise

The upper airways narrow on inspiration, whereas the lower tract expands. Thus, narrowing of an upper airway causes increased noise on inspiration. The narrowing may be caused by a foreign body, exudates, tumors, enlarged or constricted normal structures (elongated soft palate, hypoplastic trachea, etc), paralysis (toxic, infectious, traumatic), or impingement on airways (tumors).

Supportive care involves use of decongestants, antibiotics, antihistamines and/or antiinflammatories to help clear the airways. Surgery to correct structural defects or remove occluding structures may be necessary.

Coughing

Coughing occurs with irritation and stimulation of cough receptors in the pharynx, larynx (voice box), trachea, bronchi (primary and secondary), pleura, pericardium and diaphragm. Many diseases cause similar coughs. Coughs can be categorized as wet or dry. Wet coughs are productive, that is, they sound like material is being expelled from the respiratory system, usually into the pharynx, to be swallowed. Dry coughs are harsh and may be followed by a gag at the end. Coughs may also be loud, soft, paroxysmal (several in quick sequence), intermittent, accompanied by expulsion of blood (hemoptysis) or caused by eating or drinking. A description of the character of the cough provides diagnostic clues to the veterinarian. Coughs may be caused by infections, parasites, foreign objects (*eg,* hairballs), tumors, heart disease, allergies and other factors.

Supportive care involves use of expectorants if the cough is wet, or antitussives (cough suppressants) if the cough is dry (wet coughs usually should not be suppressed). Most coughs resolve if the underlying cause is removed.

Sneezing

Sneezing is associated with disease of the nasal cavity and sinuses, though it may be associated with concurrent disease of the lower respiratory tract. Sneezing is a reflex initiated by irritation of the cilia of the upper respiratory tract. It is usually accompanied by a nasal discharge that may vary in character and volume. The character, such as serous (watery), purulent (containing pus), mucoid (mucus-like), mucopurulent (mucus mixed with pus) or hemorrhagic (bloody), volume and general consistency should be noted. Causes include infection, foreign objects, allergy, tumors, trauma and parasites. Supportive care involves elimination of the underlying cause. The reverse sneeze is a sudden, deep snort (or snore) on inspiration.

Expiratory Noise

Pulmonary emphysema, an abnormal accumulation of air in the lungs caused by pathologic processes, is a cause of expiratory noise. Emphysema may be caused by loss of lung elasticity or destruction of the walls separating the alveoli (air sacs). Causes include infection, allergy, irritant gases and parasites.

Supportive care usually involves rest, decreasing the amount of environmental dust (moisten feed or the stall floor for large animals), and use of decongestants, antihistamines and/or bronchodilators.

Pneumonia

Inflammation of the lung tissues (pneumonia) can be a direct result of microbial action or secondary to other disease or injury (*eg,* parasites or inhaled foreign materials) that allows invasion. It is especially severe in young and very old animals, and may be caused by bacteria, viruses, fungi, parasites, allergies or toxins. Systemic signs are also often seen (fever, depression, etc).

Supportive care generally requires antibiotics, antitussives (cough suppressants), expectorants, antihistamines, decongestants and O_2 therapy.

Cardiovascular System

Diseases affecting the heart and blood vessels involve all other systems in the body because adequate circulation is required by all tissues. The technician must be especially diligent in monitoring the cardiovascular status.

Inadequate circulation causes loss of cells due to hypoxia, resulting in myocardial infarction, cerebral aberrations, syncope (fainting), stroke or death. Care of chronically affected animals is rarely attempted in food animals, as their value is in production of meat and milk. Companion and performance animals are the primary recipients of nursing care. Affected animals are first stabilized and then maintained in a manner to reduce further damage (*eg,* as from pulmonary edema) while working toward rehabilitation of this vital system.

Venous Engorgement

Engorgement (especially of the jugular vein) is seen when the central venous pressure is elevated (Fig 13). Inadequate cardiac output causes blood to collect in the vessels. Causes include congestive heart failure, hypernatremia (excessive sodium in the blood), renal failure, vasoconstrictive shock, pericarditis, myopathy (as in selenium deficit), or impingements (*eg,* tumors) or constrictions of major arteries (stenosis).

Supportive care includes reduction of dietary sodium (salt) intake and use of diuretics or bleeding to reduce blood volume. Some drugs (furosemide, digoxin) are effective in long-term therapy.

Fibrillation

Fibrillation (flutter) in the upper chambers of the heart (atria) may not result in signs of disease, but fibrillation of the larger, lower chambers (ventricles) may cause death. Causes of fibrillation are hypoxia, electrocution, toxins and heart disease.

Chronic care usually involves use of precisely timed doses of cardiac drugs (digitoxin or quinidine) and control of activity.

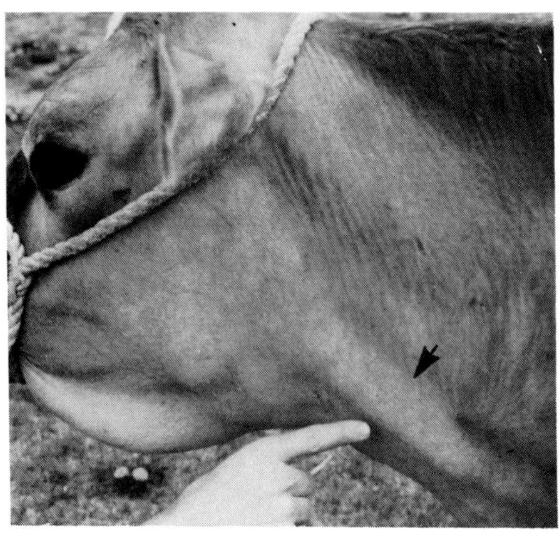

Figure 13. Jugular vein distention in a cow, caused by traumatic reticulitis and atrial fibrillation.

Bradycardia

Bradycardia (abnormally slow heart rate) is normal in athletic animals at rest but is a sign of disease in unconditioned animals. Many toxins and depressant drugs (anesthetics, hypnotics) slow the heart and can cause circulatory collapse or shock.

Supportive care involves use of fluid and O_2 therapy, stimulants or hormones.

Cyanosis

A blue cast to the tongue and other mucous membranes (cyanosis) indicates a large amount of the animal's hemoglobin is not carrying O_2. Arterial blood O_2 has been reduced by high cell demand for O_2, inadequate exchange of gases in the lungs or low pulmonary blood supply (perfusion). Causes of cyanosis include airway obstruction, a barrier to diffusion of O_2 from lungs to blood (emphysema, effusions, allergy), hypoventilation or mismatched ventilation:perfusion ratio. Anemia does not cause cyanosis, as the hemoglobin is fully saturated with O_2 though reduced in amount. Reduced ability of the blood to carry O_2 can also prevent normal mucous membrane color (*ie,* blood drawn into a tube remains brownish when shaken), as in cyanide poisoning. Cyanosis is a sign requiring immediate notification of the doctor. Transfusions, fluid and O_2 therapy, and antiinflammatory drugs may be used to correct cyanosis.

Syncope

Syncope (fainting) may be caused by circulatory or neurologic impairment, hypoxia, hypoglycemia, toxins, epilepsy, narcolepsy and metabolic disease.

Supportive care for syncope depends upon the cause. Protecting the animal from injury (removing obstructions from the area) and use of circulatory or nervous system stimulants are beneficial.

Tachycardia

Tachycardia is an abnormally high heart rate. Disease occurs when the heart rate is so rapid as to prevent effective pumping of blood. Mild to marked increases in heart rate are normal during fear, heavy exercise and excitement. Impaired circulation to the brain or skipped beats may be dangerous to the animal's health. Causes include intoxications, pain and heart disease.

Supportive care is directed at maintaining an adequate supply of blood to the body tissues, especially the brain, and reducing the heart rate. Adjustments in environmental conditions (reducing stress), and analgesics or mood-altering drugs are used in therapy.

Neurologic Disease

The nervous system is a communication network for response to stimuli and coordination of internal and external body functions.

The center of the nervous system is the brain and spinal cord (central nervous system or CNS), which are involved in conscious thought, processing sensory information and maintaining autonomic functions. Specific areas of the brain are devoted to different tasks. The brain and spinal cord are enclosed in a fluid medium (cerebrospinal fluid or CSF), much like plasma, for protection. The CNS is richly supplied with blood vessels, but the capillaries are not as freely permeable as elsewhere in the body and form a barrier between the blood and CNS (blood-brain barrier) that helps keep microorganisms, toxins, etc, out.

The spinal cord is a collection of descending tracts from the brain and ascending tracts from the periphery of the animal. Major nerve trunks exit and enter between the vertebrae (spinal column). The spinal cord terminates as a bundle of nerves supplying the tail and rear quarters of the animal.

The peripheral nervous system is composed of all nervous tissue not in the CNS and includes spinal nerves for sensory input and motor (muscle or organ action) output. The autonomic system, a part of the peripheral nervous system, has sympathetic and parasympathetic components that control visceral (organ) functions of the body not under conscious control, such as the cardiovascular, respiratory and digestive systems.

The nervous system is highly complex and neurologic damage may result in various abnormalities. Nervous diseases may be treated medically; however, most nervous system tissue does not regenerate or regenerates very slowly. The nervous system is evaluated by a systematic neurologic examination done by the veterinarian.

The brain is divided into 3 main parts: the cerebrum (main part of the brain, involved in thought, sensory integration, etc); the cerebellum (involved in coordination of incoming and outgoing impulses); and the brainstem (cranial nerve and autonomic nervous system function control). Lesions in the cerebrum can be manifested as behavior and/or personality changes, such as loss of housetraining, atypical aggression or docility, disorientation, avoidance of a favorite pastime, failure to recognize people, aimless wandering, loss of interest in life, head pressing, excessive excitement, abnormal performance of a learned task and hiding.

Seizures may occur with bursts of electrical activity from the brain, resulting in uncoordinated muscular contractions. Epilepsy, characterized by repeated seizures, usually responds well to drug therapy.

Stupor (animal requires a painful stimulus to arouse it), semiconsciousness or coma (animal cannot be aroused) may occur with lesions of the cerebrum. Pain occurs with certain cerebral diseases or when the membranous coverings of the CNS (meninges) are inflamed.

Delicate tremors and inability to correctly judge distances are signs of cerebellar disease.

Cranial nerve deficits may indicate brainstem injury or peripheral damage of the cranial nerves. Involvement of more than one cranial nerve or abnormal autonomic function is a more definite indication of brainstem disease.

Brain injuries should be handled as emergencies, especially if the signs progressively worsen. A common result of brain injury is edema (due to increased production of CSF, hemorrhage or obstruction of CSF outflow tracts). Because the brain is encased in the skull, it cannot swell (as other tissues do when they are inflamed) without the increased pressure permanently damaging nervous tissue. Progressively worsening signs indicate continuing brain damage and warrant immediate attention.

Supportive care for neurologic disease may include use of osmotic agents (*eg,* mannitol), antiinflammatories, cage or stable rest, fluid therapy, and antimicrobials that can cross the blood-brain barrier. Given time, the brain has an amazing capacity to recover from injury, and certain types of neurologic surgery have been very successful.

Vestibular Apparatus

The vestibular system is part of the inner ear and functions to maintain balance and the animal's perception of its orientation in space.

Signs of vestibular damage may include loss of balance, a head tilt, walking in tight circles, falling or rolling, dizziness or vertigo (animal appears disoriented, excited or restless), nystagmus (eyes move rhythmically from side to side, up and down or in a circle) and/or nausea (like "sea sickness").

Vestibular disease may result from trauma, severe ear infections, stroke, tumors, intracranial infections or damage to the eighth cranial (vestibulocochlear) nerve.

Supportive care may involve use of antiinflammatories, antimicrobials and diuretics. Animals should be protected from injuring themselves (remove protruding objects and confine in a safe area) and assisted with normal body functions (eating, urination, etc) with gentle support. Many animals with mild vestibular damage eventually regain their balance even though a head tilt may remain.

Cranial Nerves

Olfactory: The first cranial nerve (olfactory) is involved with the sense of smell. An animal's sense of smell is difficult to evaluate, but anorexia, refusing some foods, and a decrease in sniffing behavior may be clues. Conditions causing loss of the sense of smell may be canine tooth abscesses, tumors, upper respiratory infections and damage to the olfactory nerve.

Optic: The second cranial nerve (optic) is necessary for vision. Animals with optic nerve damage may bump into things or fail to avoid objects in their path. Other causes of blindness include damage to the retina (light-sensitive lining of the eye), intraocular infection, brain damage, tumors and congenital (birth) defects.

Oculomotor: The third cranial nerve (oculomotor) and the sympathetic nervous system control the size of the pupil. Abnormal pupillary dilation or constriction, lack of response to light, and unequal pupil sizes (anisocoria) are signs of cranial nerve or brain damage and should be reported to the veterinarian.

Trochlear, Abducens: With the third cranial nerve (oculomotor), cranial nerves IV (trochlear) and VI (abducens) control eye position and movement. The position of the pupils can be used to determine if the eye is tilted.

Trigeminal: Damage to cranial nerve V (trigeminal) may result in a dropped jaw, inability to chew, a protruding tongue, drooling, shrinking (atrophy) of some of the cranial muscles, loss of skin sensation to the ear, eyelid and/or lower lip, and food impaction in the cheeks.

Facial: Cranial nerve VII (facial) innervates the muscles of facial expression, the tear glands and certain salivary glands. Drooping of the ear, eyelid and/or upper lip and drooling are signs of facial nerve damage.

Vestibulocochlear: The vestibular apparatus and sense of hearing are supplied by cranial nerve VIII (vestibulocochlear). Loss of hearing is difficult to assess in animals unless both ears are involved. Severe inner ear infections and space-occupying masses may also cause loss of hearing.

Glossopharyngeal, Vagus, Accessory: Cranial nerves IX (glossopharyngeal), X (vagus) and XI (accessory) are all involved in innervation of the throat. Dysphagia (loss of swallowing ability) and/or a change of voice occur when they are damaged. The vagus nerve also innervates the heart and viscera.

Hypoglossal: The tongue musculature is innervated by cranial nerve XII (hypoglossal). Injury to the hypoglossal nerve results in loss of muscle tone and impaired movement of the tongue.

Supportive care for cranial nerve damage is symptomatic. Animals adjust rapidly to loss of a sense (hearing, vision, etc).

Spinal Cord

Damage to the spinal cord is manifested as a neurologic abnormality caudal to the lesion. Signs include limb paresis (weakness), paralysis (inability to move), rigidity or pain, loss of proprioception (ability to determine position in space), urinary or fecal incontinence (inability to control urination or defecation), ataxia (poor coordination in moving the limbs and body), and cutaneous anesthesia (loss of perception of pain in the skin) (Figs 14-16).

Spinal cord damage can result from compression of the cord due to intervertebral disk herniation, space-occupying masses (tumors), swelling due to inflammation, edema or hemorrhage, and bruising or tearing of the cord from trauma (*eg,* spinal fracture).

Supportive care involves restricting movement of the animal and use of antiinflammatory drugs or surgery to reduce pressure on the cord. Many animals with spinal cord injury cannot voluntarily urinate or defecate. In such cases, the bladder should be manually expressed 2-3 times a day (even if the animal dribbles) and enemas administered as needed. Animals should be cared for as if debilitated, with frequent turning, easy access to food, etc.

Figure 14. Injury to the spinal cord between segments C5 and T2 can result in tetraplegia (paralysis in all 4 limbs), with inability to perceive pain in the skin caudal to the spinal cord lesion (wound).

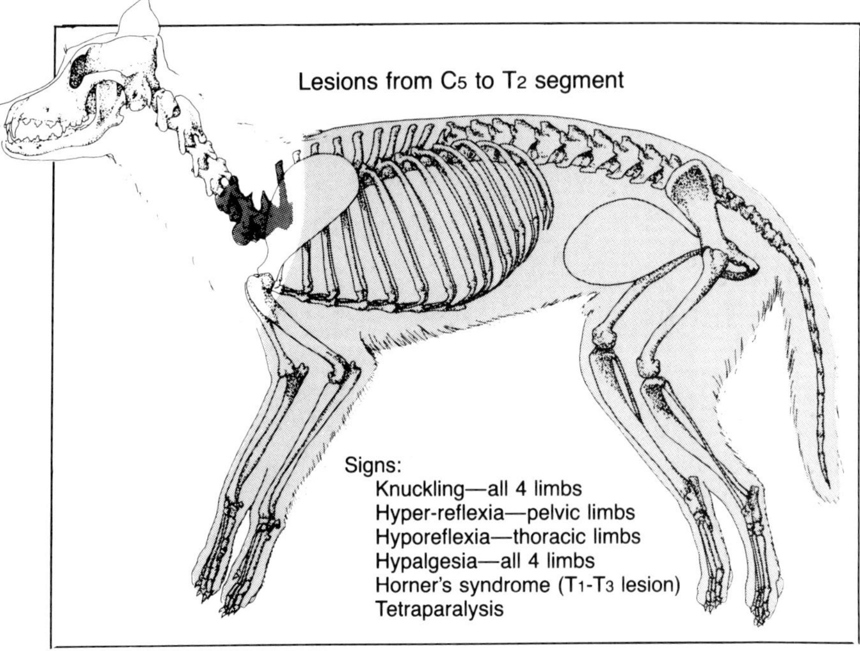

Lesions from C5 to T2 segment
Signs:
Knuckling—all 4 limbs
Hyper-reflexia—pelvic limbs
Hyporeflexia—thoracic limbs
Hypalgesia—all 4 limbs
Horner's syndrome (T1-T3 lesion)
Tetraparalysis

Peripheral Nerves

Damage to peripheral nerves, as from trauma or improper injections, results in loss of sensation and/or loss of function. The affected area becomes flaccid (limp) and atrophied (muscles shrink with time). Supportive care includes protection of the limb from damage (self-mutilation, dragging on the ground, etc), physical therapy and surgery.

Ocular Disease

Inflammation

Eye inflammation, either on the surface or inside the eye, can manifest itself as redness, pain (seen as tearing or rubbing the eyes) or an ocular discharge (may be watery or thick and yellowish, gray or white). Inflammation can be caused by infection (*eg,* canine distemper, *Chlamydia*), allergy, parasites (*eg, Thelazia californiensis* or flies), chemicals, drugs, foreign objects, trauma or other eye

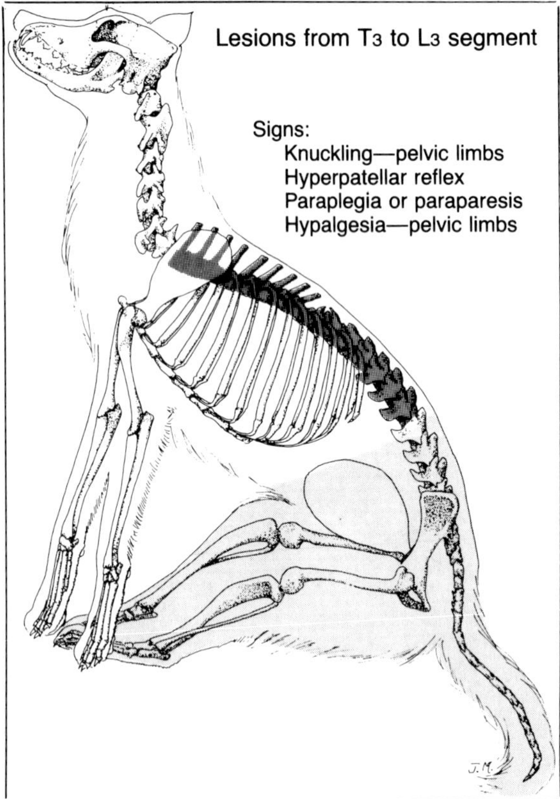

Lesions from T3 to L3 segment
Signs:
Knuckling—pelvic limbs
Hyperpatellar reflex
Paraplegia or paraparesis
Hypalgesia—pelvic limbs
J.M.

Figure 15. Spinal cord injuries between segments T3 and L3 usually cause hind limb paralysis and decreased skin sensation. Respiration and urination may also be affected.

Figure 16. Spinal cord damage in segments L4 to S3 causes paraplegia (rear limb paralysis), with possible inability to urinate and loss of anal sphincter function and skin sensation.

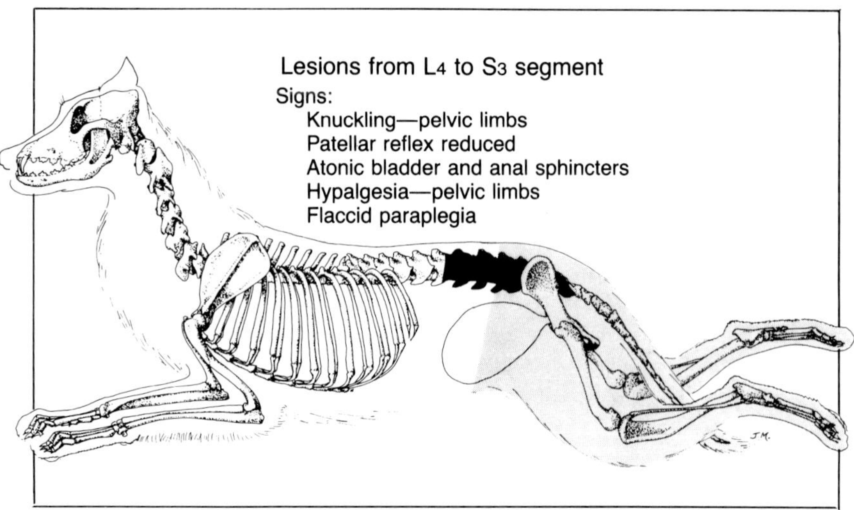

diseases. Thick, purulent discharges (pus) indicate infection. Obstructed tear ducts cause tearing without inflammation.

Supportive care may include flushing the eye and use of antimicrobial or antiinflammatory drugs. Application of an Elizabethan collar or neck cradle may be necessary to prevent the animal from rubbing its eyes. Only sterile material labeled for use as an ophthalmic should be applied to the eyes.

Ocular Opacity

Opacification (cloudiness) of various parts of the eye (*eg,* cornea, lens) can prevent the light transmission necessary for vision. The cornea may become dry, cloudy and ulcerated, the lens may gradually become cloudy with age (cataract), and the normally transparent fluid between the lens and the cornea (aqueous humor) may fill with debris from inflammation (anterior uveitis) (Fig 17). Treatment for corneal lesions includes topical application of antimicrobials and antiinflammatories. Cataracts can be removed surgically. Anterior uveitis is often treated with topical atropine and corticosteroids, but systemic medication may be used, depending on the causative factors. Lacerations of the cornea can be repaired surgically, treated with an antibiotic-soaked contact lens, or treated by suturing the nictitans across the globe until the corneal lesion has healed.

Glaucoma

The eye is a fluid-filled structure, with intraocular pressure maintained within close limits by various physiologic mechanisms. A group of diseases, collectively called glaucoma, result in an elevated intraocular pressure with resultant damage to the delicate internal structures necessary for vision. Certain breeds are prone to glaucoma. The condition can occur secondary to trauma or infections.

Acute glaucoma is an emergency that must quickly be treated with drugs to decrease intraocular pressure and so reduce pain. Glaucoma commonly results in blindness, regardless of the treatment. Glaucoma is painful, and removal of the eye is sometimes the kindest option, especially when frequent treatment is not feasible.

Urogenital Disease

Diseases of the reproductive and urinary tracts are closely linked and result in a variety of problems, from reduced fertility to death from systemic accumulation of metabolic wastes.

Persistent Hymen

The hymen, which normally covers the opening into the vagina in females that have never been bred, may be retained and so result in vaginitis or failure to breed. Pathogenic organisms may penetrate the cervix and cause infections that may lead to permanent

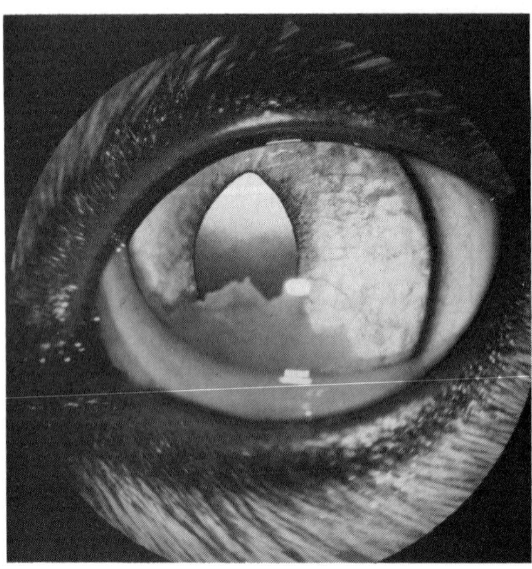

Figure 17. Anterior uveitis in a cat's eye.

sterility. Surgical correction is usually simple and supportive care involves treating any infection with antimicrobials. This can be a problem in maiden mares.

Masculinization in Females

Masculinization of females involves an imbalance of sex hormones. It can occur with male and female twin calves. Masculinization of the heifer calf is caused by the bull calf's sex hormone (testosterone). Such masculinized heifer calves are known as "freemartins." Masculinization can also occur as a side effect of various drugs (*eg,* anabolic steroids) and in some forms of neoplasia (cancer).

Supportive care involves therapeutic use of hormones. Use of estrogen (female hormone) and related compounds, such as diethylstilbestrol (DES), may be helpful but often requires long-term medication to maintain the effect and does not reverse all masculine changes. Surgery may be necessary to remove a masculinizing tumor.

Nymphomania, Satyriasis

Nymphomania and satyriasis refer to an excessive degree of sexual desire in females and males, respectively. They are expressions of abnormally high levels of sex hormones that may come from drug therapy, or ovaries that contain abnormal or cystic follicles. Affected females continually display signs of estrus (heat) and stand for repeated matings. Affected males attempt to copulate excessively or with inappropriate objects (masturbate).

Care involves reducing the level of sex hormone by surgical, mechanical (rupture of cystic follicles) or hormonal means.

Homosexuality

Homosexuality (sexual attraction between animals of the same sex) is "normal" in male populations with limited or no access to females. It is also an expression of dominance between alpha (socially high ranking) males and submissive males. "Bulling" occurs when cows mount each other and is used by herd managers to detect heat. Endocrine disturbances may influence homosexual behavior but are not a consistent cause. Homosexuality in breeding males is undesirable because it leads to a reduced sperm count.

Retained Placenta

The placenta may be retained when the afterbirth does not detach from the uterus during parturition (birth). It may protrude through the cervix or be held in the uterus. Placental retention may result from infection during gestation, scar tissue from a cesarean section, abortion, mummified fetuses (dead, dehydrated and partly resorbed), or poor uterine tone. Natural detachment may occur in a few hours or days, or may be accomplished mechanically (rectally in large animals and surgically in small animals), with infusion of hypertonic solutions of salt, or with hormones (*eg,* oxytocin, estrogen).

Prolonged Gestation

Endocrine imbalances in the dam or fetus can result in an abnormally long gestation period (duration of pregnancy) (breeding date must be known). Other causes include an overly large fetus, fetal death, fetal monstrosities (congenital defects), twinning, and adverse drug reactions.

Supportive care involves isolation of the dam in a comfortable environment similar to that for normal parturition. Often this alone relaxes the dam enough so that parturition occurs without assistance. Use of drugs to induce labor, or cesarean section may be necessary.

False Pregnancy

Pseudocyesis (false pregnancy) is fairly common in the bitch and is often recurrent and associated with endocrine disturbances. The female may display various signs of pregnancy, including a watery (serous), milk-like secretion from the mammae. Affected females often seek isolation, build nests and may "adopt" toys as offspring.

Treatment is normally with ovariohysterectomy (spay) or use of hormones. Mechanically stimulating cats to ovulate to stop a heat cycle frequently results in a false pregnancy.

Vaginal or Uterine Prolapse

Protrusion of the vagina and/or uterus through the vulva usually occurs after dystocia (difficult birth) (Fig 18). Replacing the organs or surgical removal is required.

Supportive care involves keeping the tissue clean and protected. Antimicrobial and antiinflammatory drugs are used during convalescence.

Abortion

Expulsion of a fetus at less than the full term of pregnancy is called abortion. Abortion can be induced with drugs or instruments to terminate any unwanted pregnancy. Abortion may indicate an immunologic incompatibility between the dam and fetus or infection by viral (IBR, BVD), chlamydial (foothills abortion), bacterial

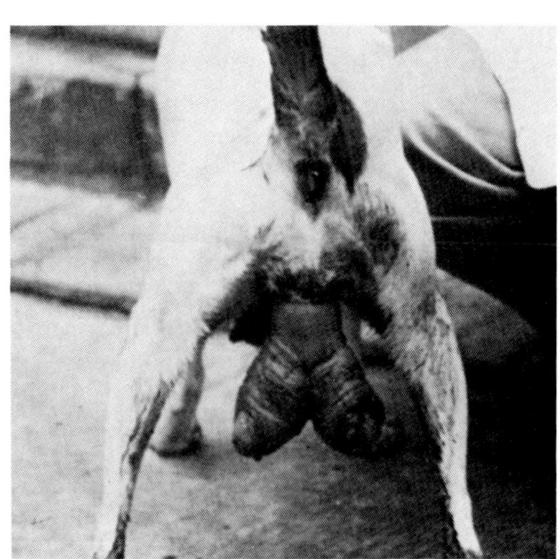

Figure 18. Uterine prolapse in a bitch.

(*Brucella, Campylobacter*) or protozoal (*Toxoplasma*) agents. Toxins and drugs (locoweed, corticosteroids) may also cause abortion. Frequently the cause of an abortion cannot be determined.

Preventive care is aimed at keeping the fetus, if viable, and the mother healthy. The dam may also be isolated, rested and protected from stress. Unless the fetus is close to term, the prognosis for survival is poor.

If an abortion has already occurred, supportive care is directed at returning the uterus to normal, or spaying the animal. Drugs that help clear out the uterus (prostaglandins, oxytocin, estrogen) and antimicrobial therapy may be started.

Savaging of Offspring

In some species the dam (mother) may destroy ill or deformed offspring; however, savaging (attacking and perhaps killing) normal offspring is abnormal and undesirable. It occurs most often with first-time dams. Restraint and mild tranquilizers may quiet the dam, but if the dam still refuses to care for her young, they must be raised as orphans or placed with a foster dam. The dam should be eliminated from the breeding population, unless the reason for the behavior is corrected, or all future offspring fostered.

Mastitis

Mastitis (mammary gland inflammation) is a serious problem in the dairy industry as it reduces profit (loss of milk sales) and can increase death of newborn animals. It is frequently manifested as unusual milk consistency and content (clots, fibrin shreds, mucus) and abnormal color (pinkish, greenish, etc) or odors (ketones).

Causes for mastitis are often related to milking management. Keeping milking machines properly adjusted (correct vacuum and pulse ratios), scrupulous attention to hygiene (use of teat dips, hand washing, etc), and good bedding practices all are necessary to control the primary or secondary microbial invaders of mammary tissue. Trauma is another cause, as from the teeth of the young (milk teeth in piglets) or being trampled. Milk from cows with mastitis is unfit for human consumption. If infectious organisms (*Salmonella,* coliforms, *Staphylococcus*) are present, the milk should not be fed to calves.

Supportive care in mastitis should be directed toward prevention. Repeat infections may occur in a herd as most animals in a given herd are managed similarly. Sanitation, antimicrobial therapy, elimination of irritants and toxins, and use of soothing or cooling applications are beneficial. Damaged mammary glands usually will not produce high levels of milk again, so the animal may have to be culled from the herd.

Penile Problems

Phimosis (inability to extrude the penis from the sheath) or paraphimosis (inability to retract the penis into the sheath) may be caused by penile inflammation (stallion kicked while breeding or dog with fractured os penis), or the opening into the sheath may be too small (pizzle rot of sheep). Inflammation, infection and fly strike (maggots in the sheath) may complicate these problems.

Repeated application of cold packs or soaking the penis in cold water, cleaning the area scrupulously or surgical measures (splitting the sheath) may aid the animal. Paraphimosis is an emergency, as the penis quickly dries and becomes inflamed.

Vulvar Discharges

Discharges from the female reproductive and urinary tract may be normal (during estrus or after parturition) or related to disease. Causes of abnormal vulvar discharges include infection (metritis, vaginitis), tumors and foreign bodies.

Supportive care includes reducing damage to the reproductive tissues with cleansing and disinfecting solutions. Active lesions may be cauterized (chemical or heat) or surgically removed. An infected uterus (metritis, pyometra) can be very toxic to the animal, resulting in kidney damage, shock and death. The best treatment is removal of the uterus (spay).

Udder Edema

Fluid accumulation (edema) in the udder may be caused by ascites (see Digestive Disease), mastitis or a genetic condition. Some females produce milk and develop udder edema before parturition and may have to be milked to reduce the pressure. "Waxing" and "bagging up" are signs of impending foaling.

Other supportive care may include massage, a reduction in fluid intake, use of diuretics to increase urine production and decrease body fluid, and use of corticosteroids to decrease any inflammation.

Agalactia

There are many causes for agalactia (failure to produce milk), including hormonal imbalances, surgery, stress, toxins (ergot), and low blood calcium levels (eclampsia). In some animals (mostly swine), the cause is unknown.

Offspring should be raised as orphans or placed with a foster mother. Nursing and handmilking may encourage milk production, but oxytocin administration has no effect on milk production, only on milk letdown. Hormones that influence milk production may be employed.

Incontinence

Inability to control urination or defecation is called incontinence. The usual sign reported is wet spots where the animal sleeps, but dribbling and dropping feces are also seen.

The causes are varied and in some cases poorly understood. Low levels of estrogen, loss of reflex control of the sphincters (spinal cord damage), masses (tumors) impinging on the bladder, developmental defects or behavior problems are causes.

Supportive care is directed at keeping the diet and fecal and urinary output as normal as possible, modifying inappropriate behavior and providing ample opportunities to void. Debilitated and old animals may lose control of elimination and require nursing care, such as providing deep bedding, frequent turning if recumbent (as often as every 30 minutes), or catheterization. Urine scalding and fly strike often occur, so such animals may need to be euthanized.

Urination Problems

When an animal assumes the posture of urination without producing urine, remains in position long after urine flow has stopped or urinates in appropriate places, there may be a urinary tract infection or obstruction.

In the normal urination posture for horses, the animal presses forward, slightly spreads its legs and either drops its penis (stallions, geldings) or lifts its tail (mares). Mild groaning is not a sign of pain. Recumbent horses do not urinate. Mares in heat urinate frequently and "wink" the vulva.

Normal cows arch their back and draw their legs up under themselves to urinate. Bulls and steers may dribble or produce short pulsations. Cattle are not particular where they urinate and, unlike horses, void while walking, eating or lying down.

Normal sows urinate in a posture similar to that of cows, but young pigs and boars may pulse or spray urine to the right or left.

Normal cats squat to urinate, though sexually active males and females may spray urine behind them to mark objects (Fig 19). The tail quivers and the hind legs tread up and down during spraying.

Female dogs also squat to urinate, but void only small volumes each time if they are in estrus. Adult male dogs raise one leg to direct a stream of urine against an object. Male puppies squat, but as they mature, gradually begin to lift their legs (males neutered early may always squat to urinate).

Causes for unusual urination behavior include cystitis (bladder infection), calculi (stones) or tumors blocking the urinary tract, and kidney disease (nephritis, renal failure). Additional causes or contributing factors include a high-mineral diet, use of certain drugs (cyclophosphamide) and various developmental anomalies (patent urachus in foals).

Treatment involves ensuring urination by catheterization, cystocentesis or surgical correction of the cause, and maintaining the animal with an appropriate diet and/or IV fluid administration.

Figure 19. Spraying of urine by male cats is genetically based behavior, the expression of which is influenced by numerous stimuli. (Courtesy of *California Veterinarian*)

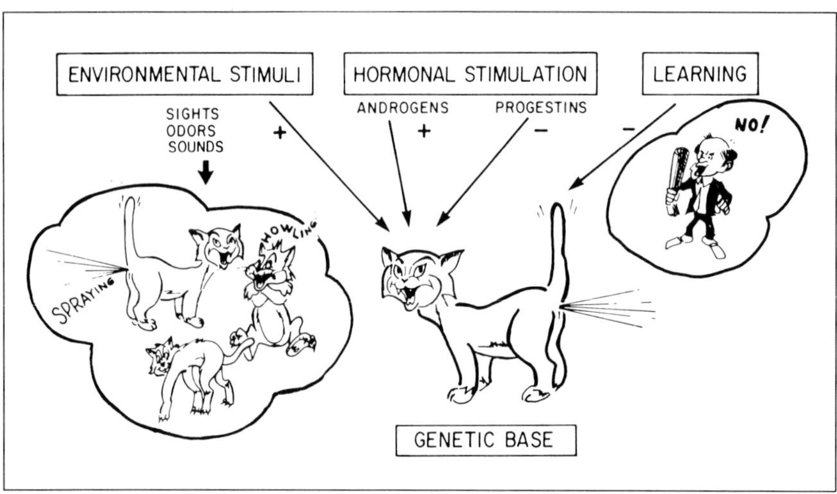

Polyuria

An increased volume of urine (polyuria) or frequency of urination may signal a problem. Urine production normally reflects fluid intake; however, regardless of fluid intake, diuretics and some diseases can cause polyuria, including diabetes (insipidus or mellitus), and renal, liver, adrenal, uterine or thyroid disease.

Supportive care is directed toward balancing body fluids, electrolytes and pH. Any losses of protein (albuminuria) and glucose (glycosuria) are also considered in selecting treatment. Maintaining hydration and meeting caloric requirements may be difficult in patients losing protein or glucose.

Anuria

Anuria (lack of urine production) and oliguria (production of only a small volume of highly concentrated urine) are caused by dehydration or low renal blood flow (perfusion) due to heart failure, shock, acidosis (excessive levels of acids), hyperkalemia (high blood levels of potassium) and a variety of infections. Obstructions in the urinary system can cause renal failure if not corrected rapidly (Figs 20, 21). Accumulation of waste products in the blood (urea, creatinine, etc) causes toxic signs, such as vomiting and diarrhea (uremic syndrome).

Supportive care depends on the duration and severity of the problem. Acute episodes can usually be managed by providing wholesome drinking water and use of diuretics. Chronic cases may require extended, aggressive fluid therapy and dialysis or surgical measures. If anuria is related to severe kidney damage, euthanasia may be the only option.

Abnormal Urine

Red to brown urine may be caused by the presence of whole RBCs, hemoglobin or the muscle pigment, myoglobin (Monday morning sickness in horses).

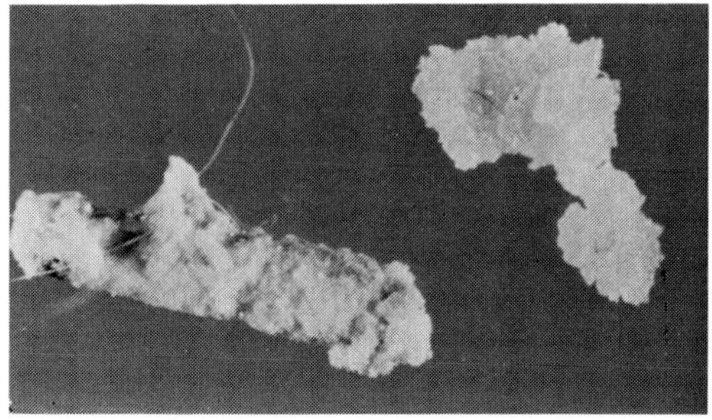

Figure 20. Obstructive debris removed from the distal urethra of a male cat with the feline urologic syndrome.

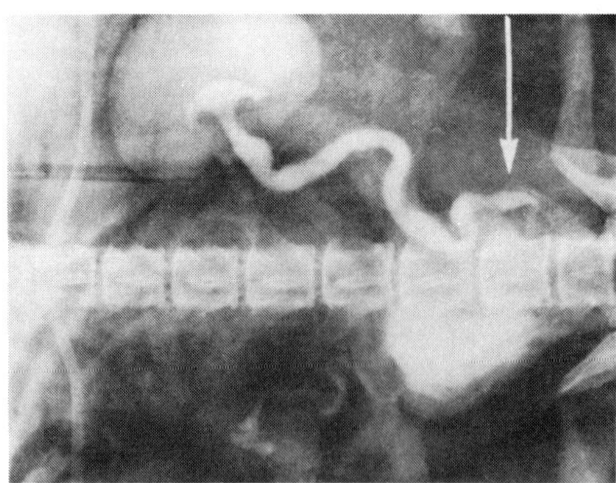

Figure 21. Urogram (contrast radiograph) in a dog reveals a distended ureter, obstructed by a ureteral calculus (arrow).

Because normal urine may turn brown (horse) or cloudy upon standing at room (or lower) temperature, gross observations should be made on freshly voided urine. Some drugs (methylene blue, epinephrine) cause production of colored or highly concentrated urine that appears cloudy. Mucus and excessive numbers of cells (WBCs in bladder infections) result in thick, translucent urine.

Supportive care involves maintaining urine output and hydration status. Antimicrobial drugs may be given, but long-term use may allow resistant organisms to overgrow.

Alimentary Tract Disease

Failure To Eat

Failure to eat is a common sign of digestive tract disease and results in progressive starvation. It may be caused by dental problems (sharp teeth, teething, misalignment, etc), anorexia (inappetence), foreign objects, pain or systemic diseases.

Supportive care involves management of any wounds, correcting dental problems, providing a soft, palatable diet, appetite stimulation, and general attention to the animal's overall health (parasite control, foot care, etc). Forced feeding is often used; however, if vomiting occurs, it may be necessary to use IV feedings.

Dysphagia

Dysphagia (failure to swallow) may be a signal of paralysis of the throat caused by nerve damage, infectious disease (rabies) or poisoning. It also is associated with pharyngeal and/or esophageal trauma caused by foreign objects or caustic chemicals (*eg,* bone slivers, lye) and may produce excessive salivation. Animals with suspected infectious disease should be quarantined for observation.

Failure To Ruminate

Failure to ruminate ("make cud") is cause for concern in any mature ruminant. Various drugs, infection, foreign bodies, bloat, milk fever (hypocalcemia), ketosis or GI obstruction can reduce rumination. Ingestion of low-fiber feeds lowers the frequency of rumen contraction but does not totally eliminate rumination.

Supportive care involves meeting fluid and energy needs, and correcting any deficits in muscle activity with drugs. Transfaunation, usually done after antimicrobial therapy or starvation has killed off the normal rumen flora, involves transferring rumen contents or a cud from a normal animal to the nonruminating patient. Once the microflora in the rumen return to normal, the rumen resumes its role in digestion. Increases in digestible protein and energy in the feed should be considered in long-term management of poor rumen activity.

Regurgitation and Vomiting

Vomiting (expulsion of stomach contents) can be caused by GI inflammation, infection or obstruction, uremia, motion sickness, and a variety of other conditions. Vomiting is preceded by retching, whereas regurgitation is not. Continual vomiting results in alkalosis, dehydration and electrolyte imbalances. Regurgitation (expulsion of undigested food) may be caused by esophageal malformation or stricture and neurologic damage. Inhalation pneumonia is often a result, particularly in comatose ruminants that are recumbent.

Supportive care is directed at stopping the losses of body fluids and electrolytes, and compensating for the lack of nutrition. Protectants (Kao-Pectate, Pepto-Bismol), antiemetics and lubricants (for hairballs) may be used to soothe gut tissues. Activated charcoal may be given to adsorb toxins. Because vomiting is an early sign of many infectious diseases, the animal should be monitored for other signs of disease.

Bloat

Bloat is distention of the GI tract with gas and is caused by excessive gas production or an inability to eructate (belch). Ruminal tympany (bloat) is common in ruminants on lush spring pastures or in some feedlot operations.

Monogastric animals (nonruminants) can become bloated when the gut twists (torsion) or telescopes back on itself (intussusception), allowing accumulation of gas and causing great pain.

Prevention of bloat involves prefeeding animals turned out to pasture, limiting access to grain or water, top-dressing rations with oils and feeding antifoaming agents (poloxalene). A plastic one-way valve can be placed in the rumen of chronically affected animals to allow gas to escape.

In nonruminants, avoiding heavy meals before strenuous exercise, good parasite control and soaking dry feeds with water help prevent GI distention.

Maldigestion

Maldigestion, manifested as recognizable food material in feces, results in poor feed efficiency, malnutrition, and poor growth rates or performance. Unground or otherwise unprocessed grains are found in the feces of normal animals, but passage of normally easily digested materials (meat fiber, starches, etc) signals a problem. Hypermotility of the gut is a common cause and may be associated with toxins, infections (*eg,* parvovirus infection), parasitism (*eg,* coccidiosis) or allergy.

Supportive care involves meeting the animal's caloric and nutrient requirements, generally by IV. Adequate water and electrolyte balance is critical as usually the patient has been off food and water for a day or more. Protection of the gut and reducing hypermotility are primary goals. Frequently feeding small amounts of high-quality food may help restore normal gut activity. The normal microbacterial population may be augmented by feeding yogurt or a commercial bacterial culture (some are freeze dried). Long-term use of digestive enzymes may be needed in some cases.

Malabsorption

Malabsorption has many characteristics of maldigestion. Food is digested but the nutrients are not absorbed from the gut, resulting in progressive loss of weight, condition and performance. Signs of malabsorption are a foul fecal odor, fat, mucus or glycogen in the stool, and unusually colored feces. Causes of malabsorption include bile duct obstruction, allergies, a poor diet and chronic intoxications (paint, molds, etc). Some changes in gut thickness caused by inflammation, tumors or other diseases can also affect absorption.

Treatment is often only supportive. The animal's nutritional needs must be met, usually by artificial means, until the problem is resolved. Predigested foods, digestive enzymes (trypsin, etc) and vitamin-mineral supplements are used when indicated.

Ascites

Ascites (accumulation of fluid in the peritoneal cavity) is seen in a variety of disorders and is usually a sign of an underlying problem in fluid balance. Hypoproteinemia, electrolyte imbalances, infection, toxic conditions (endotoxic shock, etc), migration of parasite larvae, congestive heart failure (from stenosis myopathy, anemia, etc), neoplasia, trauma and septicemia (bacteria in the blood) are common causes of ascites. Overtransfusion or overhydration is usually noted first as pulmonary edema but may subsequently cause ascites.

Supportive care involves maintaining hydration while preserving the osmotic balance between the tissues, body cavities and vessel spaces. Blood protein levels and the PCV can be monitored and fluids and/or colloids given accordingly. Removing fluid can be stressful because of protein and electrolyte loss and may not be useful if the underlying cause of fluid formation is not corrected.

Flatulence

Excessive gas in the GI tract (flatulence) can be rather uncomfortable but is rarely of concern. It is caused by feeding highly fermentable feed or upsets in the intestinal microbial populations. Bicarbonates in feed can increase intestinal gas production.

Management is directed at a gradual diet change, feeding bacterial cultures, such as yogurt, and use of certain drugs.

Diarrhea

Diarrhea (abnormally frequent defecation or abnormally liquid feces) can be caused by inflammation (enteritis, gastritis, etc), infection, parasitism (hookworms, coccidia, strongyles, etc), allergies (*eg,* milk) and irritants. A variety of drugs and toxins adversely affect the gut, including lead, bacterial enterotoxins (*eg,* from *Clostridium perfringens*), digitalis and some antibiotics (tetracycline, ampicillin, neomycin), as they kill normal gut flora.

Abnormal stool color may be caused by feed additives (*eg,* artificial colors in some pet foods), drugs, bile, GI bleeding, and some diseases (*eg,* pancreatitis may cause tan stools). Normal neonatal (newborn) animals may have a yellow to orange stool.

Supportive care starts with replacing the fluids and nutrients lost from the intestine. Mild diarrhea may resolve when food intake is reduced or eliminated for 8-48 hours to rest the gut. Increasing the dry matter content of the feed may aid long-term management of diarrhea. More severe or chronic cases may require a complete evaluation of the animal's condition, as diarrhea is often secondary to other problems. Anticholinergic drugs (Lomotil, atropine) or manipulation of the microflora (with antibiotics, antifermentives or live cultures) have been used with mixed success. In many cases, continuous use of protectants and absorbents is impractical for chronic care. Use of bland diets (Hill's i/d or rice, cottage cheese and chicken mixtures) after the intestine has been rested and then gradually returning the animal to normal feed are most often successful. Feline idiopathic bowel disease is a frequent cause of chronic or intermittent diarrhea in cats. It is treated with sulfasalazine or prednisolone.

Anal Irritation

"Scooting," or rubbing and licking the anus, is often caused by distention of the anal sacs under the skin, on either side of the anus, in dogs and cats. *Oxyuris equi,* the equine pinworm, can cause mild anal irritation and provoke tail rubbing. Diarrhea can cause anal irritation but does not last long after defecation. Some animals scoot anytime they feel something touching the anus, such as tapeworm segments or grass.

Supportive care is limited to care of the perianal region, including cleansing and lubricating, emptying the anal sacs, and increasing the roughage content in the diet of affected dogs and cats. Horses with pinworms should be dewormed. Surgical intervention may be needed to remove anal sacs, obstructions, serious impactions and tumors (Fig 22).

Constipation

Constipation (infrequent or difficult passage of dry feces) is frequently accompanied by straining (tenesmus). The posture of the animal may be the same as in animals with cystitis. Causes of constipation include dehydration, gut hypomotility (slow rate of fecal passage), or bowel obstruction. Meconium (first stool of neonates) impaction, especially in foals, may necessitate use of enemas to clear the bowel. Other causes of constipation are use of certain drugs (diuretics, anticholinergics), toxins (*eg,* nightshade), diet and intestinal problems (colic). Some house-trained dogs become constipated if confined in a cage for long periods.

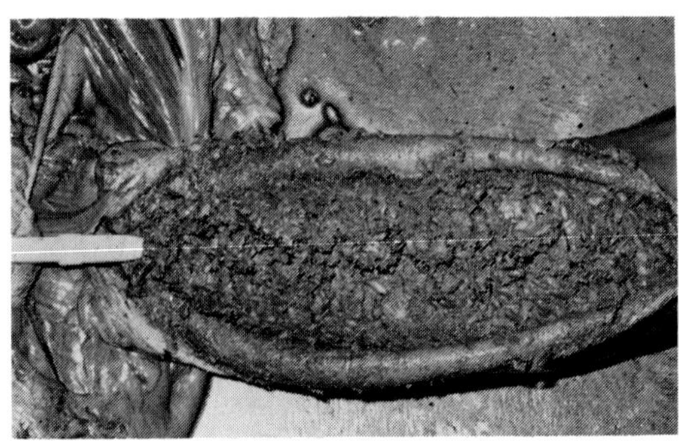

Figure 22. Intestinal impaction in a horse, caused by ground corn cobs.

Treatment of constipation may require long-term care. Changes in feed (type, amount of moisture) and feeding frequency may be helpful.

Agents that promote evacuation of the bowel include Epsom salt, phenolphthalein, bran, soapy water, mineral oil and petroleum jelly.

Mechanical removal of stools per rectum, colotomy (colonic surgery), anorectal massage, stool softeners, and repeated enemas may be necessary in severe cases. Some enema compounds liquefy the feces by drawing water from the body causing dehydration. Therefore, ask the doctor before selecting an enema solution.

Skin Disease

The largest organ in the body is also the most easily observed, accounting for the high number of skin conditions treated. The skin reflects both the general state of health (glossy, plush coat over supple, flexible skin) and specific disease processes. Some infectious diseases cause specific skin lesions (*eg,* diamond-shaped lesions in swine erysipelas), but most cause nonspecific lesions. The skin is covered with opportunistic organisms that, upon injury to the skin, can gain entry to deeper tissues to cause infection and further irritation.

Pruritus

Pruritus (itchiness) is usually a sign of inflammation but also may be behavioral in origin. It can be caused by allergies (flea-allergy dermatitis) or central nervous system disorders (scrapie of sheep).

Supportive care involves use of antiparasitics, soothing baths, soaks, flushes or topical medication (lotions, salves). Reducing the perception of itchiness with drugs (narcotics, sedatives) helps prevent self-trauma but may mask a systemic problem. Injectable and oral antiinflammatories, such as prednisolone, are commonly used in treating pruritic skin conditions.

Eruptions

Any change in surface skin may be considered an eruption, including blisters (vesicles), crusts (scabs), abscesses (pustules), masses (warts) or fluid pockets (hematomas, seromas). Each eruption should be classified as to the area affected and extent, and this information added to that obtained from the history and physical examination.

Causes of eruptions include allergy (fleas, bee sting, plants) hormonal imbalances (hypothyroidism), infections (foot and mouth disease, erysipelas), autoimmune disease, chemical irritations (battery acid), parasites (bots, mites, warbles), photosensitivity (phenothiazines) and acne (Fig 23).

Supportive care is directed at removing the cause and symptomatic treatment, such as removing hair, debriding and flushing or bathing. Various drugs (antihistamines, antiinflammatories, antibacterials, antifungals) are used for specific skin disorders. Surgical, chemical or thermal (cautery, cryosurgery) removal of affected tissue may be necessary.

Alopecia

Alopecia (hair loss) is a common problem in animals. The causes are sometimes obscure, but infections (ringworm, bacteria), parasites (fleas, mites, ticks), toxins (heavy metals, molds) and nutritional deficiencies may be involved (Fig 24). Bored or stressed dogs or cats often groom themselves excessively, causing hair loss.

Supportive care may include a dietary change, medicated baths and drug therapy (parasiticides, corticosteroids). Application of bad-tasting compounds, restraint collars and behavioral modification may also be tried.

CARE OF OLD OR DEBILITATED ANIMALS

Senile changes (changes associated with aging) involve all body systems. Specific changes in the function of the nervous system in-

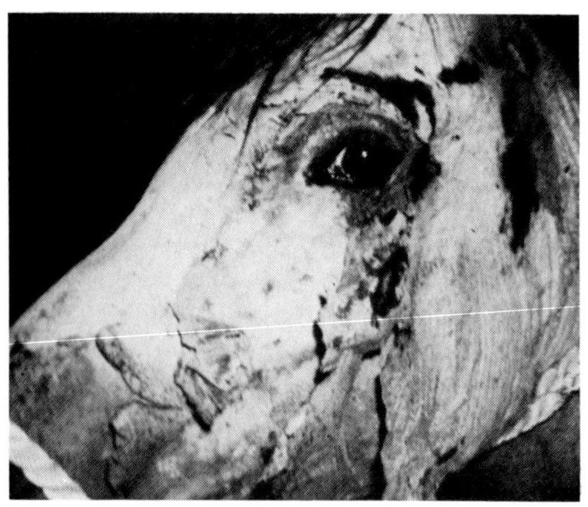

Figure 23. Sloughing of skin in a horse with severe photosensitization.

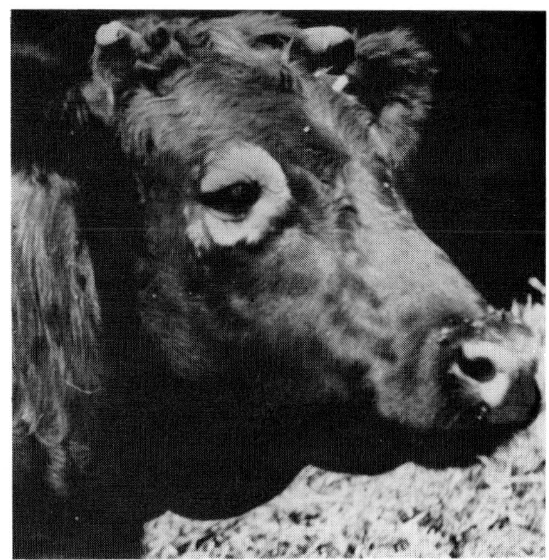

Figure 24. Ringworm lesions around the eye of a steer.

clude reduced sensation (taste, smell, sight), altered sleep patterns, and reduced intelligence and coordination. Changes in the pulmonary and cardiovascular systems reduce pulmonary gas exchange and perfusion, vascular elasticity and cardiac output. Control of blood pH, renal filtration and liver function may also be impaired. In the GI tract, the ability to digest proteins and absorb calcium is reduced. Metabolic changes hinder the animal's ability to respond to its environment and to resist disease. This is most evident in the immune system, in which impaired function results in an increased incidence of neoplasia and reduced resistance to infection.

Activity decreases with age due to reduced musculoskeletal function. Moderate exercise is beneficial as it slows senile changes and increases longevity. Because older patients do not adapt to environmental changes as well as younger animals, their environmental temperature and humidity should be kept within the optimum range. The decline in the appearance of some old animals may decrease the amount of attention they receive and can result in personality changes. Owners should be advised to make play and affection time available to old animals that are dependent on them.

Debilitated and aged animals have many similar needs. A balance should be struck between the patient's need for rest and its requirement for exercise. Both are necessary and movement of body parts is essential, even if it is passive physical therapy (see Chapter 4). Pain relief aids healing and rehabilitation and should be provided from a humanitarian viewpoint. Bedding should be thick and clean. Frequent turning is necessary for recumbent animals, and the environment comfortable and draft free. Most debilitated animals require extra warmth. In debilitated cats and dogs, reduced grooming can cause flea numbers to increase, further stressing the weakened animal.

Because debilitated animals may refuse to eat their usual ration, increasing the palatability (top-dressing hay with molasses or adding flavoring agents) and aroma (adding onion or garlic) of their feed may stimulate their appetite. The ration should be nutritious, easy to digest and geared to the patient's special needs. Geriatric animals should have a diet with high-quality protein and increased calcium content. Fluid and electrolyte levels should be monitored carefully, as debilitated animals rarely drink adequate amounts. Special diets may be needed if kidney or heart function is impaired.

Moistening the ration can aid both food and water intake. Supplemental forced feedings may be required in some cases. Because debilitated or geriatric animals may lose control of urination and defecation, they may require assistance in the form of support while defecating or urinating, genital massages, catheterization, enemas, frequent changes of bedding and bathing. Many aged animals build up tartar on their teeth at an accelerated rate and may also require frequent claw or hoof trimming.

The result of nursing care can vary from prolonging the life of a terminally ill animal to complete rehabilitation and a return to normal health. The expectations for each animal must be realistic. Success may depend upon the quality of care given and the communication between the veterinarian and owner or attendant. Often the owner is in a better position to provide intensive nursing for a debilitated animal than is a technician. Also, the curative power of the bond of trust and affection between the owner and animal cannot be underrated. Cats particularly respond well to nursing care in their own home.

Death and Dying

Death is the final equalizer for all things. Rarely does one body system dictate an animal's life span. Rather, there seems to be a "concerto of decline" in which all systems play a part. Theories of aging hypothesize a gradual accumulation of toxins (free radicals, dimers, autoantibodies) or mutations, or a depletion of essential substances (hormones, etc) that causes the body to decline. Each body system has limits beyond which it cannot compensate and begins to fail.

Death must be dealt with on a clinical and personal level. There are times when euthanasia is the most loving and responsible decision. In food animal production, death is a prerequisite to human consumption. We have a humane obligation to see that the animal dies quickly, with a minimum of pain. Methods that destroy the brain or its communication with the environment have maintained their "popularity" in capital punishment of criminals and should be the yardstick to judge the "relative experience" of dying. The method used to kill food animals depends on what product the animal's body will produce (*eg,* meat), as food products cannot be contaminated with toxins. Pets should have a quiet, dignified death.

Euthanasia is the painless, merciful killing of terminally ill, injured or unwanted animals, usually with lethal injections. Because there is no use for the body of an animal killed by injection (except where a rendering plant can make fertilizer or meat and bone meal), the bodies of most euthanized animals are buried or cremated.

Food animals are usually slaughtered, after stunning, by shooting (often with a captive-bolt device), CO_2 gas, electrocution, or with a blunt instrument (hammer, etc). Killing after stunning involves exsanguination (bleeding out) by cutting the major vessels in the throat. The animals are often blinded with bright light so they cannot see the hand of the stunner. In certain religious communities (Jewish, Islamic), unstunned animals must be exsanguinated and the kill must be supervised or carried out by a designated person. The carcass is then inspected for wholesomeness.

Grief

In companion animal practice, the technician may be required to deal with the client's grief and bereavement after loss of a pet. The overt expression of the love, fear, guilt, anger and suspicion that accompanies a pet's death or terminal illness is often embarrassing to all concerned. The technician should take steps to legitimize the client's feelings, as they are a healthy expression of the emotional bond with a pet.

Client response to a pet's death may vary from "It's only a cat," to threats of suicide. Denial of death (or impending death) is the first step and may be a protective mechanism for the owner. The client may insist that there has been some error and that the animal is not dying or dead. In some cases, the animal may have to be discharged from the hospital to give the owner time to accept the situation. Going along with the idea that an error might have been made regarding the severity of the pet's condition may give the client time to accept the situation.

Anger often replaces denial and may be expressed toward himself/herself, the doctor, the technician or other members of the client's family. This anger is often unjustified and is frequently followed (sometimes much later) by an apology, "I just lost my head for a time."

The third stage of grief is the verbal or physical expression of the loss or impending loss. This process may be smoothed by enlisting the owner's help in caring for the pet or with explanations of the animal's condition.

Resolution is the final stage, a kind of "positive submission" to the fact of death in which an inner peace and serenity complete the pattern of loss and allow healing of the emotional scars. The memory remains but the pain subsides. Condolence notes and calls can do much to further the resolution of grief so that the client is free to love another pet.

QUARANTINE

Controlling contagious disease by enforced isolation (quarantine) of animals, goods, supplies, property or people is part of state and federal law. Enforcement is charged to the sheriff or militia (National Guard). This is the only time, other than during a war or other major disturbance, when personal and civil rights can be suspended in America. The state veterinarian acts as judge, jury and executor to limit the freedom and disposition (condemnation, etc) of animals. The purpose of quarantine is to reduce exposure to disease, eliminate certain infections and preserve public health and safety. Providing quality animal products (meat, milk, fertilizer), preserving profits for food producers and reducing animal suffering and stress are additional goals.

Prevention of disease and the spread of disease (prophylaxis) can be greatly assisted by the technician. Places where animals congregate, such as race tracks, shows, parks, animal shelters and veterinary hospitals, tend to become sources of infectious diseases. Veterinary hospitals and many producers use large amounts of antibiotics that may encourage the growth of resistant pathogens. Vaccination, isolation of new or sick animals, and good hygiene practices are the foundations of animal health and husbandry.

Quarantine Procedures

Animals and people can be protected from infection by a variety of methods, depending upon the disease(s) and the species involved. Many diseases are species specific, so moving animals of a different species into an area of microbial contamination may be acceptable. Most animals diseases are no risk to people, but some are common to people and animals (zoonotic), such as salmonellosis, rabies and ringworm.

Some infections require only standard medical nursing to control, as they are not contagious. Diseases that are difficult to transfer (*eg,* botulism, histoplasmosis) can be treated without isolation of infected animals. Some conditions diagnosed by response to therapy must be treated as suspect infections until the final diagnosis is made.

When a potentially contagious disease occurs, isolation is an effective means of control. The period of quarantine may be defined legally, as in rabies, or established by the veterinarian through testing or experience with the disease. Sometimes animals may safely be returned to the group when clinical signs are no longer seen. Most veterinary hospitals are excellent quarantine areas as they are equipped to deal with disinfection. Moving healthy animals to a clean area and keeping infected ones confined in the area of outbreak help control disease spread, assuming that no currently healthy animals are harboring or just developing infection.

Test and slaughter is a more radical form of preventing spread of some very serious diseases. In this method, all animals in a suspect area are tested. Infected animals are slaughtered so healthy individuals cannot be exposed. Test and slaughter is effective and is practiced routinely with brucellosis, tuberculosis, feline leukemia virus infection and other diseases. It has been responsible for elimination or near elimination of several serious diseases. Owners of economically important animals are compensated for the loss of animals (market price).

Control of highly infectious diseases necessitates drastic measures, such as the destruction of any animal that has potentially been exposed. Eradication campaigns have been waged successfully in this country against foot and mouth disease and hog cholera. Though thousands of animals in a given area may be killed, protection of millions more justifies the method.

Milk and Meat Inspection

Meat inspection is also a form of disease control, as it maintains the wholesomeness of the food supply by preventing the spread of zoonoses and residues of harmful substances. Veterinary inspectors control the use of animal parts by condemning, diverting for nonfood use (rendering), or passing for alternative food use any part or all of a carcass.

The inspection starts with preslaughter observation of live animals. Any showing signs of disease may be held for observation or rejected. After slaughter, the internal organs are palpated or sectioned and visually inspected for abnormalities. Milk is tested for residues of drugs and numbers of cells or bacteria.

Carcass Disposal

Disposing of hazardous materials, such as contaminated bedding, bandages and carcasses, is of utmost importance in control of infectious diseases.

Toxic materials (heavy metals, pollutants, radioactive material) must be handled by toxic waste management authorities. Infectious wastes may be cremated, buried where the animal died (if this does not pollute water or soil) or turned over to a licensed rendering agent. If the dead animal must be moved, the carcass must be elevated from the ground during carcass removal to prevent a trail of contamination. Any contaminated bedding or soil should be saturated with oil and burned or turned under deeply. In some diseases (anthrax, vesicular stomatitis, exanthema), bodies must be buried with lime (though there is little evidence that this controls infection) or handled in specific ways established by law (Fig 25).

Disinfection of Contaminated Premises

Contaminated barns, buildings, pastures and equipment used on infected animals must be made safe for susceptible animals. All litter, feces and other debris are removed. Then, the area is thoroughly swept, controlling dust with moisture. After all surfaces are cleaned with steam, detergents and scrubbing, disinfectant solutions (2% lye, phenolics, formalin, etc) are applied. Drainage of wash water must be considered. New bedding or soil (placed over plastic sheeting) is brought in to replace what is removed. All utensils, tools and feed or watering apparatus must be scrubbed and disinfected. Chlorine solutions (1:20) in water are effective against many infectious agents.

Figure 25. Cattle exposed to foot and mouth disease were slaughtered and burned during an outbreak in England in 1967-68.

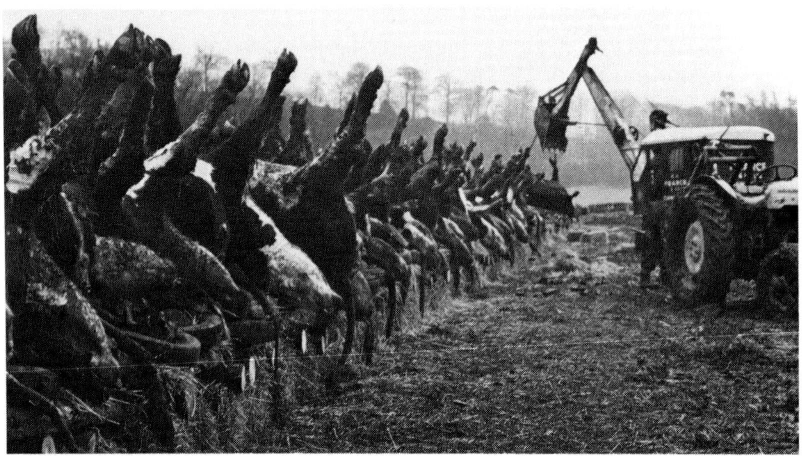

In-Hospital Isolation

Hospitalized animals with, or suspected of having, a contagious disease should be isolated from other animals within the hospital to prevent spread of the disease. The isolation unit should be completely separate from areas where other animals are housed and the air supply should not mix with that of the rest of the hospital.

Technicians should care for the isolated animals after other patients. A separate set of coveralls or change of clothing should be available in each isolation unit. Clothing should be laundered regularly and not allowed to contact other animals. Rubber boots must be worn in stalls or kennels and thoroughly scrubbed and disinfected between uses. Boots must be clean before most disinfectants are effective. Disposable or sterilizable bedding, litter boxes, feeding supplies, and food and water containers should be used. Paper towels for handwashing and cleaning are helpful.

No visitors should be allowed into the isolation unit. Disease vectors, such as flies and mice, should be eliminated from the isolation unit. All cleaning must be done with a wet mop, cloth or sponge to prevent spread of disease through contaminated dust. Cages should be carefully disinfected regularly and all bedding and disposable equipment burned or tightly bagged. Reusable equipment must be autoclaved or otherwise sterilized before other animals come into contact with it.

Technicians should wash their hands, arms and other contaminated body surfaces before and after entry to the isolation unit. Between occupants, all surfaces in the isolation unit must be cleaned and sprayed with an appropriate disinfectant (not all organisms are killed by a single disinfectant).

INFECTIOUS DISEASES

An infectious disease is one that can be transmitted from one animal to another. Contagious diseases are infectious diseases spread by direct contact between animals. Additional means of disease transmission include fomites (inanimate objects that carry microorganisms), food, water, soil, air, etc. Infectious diseases may be caused by bacteria, viruses, protozoa, rickettsiae, mycoplasmids, molds, yeast, helminths (worms) or arthropods.

Whether an animal becomes sick or not depends upon its resistance to disease, the virulence (potency) of the microorganism, number of invading organisms, route of infection, ability of the pathogen (disease-causing agent) to propagate in tissues, and the formation of toxins. The animal's response to the pathogen is manifested as fever, anorexia and various other clinical signs. Some diseases have characteristic signs, whereas others produce nonspecific signs and must be recognized by other means (*eg,* laboratory tests, exploratory surgery). The disease may last for only hours (peracute), through days (acute), to years (chronic).

Animals may clear their bodies of a pathogen and become immune or susceptible to reinfection, harbor the disease at low levels and reactivate the infection at a later date (latent infection), or appear recovered but shed the organism and infect other animals (carrier infection).

Bacterial Infections

Bacteria are very small (the oil-immersion objective must be used to see them with a microscope), one-celled organisms with a less complex cellular structure than either plants or animals. They can be motile (capable of movement) or nonmotile, and require either O_2 (aerobic) or lack of O_2 (anaerobic) for growth. Because they multiply by cell division, signs of infection usually take some time to appear, unless a toxin is present, such as botulinus toxin. The virulence of bacteria varies greatly; most do not cause disease.

Living organisms have good defenses against bacterial invasion, including antibody production (large molecules that enhance or activate internal defenses) and phagocytosis by WBCs (engulfing and destroying the organism). However, some bacteria can circumvent these mechanisms. Good vaccines are available to protect against many bacterial pathogens (bacterins) and toxins (toxoids). Many effective antibacterial drugs (antibiotics, disinfectants) are now in common use.

Bacterial infections may be spread through the blood (bacteremia or septicemia), or may be localized to a tissue or organ. Bacterial diseases are not as specific regarding host and target tissue (area of the body primarily affected) as viral infections.

A classification scheme has been developed to separate one type of bacterium from another as an aid in recognition of pathogens and their association with specific diseases.

Bacteria are grouped by shape (rod, spiral, sphere) and by Gram-staining reaction (blue indicates Gram positive, pink indicates Gram negative). Many bacteria growing in a clump make a visible spot (colony) on culture media and may be classified by colony morphology (appearance) and reactions with various types of media, stains, chemicals, etc. Because many bacteria are similar, multiple tests are usually required to distinguish them.

Gram-Negative Bacteria

Pseudomonas: This motile, rod-shaped organism (bacillus) is usually involved in suppurative (pus-forming) processes. The pus is frequently greenish and has a sweetish odor. It is an opportunist that invades after other processes have impaired body defenses.

Diseases caused by *Pseudomonas* include green wool, rhinitis and pneumonia in swine, abscesses, bovine mastitis, genital infections, otitis in dogs, respiratory disease in horses, and cystitis in small animals.

Supportive care involves debridement (excision of dead tissue) of infected areas and use of topical or systemic antibiotics. Because *Pseudomonas* can cause endocarditis, meningitis, pneumonia and otitis in people, especially if they are immunosuppressed or taking antibiotics to which the organism is resistant, latex gloves should be worn when handling infected tissue or debris.

Escherichia coli: This organism is a normal inhabitant of the large intestine of all mammals. It varies from a short, plump rod to filamentous in form. Certain strains are enteropathogenic (capable of causing intestinal disease) due to a toxin found in them (enterotoxin). These strains are usually species specific and cause disease in young animals. Signs of *E coli* infection include anorexia, diarrhea, fever and depression. The organism causes edema and death in pigs, mastitis in cattle, abortions in horses and septicemia in neonatal (newborn) animals. Supportive care includes good hygiene to reduce the number of organisms to which the animal is exposed (fecal contamination), and antibiotic and fluid therapy. Some vaccines are available.

Salmonella: This organism is a short rod with a variety of serotypes (subspecies classification based on surface structure of the organism) that may or may not be species specific. Young and stressed animals are more prone to infection than others. Disease usually occurs from fecal contamination and is often an enteric (intestinal) infection but may become generalized with septicemia and internal abscesses. Salmonellosis is a highly contagious disease that is hard to eliminate once animal quarters are contaminated. Supportive care includes quarantine of infected animals, use of scrupulous hygiene and antibiotic and fluid therapy. In some cases, a vaccine may be available.

Hemophilus: This bacterium is a small or medium-sized, filamentous or pleomorphic (variable shapes in one microscopic field) bacillus (rod). It typically infects the mucous membranes and usually only causes disease when the animal's resistance to infection is decreased, resulting in genital (horses), respiratory (swine) and CNS (cattle) diseases. Vaccination and antibiotic therapy are used in prevention and treatment, respectively.

Pasteurella: This small, ovoid rod often stains lighter in the center than at each end. The organisms are carried as normal flora of the mouth and throat and can cause disease when the animal is stressed. General signs may include fever, respiratory distress, edema, hemorrhages on membranes, and fluid in body cavities. *Pasteurella* is a common cause of abscesses in cats and severe mastitis in sheep. Many cases in people result from animal bites. Such bite wounds are slow to heal and have a watery discharge. Bacteremia and CNS and respiratory infections may also occur in people. Treatment includes use of antibiotics, such as penicillin, and vaccination with a bacterin.

Bordetella: This organism is a motile rod that is an important contributor to bronchopneumonia after viral infection (*eg,* kennel cough, canine distemper) and atrophic rhinitis in pigs. Culling of carrier animals in swine herds, vaccination, administration of serum from immune animals, and antibiotic therapy are all involved in treatment.

Moraxella bovis: This organism is a short, curved rod found in pairs. It causes pinkeye in cattle, which starts as simple conjunctivitis that may progress to blindness. Supportive care involves vaccination, use of ophthalmic preparations, and minimizing such predisposing causes as dust and bright sunlight.

Actinobacillus: These pleomorphic organisms are found in small granules in pus from infected areas. They are part of the normal mouth flora of sheep and cattle but can form large abscesses in soft tissue when introduced into deep oral tissue (foreign body penetration often introduces them). These masses often occur in the tongue (wooden tongue) but can form in the limbs and internal organs. The bacteria also cause bacteremia in foals and young pigs. Treatment involves use of a systemic iodine compound and antibiotics.

Fusobacterium and Bacteroides: These bacteria are anaerobes and are differentiated by gas chromatographic analysis. *Fusobacterium* normally occurs as long rods, invades damaged tissue and causes necrosis, abscesses and a foul odor. It invades the liver, mouth and throat of young calves (calf diphtheria), as well as the udder, rumen wall and hooves of adults. Sulfonamides may be an effective treatment.

Bacteroides is also involved in "foot rot" (paronychia) in cattle and sheep, and may be the primary disease agent. Supportive care includes paring the hoof to expose diseased tissues to O_2, use of a topical antibiotic or disinfectant foot dip (*eg,* formalin), and vaccination.

Gram-Positive Bacteria

Staphylococcus: These cocci (spherical shape) are found arranged in grape-like clusters (in a fluid culture they may be single, in short chains or small groups). They are very resistant to drying, heat and disinfectants, and thus are often responsible for infections acquired in hospitals (nosocomial). They can be carried as normal flora of skin and mucous membranes of people and animals.

Staphylococci produce many extracellular toxins (exotoxins) and enzymes damaging to cells. Infections caused by *Staphylococcus* include many suppurative diseases, such as mastitis, equine botryomycosis, eye infections, canine pyoderma, urinary tract infections and greasy pig disease. Supportive care involves flushing of lesions if possible and antibiotic therapy based upon sensitivity test results, as many of these organisms are resistant to common antibiotics and disinfectants.

Streptococcus: These bacteria arrange themselves in chains of various lengths. They are found on mucous membranes and are opportunistic invaders. Frequently appearing in milk and milk products, they cause suppurative diseases of the udder, umbilicus, CNS, respiratory tract, uterus and joints. *Streptococcus* causes equine and porcine "strangles," when it invades lymph nodes and the upper respiratory tract. Abscesses and bacteremia often result from infection. Some diseases caused by *Streptococcus* are prevented by herd vaccination and isolation of infected animals. Antibiotics and symptomatic therapy are also given.

Erysipelothrix rhusiopathiae: This organism is a short, slender rod that causes swine erysipelas (diamond skin disease) and polyarthritis in calves and lambs. Healthy animals carry the organism in their tonsils and stress activates the disease. It is spread in urine, feces, saliva and vomitus and lives for long periods in the environment, so good hygiene is an important part of supportive care. People with small wounds have been infected by handling infected animals and tissues; therefore, latex gloves should be worn in such situations. Vaccination, immune serum (serum from recovered animals) and antibiotic therapy are used as disease control.

Clostridium: These organisms are anaerobic, spore-forming rods (spores are like plant seeds that allow the organism to resist adverse environmental conditions for long periods and germinate when conditions are right). Two organisms produce powerful endotoxins and cause tetanus (*C tetani*) (Fig 26) and botulism (*C botulinum*). Other species of the organism invade tissue and produce toxins of less potency, causing yellow lamb disease, lamb enteritis and enterotoxemia in sheep (*C perfringens*), red water in cattle (*C hemolyticum*), black disease in sheep (*C novyi*), and black leg (*C chauvoei*) and malignant edema (*C septicum*) in ruminants. Because of the seriousness of most of these diseases, vaccination with bacterins and toxoids is widely used.

Supportive care involves use of antitoxins, transfusions, fluids, antibiotics and purgatives, reducing feed (enterotoxemia) and wound care. Spores in the environment are difficult to eradicate.

Listeria monocytogenes: This bacterium is a small rod with slight clubbing at one end. Coccoid (spherical) forms can be seen. Low pH favors its survival, especially in high-moisture silage feeds. It causes meningoencephalitis (circling disease) and septicemia in horses, ruminants, rabbits, rodents and people. Treatment involves antibiotic therapy.

Corynebacterium (Rhodococcus): These organisms are pleomorphic, straight to slightly curved rods with frequent clubbing and irregular staining. They produce pus and are found in abscesses, especially of the lymph nodes, in ruminants, swine and occasionally other animals. Diseases caused include summer mastitis, pneumonia, arthritis, pseudotuberculosis, endocarditis, and genital and urinary tract infections.

Supportive care includes draining abscesses, isolation of infected animals, prevention of wounds, and good hygiene to prevent spread. Antibiotics have been useful in some cases.

Actinomyces: These bacteria produce a mycelium (mass of thread-like processes) that may branch and fragment into rods. It is the cause of lumpy jaw in cattle and abscesses in cats and dogs, and may invade the bone. Treatment includes use of antimicrobial agents, such as Lugol's iodine and penicillin. Treatment may be extended over many weeks and sometimes is not successful.

Nocardia: This organism also produces a long, filamentous, branching mycelium that breaks up into coccoid or rod forms. It causes bovine mastitis and granulomatous (proliferative, tissue-like) lesions of the skin and thoracic organs of dogs and cats. Abscesses may drain pus to the bodies' surface and contain granules. Thoracic fluid from affected animals resembles tomato soup. Antimicrobial agents are used to treat nocardiosis. Needles used for intramammary infusion may be a source of spread unless disinfected between uses.

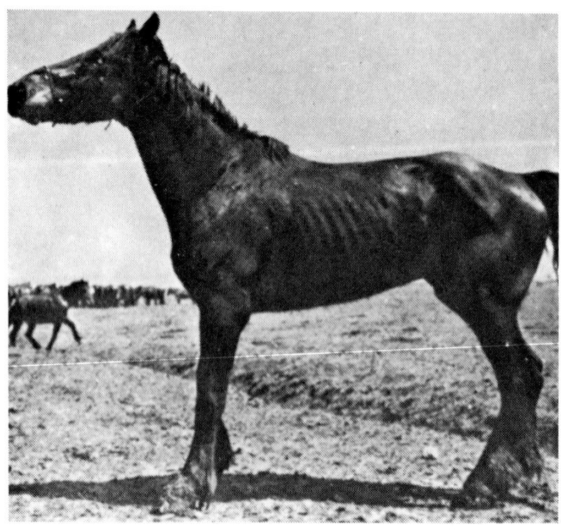

Figure 26. A horse with tetanus.

Dermatophilus congolensis: Narrow, tapering filaments, with branching at right angles to the main stem, characterize this organism. It causes streptothricosis, strawberry foot rot and greasy heel disease. Supportive care involves use of antimicrobials.

Mycoplasmas

These organisms are the smallest and simplest cells capable of self-replication. Pleomorphic (variably shaped) in form, they may appear coccoid, filamentous, spiral, or as rings, granules or globules. They cause contagious bovine and caprine pleuropneumonia, mastitis, vulvovaginitis, arthritis, conjunctivitis, bronchopneumonia, and polyserositis and enzootic pneumonia of swine. Some forms are sensitive to antibiotics; however, in others, growth may be enhanced by these drugs. Vaccination is practiced in some areas as a control measure. Mycoplasmas require special media and conditions to grow, so suspect samples are often sent to an outside laboratory for culture and identification.

Rickettsiae

These are a group of small rod-shaped coccoid or pleomorphic organisms that must live inside host cells. They are true bacteria and are usually associated with reticuloendothelial (macrophage-like), vascular or blood cells.

Arthropods (*eg,* fleas, ticks) often act as vectors, transmitting the rickettsiae with their bite. Some diseases are species specific, but many are not, and a few are zoonotic. Diseases caused by rickettsiae include tick-borne fever, benign bovine and ovine rickettsiosis, bovine petechial fever and contagious ophthalmia in ruminants, equine ehrlichiosis, canine ehrlichiosis, borreliosis (Lyme disease), feline hemobartonellosis, and salmon poisoning in dogs.

Supportive care involves elimination of arthropod vectors and use of antimicrobials, transfusions and fluid therapy. Infected animals may be carriers for long periods and in some cases should not be used as blood donors.

Anaplasmas

These organisms are found on or within RBCs and are transmitted by blood-sucking arthropods, transfusion or contaminated instruments. The course of the disease depends upon the number of organisms present and the health of the animal. Ruminants are tested and animals with anaplasmosis are slaughtered. In pets, hemobartonellosis and eperythrozoonosis may respond to antimicrobial therapy. Supportive care involves use of transfusions and reduction of stress. Sometimes the disease is chronic. If the animal is immunocompromised, such as from concurrent feline leukemia virus infection, the prognosis is poor.

Chlamydiae

Chlamydiae are probably bacteria that lack cellular machinery for extracellular existence. Included in this group are agents that cause psittacosis (parrot fever) and ornithosis in birds, pneumonitis and conjunctivitis in cats, encephalomyelitis, polyarthritis, placental disease and enteritis in cattle, and enzootic abortion in sheep and cattle. Antibiotics are useful but sometimes unable to clear infection; carrier animals should be culled. Vaccines are available for protection against some disease caused by chlamydiae. Some of the infections in this group are transmissible to people. Always wear a mask and wash your hands when exposed to the fecal material of infected birds. Psittacosis in people causes flu-like symptoms, with respiratory involvement and fever, but it can also produce meningitis, with permanent destruction of brain cells.

Fungal Infections

Fungi are filamentous or unicellular organisms with chitinous cell walls. The major pathogenic groups are molds and yeasts. Molds are composed of mycelia (stem-like processes), and reproduce by spores. Yeasts are single-celled fungi that reproduce by budding. Identification is based on morphology (physical appearance).

Two yeasts that cause superficial infections of animals are *Candida* and *Malassezia* (formerly called *Pityrosporum*). *Candida* invades mucosal surfaces, especially when the animal is stressed or on prolonged antimicrobial therapy. The superficial disease causes caseous (cheese-like), round lesions and is called thrush; the organisms may also produce mastitis, genital tract infections and systemic disease.

Malassezia can invade the ears of dogs and cats, causing inflammation (otitis) and a thick, brown exudate.

Treatment includes thorough cleaning of involved areas and long-term chemotherapy.

Mold-like organisms, including *Sporothrix, Aspergillus* and *Rhinosporidium,* cause granulomatous, necrotic and suppurative reactions (Fig 27). Therapy includes use of antifungal medications and surgical removal of infected tissues. Unfortunately, long-term treatment is required and often is not successful in eliminating the organism. Chronic debilitation is the frequent result of systemic mycoses.

Dermatophytes are organisms causing superficial fungal infections, often called "ringworm." They feed on keratin in dead skin and hair shafts, causing peripherally expanding circular lesions; hence the name ringworm. Some animals can carry infectious spores after apparent clinical cure. Also, dermatophyte spores can survive in the environment for long periods.

Protozoal Infections

Only a few of the numerous types of protozoa cause disease. These one-celled animals are larger than bacteria, frequently motile and often have complex life cycles.

Trypanosomiasis and babesiasis are transmitted by arthropods and are found in the blood stream. Signs vary and may include chronic wasting, caudal paralysis, jaundice and infertility. Many effective systemic drugs are available for treatment, but decreasing the numbers of the arthropod vector is essential to controlling the protozoa.

Trichomoniasis is a contagious venereal disease, principally of cattle, that causes sterility, pyometra and abortion. Slaughter of bulls and artificial insemination of cows are recommended for control.

Sarcosporidiosis occurs when the muscle of an animal is invaded by the protozoan, *Sarcocystis.* Unless animals are heavily infected, no clinical signs are seen and affected areas of tissue are trimmed after slaughter.

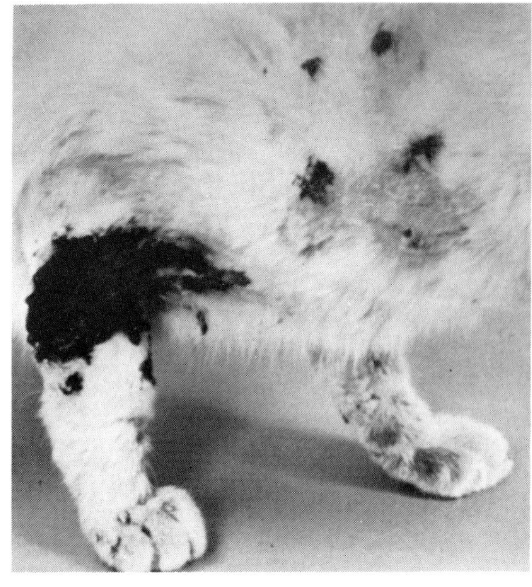

Figure 27. Cat with sporotrichosis, showing scattered skin lesions and a large necrotic area on the foreleg.

Coccidiosis is an acute infection caused by the invasion of intestinal mucosa by *Eimeria* or *Isospora,* resulting in bloody diarrhea. It is an important disease of all domestic animals except the horse. Because animals acquire the disease through contact with infected feces, good hygiene is important in control of the disease. Sick animals should have minimum stress, clean quarters and adequate supportive care. Use of coccidiostatic or coccidiocidal drugs and symptomatic therapy for diarrhea are indicated. Immunity to infection usually develops as animals mature. Rabbits can be fed pellets mixed with a coccidiostat at periodic intervals to control rather than eliminate the protozoa.

Parasitic Infections

A parasite is an organism that lives in or upon and at the expense of another organism, called the host. Internal parasites are found inside the host and external parasites inhabit the surface of the host. They are typically multicelled, except protozoa, and usually visible to the naked eye.

Internal Parasites

Internal parasites, except protozoa, are helminths (worms) and are divided into 3 groups: flatworms (trematodes), roundworms (nematodes) and ribbon-like worms (cestodes). Internal parasitism is diagnosed by seeing the worms grossly or the eggs microscopically (in feces, vomit or tissue).

Trematodes: Trematodes are leaf-shaped flatworms of various sizes. They usually have a complex life cycle involving one or more intermediate hosts (a host, other than the primary, that is necessary for completion of the life cycle); often a snail is involved. Trematodes mature in body tissues (liver, lung), cause necrosis and inflammation, and interfere with body function.

In large animals, *Fasciola* is an important species that lives in the bile ducts (Fig 28). In small animals, *Nanophyetus salmincola* carries the rickettsia that causes salmon poisoning; *Paragonimus* encysts in the lungs.

Supportive care includes use of anthelmintics, therapy to aid the animal while affected tissues heal, and protection from reinfection by elimination of contact with the intermediate hosts (snails, fish, etc). Only a few drugs are effective against flukes.

Nematodes: Nematodes are spaghetti-like roundworms, often pointed on the ends, and may be microscopic to many inches in length. Typically, they have a direct life cycle (only a primary host is involved) and migrate within body tissues before completing their life cycles in the digestive, vascular or respiratory system. Eggs from fecal contamination are the usual source of infection, but penetration of the skin and transplacental transfer may also occur in some species. Typically the eggs survive in the environment for long periods.

Ascarids are roundworms that occur in most nonruminants and look like large, white, rubbery earthworms. Their life cycle involves migration throughout the body (especially the liver and lungs) before adults develop in the intestine. Disease occurs by physical blockage of the intestine, competition for nutrients with the host, tissue destruction during migration, and interference with digestion (Fig 29). Affected animals are usually thin, with a rough haircoat and a pot belly. The diarrhea and vomitus of affected animals may contain worms. Because young animals are often infected before birth or from the dam's milk, mature worms may occur in animals as young as 4 weeks of age. Treatment involves deworming with an anthelmintic, followed by provision of a good diet to return the animal to good condition. To avoid impaction of the intestine with dead worms in a heavy infection and to kill migrating larvae, a series of dewormings is used. Because ascarids pose a public health hazard, puppies should be checked for worms at an early age.

Large strongyles (bloodworms) in horses and *Dirofilaria* (heartworms) in dogs live in the vascular system (Fig 30). Large strongyles invade artery walls and are a common cause of colic when they compromise the blood supply to the intestinal tract. Horses

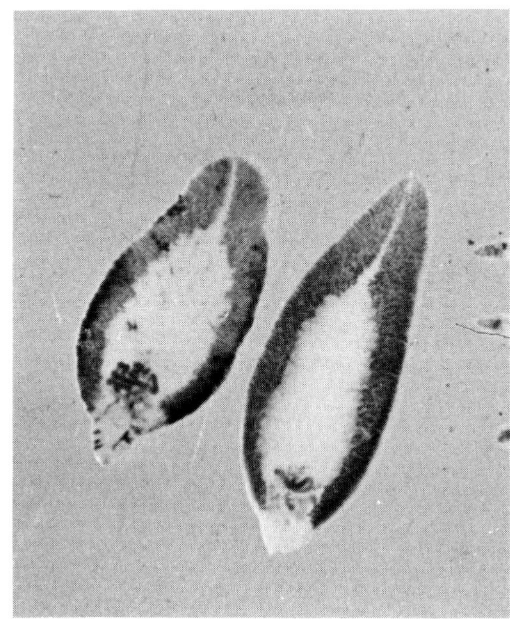

Figure 28. *Fasciola hepatica,* the common liver fluke of cattle.

should be dewormed about every 6-8 weeks. *Dirofilaria* interferes with the blood supply to the lungs and may cause dyspnea. Heartworms are transmitted by mosquitoes. Treatment involves use of drugs to kill the adults and microfilariae (larvae). People bitten by infected mosquitoes may develop granulomatous lesions in their lungs.

Hookworms (*eg, Ancylostoma*) attach to the intestinal lining and suck large quantities of blood. Infection causes melena (blood in the stool), anemia and weight loss. Heavy infections may require transfusions after deworming. Larvae may be ingested or penetrate the skin to gain entrance to the host, so good hygiene is essential to prevent transmission. Larvae that penetrate human skin do

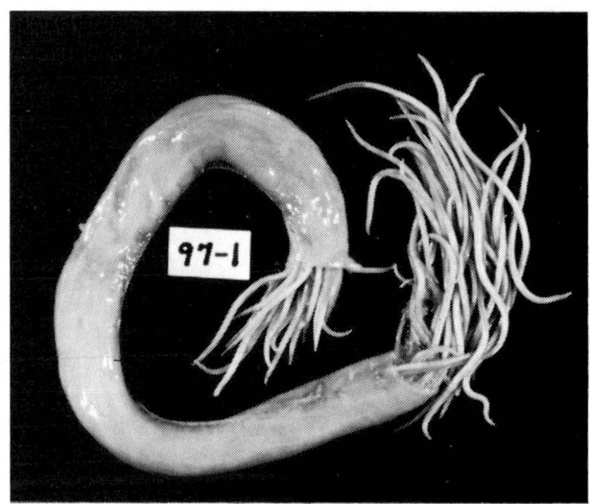

Figure 29. Impaction of the small intestine of a foal by roundworms (*Parascaris equorum*).

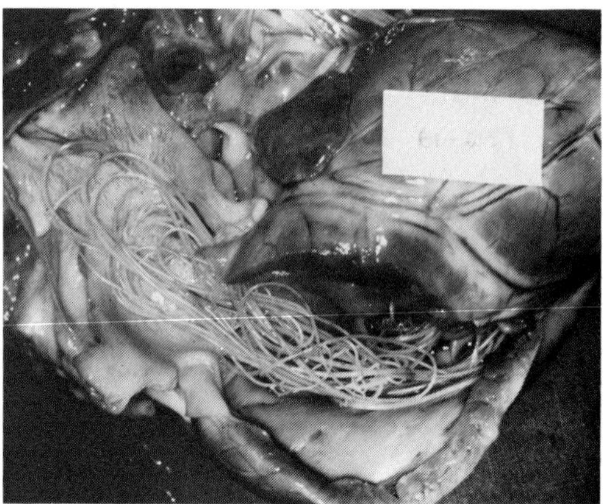

Figure 30. Adult heartworms in the heart of a dog.

not complete their life cycle but travel subcutaneously, causing a rash and itching (creeping eruption or cutaneous larva migrans). People can become infected by walking without shoes in contaminated areas.

Whipworms (*Trichuris*) live in the large intestine and, in heavy infections, cause loss of weight, diarrhea and fresh blood in the stool. Affected animals should be treated with an anthelmintic. Because eggs are susceptible to drying, cleanliness and elimination of damp areas in the animal's environment are helpful control measures.

Pinworms (*Oxyuris*) occur in horses and are not transmissible to people. Females lay their eggs around the horse's anus, causing intense itching. Inspecting the anal folds, cleaning the perineal area and routine anthelmintic therapy constitute a good control program. Pinworms do not occur in dogs and cats.

Ruminants have a variety of small roundworm parasites (*Hemonchus, Ostertagia,* etc) that live in various portions of their digestive tracts. Depending on the number of parasites and the species, signs vary from none to weight loss, anemia and diarrhea. Good hygiene (pasture rotation, use of feed bunks, providing good drainage, manure removal) and regular deworming are necessary for control.

Lungworm infections occur in cattle and horses (*Dictyocaulus*), swine (*Metastrongylus*) and cats (*Aelurostrongylus*). The eggs are coughed up and swallowed by the host. Signs include coughing, weight loss and dyspnea. Use of anthelmintics, moving dewormed animals to a clean pasture or stall, and providing a high level of nutrition are important.

Cestodes: Tapeworms are composed of a series of identical reproductive segments (proglottids) in a chain extending from a head (scolex) that is anchored in the intestinal wall. Their life cycle involves an intermediate host. In small animals, typical intermediate hosts are fleas, mice or birds. They are usually well adapted to their host and cause little damage other than competition for nutrients. The passing of tapeworm segments can be distressing to the client and several types are transmissible to people through the intermediate host. Weight loss may be seen. Elimination of the intermediate host to break the life cycle or regular deworming is essential to clear this parasite.

External Parasites

External parasites include fleas, flies, ticks, mosquitoes, lice and mites. The first 4 of these parasites spend at least part of their life cycle off the host and the last 2 remain continuously on the animal. Damage to the host includes blood loss, skin irritation, spoiling of the haircoat, transmission of disease and destruction of tissues. External parasites are often a seasonal problem and require diligence to eliminate an infestation.

Ticks: Ticks are arachnids (8-legged arthropods) and come in a variety of sizes, shapes and colors (some look like beetles, others like spiders). The female requires a blood meal for egg development and some species need a blood meal before every molting cycle (2-3 times). They are a particular problem in rural areas and may transmit a variety of diseases to animals and people (*eg,* Rocky Mountain spotted fever, tick fever, borreliosis).

Ticks attach themselves to the host and engorge themselves by burying their head in the host's skin to consume blood and tissue fluids. A variety of compounds can be applied to kill them. Individual ticks can be removed with the fingers or forceps, grasping the tick at the base of the head and using gentle traction. Wear gloves when removing ticks to prevent disease transmission. Ticks prefer to attach themselves where the skin is thin and moist. Infestation may be prevented with collars, dips, powders and sprays, though many species of ticks have built up resistance to them.

Heavy infestations may cause anemia from blood loss. Ticks that attach near the spinal cord may cause ascending paralysis (tick paralysis) that can kill the animal when the respiratory muscles are paralyzed. Removal of the tick causes a rapid return to normal. A neurotoxin in the tick's saliva is the apparent cause; only certain ticks cause the disease.

Flies: Flies have 3 parts to their life cycle. Adults lay eggs that hatch into larvae (maggots), which pupate (usually on the ground) and hatch into adults. Adult flies are pests that irritate animals and may spread disease, but most damage is caused by the larvae. Larvae developing in wounds produce an enzyme that liquefies tissue so they can consume it. Because the enzyme dissolves both dead and healthy tissue, maggots enlarge existing wounds or create new ones when eggs are laid on matted hair contaminated with feces or wet wool.

Some types of flies (bots in horses, warbles) have modified life cycles. The larvae live inside the animal's body, protected from environmental conditions, and are released when the environmental temperature is right for pupation. Such flies destroy tissue (meat), spoil hides and, in large numbers, interfere with normal body functions.

Treatment is aimed at preventing contact between the host and fly (stabling, clipping matted hair, etc), killing adult flies with insecticides, removing eggs by flushing wounds or scraping eggs off the hair, removing maggots from wounds, and using internal insecticides. Good hygiene, especially proper manure disposal and protecting open wounds in summer, is an important control measure.

Mosquitoes: Mosquitoes are flying pests that must breed in standing water. Females require a blood meal before egg production (males generally do not suck blood). The female may visit several hosts in search of blood and her proboscis (mouthparts) often transmits disease.

Control measures include draining, treating (such as adding a layer of oil to the surface) or screening standing water, using mosquito repellents to prevent bites, and using medication to prevent disease once a bite has occurred.

Fleas: Fleas are the bane of mammals in humid, temperate areas, especially in late summer and fall. Their life cycle is similar to that of flies, but adults live most of their life on the host and cause irritation with their bites. Eggs are resistant to insecticides. The larvae eat organic debris and pupate in rugs and crevices.

In animals that develop an allergy to flea saliva, one bite is enough to cause rashes, hair loss and extreme discomfort. Adult fleas can live for months without a blood meal.

Successful control involves killing the adults and larvae on the animal, in the house (or animal's sleeping quarters), and outdoors around the yard or other premises with insecticides. The process must be repeated at intervals to kill newly hatched larvae and immature fleas until all the eggs are hatched. Eggs hatch 3-14 days after being laid, depending on the environmental temperature and humidity (increasing both speeds up the life cycle). Poor control results are obtained if any facet of environmental control is missed (only killing fleas on the animal is not enough), if newly hatched fleas mature and lay fresh eggs, or if the animal contacts fleas on another animal or area. In addition, fleas have become resistant to many insecticides on the market.

Some insecticides have residual activity or interfere with adult development to prevent reinfestation between applications. Ultrasound generators have been used to drive fleas away, but they are not effective. Internal insecticides may be useful in some cases but they may cause side effects.

There are a variety of products for flea control on the animal, including dips, powders, sprays, systemic drugs, collars and baths. Heavy flea infestations can kill an animal through blood loss. Debilitated, young or old animals are especially prone to this problem as they have difficulty grooming themselves and a limited ability to respond to blood loss.

Animals allergic to flea bites (flea-bite dermatitis) should be kept as free of fleas as possible, as one bite is enough to set off a violently pruritic (itchy) reaction. If it is impossible to eliminate flea contact, the allergic reaction can be reduced with corticosteroids, but there can be undesirable side effects. Killing the flea after it has bitten the animal does not prevent the allergic reaction.

One type of tapeworm (*Dipylidium*) is carried by fleas and may infect both animals and people if fleas are consumed.

Lice: Lice are small insects, visible to the naked eye, that cement their eggs (nits) to the host's hair. The adults produce irritation by biting and sucking out tissue fluids. Heavy infestations result in loss of condition and anemia.

Control measures include periodically dusting the animal with an insecticide. Because they spend all of their lives on the animal, lice are fairly easy to control. They can be transmitted directly by close contact between animals or indirectly from grooming brushes, blankets, etc.

Mites: There are a variety of sizes and shapes of mites, but most are microscopic. They may live on normal animals without producing disease (*Demodex*) or they may burrow into the skin, consuming tissue and fluids, and causing intense irritation (Fig 31). Some mites live on the skin surface (*Cheyletiella*), while others live in the ear canal (*Otodectes, Notoedres*). A mite infestation is called mange.

Control measures include use of acaricides (baths, dips or pour-ons that kill mites), worked well into the skin, with use continued until all eggs hatch. In cases of otodectic mange (ear mite infestation), scabs or ear wax should be removed before instilling an acaricide in the ear to allow the medication to contact the mites. Some types of mange may not respond to treatment if the disease

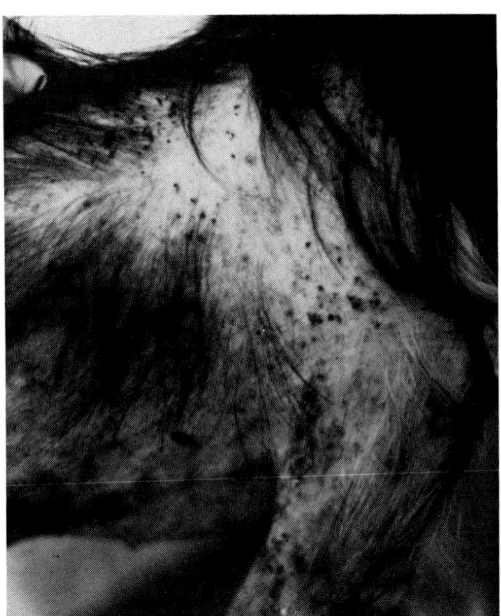

Figure 31. Severe sarcoptic mange in a dog.

has manifested itself because of concurrent disease or immunosuppression. Ivermectin is effective against several types of mange.

Viral Infections

Viruses are composed of genetic material that may be encased in a protective coat. They reproduce by inserting their genetic material into the host cell and commanding the cell's reproductive machinery to make virus particles instead of cells. Infected cells usually die when their nutrients are exhausted, waste products build up, or the virus particles rupture the cell membrane.

Viruses are extremely small (with a few exceptions) and the light microscope can only be used to visualize cell death caused by infection. Most can be seen with the electron microscope. Because they can only be cultured in living cells (eggs, tissue culture), viral diseases are often diagnosed by their effect (signs, antibody titer rise, etc), rather than by finding and culturing the organism, as in bacteriologic procedures.

Viruses are classified as either DNA or RNA viruses, depending on the nucleic acids (genetic material) they contain, similar to the classification of bacteria into 2 groups by their Gram stain reaction. No virus contains both DNA and RNA. Further classification is based upon the protein coat (capsid), which protects the virus particle from enzyme degradation. The coats are described by their symmetry (icosahedral, helical, etc), size, number of units making up the protein coat (capsomeres) and sedimentation rate.

Control of Viral Infections

Most viruses are inactivated by heating at 56 C (132.8 F) for 30 minutes, and so are inactivated by boiling water. Enveloped viruses are less stable than unenveloped viruses, as the envelope is very susceptible to degradation, especially by lipolytic agents.

Many viruses are preserved by drying or cooling on dry ice. Practically all viruses are inactivated at a pH above 9 and below 5, so acids and bases are good disinfecting agents. Enveloped viruses are inactivated by most disinfectants including phenol, detergents and formaldehyde. Certain unenveloped viruses (*eg,* parvoviruses, caliciviruses) are resistant to all common disinfectants except a 1:20 bleach solution (*eg,* Clorox).

With few exceptions, antibiotics have no effect on viruses, as they are protected inside living cells for most of their existence. Drugs powerful enough to kill viruses often kill host cells too.

Interferon is a natural substance produced by a virus-infected cell that prevents infection of surrounding cells by other viruses.

Commercially produced interferon is available to treat some viral infections.

Disease Production

Most viruses are specific for a species (with some notable exceptions, such as rabies) and may even require a specific cell type for replication (reproduction).

Viruses generally first attack body surfaces, especially mucous membranes, and replicate locally. They may remain local or spread to other tissues, often via the blood or lymph. In other cases, viruses may enter mobile body cells (*eg,* WBCs) and are distributed throughout the body. Some viruses cross the blood-brain barrier and many infect the fetus *in utero.* The same virus may produce different clinical signs in animals of varying ages.

The course and manifestation of disease are determined by the number of viruses involved, the type and number of host cells infected, and the nature of viral replication within the cell. The infection may cause no clinical signs, serious disease or sudden death. In some cases, clinical signs do not appear until late in the infection. Secondary bacterial (and fungal) infections often complicate viral diseases, as the virus reduces the body's resistance to bacterial invasion. This is especially true of respiratory and skin infections.

Some viruses can also change the genetic make-up of normal body cells, resulting in tumor production. Certain viruses cause chronic disease or persist in the host and are reactivated when body defenses are reduced from stress (latent infection).

Usually the mechanisms that lead to signs of disease and death are unknown; however, vascular shock, toxicity (viral toxins or cellular metabolites) and failure of organ systems may account for disease.

Certain diseases have a seasonal prevalence and may cause explosive outbreaks in a susceptible population. Reduction of the number of susceptible animals below a certain level may terminate an outbreak of a viral disease. Many viral diseases are transmitted by vectors, such as arthropods, or contaminated material or instruments (fomites).

Immunity in most natural viral infections is absolute and relatively long lasting (as opposed to that in bacterial diseases). Serum from immune animals can be given to susceptible animals before infection occurs or before the virus is widely disseminated to produce effective but short-lived (1-2 weeks) immunity. The dam (mother) usually passes immunity to its offspring across the placenta and/or in the colostrum (first milk), so it is very important that neonatal animals nurse within the first few hours of life. Maternal antibody protection usually wanes at about 6-12 weeks of life.

When newborn animals fail to nurse or do not receive good-quality colostrum, plasma from donor animals or commercially available hyperimmune serum can be infused IV to provide temporary protection.

Vaccination with a modified live virus (altered so it cannot produce disease) or a killed virus confers variable immunity, depending on the virus type and immunocompetence of the host. Agents that boost the immune response, called adjuvants, are sometimes added to killed vaccines. Modified-live-virus vaccines usually give better protection, as the virus actually multiplies within the host tissue. Regular boosters are usually recommended to keep immunity at a protective level. The manufacturer's recommendations should be closely followed when using any vaccine.

DNA Viruses

Parvoviridae: This group contains viruses that cause feline panleukopenia, canine, porcine and bovine parvovirus infections, and hemorrhagic encephalopathy. They are very small viruses with a protein coat arranged in a many-sided geometric figure. The viruses do not have envelopes and so are resistant to disinfectants, heat and lipid solvents.

Papoviridae: This group of viruses contains 2 genera, *Polyomavirus* and *Papillomavirus.* They are icosahedral in shape (20-sided), more than twice as big as parvoviruses and do not have an envelope. Some can cause growths (warts or papillomas), but most cause inapparent infections (Fig 32).

Adenoviridae: The genus *Adenovirus* contains a number of pathogenic organisms, including those causing infectious canine

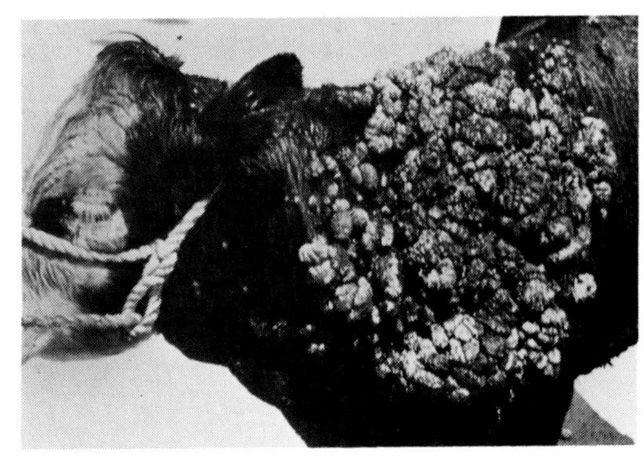

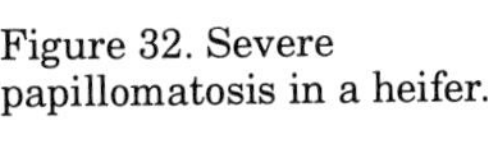
Figure 32. Severe papillomatosis in a heifer.

hepatitis and respiratory disease in dogs, conjunctivitis, pneumonia, diarrhea and polyarthritis in calves (weak calf syndrome), pneumonia in foals, and diarrhea and/or meningoencephalitis in swine. Adenoviruses are larger than papovaviruses but have the same geometric shape; however, they have fine, filamentous projections on some corners. They do not have an envelope.

Iridoviridae: African swine fever is caused by a virus from this group. *Iridoviridae* are enveloped and large, and their protein coat is composed of complex particles.

Herpesviridae: This family contains many viruses causing a variety of catarrhal (weepy), chronic and even neoplastic conditions. Diseases they may cause include pseudorabies, infectious bovine rhinopneumonitis (IBR), equine rhinopneumonitis, malignant catarrhal fever of cattle, bovine ulcerative mammillitis, feline rhinotracheitis, canine herpesvirus infection, and porcine inclusion-body rhinitis. Almost every animal species is plagued by one or more herpesvirus infections.

A herpesvirus is larger than an adenovirus but has the same icosahedral symmetry. Because it has a lipid envelope, it is quite sensitive to disinfectants and environmental conditions.

Poxviridae: Viruses in this group cause cowpox, swinepox, horsepox, lumpy skin disease, bovine papular stomatitis and pseudocowpox. There are no pox virus infections of dogs or cats but livestock pox viruses cause fatal and economically serious losses.

Pox viruses are very large (just visible with the light microscope) and have a complex structure composed of ovoid or brick-like components. Some have an envelope.

RNA Viruses

Picornaviridae: Diseases caused by the genus *Enterovirus* are various forms of intestinal disturbances ranging in severity. The rhinoviruses are the agents of bovine and equine upper respiratory disease; aphthoviruses cause foot and mouth disease. All picornaviruses have an icosahedral shape and are not enveloped.

Caliciviridae: Viruses in this group cause vesicular exanthema of swine and feline calicivirus infection. They are icosahedral and unenveloped. Some types are zoonotic.

Reoviridae: Three serotypes of this group have been associated with respiratory and enteric diseases of animals, but most infections are inapparent. They are icosahedral and unenveloped, and the only group with double-stranded RNA. An important genus, *Orbivirus,* causes African horsesickness, bluetongue and Colorado tick fever.

Togaviridae: These viruses are isometric and enveloped. They cause Western, Eastern and Venezuelan equine encephalomyelitis and louping ill. The genus *Pestivirus* causes bovine virus diarrhea and hog cholera.

Orthomyxoviridae: Viruses in this group are spherical, elongated or filamentous and have an envelope. They cause hemagglutination (cause RBCs to stick together) and are sensitive to dactinomycin. Diseases caused include porcine and equine influenza.

Paramyxoviridae: These viruses are spherical or pleomorphic and enveloped, and cause hemagglutination but are resistant to dactinomycin. Diseases caused include Newcastle disease, parainfluenza, canine distemper and rinderpest.

Rhabdoviridae: Rhabdoviruses are "bullet shaped" and have an envelope. Some types can cause hemagglutination. Rabies and vesicular stomatitis are caused by viruses in this group.

Retroviridae: Retroviruses are complex and enveloped. Members of the subfamily Oncovirinae cause feline leukemia and sarcoma, mammary carcinomas, and many other neoplastic diseases.

Bunyaviridae: This virus particle is spherical and enveloped, and causes Rift Valley fever.

Coronaviridae: These viruses are spherical or pleomorphic and enveloped, with bulbous projections forming a crown (corona). They cause GI disease in cattle, pigs, dogs and possibly horses, infectious peritonitis in cats, and encephalitis in pigs.

Arboviruses: "Arbovirus" is a term for virus carried by arthropods. Most have been reclassified into RNA virus groups.

Unclassified Viruses: Scrapie, ulcerative stomatitis, bovine papular stomatitis, contagious pneumonia of calves, proliferative stomatitis, ocular squamous carcinoma of cattle, and transmissible venereal tumor and mastocytoma of dogs are caused by various unclassified viruses.

Zoonoses and Public Health

Zoonotic diseases (zoonoses) are infections transmitted from animals to people, under natural conditions. They are of particular concern in veterinary medicine because animal handlers are a high-risk group for such diseases. Veterinarians and their co-workers must educate the general public on zoonoses.

In most cases, people are accidental hosts of zoonoses, as outbreaks are usually propagated by animal-to-animal spread; person-to-person transmission is very rare. Many zoonoses must be reported to public health authorities so that steps can be taken to contain the infection and the human medical community can be alerted.

Technicians are not qualified to advise clients regarding human health matters, but they can indicate steps necessary to reduce the risks of zoonotic disease to animal owners.

Bacterial Zoonoses

Leptospirosis: Leptospira is a slender, spiral organism that infects dogs, cattle, pigs, sheep and horses. Most infections are subclinical, but jaundice, fever, hemoglobinuria (hemoglobin in the urine), abortion and death can occur. Organisms are shed in the urine of infected animals for months or years, and so may contaminate water supplies.

The disease is contracted through contact with infected urine (enters through skin wounds), ingestion of contaminated water, or by splashing infected material onto the mucous membranes. Most outbreaks are self-limiting but may be perpetuated by rodents.

Wearing gloves when handling urine and avoiding potentially contaminated water supplies for drinking are recommended, as 5% of human cases are fatal. Serologic tests, urine cultures or tissue biopsy can be used to diagnose leptospirosis. Antimicrobials are used in control of the disease. Vaccination prevents clinical signs in animals but does not eliminate the carrier state, in which organisms are shed in the urine.

Plague: Bubonic plague is caused by *Yersinia pestis,* a Gram-negative rod. Plague is not a disease of people but a natural infection of rodents (rats, ground squirrels, etc) that is spread by the rat flea. In people, *Yersinia* infects regional lymph nodes and may become systemic. The pneumonic form of plague can be spread by aerosol (droplets in the air) and is especially serious. Veterinarians have developed plague after treating abscesses or respiratory infections (cats can carry plague, as diseased rats are easy to catch).

Diagnosis is by culture or inoculation of rodents. People may be vaccinated against plague and antimicrobial therapy is useful; however, the main method of control involves reducing the rat populations.

Tularemia: Tularemia is an infectious disease of rodents, especially rabbits, caused by *Francisella tularensis,* a Gram-negative, pleomorphic organism. Transmission to domestic herbivores is by blood-sucking arthropods. In lambs, calves, piglets and foals, tularemia causes weakness, depression, coughing and diarrhea. The infection may remain latent for long periods.

Transmission to people occurs through contact with tissue or blood from infected animals, inhalation of aerosol, bites of blood-sucking insects, or the bite of animals (cats, dogs, skunks, non-poisonous snakes) that have fed on infected carcasses. Cats do not usually display signs of illness.

Infected rabbits caught by dogs and cats should be burned or buried. People should avoid sick, wild rabbits and rubber gloves should be worn when such animals are necropsied.

The disease can be diagnosed by blood culture or serologic analysis. Supportive care is based on therapy with streptomycin or other antibiotics.

Brucellosis: Brucellosis affects cattle, swine, goats, dogs and people. The *Brucella* organism is a small, Gram-negative rod. Brucellosis is characterized by infertility, abortion and testicular infection. In horses, it is associated with fistulous withers and poll evil. In people, brucellosis causes a protracted, debilitating disease called undulant fever (fever waxes and wanes).

The organism is transmitted venereally in dogs and is contained in infected fetuses, placentas and birth fluids of all affected species. Raw milk or milk products and aborted material from infected animals are the primary sources of infection in people.

Milk and cattle are tested for brucellosis in an effort to trace infected herds. Adult cattle that test positive are slaughtered, as there is no effective treatment in animals. Antibiotic therapy is used to treat infections in people, but relapses are common. Diagnosis is based on serologic examination and culture of the organism.

Technicians can reduce their chance of infection by not drinking raw milk, wearing gloves when handling dead fetuses, placentas or birth fluids, and careful handling of the strain-19 brucellosis vaccine (this vaccine is not attenuated for people and splashing it in the eyes or injection into the skin can cause the disease).

Vibriosis: Campylobacter (formerly called *Vibrio*) is a short, curved Gram-negative rod. *Campylobacter fetus jejuni* causes hemorrhagic enteritis in dogs and people, and winter dysentery (black scours) in cattle.

The diarrhea of infected dogs may infect people. Contaminated pork and chicken are a source of disease for people and dogs.

Diagnosis is by stool cultures or microscopic examination of fecal smears. Most strains are sensitive to antibiotics. Washing the hands after handling dogs with diarrhea or raw meat is recommended to help prevent infections.

Anthrax: Bacillus anthracis, a Gram-positive, nonmotile, spore-forming rod, causes anthrax, an acute, febrile disease that can affect all species. The most common disease form consists of septicemia, with a rapidly fatal course; local and pulmonary forms are also seen.

The carcasses of infected animals often have blood oozing from the anus and nostrils and become bloated. Such carcasses should not be opened, as the organism forms spores when exposed to the air; these spores can remain viable in soil for 20-30 years. People become infected by inhaling spores, especially from raw wool, hides or horse hair (wool sorter's disease), ingestion of poorly cooked meat or contact with infected tissues.

Diagnosis is based on culture, microscopic examination of tissues and blood, clinical signs and rodent inoculation. Sick animals may be treated with antimicrobials and contact animals vaccinated, but infected premises are quarantined and disinfected by state authorities.

Botulism, Tetanus: Botulism and tetanus are both caused by powerful neurotoxins elaborated by the anaerobic bacterium, *Clostridium.* All animals are susceptible to the diseases caused by this spore-forming rod.

Tetanus occurs when the organism is introduced into a wound, especially puncture wounds, and causes prolonged contraction of muscles (lockjaw). The organism is naturally found in soil, especially where horse manure is present. Toxoids, antibiotics and antitoxins are used as therapy. Puncture wounds should be made to bleed freely to help eliminate an anaerobic environment. When large numbers of animals are castrated or docked, instruments should be sterilized frequently. Iodine or chlorine application to wounds kills spores.

Botulism occurs when spoiled food (meat, bones), containing the toxin, is ingested. Paralysis progresses until death is caused by respiratory collapse. Antitoxin has been used with variable success. Control involves avoiding spoiled feed and elimination of old carcasses.

Tuberculosis: Tuberculosis, caused by a mycobacterium, is a chronic disease affecting almost all vertebrates. There are 3 main types: human, avian and bovine tuberculosis. The bovine form is responsible for human disease caused by ingestion of infected raw milk or milk products and inhalation of infectious aerosol. Pasteurization of milk kills these bacteria. Wherever the organism becomes localized (usually the lungs), large masses form. Animals can also contract infections from infected people.

An intradermal skin test is used to detect the infection, along with radiographs and cultures (Fig 33). The usual control measures involve test and slaughter, but chemotherapy has also been used; however, infected animals are a health hazard to people and other animals. Infected animals shed organisms in their feces, and dust particles, food and water may become contaminated.

Salmonellosis: Salmonella organisms inhabit the intestinal tract of many birds, reptiles and mammals, and quite a few species can cause GI disease in people. Infection occurs through ingestion of contaminated food. Direct infection from animals is uncommon.

Cats are seldom involved in this zoonotic disease, but poultry and many reptiles carry *Salmonella* as normal gut flora.

Ornithosis-Psittacosis (Chlamydiosis): This is an acute or chronic disease of birds caused by *Chlamydia psittaci* (in people and psittacine birds, it is called psittacosis, in other birds ornithosis). In birds, it causes weight loss, nasal discharge and diarrhea, and in people, flu-like symptoms.

Pet birds should come from an aviary free of disease, as an inapparent carrier state can occur. Screening aviaries against wild birds is necessary. Tetracycline-coated seeds or granules may be fed; however, some resistance is developing to this drug. Doxycycline is often effective. Thorough disinfection of the premises is essential for control.

In people, the disease occurs after exposure to infected aerosol or dust. When necropsying birds, the feathers should be moistened with a disinfectant to prevent spread of the disease. Live birds can be examined using a surgical mask or transparent container (glove box).

Outbreaks of the disease must be reported to public health authorities. An enzyme-linked immunosorbent assay (ELISA) is available for rapid diagnosis of chlamydiosis.

Cat-Scratch Fever: This is a disease of people, thought to be caused by introduction of an infectious agent into the body via a cat scratch or bite. The disease occurs about 4 weeks after a cat scratch has healed. The lymph node draining that region becomes inflamed and may develop an abscess. Fever, weakness and headache may accompany lymph node enlargement. It is a self-limiting disease. More reports of this disease have been from wire fence scratches than from wounds caused by cats.

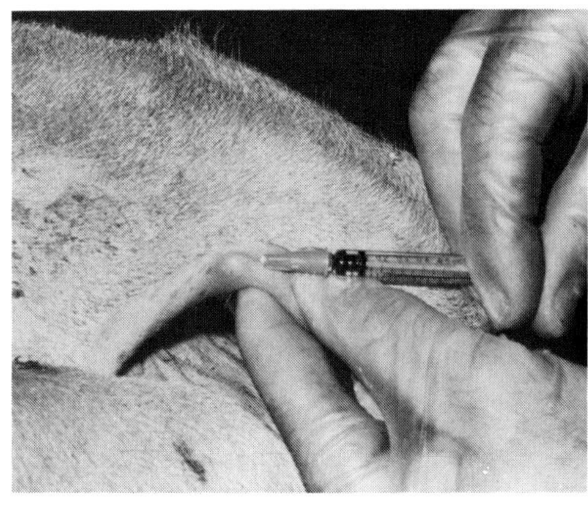

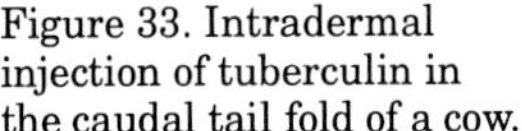
Figure 33. Intradermal injection of tuberculin in the caudal tail fold of a cow.

Rickettsial Zoonoses

Rocky Mountain Spotted Fever: Rickettsia rickettsii causes Rocky Mountain spotted fever in people and inapparent infections in animals. The disease consists of fever, severe chills, headache, muscle pain and a rash in people, and is transmitted by the wood tick (*Dermacentor andersoni*) or the dog tick (*D variabilis*). The tick must be attached to the skin for several hours for transmission of the disease.

The disease is diagnosed by symptoms, isolation of the organism, serologic examination, or inoculation of rodents. It is treated with antimicrobials, though 5-10% of affected people die. Rocky Mountain spotted fever can be prevented by avoiding ticks (protective clothing), vaccination, and frequent inspection of the body. Ticks on people should be removed with forceps or with fingers protected by paper or gloves. Care should be taken not to rupture ticks during removal, so as to prevent spread of the disease.

Q Fever: Q fever is caused by *Coxiella burnetii* and causes abortion in sheep and goats, and an influenza-like disease and chronic endocarditis in people. It is carried by a variety of ticks that must feed for several hours for transmission of the disease. Contamination of the mucosae or wounds with crushed ticks or tick feces may also cause the disease. Diagnosis is based on isolation of the organism or serologic examination.

Vaccination of people reduces the severity of clinical signs but does not eliminate infection. Killing ticks with insecticides and clearing of brush that can house ticks are recommended.

Borreliosis (Lyme Disease): Borreliosis is caused by the spirochete, *Borrelia burgdorferi,* and is transmitted by *Ixodes* ticks. Infected dogs, horses and cattle may show lameness, fever, lethargy, inappetence and joint pain. There is no specific test for diagnosis, but a blood titer higher than 1:64 is considered positive. Early treatment with amoxicillin, doxycycline or cephalexin is effective. Nonsteroidal antiinflammatories can be used to reduce musculoskeletal pain. Prevention involves tick control with topical sprays and dips.

Viral Zoonoses

Rabies: Rabies is a viral disease that affects all warm-blooded animals, though some are more resistant than others. It is usually transmitted by the bite of an infected animal, but it has been transmitted by inhalation of aerosol in bat-infested caves. The disease is propagated by wild animals, especially skunks, bats and foxes.

The virus travels up nerve trunks to the brain and then enters the salivary glands, where it can be transmitted in the saliva by biting. Therefore, clinical signs occur before the virus is present in the saliva.

The furious form presents a picture of the typical "mad" animal and the dumb form is characterized by progressive paralysis. Pharyngeal paralysis may cause the animal to act as if it has an obstruction in its throat. This is particularly hazardous for veterinarians and technicians examining an affected animal's mouth and throat for a suspected foreign body.

Domestic animals that have bitten people should be quarantined for 10-12 days and watched for clinical signs. If signs of rabies appear within that time, there is a possibility the virus was in the saliva at the time of the bite and treatment of the bitten person should begin. If no signs are observed, the virus was not transmitted at the time of the bite, though the animal could still be incubating rabies. Wild animals that, without provocation, have bitten people are killed and their brain is examined microscopically for the disease. Animals that have bitten other animals must be quarantined for longer periods, as the incubation time is variable. If the biting animal has a current rabies vaccination, it is revaccinated and confined for 90 days. If the biting animal was not vaccinated, it must be placed in strict isolation for 6 months and revaccinated 1 month before release. Suspect livestock should be slaughtered or observed closely for 6 months.

Control measures include vaccination of pet animals, stray animal control and education of the public.

Rabies vaccination is recommended for all technicians.

Encephalitis: A number of viral zoonoses cause encephalitis (inflammation of the brain), including Eastern, Western and Venezuelan equine encephalitis, Rift Valley fever, Ross River disease, Japanese encephalitis, St. Louis encephalitis, West Nile disease, louping ill and California encephalitis. All are transmitted by mosquitoes or ticks.

The equine encephalitides are a similar group of diseases characterized by CNS disturbances. They are propagated in nature by birds or rodents and transmitted by mosquitoes. The diagnosis is based on clinical signs, geographic area and season (fall and summer) of infections, and serologic examination. Fever, convulsions, cyanosis, drowsiness and increased intracranial pressure occur in infected people. Eastern encephalomyelitis is fatal in 50% of affected horses and Western encephalomyelitis in 5-15%, as there is no effective treatment. Diagnosis is by serologic examination.

Vaccination of horses and mosquito control are used to combat spread of the disease.

Mycotic Zoonoses

Dermatomycoses: Infections by *Microsporum* and *Trichophyton,* both fungi termed dermatophytes, are commonly known as "ringworm." The organisms feed on keratin found in the skin, hair and nails. Lesions grow centrifugally (in a circle) and result in hair breakage and thickened, scaly skin. Long-haired cats may carry dermatophytes without showing clinical signs. Lesions in people may occur on exposed areas, such as the arms, and appear as red, circular or blotchy patches that slowly enlarge.

Therapy includes topical or systemic antifungals (*eg,* griseofulvin). Because fungal spores remain viable in the environment for several months, infected animals should be confined to an area where thorough cleaning is possible. Contaminated brushes, collars, bedding and other items should be sanitized or replaced.

Systemic Mycoses: Such diseases as histoplasmosis, blastomycosis, coccidioidomycosis and cryptococcosis are not directly transmissible from animals to people. However, infected animals contaminate the environment and may increase the likelihood that people, especially very young, old or immunosuppressed people, will contract these potentially serious infections.

Yeast Infections: Yeasts are a type of fungi that tend to proliferate after antibacterial treatment. The mucosae (*eg,* vagina) and ear canals are common sites of yeast infection, which is characterized by inflammation and exudation. Microscopic examination of exudate smears reveals the characteristic budding or branching yeast organisms. Treatment is with systemic and topical antifungals.

Parasitic Zoonoses

Cestodes: A variety of tapeworms are transmissible to people, including *Taenia saginata* in undercooked beef, *Taenia solium* in undercooked pork and *Diphyllobothrium latum* in raw fish. *Hymenolepis nana* does not require an intermediate host and infects people through food contaminated by infected rodents. *Dipylidium caninum* infects people when fleas are accidentally consumed. These parasites mature into adult tapeworms in the human intestinal tract, where they cause mild enteritis, compete with the host for nutrients and produce proglottids (tapeworm segments), but no serious disease.

Echinococcus, on the other hand, may follow a similar pattern when undercooked meat is eaten; however, if an egg is consumed (from fecal contamination), a hydatid cyst develops in the liver, lungs, kidneys, spleen, heart, skeletal muscles, brain or bone marrow. The cyst is filled with fluid and scoleces (worm heads) and can grow very large.

Control is by fecal examination for animals, elimination of intermediate hosts and careful food preparation (well-cooked meat).

Trematodes: Fasciola hepatica, a fluke that inhabits the liver and bile ducts, is transmitted to people when contaminated raw greens (*eg,* watercress) are eaten. It is found where snails, moisture and herbivorous animals are combined. Cooking of wild greens and treating infected animals are recommended control measures.

Nematodes: The roundworm of swine (*Ascaris suum*) can infect people through ingestion of food or water contaminated with the feces of infected swine. The roundworm then completes its life cycle as in the natural host.

Toxocara (roundworm of dogs and cats) also infects people in a similar fashion but does not complete its life cycle (people are an aberrant host). Instead, it wanders throughout the tissue (especially damaging to the brain or eye), causing damage until the worm dies (larva migrans).

Hookworms (*eg, Ancylostoma*) and *Strongyloides* penetrate the skin and migrate subcutaneously, causing itching, inflammation and a rash (cutaneous larva migrans or creeping eruption). *Strongyloides* has a free-living cycle and can heavily contaminate the environment. It may cause enteric disease in people and, if the infective stage is activated internally, can penetrate the colon or skin around the anus with fatal results in a person with an immunodeficiency.

Domestic animals, especially young puppies, should have a fecal sample examined routinely to reduce the public health hazard of these parasites.

Trichinella spiralis encysts in the muscle of pigs and may be consumed in undercooked pork. In people, the parasite prefers highly active muscles, such as the tongue and diaphragm, where the cysts cause pain and even death.

Heartworms (*Dirofilaria*) cause granulomatous lung lesions in people bitten by infected mosquitoes.

Protozoa: Consumption of water contaminated by *Entamoeba* and *Giardia* can lead to enteritis (diarrhea) and weight loss.

Toxoplasmosis (*Toxoplasma gondii*) is a protozoal infection of domestic animals and many birds. The sexual phase of its life cycle takes place only in the intestinal tract of cats. Ingestion of oocysts in cat feces leads to cyst formation in other species (eating cysts in undercooked meat causes cyst formation in the new host). Cyst formation is of particular concern to pregnant women, as it can cause serious deformities in the fetus. Clinical disease in people resembles influenza or infectious mononucleosis; chronic disease can result in ocular abnormalities.

Table 1. Zoonotic parasites.

Parasites in Food and Water

Taenia solium (pork tapeworm)
Taenia saginata (beef tapeworm)
Diphyllobothrium latum (broad fish tapeworm)
Trichinella spiralis
Entamoeba histolytica
Toxoplasma gondii

Parasites of Dogs

Echinococcus granulosus
Toxocara canis (dog roundworm)
Dipylidium caninum (flea-transmitted tapeworm)
Ancylostoma braziliense (hookworm)
Dirofilaria immitis (heartworm)
Strongyloides canis
Trypanosoma cruzi
Ctenocephalides canis (dog flea)

Parasites of Cats

Toxocara cati (cat roundworm)
Toxoplasma gondii
Ctenocephalides felis (cat flea)
Sarcoptes (sarcoptic mange mite)
Notoedres (notoedric mange mite)

Miscellaneous Parasites

Strongyloides
Cryptosporidium
Giardia
Sarcocystis
Ascaris suum (swine roundworm)
Fasciola hepatica (liver fluke)
Hymenolepis nana
Balantidium coli
Echinococcus multilocularis
Cheyletiella

Precautions involve completely cooking meat, washing hands after handling raw meat, avoiding cat litter pans when pregnant, and covering children's sandboxes when not in use.

Cats usually pick up the infection through hunting and may be tested for toxoplasmosis. People with prior exposure may have protective antibody levels.

Ectoparasites: Flies, fleas, ticks and mosquitoes may transmit a variety of diseases through their bites. *Sarcoptes, Notoedres, Demodex* and *Cheyletiella* are mites that can cause rashes in people. Direct contact with infected animals is necessary for transmission. Bright-red, itchy papules are formed, especially in areas where clothing fits tightly. Elimination of infestation on animals often clears the rash on people, but topical insecticides may be required.

Recommendations

Prevention of zoonotic disease involves some very simple measures. Do not eat, drink or smoke unless your hands have been thoroughly washed. Do not eat undercooked meat or drink contaminated water or unpasteurized milk. Protect open wounds from animal waste, saliva, pus and other contaminants. Wear rubber gloves when handling dead animals, aborted fetuses, placentas or birth fluids and wash hands well after cleaning up animal waste or vomit. Get vaccinated for tetanus and rabies. Educate clients regarding the value of fecal examinations and vaccinations in preventing zoonotic diseases. Finally, encourage owners to obey leash laws, control stray animals and clean up after their pets in public areas.

Recommended Reading

Allen DG *et al: Small Animal Medicine.* Lippincott, Philadelphia, 1991.

Colahan P *et al: Equine Medicine and Surgery.* 4th ed. American Veterinary Publications, Goleta, CA, 1991.

Colville J: *Diagnostic Parasitology For Veterinary Technicians.* American Veterinary Publications, Goleta, CA, 1991.

Howard JL: *Current Veterinary Therapy, Food Animal Practice 3.* Saunders, Philadelphia, 1993.

Ikram M and Hill E: *Microbiology For Veterinary Technicians.* American Veterinary Publications, Goleta, CA, 1991.

Kirk RW *et al: Handbook of Veterinary Procedures and Emergency Therapy.* 5th ed. Saunders, Philadelphia, 1990.

Kirk RW and Bonagura JD: *Current Veterinary Therapy, Small Animal Practice XI.* Saunders, Philadelphia, 1992.

Leman A: *Diseases of Swine.* 7th ed. Iowa State Univ Press, Ames, 1992.

Pedersen NC: *Feline Infectious Diseases.* American Veterinary Publications, Goleta, CA, 1988.

Pratt PW: *Laboratory Procedures for Veterinary Technicians.* 2nd ed. American Veterinary Publications, Goleta, CA, 1992.

Robinson NE: *Current Therapy in Equine Medicine 3.* Saunders, Philadelphia, 1992.

Smith BP: *Large Animal Internal Medicine.* Mosby, St. Louis, 1990.

Notes

4

Treatment Techniques for Dogs and Cats

C.B. Waters, J.C. Scott-Moncrieff, P. Phegley

Routes of Drug Administration

Numerous routes are available for administration of drugs, vaccines and fluids in small animal medicine. These include alimentary (gastrointestinal tract), topical, aerosolized and parenteral routes. The most appropriate route depends upon the specific characteristics of the medication itself, the relative size of the patient, and the medical requirements of the patient.

Medications given via the alimentary route are usually given *orally* (*per os*). In some cases, medications may be given through a feeding tube that bypasses the oral cavity and is inserted into the esophagus, stomach or intestine. *Rectal administration* of a drug or enema is another form of alimentary administration.

*Topical route*s include direct administration onto the skin (dermal), into the nasal cavity (intranasal), into the ears (otic), or on the eyes (ophthalmic). Aerosolized medications are first inhaled and then absorbed in the lungs. *Parenteral administration* refers to injection of drugs or fluids. Parenteral routes include intradermal (into the skin), intralesional (into the lesion), subcutaneous (under the skin), intramuscular (into the muscle), intravenous (into the vein), intraperitoneal (into the abdominal cavity), and intraosseous (into the bone).

Oral Route

The oral route is readily accessible, and all but the most intractable patients can easily be medicated by this route. It is the route of choice for most systemic medications. The oral route should not be used in patients that are persistently vomiting (oral medication may exacerbate vomiting), weak or moribund patients (oral medications may not be swallowed or, even worse, may be aspirated into the lungs) and patients in which gastrointestinal absorption may be compromised. Medications for oral administration may be formulated as tablets, capsules, elixirs or solutions. Fluids, such as balanced electrolyte solutions or water, may also be administered orally.

Tablets and Capsules: Tablets and capsules are administered to both cats and dogs using a similar technique. In most cases, only one person is required to administer to medication; however, 2 people may be necessary in less cooperative patients (one to hold the animal and one to administer to drug). The animal's muzzle is grasped and the nose is pointed toward the ceiling. This causes the jaw to relax. The jaw is pulled downward and the pill is placed at the base of the tongue (Fig 1). For cats, it is safer to drop the pill

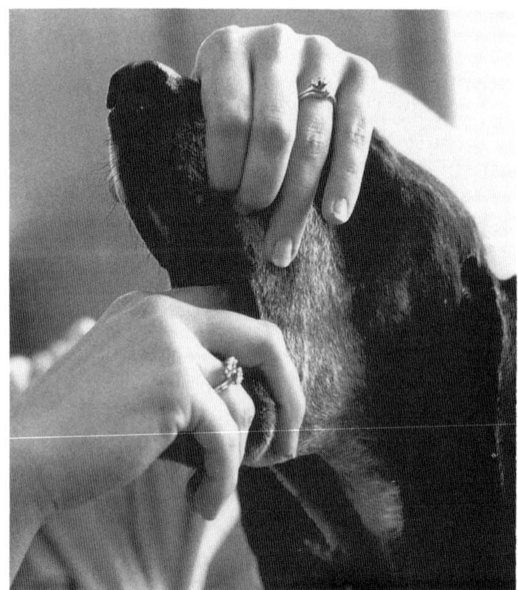

Figure 1. Oral administration of a tablet or pill to a dog.

into the back of the throat, rather than relying on placement with the fingers.

The mouth is closed and the head is lowered until the animal swallows. If the animal does not swallow, lightly stroking the pharyngeal region of the neck or blowing on the nose helps to elicit a swallowing reflex. It may take 1-2 minutes for swallowing to occur. Once the animal has swallowed, the mouth should be inspected to ensure that the pill has been swallowed. Some animals become adept at hiding the pill in the cheek pouches.

If the cat or dog will not hold still, an assistant should restrain the animal. Cats are easier to pill if they are on a table, giving the assistant more control than if the cat is on the floor. The assistant should hold the cat's front feet to prevent scratching of the person giving the pill. Dogs may be restrained by placing one arm around the dog's neck and the other around its body.

Occasionally, a fractious cat or dog will make oral administration very difficult and may present a danger to the individual giving the medication. One solution is to use a pill gun, which is a plastic device with a soft rubber applicator tip. The pill gun lengthens the distance between one's fingers and the animal's teeth. The pill is first inserted into the rubber applicator. The applicator, instead of the fingers, is then placed at the base of the animal's tongue. The pill is released by pushing the plunger. The mouth is then kept closed until the animal swallows.

We have seen hemostats used in a similar manner as a pill gun. However, the hard metal of the hemostats may cause considerable damage to the oral cavity or the pharynx, especially if the animal is vigorously struggling; therefore, this technique is not recommended.

Another way to administer medication to cats and dogs that are difficult to pill is to hide it in their food. Most dogs will readily eat a small meatball of canned food with the pill embedded in the center. Cats tend to be more selective, however, and usually will not eat medicated food. It is important to be sure that the pill has been swallowed if this technique is used.

Elixirs, Solutions and Fluids: Liquid medications, such as elixirs, solutions, oral electrolyte solutions and water, should be administered with a syringe or dropper. A dosing syringe is a more practical choice when large volumes of fluid are required. When administering liquid medications, the animal's mouth does not need to be forced open (as when administering a pill). The folds of the lips should be lifted up on one side of the face and the syringe or dropper is gently inserted between the canine and premolar teeth (Fig 2). Small amounts of liquid are injected into the oral cavity, allowing the animal sufficient time to swallow between each bolus. Generally, a cat or small dog can comfortably swallow 0.5-2 ml at a time, while a large dog can swallow 3-5 ml at a time. If the animal struggles excessively, an assistant should restrain the animal. It is important not to inject the liquid too quickly. This may result in aspiration into the lungs, with serious consequences, such as pneumonia.

Large amounts of fluid, such as water, electrolyte solutions or pureed food, can also be administered *per os.* This can be time consuming and the animal may become increasingly more reluctant to accept the fluid. Tube feeding may be a better alternative in this case.

Some cats and dogs tolerate liquid medications better than tablets or capsules, while others are easier to pill. Medications may come in either form (*eg*, amoxicillin is formulated as both a tablet and a solution), providing alternative ways to administer drugs. However, most drugs have only one formulation. If liquids are easier to administer than pills, the pills can be crushed and mixed with a small amount of water. Likewise, the contents of capsules can be dissolved in water and administered as a liquid. However, it is very important to check the drug package insert first, as some drugs may lose their activity if not administered in their original form.

Client Education: Before a cat or dog goes home with oral medication, the owner should be shown how to administer the medica-

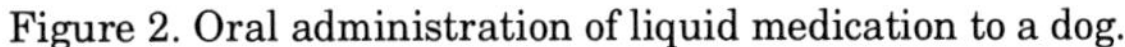

Figure 2. Oral administration of liquid medication to a dog.

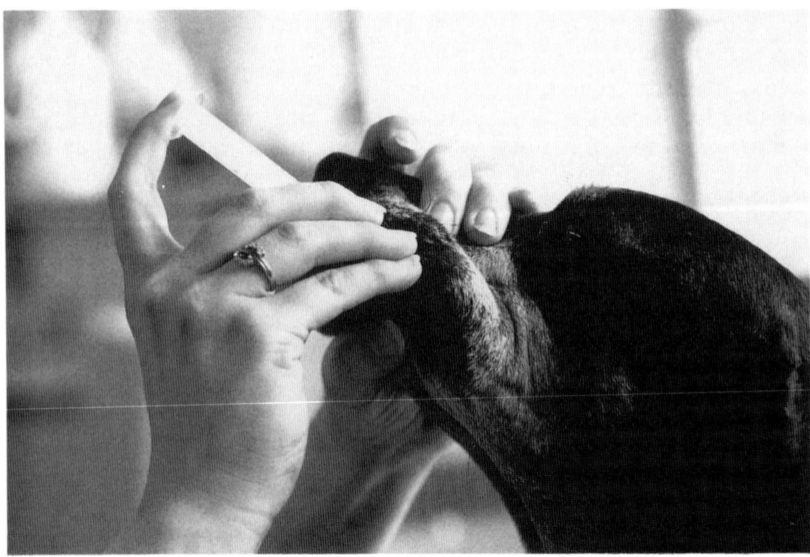

tion in order to ensure owner compliance. Unfortunately, many animals never receive the prescribed amount of medication because of the owner's uncertainty, lack of skill or fear of getting bitten. A client may think that s/he has successfully administered medication, but, unbeknownst to him or her, the pet has spit out the pill behind the couch. Emphasis on the proper technique, including an oral examination for potentially unswallowed pills after giving the medication, is very important.

Topical Route

Dermal: Ointments, liquids, powders, gels and sprays may be applied topically to the skin. Ideally, the skin surface should be clean and dry before medication is administered. The haircoat may need to be clipped. The drug information sheet should always be consulted for the proper way to administer topical medications.

Some drugs are specifically designed to be absorbed through the skin to affect an internal organ (*eg*, nitroglycerin is a topical ointment that affects the heart and blood vessels). While most topical drugs are designed to exert a local effect on the skin, they may result in undesirable systemic side effects caused by their absorption (*eg*, topical corticosteroids can cause hyperadrenocorticism and organophosphate flea preparations can cause systemic organophosphate toxicity). Clients should be advised if a topical preparation contains potentially harmful ingredients that may be absorbed through their own skin. For example, a client applying nitroglycerin ointment to an animal should wear gloves for each application.

Intranasal: The intranasal route is commonly used in veterinary medicine for administration of respiratory vaccines (*eg*, *Bordetella* vaccine for kennel cough). The vaccine is usually administered with a syringe or nasal applicator attached to a syringe. The patient's nose is raised toward the ceiling to prevent the vaccine from dripping out of the nose (Fig 3). The vaccine is injected in equal parts into each nasal cavity. The patient's nose is maintained in an elevated position for a moment to allow the vaccine to drain into the rest of the upper respiratory tract.

Other medications that are occasionally given intranasally include phenylephrine drops (Neo-Synephrine: Sanofi Winthrop) in cats with severe upper respiratory infections and aqueous vasopressin in patients with antidiuretic hormone insufficiency. The same method described for administering intranasal vaccination is used.

Aerosolized Route

Some drugs can be directly administered to the pulmonary tissue by aerosolization. This route enables treatment of lung disease, while avoiding a systemic route. Examples of pulmonary medications include gentamicin (to treat bacterial pneumonia) and acetylcysteine (to dissolve mucous secretions in the airways). In people, inhalers are used to administer aerosolized drugs. However, cats and dogs do not tolerate inhalers. Therefore, these drugs are usually administered with a mask and nebulizer. Water vapor, to moisten dry respiratory tissues, may also be administered with a nebulizer.

Parenteral Route

Intradermal: The intradermal route is commonly used in intradermal skin testing for skin allergies. Adequate patient restraint is necessary for accurate injection. The cat or dog may need to be sedated before starting the procedure. A large area is clipped on the animal's side. Multiple sites are numbered with a felt-tipped pen. Allergens are individually injected at different sites with a small needle (typically, 25 gauge). A small amount of allergen is deposited within the dermal layer, forming a bleb. The animal's skin is observed for a wheal and flare reaction at each site, suggesting possible hypersensitivity. It is important to inject the allergen intradermally, as adequate bleb formation will not occur with subcutaneous injection.

Figure 3. Intranasal administration of a drug or vaccine to a dog.

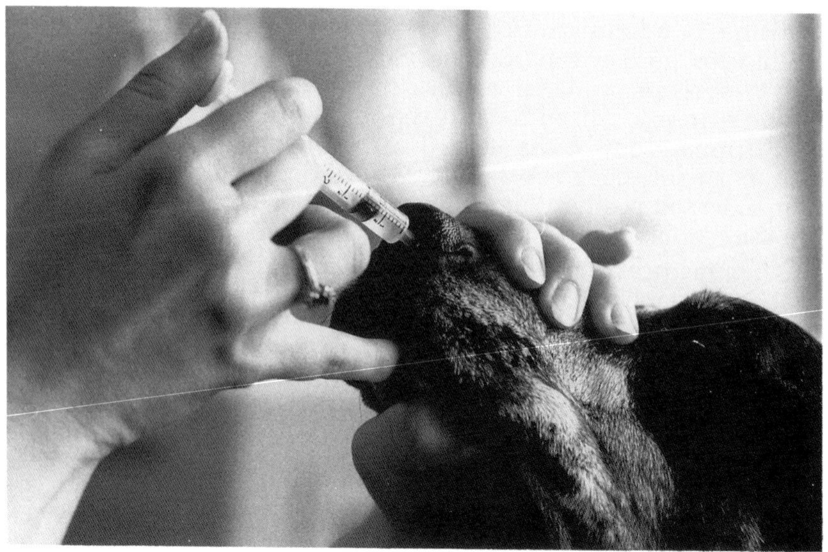

Intralesional: The intralesional route is primarily used for injection of corticosteroids into an inflammatory lesion or into a cutaneous tumor. Intralesional injection is not an efficient mechanism for administering drugs systemically. Patient preparation before intralesional injection may include clipping the hair and prepping the injection site with a surgical scrub. A separate, sterile needle should be used at each injection site. The injection may cause discomfort, so proper restraint is important to ensure that the full dose of medication is delivered to the correct site. Small needles, usually 22 or 25 gauge, are used. Only a small amount of medication is injected in each site.

Subcutaneous: The subcutaneous route is used for administering medication, fluids and vaccinations under the skin. If the patient is severely dehydrated, the subcutaneous route is a poor choice for drug or fluid administration, as systemic absorption is diminished. Many drugs can be administered via the subcutaneous route. The instructions on the drug package insert should always be consulted to determine if the subcutaneous route is an appropriate way to administer a specific drug or vaccine.

Medication and vaccines are administered subcutaneously in a similar manner. Restraint of the animal with the aid of an assistant may be necessary. The loose skin at the back of the neck is gently, but firmly, grasped and lifted upward to form a skin fold or tent. The needle (attached to the syringe filled with medication or vaccine) is placed through the tented skin and into the subcutaneous space (Fig 4). The syringe barrel should be partially withdrawn to ensure that the needle has not entered a blood vessel. If no blood is aspirated, the drug or vaccine is injected and the needle is then withdrawn. If blood is aspirated, the needle is withdrawn without injecting and a different site is used. When multiple injections

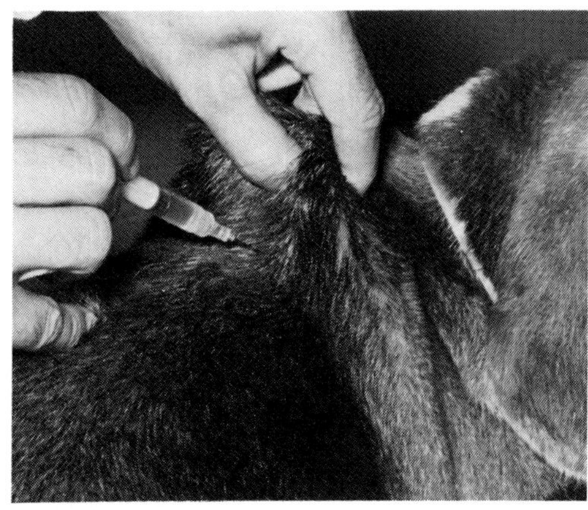

Figure 4. Needle placement for subcutaneous injection.

must be given, a number of sites on the dorsal neck and back should be used.

Occasionally, improper placement or animal movement can result in inadvertent administration of medication or vaccine through the skin fold and out through the opposite surface of the skin. Vaccination should be repeated if this happens, in order to ensure adequate immunization of the animal. However, administration of some medications, such as insulin, should never be repeated, as some of the drug may, in fact, have already been absorbed and estimation of the exact amount administered is impossible.

Subcutaneous administration of fluids is an easy, economical way to rehydrate slightly to moderately dehydrated animals, especially cats and small dogs. Subcutaneous fluids are not practical for rehydration of large dogs, nor is their use recommended for severely debilitated animals. Only sterile, isotonic solutions should be used. Solutions containing glucose should not be administered subcutaneously, as the glucose can irritate subcutaneous tissue and promote development of an infection. A sterile needle should be used for each injection site. Multiple injection sites may be needed, as not more than 50-100 ml should be administered at each site.

An 18- or 20-gauge needle is inserted into the subcutaneous space as described above. The needle is attached to a large syringe or an intravenous fluid administration set. If a syringe is used, the fluid is infused manually. If a fluid administration set is used, the bag or bottle of fluids may be hung from a hook or fluid stand, allowing gravity to assist flow into the subcutaneous space. We prefer to use an intravenous fluid administration set because it allows for greater range of animal movement, is less painful for the animal (fluids are not forced into the tissue), and frees a hand for restraint. After an appropriate amount of fluid has been administered at an injection site, the skin surrounding the injection site is gently pinched for one minute after withdrawing the needle. This helps prevent fluid leakage through the hole created by the needle.

Infection at the injection site rarely occurs as a sequel to subcutaneous administration of medication or fluids. Infection may be secondary to contamination of the needle or syringe (*eg*, using the same needle at multiple injection sites when administering subcutaneous fluids) or from contamination of the drug or fluids. If abscessation occurs, treatment should include clipping the area and lancing the abscess.

Clients may be taught how to give subcutaneous injections or fluids at home. Situations in which this may be necessary include administering insulin in the diabetic animal or fluid therapy in a patient with chronic renal failure. It is important to spend sufficient time showing the client how to withdraw medication into a syringe and allow them to practice administering saline injections to an inanimate object (an orange works well). Once they feel comfortable handling a needle and syringe, they should master giving subcutaneous injections of sterile saline to their pet before being sent home to administer medication.

Intramuscular: The intramuscular route is used to administer certain vaccines and small amounts of drugs (usually less than 3 ml). It is never used for fluid therapy. The intramuscular route allows for faster systemic absorption than the subcutaneous route and is easier than administering drugs via the intravenous route. This route is a poor choice for drug administration in an animal with a bleeding disorder, as muscle is very vascular. Intramuscular administration can result in severe hemorrhage in a dog or cat with a coagulopathy.

Several sites are available for intramuscular injection. The semimembranosus/semitendinosus muscle group (the hamstring) of the caudal thigh is commonly used. The advantage of this site is that it is readily palpable, even in small dogs and cats. However, care must be taken, as permanent sciatic nerve damage, with subsequent leg dysfunction and muscle atrophy, may result from improper administration of intramuscular injections.

Other intramuscular sites include the quadriceps muscles on the cranial thigh, the lumbar paraspinal muscles on the caudal back, and the shoulder muscles. These sites are easier to palpate on large dogs. When giving multiple intramuscular injections, rotation between the left and right sides is recommended to prevent muscle soreness. The intramuscular route is not a good choice when frequent injections are necessary, as the animal may become lame with repeated administration.

After the muscle group has been palpated and stabilized, the needle, attached to the syringe, is inserted into the muscle belly. When using the hamstring muscle group, the needle is inserted laterally and directed caudally to avoid the sciatic nerve (Fig 5). The syringe barrel is partially withdrawn to determine if the needle has entered a blood vessel. If blood is observed in the syringe after aspirating, the needle should be withdrawn and placed in another site. If no blood is observed, the medication or vaccine should be injected into the muscle and the needle withdrawn. Intramuscular injections are more painful than subcutaneous injections. It is important to have adequate restraint to prevent injury to the animal or technician and to ensure adequate delivery of the drug to the intramuscular site.

Intravenous: The intravenous route is frequently used to administer drugs and fluids. Vaccines are never administered intravenously. Intravenous administration is the fastest way to deliver drugs and fluids to the systemic circulation. Large volumes of fluid may be infused in a short time. To be proficient at administering drugs via this route, one must first be proficient at venipuncture. Venipuncture is an indispensable clinical skill in small animal medicine. Venipuncture may be used to collect blood samples, administer intravenous injections, and place intravenous catheters for medical and fluid therapy.

Common sites of venipuncture in dogs and cats include the cephalic veins, the jugular veins, and the saphenous veins (lateral saphenous in the dog, medial saphenous in the cat). Occasionally, the femoral veins or, in an unconscious or anesthetized animal, the lingual vein are used. The ideal selection site for venipuncture is dependent upon a number of factors. For collecting large volumes of blood (more than 1-2 ml), particularly in cats and small dogs, the jugular vein is easiest to use. Smaller volumes of blood can readily

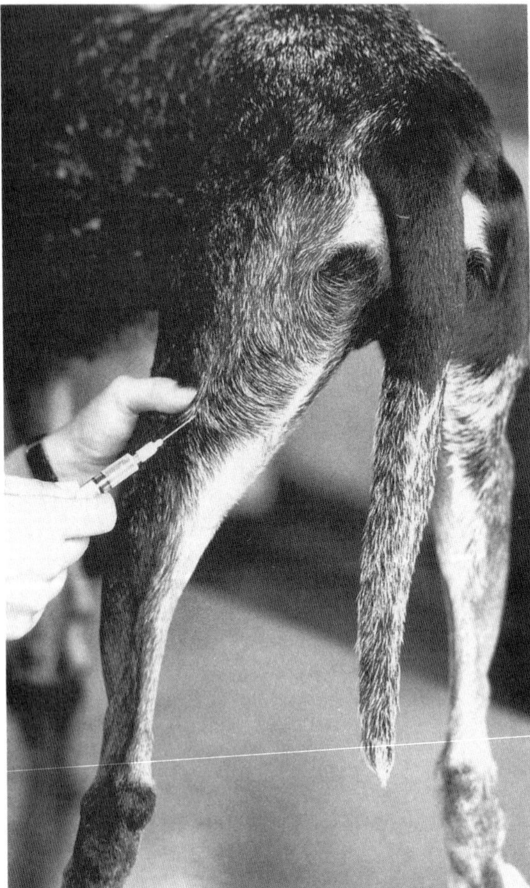

Figure 5. Intramuscular administration into a dog's semimembranosus/ semitendinosus (hamstring) muscle group.

be obtained from the cephalic or saphenous veins, especially from large dogs.

The cephalic and saphenous veins are used to administer intravenous injections with a needle and a syringe. The cephalic, saphenous and jugular veins are used to administer intravenous medications or fluids with indwelling catheter. Advantages of a jugular catheter include the large volume of fluid that can be infused in a short time, a readily accessible port for collecting blood samples in a patient that requires intensive monitoring and frequent blood sampling, and a central venous line for administration of parenteral nutrition and measurement of central venous pressures. However, a jugular catheter used for total parenteral nutrition should always be a dedicated line that is not used for blood sampling or concurrent fluid administration.

For intravenous administration, the cat or dog is placed on a table in lateral or sternal recumbency or allowed to sit. The animal's position depends on how the animal feels most comfortable and the preference of the person performing venipuncture. Adequate patient restraint by a trained assistant is crucial to successful placement of a needle or catheter into the vein.

The venipuncture site may be clipped first to aid visualization of the vein. If an intravenous catheter will be placed, the injection site should always be clipped to remove all hair at the site and a diligent surgical scrub (triple scrubs with alcohol and povidone-iodine or chlorhexidine) should be performed. If an intravenous injection will be performed, the venipuncture site is prepared with alcohol applied directly to the skin. In addition to its disinfectant properties, alcohol helps to visualize the vein.

An assistant is usually necessary to occlude and stabilize the vein, though a tourniquet may also be used (Fig 6). A tourniquet should never be used on the jugular vein. The vein should be raised and filled with blood by holding off the vein proximal to the site of venipuncture (at the elbow for the cephalic vein, at the knee for the lateral saphenous vein, at the medial thigh for the medial saphenous vein, at the thoracic inlet for the jugular vein). Adequate light is essential to help visualize the vein. However, obese dogs or unclipped animals with long hair may have veins that are difficult to see. In any case, the vein should always be palpated before venipuncture is attempted.

The needle or catheter is pointed proximally (toward venous return to the heart) and advanced through the skin over the venipuncture site. The needle or catheter is then inserted into the lumen of the vein and advanced slightly.

If a needle and syringe or butterfly catheter is used, the needle is threaded into the vein (Fig 7). Gentle aspiration of the syringe, while the vein is still occluded, should result in back flow of blood into the syringe. The drug is injected into the vein (the assistant should be reminded to release pressure on the vein before the drug is injected). After the injection, the needle is withdrawn and pressure is applied to the puncture site for one minute to prevent extravascular bleeding and hematoma formation.

If an over-the-needle catheter is used, the catheter is advanced steadily into the vein and the stylet is withdrawn. The intravenous fluid administration set or injection cap is attached to the catheter. The catheter should be flushed with heparinized saline to ensure patency. A sterile pad, with or without sterile ointment (*eg*, povidone-iodine) should be placed over the catheter entrance into the skin.

The catheter is carefully, aseptically and securely taped into place. Folding over the ends of the tape edges is a useful trick, as it

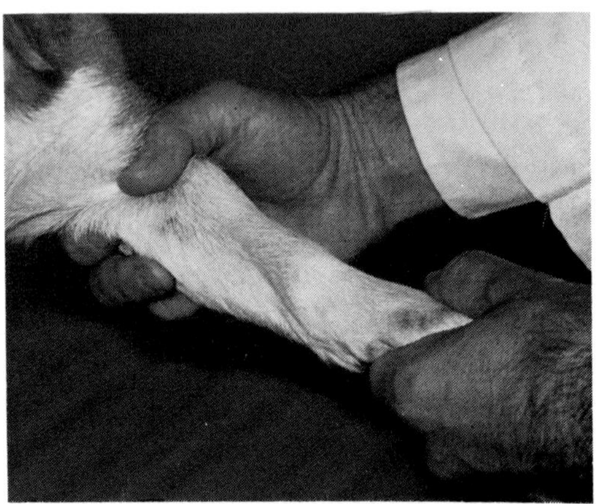

Figure 6. Extending the leg before attempting intravenous injection stabilizes the vein beneath the skin.

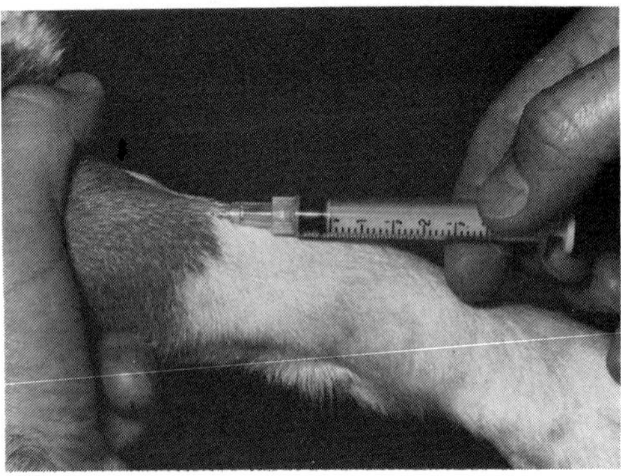

Figure 7. Proper placement of needle and syringe for intravenous injection or withdrawal of blood.

permits easier unwrapping when the catheter is eventually removed. A second flushing with heparinized saline is recommended if fluid therapy is not started immediately or if the catheter is to be used for administering intravenous drugs. A catheter should never be left in a vein for more than 72 hours and should be retaped daily so that the catheter site may be regularly inspected.

Intravenous administration of drugs and/or fluids may be required in an emergency. The urgency of the situation may make ordinarily straightforward venipuncture difficult. Further, an animal in shock may be severely volume depleted (hypovolemic), making veins difficult to visualize and palpate. Venipuncture should be performed in a calm, orderly manner. In an emergency situation, the most experienced person should perform the procedure.

When a vein cannot be visualized or palpated, a *venous cutdown* may be indicated. A cutdown is a surgical procedure involving an incision through the skin down to the vein, allowing visualization of the vein. This permits direct catheterization of the vein. A cutdown creates an open would that must be kept sterilely wrapped and the incision must be sutured close when the catheter is removed.

Complications of venipuncture include venous collapse, hematoma formation, catheter occlusion, extravascular administration of drugs or fluids, and phlebitis (inflammation and/or infection of a vein). Venous collapse may occur when blood is aspirated too quickly from a small vein. If this occurs, gentle, slow and intermittent aspiration usually corrects the problem.

Hematomas, caused by extravascular leakage of blood from the vessel, usually occur with repeated venipuncture attempts, failure to apply pressure to the vein after withdrawing a needle or catheter, or inadvertently holding off a vein after venipuncture has occurred. If a hematoma does develop, venipuncture will probably be unsuccessful if attempted distal to the site of hematoma formation. It is wise to begin venipuncture as distal as possible in case a hematoma does form; the procedure may then be attempted proximal to the hematoma site.

Catheter occlusion can occur when clots form within the catheter lumen. These clots should not be forced out of the catheter with heavy pressure. Clots are potentially thrombogenic, so flushing a clot into the vein to renew catheter patency is contraindicated.

Extravascular administration of some drugs may have serious consequences, resulting in tissue sloughin and phlebitis (*eg*, pentobarbital, and anesthetic, and thiacetarsamide, a heartworm adulticide) and even endangering the animal's limb (*eg*, doxorubicin, a chemotherapeutic drug). If a drug is injected outside the vein, the drug package insert should be consulted and appropriate measures taken immediately. Emergency measures may include injection of sterile saline or a corticosteroid preparation in the limb and application of ice packs.

Phlebitis may occur from using a contaminated needle or syringe or a contaminated drug but is more commonly associated with placement of an indwelling catheter. Strict aseptic technique should be used when placing the catheter. Additionally, the catheter should be rebandaged daily. The dermal insertion site should be inspected for swelling or redness. When a catheter is inserted into a limb vein, the leg should regularly be checked for swelling or heat.

If an animal develops a fever or other signs of systemic infection, the venous catheter should be the prime suspect as the source of infection. When phlebitis or infection is suspected, the catheter should be removed and, ideally, the catheter tip should be submitted for bacterial culture. Hot packing of the limb and antibiotic therapy may be indicated. The next intravenous catheter should be placed in a different limb. Indwelling catheters should never be left in a vein longer than 72 hours, regardless of how well asepsis is maintained.

Intraperitoneal: The intraperitoneal route is used in neonates that require fluid therapy and have veins too tiny for catheter placement. However, only a limited amount of fluid can be given intraperitoneally, and there is the risk of perforating intestines or other abdominal organs.

Intraosseous: The intraosseous route has become an increasingly popular way to deliver large volumes of fluids quickly to animals, especially young puppies and kittens. Sites of intraosseous fluid administration include the tibial tuberosity and the trochanteric fossa of the femur. The area around the intraosseous site is clipped and prepped in a manner similar to that described for intravenous catheter placement. A hypodermic needle, a spinal needle, a bone marrow needle or an intraosseous catheter is inserted through the skin and then embedded into the bone.

An intravenous fluid line is attached and fluids are infused with a fluid administration set, similar to the delivery of intravenous fluids. Drugs can also be administered via the intraosseous route (as long as they are also acceptable to administer via the intravenous route). Care of the intraosseous site is the same as with the intravenous catheter site. The site should be rebandaged daily. The needle is removed after 72 hours of use.

Tube Feeding

Debilitated cats and dogs are often too weak to consume adequate amounts of food and water. As a result of inadequate nutrition, they may become even weaker. Tube feeding has revolutionized the way in which we can support our small animal patients. However, initiation of tube feeding early in the course of anorexia is crucial for a successful outcome.

Types of Feeding Tubes

The nomenclature of feeding tubes can be confusing and warrants a brief discussion. A tube that is placed into a body cavity (*eg*, the esophagus or stomach) is referred to by the *initial cavity* it is passed through and the *final cavity* where the tip of the tube is placed. For example, a nasoesophageal tube is placed through the nose and into the esophagus.

A tube may be placed through an artificial opening, or stoma, into a body cavity. For example, a gastrostomy tube is placed through the skin and into the stomach. The stoma, in this case, is through the skin, abdominal wall and stomach wall. A jejunostomy tube is placed through the skin and abdominal wall, and into the small intestine. A pharyngostomy tube is placed through the skin and cervical musculature, and into the pharynx. An esophagostomy tube is placed through the skin and cervical musculature, and into the esophagus.

Nutritional support can be provided by using a tube that is placed at the time of each feeding (temporary feeding tube) or by using a tube that remains in place for several days to months (semi-permanent feeding tube). Oroesophageal tubes are temporary tubes, as cats and dogs will not tolerate a feeding tube in their mouth for any period of time. Nasoesophageal tubes can be temporary or semi-permanent. When sutured into place, a nasoesophageal tube can be used for up to 2-3 weeks. Jejunostomy tubes are semi-permanent and usually used for a few days post-operatively. Pharyngostomy, esophagostomy and gastrostomy tubes are semi-permanent tubes and can be used for several weeks to months.

Several types of feeding tubes are commercially available, including soft red rubber tubes, polyurethane tubes and pediatric feeding tubes (Fig 8). Tubes used for a gastrostomy or jejunostomy may have a bulb, mushroom or Foley near the tip. These devices help maintain the tube in its desired location.

The ideal size and type of tube selected and the best site for tube placement depend upon a number of factors, including the animal's primary problem, the severity and nature of the illness, the type of diet to be fed, the equipment available and the owner's financial situation.

Oroesophageal Tube Feeding

Oroesophageal tube feeding is a temporary method of alimentation. The tube is placed in the oral cavity and passed into the esophagus. This type of tube feeding is especially useful for feeding neonates (*eg*, orphaned puppies and kittens). These animals are too small to consider placing a more permanent type of feeding tube and are not difficult to intubate repeatedly. Great care must be taken not to inadvertently place the tube into the respiratory tract, as aspiration pneumonia and death will invariably result.

The length of tube necessary to reach the distal esophagus should be estimated by measuring from the tip of the nose to the eighth or ninth rib (Fig 9). This point should be marked on the tube. A 3- to-8-French pediatric feeding tube, soft red rubber tube or polyurethane nasogastric tube is recommended for tube feeding neonates. With one hand, the puppy's or kitten's mouth is gently opened. The tube is slowly passed caudally into the pharynx, allowing time for the neonate to swallow the tube as it passes. The tube is passed into the distal esophagus to the level of the eighth or ninth rib.

If the tube has been satisfactorily placed in the esophagus, the tube can usually be palpated on the left side of the ventral neck region, separate from the trachea. If the tube has been passed into the trachea, only the trachea is palpated. When the tube is inadvertently passed into the trachea, the animal may cough. However, the absence of a cough should not be relied upon to confirm tube placement. To ensure proper placement, several milliliters of air should be injected into the tube and the stomach auscultated for bubbling sounds. A small amount of water (0.5-1 ml) should also be injected into the tube and the animal observed for coughing. These methods are not foolproof; however, the small size of the neonatal larynx makes tube feeding a relatively safe procedure and most clients can be taught how to feed a litter of puppies or kittens.

Figure 8. A sample of the various feeding tubes available: soft red rubber feeding tube (top); Foley (center); mushroom tip (bottom).

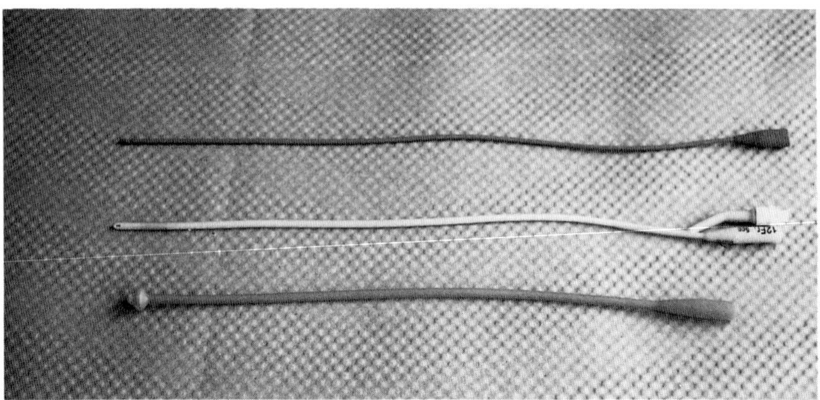

Figure 9. Measuring the feeding tube for oroesophageal placement in a puppy.

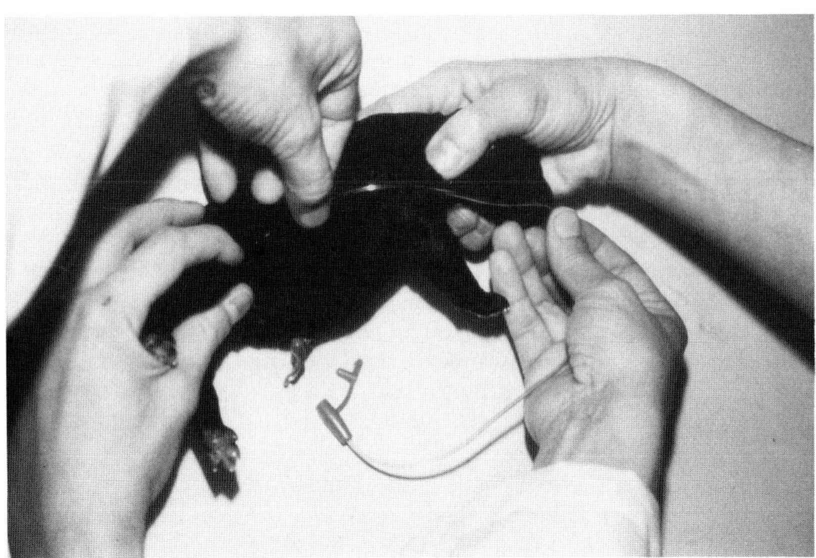

Placement of an oroesophageal tube is occasionally necessary in an adult dog or cat. Examples include administration of barium for an upper gastrointestinal radiographic study, decompression of the stomach of a dog with gastric-dilatation and volvulus, and very-short-term nutritional support. An oral speculum or mouth guard is necessary to prevent the animal from biting the tube. A roll of tape may be used, with the tube inserted through the center of the roll (Fig 10).

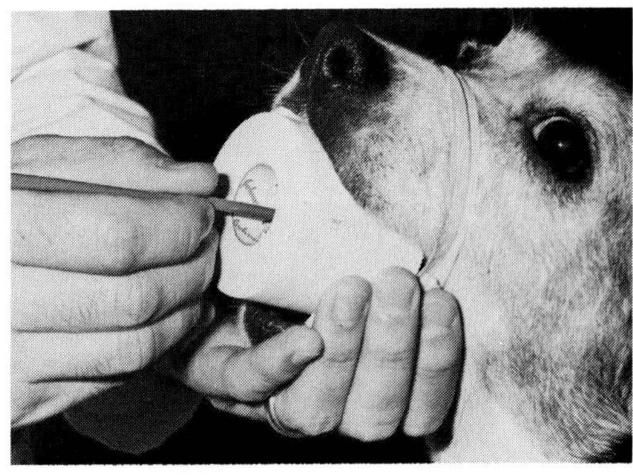

Figure 10. A roll of adhesive tape is an effective speculum when passing a tube into the esophagus.

Nasoesophageal Tube Feeding

Nasoesophageal tubes may be used as temporary or semi-permanent tubes. Nasoesophageal tubes are inexpensive and easy to place, and usually do not require general anesthesia or sedation. The animal may be sent home with the tube in place and the owner taught how to maintain the tube and administer nutrients.

The tube is premeasured for placement at the level of the eighth or ninth rib. Nasoesophageal tubes were formerly called nasogastric tubes because they were placed in the stomach. However, the current recommendation is to place the tube in the esophagus, not the stomach, to help minimize gastroesophageal reflux.

A polyvinyl infant feeding tube, a soft red rubber feeding tube, or a commercial polyurethane nasogastric feeding tube is used. A 5- or 6-French tube is the appropriate size for a cat. A large cat or small dog may tolerate an 8-French tube. An 8- or 10-French tube works well for larger dogs.

Before placing the tube, a couple drops of a topical ophthalmic anesthetic or lidocaine 2% are instilled into one nostril, holding the animal's head upward (Fig 11). This procedure should be repeated 2-3 minutes later. The tube tip is lubricated with a small amount of water-soluble lubricant (K-Y Jelly: Johnson & Johnson). The lubricated tube is gently inserted into the ventral aspect of the anesthe-

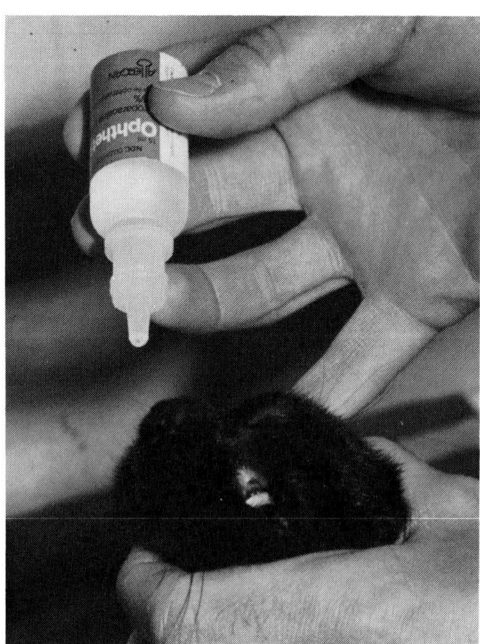

Figure 11. A topical ophthalmic anesthetic is instilled directly into one nostril before passing a flexible feeding tube.

tized nostril. In cats, the tube should readily pass into the nasopharynx and down into the esophagus. In dogs, pushing upward on the nose facilitates passage of the tube into the ventral nasal meatus. After the tube has been advanced through the pharynx, the head is held with the nose pointing downward while the tube is advanced into the esophagus. This helps prevent the tube from entering the trachea.

The patient should be observed for signs of coughing. A small amount of air and water should be injected into the tube to help confirm placement in the esophagus, as previously described. For absolute safety, a lateral thoracic radiograph may be made to confirm tube placement in the distal esophagus. This is mandatory if the operator is inexperienced with this technique.

The tube should be attached to the face using a butterfly tape (a piece of tape folded around the tube, with the ends used as suture sites) sutured to the skin on the face. This helps prevent slippage of the tube through the sutures. A suture on the muzzle and a suture on top of the head work well. An injection cap should be placed on the end of the tube when it is not in use. An Elizabethan collar placed around the animal's neck is necessary to prevent the animal from pulling out the tube.

The tube is flushed with a small amount of water before and after each feeding to ensure tube patency and to keep the lumen clean. The major disadvantage of nasoesophageal feeding, especially in cats and small dogs, is that the smaller diameter of the tube necessitates a liquid diet (pureed diets will clot the tube). An 8-French tube or larger can generally accommodate a finely strained, pureed diet.

Occasionally, a patient will sneeze or vomit up the tube. If this happens, the tube should be replaced. However, if an animal is vomiting continuously, a nasoesophageal tube is not an appropriate method of nutritional support.

Pharyngostomy and Esophagostomy Tube Feeding

Pharyngostomy and esophagostomy tube placement both require general anesthesia and surgical placement of a feeding tube directly into the esophagus through the walls of the pharynx or esophagus, respectively. In our experience, these methods of tube feeding are used less frequently because of the increasing availability of endoscopes for gastrostomy tube placement, (see below).

Gastrostomy Tube Feeding

Gastrostomy tube placement also requires general anesthesia. The tube can either be placed surgically or with the aid of a fiberoptic endoscope. Surgery is a more invasive procedure than endoscopic placement. However, endoscopic placement requires endoscopic retrieval of the tube (and a second general anesthesia) when the tube is eventually removed.

The gastrostomy tube is placed through the skin and the abdominal and stomach walls, and into the stomach (Fig 12). A specialized tip, such as a Foley or mushroom, anchors the tube in the stomach and prevents it from coming out of the stoma.

As with other semi-permanent tubes, the gastrostomy tube is always flushed with water before and after each feeding. The large diameter of the tube permits feeding a pureed diet. Some medications can also be administered through the tube. Tablets can be crushed and flushed through the tube with water.

Cats and dogs tolerate gastrostomy tubes very well. Some animals may require an Elizabethan collar to prevent them from pulling or biting the tube. A gastrostomy tube can be left in place for several weeks, and even several months, as long as the animal tolerates the tube and shows no signs of infection (*eg*, discharge, foul odor or redness around the tube exit site).

Maintenance of a gastrostomy tube requires keeping the stoma clean and dry. A bandage is placed over the stoma site to help prevent contamination. When an animal is sent home with a gastrostomy tube in place, the client should be shown the correct way to change the bandage twice a week. In addition to infection, other

Figure 12. Gastrostomy tube placement through a dog's flank.

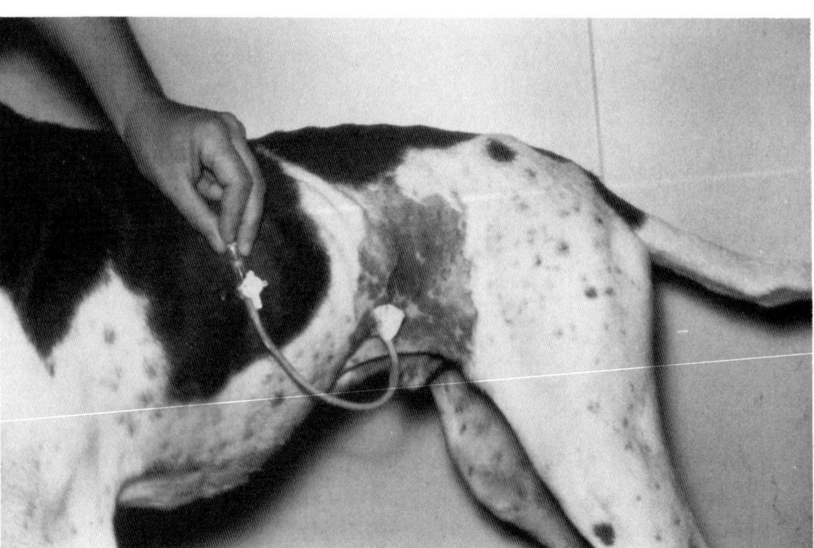

complications of gastrostomy tubes include vomiting of the tube and leakage of food into the peritoneum.

When a mushroom-tip gastrostomy tube is no longer necessary, it can be removed by cutting it off at the level of the stoma and retrieving the gastric portion with the fiberoptic endoscope. Alternatively, the tube tip may be allowed to pass into the intestines and evacuated in the feces. This should present no problem in a large dog but could cause obstruction of the intestines in a cat or small dog and is not recommended in these small animals. If a Foley catheter is used as a gastrostomy tube, the Foley bulb is deflated and the tube pulled through the skin stoma.

Jejunostomy Tube Feeding

Jejunostomy feeding requires surgical placement of a feeding tube directly into the jeunum of the small intestine (Fig 13). Unlike nasoesophageal or gastrostomy tube feeding, in which the animal is usually fed several small meals a day, jejunostomy tube feeding requires continuous infusion of a liquid diet because of the much smaller size of the intestinal lumen. Further, only special, easily digestible diets can be used. This type of tube feeding is generally reserved for referral hospitals or clinics with 24-hour care and is not appropriate for the client to manage at home.

Diets for Tube Feeding

The choice of an appropriate diet for tube feeding is dependent upon the type and size of tube used and the nutritional requirements of the individual patient. Small tube diameters preclude use of a pureed diet, as the tube may clog with food particles. Commercial liquid diets are available, including specialized diets for kidney failure and other critically ill patients. These diets may be expensive for long-term use.

Pureed diets are more economical but require more effort to prepare than liquid diets. Pureed diets are used with gastrostomy, pharyngostomy, and esophagostomy feeding tubes. A prepared, pureed commercial diet (a/d: Hill's) is now available.

Before a semi-permanent tube is used for feeding, the patient is given small amounts of water through the tube for the first 24 hours, then gradually fed increasing amounts of diet over the next 24-72 hours. The tube should always be flushed with water before and after each meal. The cat or dog is sent home with clear instructions for the owner on how to administer a maintenance diet.

Urine Collection

Collection of urine for urinalysis is very important for diagnosis of numerous diseases, including kidney failure, urinary tract infections, and urinary tract calculi ("stones," urolithiasis). A complete urinalysis should include urine specific gravity measurement, urine chemical analysis, and urine microscopic examination. Additionally, a urine sample collected aseptically should be submitted for urine culture and sensitivity testing if urinary tract infection is suspected. A 10-ml sample is ideal for a complete urinalysis.

Urine is formed in the kidneys and transported via the ureters into the bladder, where it is stored. During urination (micturition), the bladder contracts, the urethra relaxes, and urine is expelled through the urethra to the outside. There are several ways to collect urine, including cystocentesis, catheterization, manual expression, and collection during voiding. Each technique has advantages and disadvantages. One must always take into account the method used when interpreting the results of urinalysis.

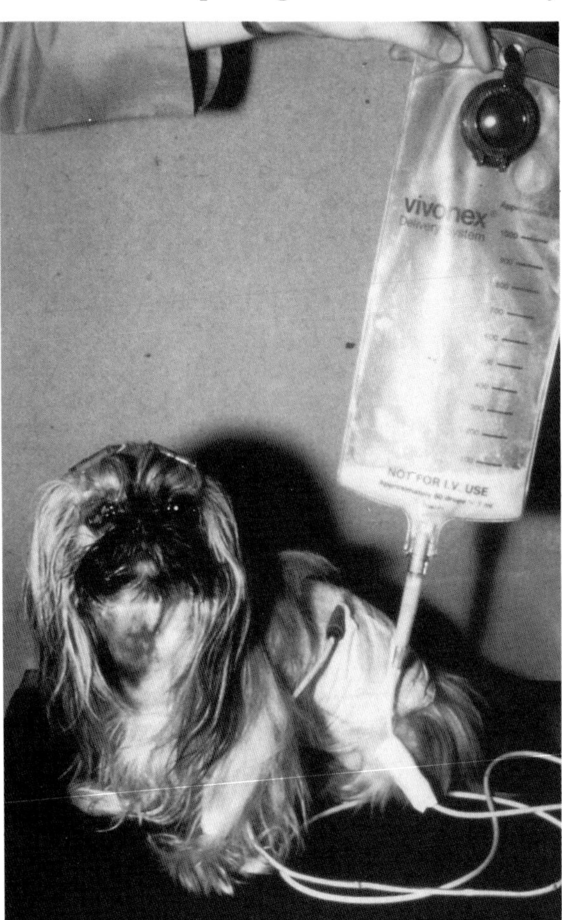

Figure 13. Jejunostomy tube placement with attached feeding bag.

Voided Urine Collection

The simplest way to collect urine is to allow the animal to void normally. If the patient is a dog, it should be walked outside. When the dog starts to urinate, a clean collecting cup should be placed under the prepuce or vulva to cath the urine flow. If possible, a midstream sample should be collected. This helps decrease contamination from the urethra and external genital organs. If the patient is a cat, plastic pellets (NoSorb: Catco) or Styrofoam peanuts can be placed in a clean, empty litter box. Most cats will readily urinate in the pellets instead of their regular litter, and the voided urine sample may be aspirated into a syringe for analysis.

Clients should be advised to store the collected sample in their refrigerator until bringing the urine to the hospital. Even refrigerated urine will decompose with time, so an effort should be made to perform the urinalysis on the same day as the sample is collected.

One disadvantage of a voided sample is the nonsterile nature of collection, which contaminates the sample with microorganisms. Another disadvantage of voided collection is that it requires the cooperation of the animal.

Sometimes a cat or dog will unexpectedly urinate onto the examination table or floor. The urine can be aspirated into a syringe for urinalysis, but the sample will be heavily contaminated by bacteria and other debris. This should be taken into account when interpreting the results of the urinalysis.

Bladder Expression

If a cat or dog has a palpable bladder, a urine sample may be obtained by manually expressing the bladder. This technique requires gentle, but firm compression of the bladder until the animal's urethral sphincter control is overridden, resulting in evacuation of the bladder. Manual expression of the bladder can traumatize the bladder and may cause gross or microscopic hematuria. Manual expression should never be used in an animal with an obstructed urethra, as bladder or urethral rupture could result.

Manual expression of the bladder is often used to help animals with decreased bladder tone (*eg*, a dog with urinary incontinence from spinal cord paralysis). The bladder should be emptied as completely as possible 3-4 times per day to help prevent bacterial accumulation in the residual urine. Clients can be taught how to perform this procedure at home if long-term management of urinary incontinence is required.

Urinary Catheterization

Urinary catheterization is an alternative method of urine collection. Indications for catheterization include obstruction of the urethra or when an immediate urinalysis is required and no bladder is palpable. In some cases, placement of an indwelling urinary catheter may be necessary to ensure that the urethra remains patent or to measure urine output.

A urinary catheter should be placed using aseptic technique; however, there is always a risk of causing a urinary tract infection. If an indwelling catheter is left in place for more than 24 hours, the tip of the catheter that was placed in the bladder should be cultured for bacterial organisms when it is removed.

Several types and sizes of urinary catheters are available (Fig 14). Rigid metal catheters may be used to collect urine from female dogs. These catheters may cause significant injury to the bladder or urethra if sufficient restraint is not used. Additionally, they are more likely to cause hematuria than other types of catheters. Polyethylene catheters are semi-rigid plastic catheters that are suitable for single-use catheterization in male dogs and cats. Finally, soft rubber catheters can be used for single-use or for indwelling catheterization. These are the last traumatic types of catheters and the best suited for use as indwelling catheters. However, because of their flexibility, they are more difficult to place than polyethylene catheters.

A modification of the soft rubber catheter is the Foley catheter. This catheter has an inflatable bulb on the end. Once the catheter has been placed with the tip in the bladder, the bulb is inflated with sterile water or saline. The inflated bulb prevents the catheter from slipping out of the bladder. Foley catheters are too large to pass through the male urethra but are ideal for female dogs and cats.

Figure 14. Various catheters available for urinary catheterization. From top to bottom: polyethylene tomcat catheter; stylet for Foley catheter; Foley catheter; rigid metal catheter; soft rubber catheter; and semi-rigid polyethylene catheter.

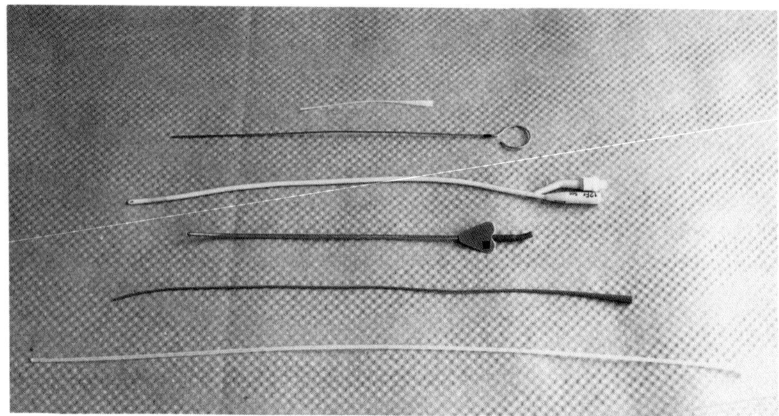

Catheterizing Male Dogs: There are numerous techniques used to place urinary catheters, depending on the species and sex of the animal. Male dogs are generally easy to catheterize and seldom require sedation or anesthesia. The dog is restrained in lateral recumbency. The penis is extruded by retracting the prepuce caudally toward the scrotum (Fig 15). The penis is held in this position during the catheterization procedure. A nonirritating surgical scrub, such as povidone-iodine or chlorhexidine, is used to clean the urethral opening and tip of the penis to remove surface bacteria and debris.

The distance from the urethral opening to the bladder should be estimated by measuring the distance from the end of the prepuce to the pelvis. The size of the dog determines the size of the catheter used (3.5 to 8 French). The catheter should be handled with sterile gloves by the person performing the procedure or the ends of the wrapper containing the catheter should be cut so that the catheter can be advanced sterilely through the catheter wrapping without contamination (Fig 16).

The sterile catheter should be lubricated with sterile water-soluble lubricant (K-Y Jelly: Johnson & Johnson), inserted into the urethral opening, and advanced along the urethra. Some resistance is usually felt at the level of the ischial arch and prostate gland, but gentle firm pressure advances the catheter past this point. If significant resistance is felt, especially when urethral ob-

Figure 15. Male dog catheterization: the penis is extruded from the prepuce.

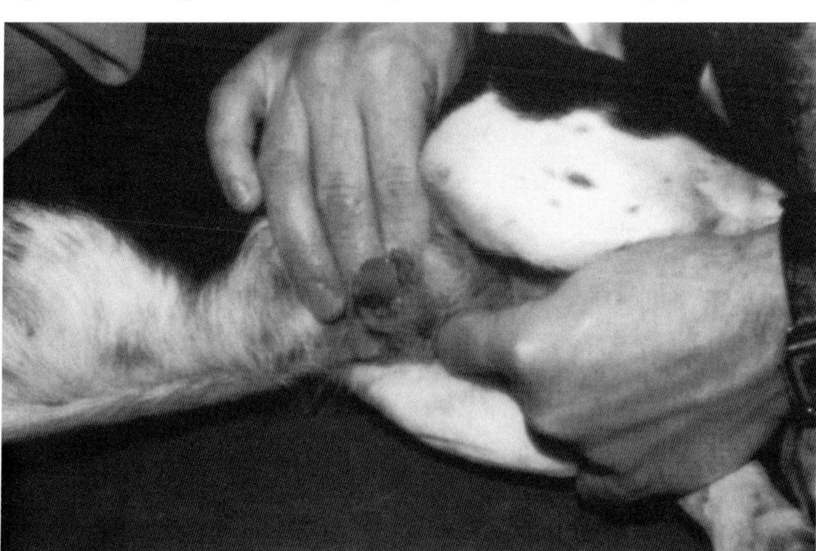

struction is suspected, the catheter should not be forcibly advanced, as this could result in urethral damage or rupture.

Once the catheter has been passed into the bladder lumen, urine usually flows freely out the end of the catheter. The catheter should never be pushed too far into the lumen, as it may damage the bladder wall or form a knot, necessitating surgical intervention to remove it. A syringe is immediately attached to the catheter for urine collection. The bladder should be completely emptied, even if only a small sample is required for urinalysis (Figs 17, 18). This decreases the risk of urinary tract infection. After all of the urine has been removed from the bladder, suction should be discontinued and the catheter withdrawn from the bladder.

If an indwelling catheter will be placed, the same technique is used. As previously mentioned, a soft rubber catheter is recommended for indwelling catheterization. The end of the catheter is connected to a sterile, closed collection system, instead of a syringe. An intravenous fluid administration set attached to an empty fluid bag works well as a collection system.

A butterfly tape (tape folded on either side of the catheter and adhered to itself, forming 2 tags) is used to attach the catheter to the animal. Sutures through the butterfly tape and skin of the ventral abdomen or prepuce secure the catheter in place. Dogs with an

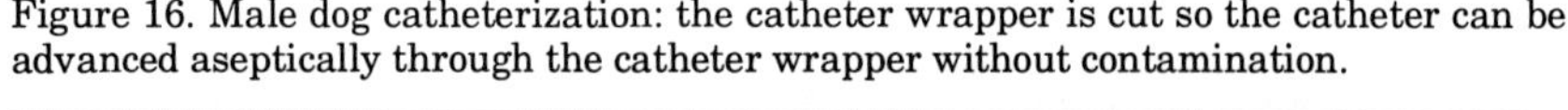
Figure 16. Male dog catheterization: the catheter wrapper is cut so the catheter can be advanced aseptically through the catheter wrapper without contamination.

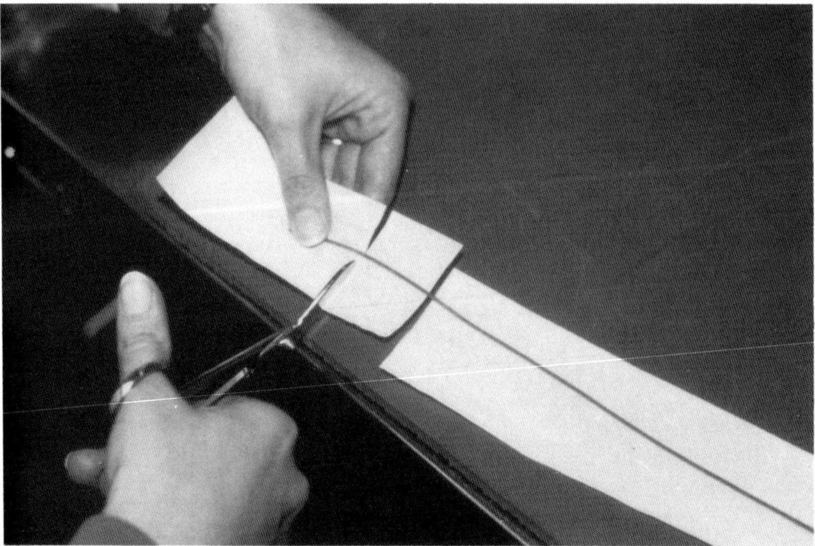

indwelling catheter should always wear an Elizabethan collar to prevent removal or damage to the catheter by the dog.

Catheterizing Male Cats: Male cats generally require heavy sedation or general anesthesia for placement of a urinary catheter. A short, polyethylene catheter (*eg*, Tom-Cat Catheter, Sherwood Medical) is used to relieve obstructions. A soft rubber catheter is less traumatic and therefore preferred if an indwelling catheter is required, but these may be difficult to place because of their flexibility and small size. Freezing the soft rubber catheter before use

Figure 17. Male dog catheterization: a syringe is attached to the catheter to empty the bladder.

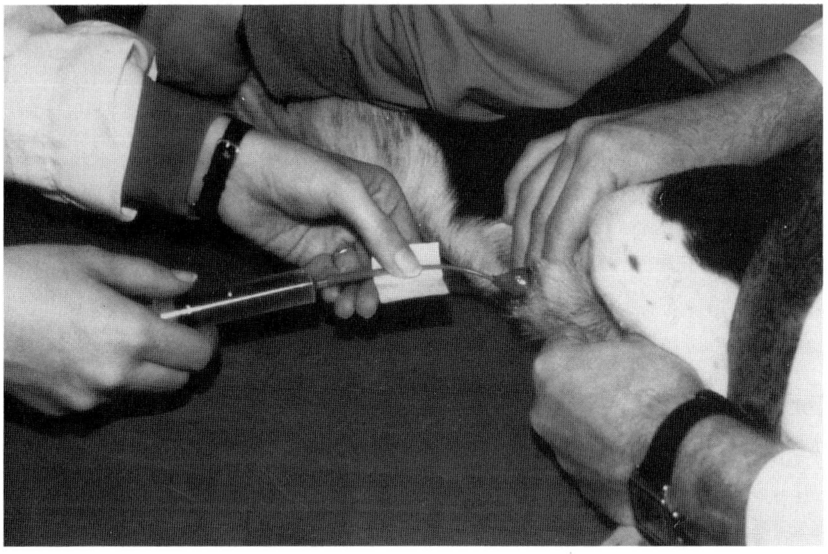

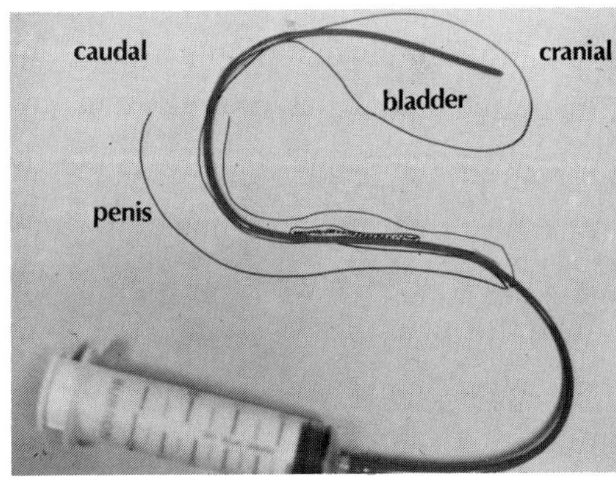

Figure 18. A soft, rubber urinary catheter is more flexible and therefore safer to use than polyethylene (plastic) catheters.

may make the catheter more rigid and easier to place. The cat is placed on lateral or dorsal recumbency. The prepuce is gently grasped ventral to the penis and then reflected dorsally. This exposes the penis and straightens the penile urethra, facilitating passage of the catheter. The catheter is placed in a manner similar to that described for male dogs. Again, aseptic technique should be employed.

Catheterizing Female Dogs and Cats: Placing a urinary catheter in a female dog or cat can present more of a challenge. Some female dogs and all female cats require heavy sedation or general anesthesia. The animal should be placed in sternal or lateral recumbency. Some female dogs may be easier to catheterize standing or, if placed in sternal recumbency, by positioning their rear limbs off the end of the table. Excessive hair should be removed from the genital area to help prevent contamination. The outer labia should be swabbed with chlorhexidine or povidone-iodine and sterile gloves should be worn.

Placement of the urinary catheter may be accomplished either by palpation or visualization of the urethral papilla. In a female dog, the urethral papilla is palpated with a lubricated, gloved finger. The urinary catheter is placed just caudal to the papilla and should glide easily into the urethra. Smaller dogs, obese dogs, and bitches in heat are harder to palpate. If the visualization technique is used in a female dog, a vaginal speculum or otoscope is used to visualize the papilla and urethral orifice (Fig 19).

In a female cat, a rigid Tom-Cat polyethylene catheter (Sherwood Medical) may be passed while the cat is in sternal recumbency. This is not a palpation technique and is considered a "blind" procedure. If the visualization technique is used, an otoscope is positioned to enhance visibility of the urethral orifice with the cat in lateral recumbency.

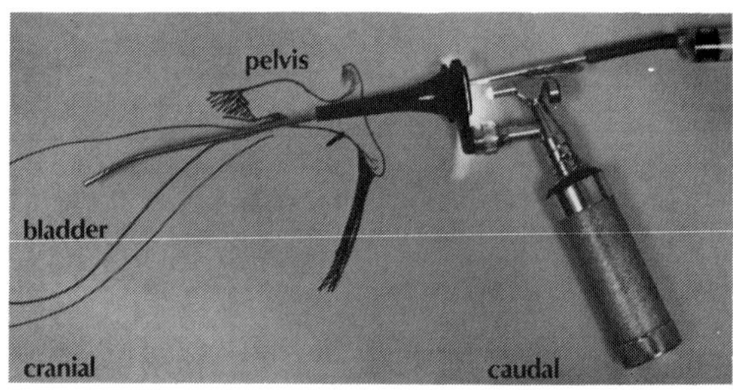

Figure 19. Use of a veterinary otoscope to facilitate urinary bladder catheterization in a female dog.

As previously mentioned, a Foley catheter is the best choice for an indwelling catheter in female dogs, as the inflated bulb retains the catheter in the bladder. Foley catheters small enough to use in female cats (5 French) are now available. A removable metal stylet fed into the catheter lumen can facilitate passage of the flexible catheter into the urethra. Once the catheter is placed in the bladder, the bulb is inflated, the stylet is removed, and the catheter is sutured to the perivulvar region. As with males, an indwelling catheter should be attached to a sterile, closed collection system and an Elizabethan collar is mandatory to prevent damage to the catheter.

Cystocentesis

Cystocentesis involves aseptic aspiration of urine directly from the bladder. Cystocentesis can easily and safely be performed in male and female dogs and cats. This procedure is the preferred technique for obtaining urine for culture, as aspirated urine is minimally contaminated during collection. A sterile 22-gauge, 1.5-inch needle should be attached to a 12-ml syringe for sample collection. Alcohol is applied to the skin.

Several techniques may be used for cystocentesis. If the bladder can be palpated, the animal is restrained in dorsal or lateral recumbency or standing. The bladder should be immobilized with one hand. If a midline entry is used in a male dog, the prepuce must be moved away from the midline before cystocentesis. The needle is inserted through the skin and into the bladder lumen. The required amount of urine, usually 10 ml, is aspirated. Aspiration should be discontinued before withdrawing the needle from the bladder. If some of the sample is to be submitted for culture, the needle on the syringe is changed or removed before transferring the urine to a sterile culture tube so as to minimize contamination from skin bacteria.

If the bladder cannot be palpated (*eg*, in an obese dog or a dog with a very tense abdomen) but a full bladder is suspected, cystocentesis may be attempted using abdominal landmarks. The animal is restrained in dorsal recumbency or standing. The pelvic bone is palpated ventrally. The needle is directed 1.5-2 inches (depending on the size of the animal) cranial to the pelvic bone on the midline. The needle is angled slightly caudal and advanced through the skin and into the urinary bladder. The required amount of urine is aspirated (Fig 20). If no urine is obtained after 1-2 attempts and appropriate landmarks have been used, cystocentesis should not be repeated for at least 1-2 hours, after more urine has accumulated in the bladder. The needle should always be changed after each attempt at cystocentesis.

Cystocentesis should never be performed on a cat or dog that is struggling. If an animal starts to struggle after the needle has already been inserted, the needle should be withdrawn immediately to minimize any damage. Though rare, bladder tears or rupture may occur if the animal is not sufficiently restrained. The other major complication of cystocentesis is infection secondary to perforation of the intestines. This is extremely unlikely if proper technique is used. Cystocentesis may result in hematuria and urinalysis results should be interpreted accordingly.

Grooming

While one of the main goals of nursing in small animal medicine is to help sick animals get better, it is just as important to keep sick cats and dogs clean and dematted. Clients appreciate the extra effort on their pet's behalf and animals unable to groom themselves may feel better when they are cleaned and brushed. More important, debilitated animals are susceptible to urine scald and decubital ulcers. Keeping these animals clean minimizes secondary infections of the skin. Of course, not only sick animals require grooming. Bathing, dipping, nail trimming, anal sac expression and ear cleaning are an integral part of day-to-day activity at most small animal veterinary hospitals.

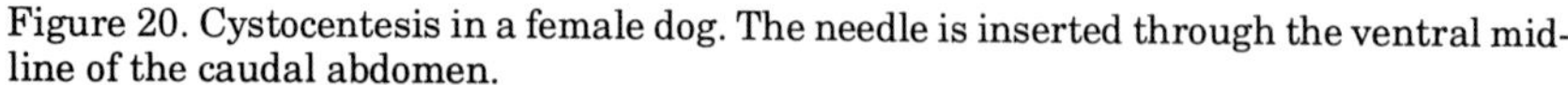

Figure 20. Cystocentesis in a female dog. The needle is inserted through the ventral midline of the caudal abdomen.

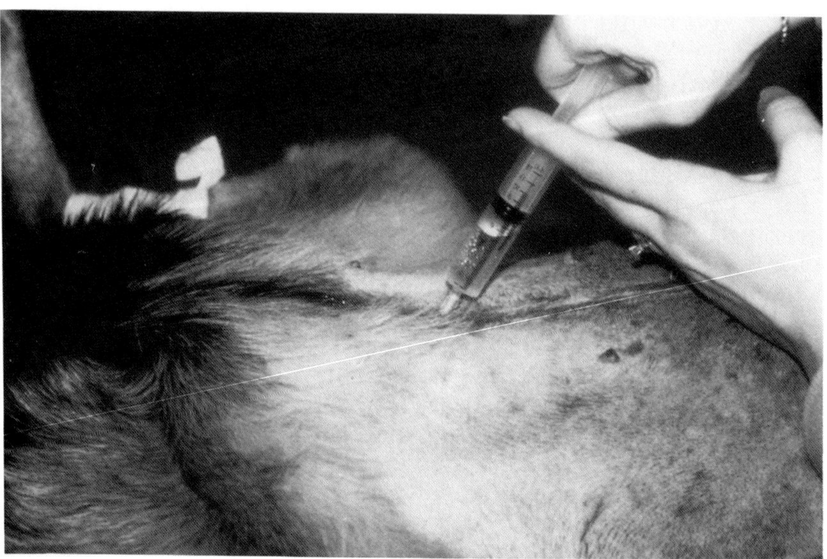

Baths and Dips

Baths are most commonly used to clean dirty animals or treat flea infestation. Dips are often used in conjunction with baths to treat flea infestation. Dips are also used to treat mite infections (*eg*, *Demodex* or *Sarcoptes*). Bathing and dipping are fairly straightforward procedures, but there are a few important guidelines to keep in mind.

Before placing the cat or dog in the bathing tub, the products to be used should be selected. Some products, especially certain dips, are toxic to cats and should never be used in this species. A waterproof apron or smock is recommended to keep the bather dry. The animal should be adequately restrained in the tub or sink. Dogs can be tied to a tub ring. A dog should never be left unattended in a tub, as it could seriously injure itself if it attempted to jump from the tub while still tied to the ring. Cats may be gently grasped around the neck while being bathed. Some cats may need to be sedated or restrained by an assistant.

Technique for Baths: Nail trimming, anal sac expression and/or ear cleaning may be performed before bathing. Doing these procedures first gets the messy procedures out of the way and ensures that the animal will stay clean after bathing.

The animal's fur should be thoroughly soaked with warm water. Shampoo is lathered over the body. Long-haired animals require extra attention to work the shampoo down to the skin. Animals with dermatitis may benefit from lightly scrubbing the affected areas to help loosen dead skin and debris.

The face, especially the ocular area, should be avoided. In the past it was recommended to instill ophthalmic ointment in both eyes to protect against soap irritation. However, this procedure is no longer recommended, as the ointment can act as an occlusive agent, sealing soap suds onto the cornea and exacerbating any potential irritation. If soap inadvertently enters an animal's eyes, sterile saline or eye wash should be used to lavage the soap from the eyes.

Some shampoos, such as flea products, should be left on the animal for 5-10 minutes for maximum efficacy. The shampoo should be thoroughly rinsed. If a dip will follow the bath, the animal is not dried. Otherwise, the cat or dog is towel dried. Cage dryers can be used to facilitate the drying process. Strict attention to the dryer setting is important to prevent the animal from becoming overheated or burned.

Techniques for Dips: When dipping an animal, gloves should be worn. The dip manufacturer's label should always be consulted for directions. Some dips are extremely toxic. Precise dilution of the dip with water is imperative. Improper reconstitution of a dip can poison or even kill an animal. The dip can be mixed with water in a sink or bathing pan and the animal directly dipped into this solution. This works well for cats and small dogs, but is impractical for larger dogs. Alternatively, the dip can be mixed in a bucket and sponged over the entire surface of the animal's coat, again avoiding the ocular area. One precaution regarding sponge dipping is that an animal with a dermatophyte infection (ringworm) or sarcoptic mange (scabies) may infect other animals if the contaminated sponge is used to dip other animals.

Dips are usually applied to a pre-soaked animal and adhere better if the coat is clean; hence, the logical sequence of first bathing, then dipping the animal. After dipping, the cat or dog is allowed to drip-dry, as towel drying removes dip from the animal. Cage dryers may be used to speed the drying process.

Complications: Dogs and cats may have reactions to shampoos or dips. This is most commonly a problem when cats are inadvertently treated with a product that is not labeled for use in cats (*eg*, many organophosphate products). If side effects, such as weakness, disorientation, vomiting, diarrhea, ptyalism (excessive salivation) or seizures, occur, the animal should immediately be rebathed (with a noninsecticide product) and thoroughly rinsed. If clinical signs persist, aggressive medical therapy may be necessary.

Comb Out: After the animal has finished drying from its bath or dip, it should be combed out before being released. Depending on the length and texture of the fur, a comb or brush is used to comb out mats and loose hairs. An excessively matted cat or dog may require clipping with scissors or electric clippers. This may be done before or after the bath. If scissors are used, care should be taken to avoid inadvertently cutting the skin. Likewise, electric clippers can cause "clipper burn," nicks and cuts if used improperly or if the blade is dull. Occasionally, an animal may require sedation for combing, especially if it is heavily matted.

Sprays, Powders and Mousses

These products are primarily used to treat flea infestation. Some products are not safe for use in cats. Certain products can be applied daily, while others should not be used that frequently. We recommend wearing gloves when applying these products to cats and dogs.

Sprays are lightly sprayed over the animal, avoiding the eyes. The product is worked into the animal's coat. Many cats dislike aerosol sprays and may struggle vigorously during their application, so adequate patient restraint is essential. A common side effect of both aerosol and pump sprays in cats is ptyalism (excessive salivation). This may be in response to inhalation of the spray.

Powders and mousses are often better tolerated by cats. Powders are sprinkled on the parted haircoat. Mousses are applied to several areas of the animal's coat and then worked into the coat in a manner similar to that for the sprays. If a cat or dog shows side effects from a spray, powder or mousse, the animal should be bathed immediately, as previously discussed.

Nail Trimming

Trimming the nails of cats and dogs accomplishes several goals. Nail trimming prevents the animal from seriously scratching its handlers and damaging its home environment (carpeting and upholstery). Trimming also prevents injury from overgrowth of nails. Unchecked nail growth can cause lameness from the nails' curling back on themselves and growing into the skin or foot pads (Fig 21). In cats, regular nail trimming is considered a humane alternative to declawing. However, some cats appear to sharpen their nails on furniture more frequently with trimming.

The toenail is an extension of the third phalanx, the last bone of the digit of each toe. The toenail is comprised of keratin, a hard,

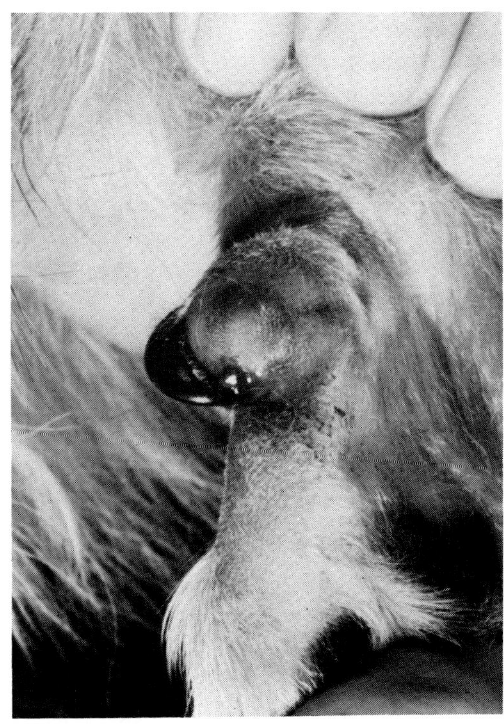

Figure 21. Neglected dewclaw nail penetrating the skin of the digit, causing painful digital infection.

horn-like material. The toenail functions to protect the vascular supply of the ungual process, defend the animal against predators and provide traction for running and climbing.

Equipment: Several instruments are available for nail trimming, including toenail scissors, guillotine clippers and human toenail clippers (Fig 22). Human toenail clippers can be used on cats and puppies but are not designed for dogs. Toenail scissors can be used on dogs but are too heavy to use on cats. Guillotine clippers (Resco) are probably the most popular nail trimmers in veterinary medicine and are suitable for use in both cats and dogs.

Nail trimming equipment should be kept clean. Blades become dull with repeated use and require sharpening or replacement. Dull blades may pinch the toe, causing pain, and crush the nail, damaging the nail tissue.

Technique: The goal in trimming nails is to remove as much nail as necessary to prevent the nail tip from extending below the level of the bottom of the foot pad. The blood vessel in the nail is referred to as the "quick" and bleeding of the nail caused by overzealous trimming is known as "quicking the nail." Quicking the nail should be avoided because it is painful to the animal and the resultant hemorrhage is aesthetically displeasing to the owner. Further, repeatedly quicking nails causes an animal to resist future efforts at nail trimming, making the procedure more difficult.

Animals with excessively long nails may have blood vessels extending to or past the level of the bottom of the foot pads. Trimming the nails to this level in these animals causes hemorrhage. This

Figure 22. Toenail clippers: scissor type (left); human toenail type (center); guillotine type (right).

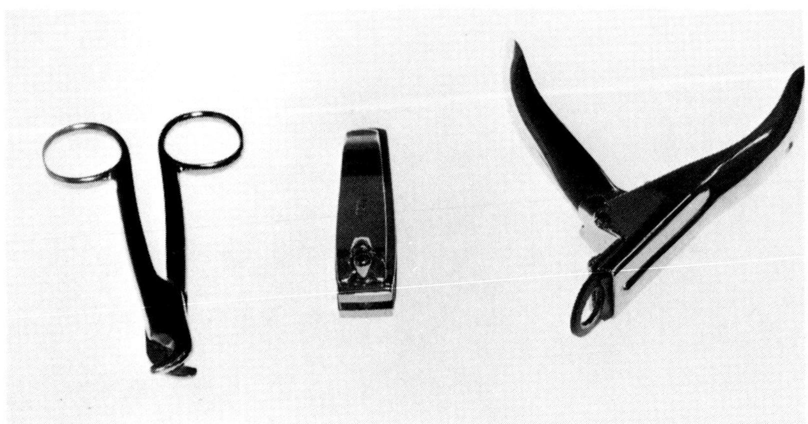

procedure should only be done under general anesthesia. Alternatively, frequent, repeated trimmings may help the quick regress so that the nails can eventually be trimmed back to the appropriate level. Excessively long nails are primarily a canine problem, as most cats keep their claws to a manageable length by sharpening them.

When trimming nails, the entire nail surface is exposed dorsally by pushing the nail bed distally (Fig 23). As cats have retractable claws, their claws must be pushed out of the foot. The nail is trimmed distal to the blood supply. Dogs with white nails and cats have clearly visualized pink-white quicks. However, dogs with black nails present more of a challenge, as the quicks are not visible. With experience, nail trimming in these animals becomes easier, though quicking the nail may occasionally occur, no matter how careful the trim. Moreover, dogs with severely overgrown nails may require trimming at the level of the quick, inevitably resulting in hemorrhage.

Silver nitrate sticks or styptic solution may be applied to the bleeding quick if direct pressure is unsuccessful in stopping hemorrhage. However, silver nitrate stings, stains clothing and discolors skin. After each nail trimming, the animal should be carefully inspected for signs of hemorrhage before release to the owner.

Figure 23. Nail trimming in a dog. The foot is extended and a guillotine clipper is used to trim the nail end.

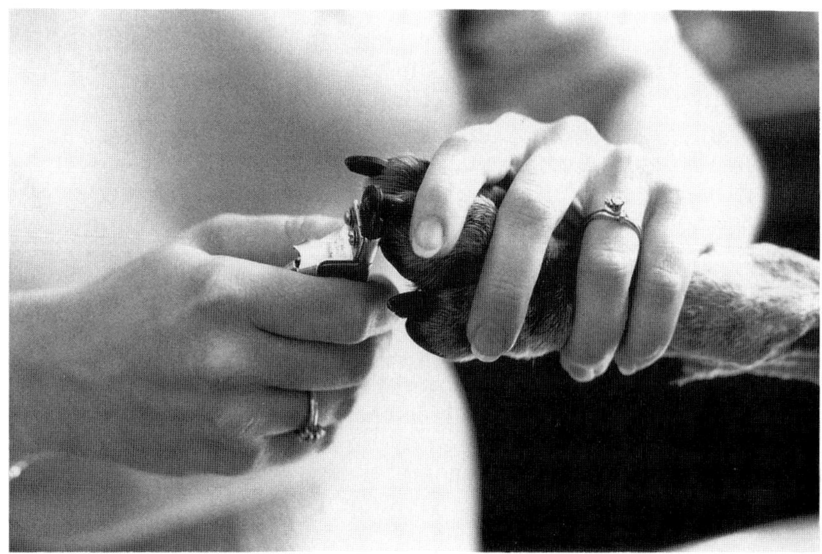

Anal Sac Care

The anal sacs, often incorrectly referred to as “anal glands,” are 2 small sacs located at the 4 and 8 o’clock positions just inside the anus. The anal sacs function as scent glands. The sacs are normally emptied when the animal defecates.

Dogs, especially those that are small to medium sized, under exercised or overweight, and, more rarely, cats, may fail to express their anal sacs naturally, resulting in impaction and sometimes abscessation of the anal sacs. Signs of impacted anal sacs include licking the anal area and rubbing the perineum against the carpet or floor (“scooting”) in an effort to relieve the pressure and pain of anal sac impaction.

Technique: Impacted anal sacs are usually easy to express. However, the procedure often causes discomfort, so adequate restraint is important. The animal is restrained in a standing position. Latex gloves are used. After raising the tail to expose the anus, a lubricated finger is gently inserted a couple of centimeters into the anal opening. One anal sac is palpated with the index finger. Firm pressure is applied with the index finger internally and the thumb externally, expressing the contents of the anal sac. The procedure is repeated with the opposite sac.

Anal sacs may also be expressed using external perirectal pressure. The anal sacs are palpated perirectally and external pressure is applied dorsally and medially, again using the index finger and thumb. We do not recommend external expression of the anal sacs, as complete expression of anal sac material is difficult with this method.

While expressing the anal sacs, the anal opening should be covered with a paper towel, cotton or gauze to collect the foul-smelling anal sac material. The anal sac material is discarded in a covered waste bin (or in another room) to minimize odor.

If an anal sac becomes abscessed, the anal sac may need to be hot-packed or drained, or may even require surgical removal. In cases of chronic, persistent anal sac impaction, surgical removal may also be indicated.

Ear Care

Dogs and cats are often presented for evaluation of ear disease. Signs of ear disease include shaking the head, scratching the ears, otic discharge, a head tilt, an aural hematoma, or an unpleasant odor. Causes of ear disease include bacterial or yeast infections, ear mite infestation, foreign bodies and tumors. A complete ear examination includes visual inspection of the outer ear and otoscopic examination of the external ear canal and tympanic membrane.

Cleaning the ears regularly should be considered a routine part of grooming cats and dogs. Additionally, ear cleaning is performed before instillation of otic medication, in order to remove dirt and debris. If excessive debris is present, ear cleaning may also be required before otic examination.

The outer ear consists of the pinna and the external ear canal (Fig 24). The external ear canal functions to collect sound. The ear canal is L-shaped, consisting of an outer vertical canal and an inner horizontal canal. The tympanic membrane (ear drum) lies at the proximal end of the inner horizontal canal. The tympanic membrane separates the outer ear from the middle and inner ear. The middle ear is comprised of tiny bones (malleus, incus, stapes) that transmit sound. The inner ear contains nerve cells for both hearing and balance (within the cochlea and semi-circular canals, respectively) and transmits information to the brain.

Rupture of or severe trauma to the tympanic membrane can damage the middle and inner ear, resulting in hearing loss, disruption in vestibular (balancing) function, and facial nerve paralysis. Signs of peripheral vestibular disease include a head tilt toward

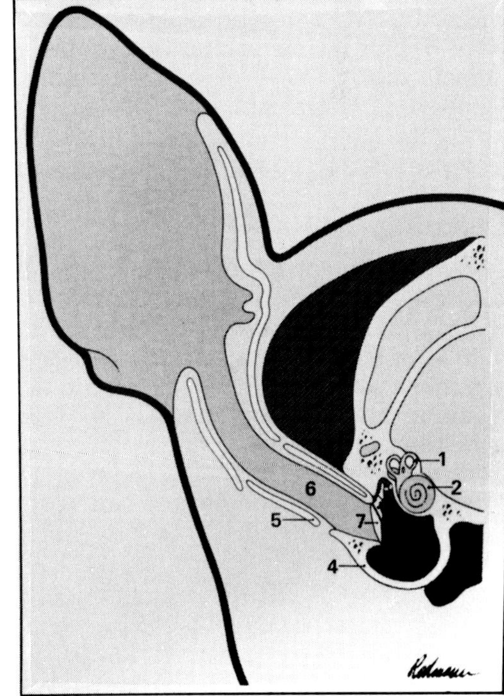

Figure 24. Anatomy of the ear: (1) semicircular canals; (2) cochlea; (3) tympanic cavity (middle ear); (4) tympanic bulla; (5) cartilage of the external ear canal; (6) external ear; (7) tympanic membrane (ear drum). (Courtesy of Jane Redmann)

the affected side, loss of balance (ataxia), incoordination and nausea. Signs of facial nerve paralysis include a lip droop and loss of the blink reflex on the affected side.

Otic Examination

A complete ear examination may be performed without anesthesia in a cooperative patient but sometimes is impossible without sedation or anesthesia. Inflamed, irritated ears are painful and an ear examination, especially with the otoscope, may be resisted by the patient. Adequate restraint by an assistant is important.

To perform an ear examination, the pinna is gently grasped and lifted to better visualize the external ear canal (vertical portion). The canal is observed for inflammation, discharge or stenosis (narrowing of the canal). If excessive discharge is present, it may prevent proper visualization of the horizontal canal with the otoscope. If this is the case, the ears must first be cleaned. Before cleaning the ears, samples for cytologic examination and bacterial culture should be obtained, if indicated.

An appropriately sized cone (speculum) is attached to the otoscope for otoscopic examination. The pinna is lifted dorsally while the otoscope cone is inserted into the vertical canal. To facilitate visualization of the horizontal canal, the pinna is pulled dorsolaterally (upward and outward) while the cone is passed through the vertical canal into the horizontal canal. This helps straighten the ear canal. The tympanic membrane is normally seen as a pearlescent structure spanning the diameter of the canal.

Cleaning the Ears

Ear cleaning products include ceruminolytic agents, dilute antibacterial solutions (*eg*, povidone-iodine or chlorhexidine), and weak acetic acid solutions. If tympanic membrane damage or rupture is suspected (*eg*, in cats or dogs showing signs of middle or inner ear disease), it is important to remember that many ear cleaning products are potentially ototoxic to the middle or inner ear. Therefore, these products may make ear disease worse and even result in permanent damage. If the canal must be cleaned before the tympanic membrane can adequately assessed, the safest product to use to clean the external ear canal is normal saline (0.9% NaCl).

Several drops of the ear cleaning product are placed in each ear and the base of the canal is massaged gently. Cotton balls should be used to remove the excess fluid and accumulated dirt and debris. Several applications of cleaning product may be necessary to achieve satisfactory results. Cotton-tipped applicators, if used very carefully, can be used to remove ear debris. They should never be used in an inadequately restrained animal, as the dog or cat may struggle, causing the applicator tip to break off within the ear canal or rupture the tympanic membrane. Further, when improperly used, applicators may only serve to push debris deeper into the canal.

The ears may be flushed with an otic cleaning solution using a bulb syringe or a 6- to 12-ml syringe attached to a small-diameter rigid catheter (*eg*, Tom-Cat Catheter: Sherwood Medical). Ear flushing requires heavy sedation or general anesthesia. Flushing the ears leaves fluid in the canal, making otoscopic examination difficult. Any remaining fluid should be gently aspirated out of the canal after flushing with the syringe and catheter.

Excessive otic hair makes ear cleaning more difficult because of accumulation of debris between the hairs. A hemostat can be used to pluck the hairs from the canal. Again, adequate restraint is crucial, as a struggling animal may harm itself if the hemostat is inadvertently pushed too deep into the canal. Hairs should be plucked only a few at a time, as plucking too many hairs simultaneously is painful and causes increased inflammation in the ear canal.

Medicating the Ears

Dogs and cats with ear disease may require otic medication. Topical medication is applied into the external ear canal after the ears are cleaned. Usually, only 1-5 drops (or a 1/4-inch strip of ointment) are instilled into each ear. Each ear is gently massaged to help disperse the drug (Fig 25).

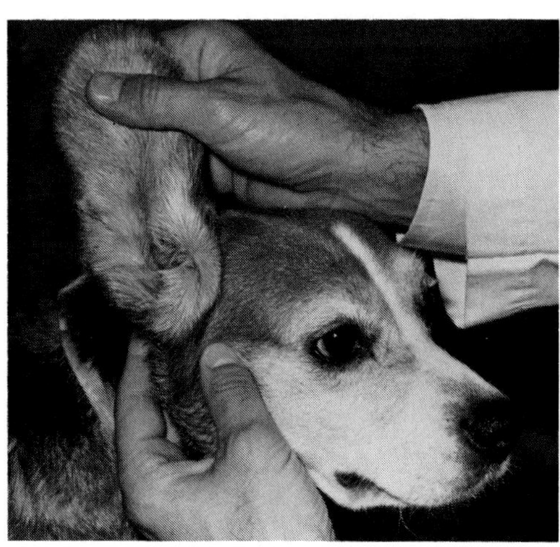

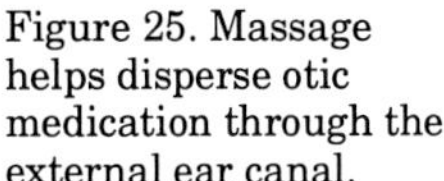

Figure 25. Massage helps disperse otic medication through the external ear canal.

Client Education: Clients can be shown how to safely and effectively clean their pet's ears and how to instill topical medication. In many cases, an ear cleaning product used daily to once weekly may be all that is necessary to maintain good ear health. Sometimes, however, aggressive topical treatment and oral antibiotics may be required. Refractory, chronic cases may require surgical intervention.

Eye Care

Numerous eye diseases require topical ophthalmic medication. Examples include conjunctivitis, keratoconjunctivitis sicca ("dry eye"), corneal abrasion/ulceration, uveitis and glaucoma. It is important that only appropriate ophthalmic products prescribed by the veterinarian, be used. A veterinarian should always be consulted before a client treats the eye with an ophthalmic medication that was previously prescribed for an eye problem. Otherwise, serious consequences, including blindness, could result.

The eye is composed of the cornea, the uvea (including the lens and iris), and the retina (Fig 26). Light rays pass through the eye to the retina, and are converted into neurologic impulses passing

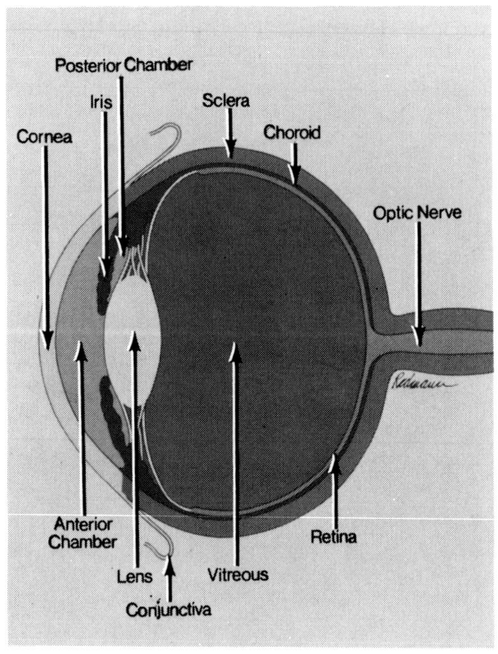

Figure 26. Basic ocular anatomy. (Courtesy of Jane Redmann)

into the optic nerve and the brain. Disruption in this pathway can result in a visual deficit or total blindness.

Accessory eye structures include: the conjunctiva, which lines the inner surface of the eyelids and surrounds the cornea; the eyelids and eyelashes, which protect the eye and disperse moisture; the lacrimal glands, which provide natural tears to lubricate the cornea and prevent corneal drying; and the nasolacrimal ducts, which serve as conduits for tears.

Medicating the Eyes

Irritated or inflamed eyes may be quite painful and many animals resent application of topical medication. Adequate patient restraint is important to prevent trauma to the animal or technician. Any debris surrounding the eye is removed before each treatment. Cotton gauze, moistened with warm water, helps loosen encrusted mucus or pus. Mucus or pus on the surface of the globe may be gently flushed away from the eye with sterile normal saline (0.9% NaCl) or a commercial eyewash preparation.

Eye medications are available as solutions and ointments. Solutions are often easier to apply than ointments because the application tube is not in direct apposition with the eye and the solution may be dripped into the eye. Solutions are less likely to leave behind residual material that can accumulate around the eye. However, ointments are often preferred by many veterinarians because they have a longer duration of action and, therefore, require less frequent application. An ophthalmic drug should never be applied directly to the corneal surface. The applicator tip could damage the cornea, especially if the cat or dog should move. The animal's own natural blinking action spreads the drug evenly over the eye surface.

In addition to providing restraint, grasping the animal's head allows the technician to move with the animal if it should move and helps prevent inadvertent injury of the eye with the applicator tip. The nose is pointed toward the ceiling.

When using an ophthalmic solution, the eyelids are spread apart and the solution is dropped onto the eyeball (Fig 27). Usually 1-2 drops are all that is required. The tip of the container should never be allowed to touch the surface of the eye or surrounding structures. This could contaminate the bottle's contents with microorganisms. The cap should be tightly replaced on the bottle during storage.

When administering an ophthalmic ointment, the lower lid is retracted ventrally, exposing the conjunctiva lining the lower lid. Ointment is deposited in the space between the lower lid conjunctiva and the surface of the eye. A small amount of ointment (a strip of about 1/8 inch) is first expressed and discarded from the tube.

Then a strip of ointment, usually 1/4-1/2 inch, is applied into the conjunctival space (Fig 28). The applicator tip should not be permitted to come into direct contact with the conjunctival surface, in order to prevent contamination. The retracted eyelid is then released.

When both a solution and an ointment must be applied to the eye, the solution is first applied and, after at least 5 minutes, the ointment is then applied.

Client Education

Clients should be shown the correct way to apply topical eye medication. The procedure is straightforward but may be technically difficult for inexperienced owners. The owner should be advised that apparent worsening of an eye problem (*eg*, increasing redness or discharge) warrants immediate reevaluation. Animals that are sent home with ophthalmic medication should also have an Elizabethan collar to prevent trauma to the eye.

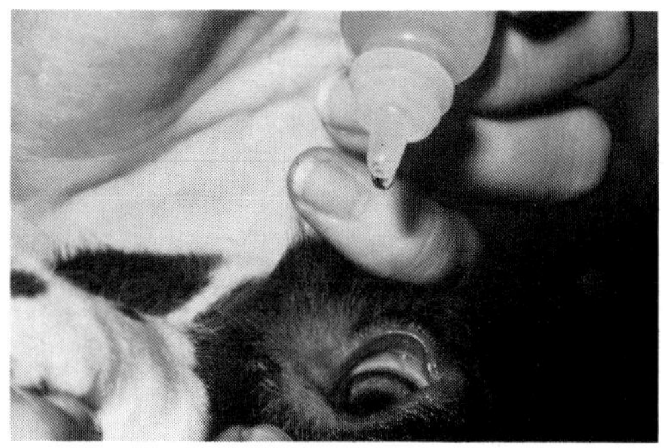

Figure 27. Instillation of ophthalmic solution.

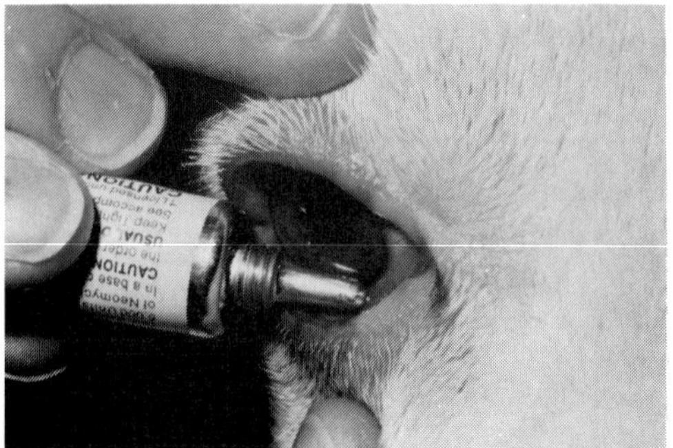

Figure 28. Medicating an eye with ophthalmic ointment.

Enemas

An enema is the introduction of fluid into the rectum through the anus. Distention and irritation of the rectum by the administered fluid stimulate colonic and rectal contractions and promotes fecal evacuation. Enemas may be performed to relieve severe constipation or obstipation. Enemas may also be given before abdominal radiography and are necessary as preparation for contrast radiographic studies of the colon and for proctoscopic examination. Less frequently, enemas may be used therapeutically (*eg*, lactulose enemas to treat hepatic encephalopathy) and diagnostically (*eg*, ammonium chloride enemas to evaluate liver function).

Enema Solutions

Various enema solutions are available. Warm-water enemas are most commonly used and are the enema fluid of choice. Commercial enema products include detergent enemas, magnesium salts and sodium phosphate salts. Mineral oil and white petrolatum enemas are also used. A warm-water enema is safe and effective, and causes the least irritation. Other enema products may irritate the lining of the rectum and colon, and do not provide any additional benefit in promoting defecation. Sodium phosphate enemas (*eg*, Fleet Enema: Fleet) are contraindicated for use in small animals and can cause death in cats and small dogs from absorption of sodium and phosphate.

Enema Administration

An enema may be an uncomfortable procedure for a severely constipated cat or dog. Occasionally, sedation or general anesthesia may be required. Adequate patient restraint is recommended, as the animal may not stand still or may try to bite the administrator. Enemas are best performed in a large sink or tub, one that preferably is not used for other functions. Alternatively, enemas may be performed outdoors, in a run, or on a drain table.

Warm water is infused into the rectum at 10 ml/lb of body weight (22 ml/kg) for each enema. When large volumes of fluid are administered, an enema administration bag with an attached tube may be used. The administration bag is hung from an elevated position and the enema solution is allowed to flow into the rectum by gravity. Smaller volumes, for cats and dogs, may be administered with a 5- to 60-ml syringe (depending on the patient's size), attached to soft red rubber tubing (*eg*, a pediatric feeding tube).

Latex examination gloves should be worn. The patient is restrained in a standing position. The tip of the enema administration tube (or rubber tubing) is generously lubricated with water-soluble lubricant (K-Y Jelly: Johnson & Johnson) and then gently inserted into the rectum and colon. The length of tubing inserted into the rectum depends upon the size of the animal. Ideally, the tip of the tube should be placed at the colorectal junction. In general, the tube should be inserted at least 5-6 cm in large dogs, 3-4 cm in small dogs and 2-3 cm in cats. The enema solution is slowly administered over 3-5 minutes. Overly rapid administration can result in vomiting, especially in cats.

Enemas may need to be repeated to ensure complete evacuation of the colon. If necessary, enemas should be repeated at least an hour apart and, preferably, should be spaced over a 24-hour period. Infusing too large a volume in a relatively short period can result in vomiting or, even worse, a "through and through" enema, in which the animal vomits its own feces. This can be a serious situation if the cat or dog then aspirates the vomitus, resulting in aspiration pneumonia.

The animal may defecate immediately after receiving the enema or may pass stool minutes to hours later. Therefore, after the enema has been administered, the cat or dog should be placed in an environment where it is less likely to soil itself (*eg*, on a cage grate or in a run).

Complications

In addition to vomiting, other complications of enemas include rectal trauma or perforation of the colon. The enema tubing should never be forced into an animal's rectum. If resistance is met on inserting the tube, additional lubrication may help. In small dogs and cats, hypothermia is another potential complication. Cold-water enemas should never be used in these animals.

Special Procedures

Enemas are routinely given to remove feces before special procedures, such as radiographic contrast studies or proctoscopic or colonoscopic examination. Three enemas are usually administered: one the night before the procedure, a second the morning of the procedure, and a third enema 1-2 hours before the procedure. A 24-hour fast is also instituted. After all of the enemas have been performed, a survey lateral abdominal radiograph should be made to ensure adequate evacuation of the colon before the procedure. If the radiograph shows residual fecal material in the colon, the procedure should be postponed while additional enemas are given.

Hyperosmotic laxatives (*eg*, GoLytely: Braintree Labs) may be used instead of multiple enemas to prepare an animal for colonoscopy or protoscopy. These drugs may be administered orally but are usually easier to administer with an oroesophageal tube because of the large volume required. Hyperosmotic laxatives are administered 2-3 times before the procedure. Again, a 24-hour fast is also instituted.

Medicated Enemas

Rectal administration of drugs is best performed in a pre-evacuated rectum. Therefore, warm-water enemas are usually administered before these enemas. Lactulose and ammonium chloride enemas are administered with a syringe and red rubber tubing, as much smaller volumes are used. These drugs are administered into the colon and should be placed 2-3 cm farther cranially than a warm-water enema.

After administering these enemas, the catheter is held in the rectum for a minute and a small amount of air is flushed through the catheter to prevent back-flow of the drug. Ammonium chloride enemas can be irritating and the animal may become agitated shortly after the enema is administered.

Dental Prophylaxis

Prevention of progressive dental disease is an invaluable service offered by small animal hospitals. With the increasing availability of ultrasonic dental scalers, dental prophylaxis, rather than tooth extraction, has become the primary focus of veterinary dentistry. Further, educating clients about prophylactic care has helped owners to take a more active role in their pet's dental health.

Routine dental prophylaxis, which includes scaling and polishing the teeth and, possibly, fluoride treatment, is not only preventive; it also offers the opportunity for a thorough dental examination to identify any potential problems.

Dental Anatomy

Dogs and cats have 2 sets of teeth: deciduous (temporary) and permanent teeth. The deciduous teeth are also referred to as "milk" or "baby" teeth. These teeth occur in young animals, become loose as the animal matures, and eventually fall out. Permanent teeth then replace the deciduous teeth. The shedding of deciduous teeth and the appearance of permanent teeth can be helpful in determining the age of a young animal. Most young cats and dogs have lost all of their deciduous teeth by 6-8 months of age. Occasionally, especially in small breeds of dogs, some deciduous teeth are retained, resulting in crowding of the permanent teeth and possible malocclusion. The dental formulae for dogs and cats are shown in Table 1.

Identifying the different types of teeth is important as a reference point for medical records, especially when diseased teeth are being described. There are 4 types of teeth: incisors, canines, premolars and molars. Teeth are described as being upper or lower arcade (maxillary and mandibular teeth, respectively) and are numbered (*eg*, right third upper premolar) (Figs 29, 30).

A tooth is composed of 3 layers: the hard outer enamel, the middle dentine layer, and the inner pulp (Fig 31). The pulp contains the nerves and blood supply to the tooth and is the part of the tooth sensitive to pain. Each tooth has a root extending below the gum line. Cementum helps adhere the root to the tooth socket, which is composed of alveolar bone.

The periodontium is composed of supportive structures surrounding the tooth, including the gingiva, the periodontal ligament and the alveolar bone. Periodontitis refers to inflammation of all of these structures, whereas gingivitis refers to inflammation of the gingiva. The goal of dental prophylaxis is to prevent periodontitis or, at least, slow its progression.

Dental Disease

In dogs and cats, dental disease usually begins with accumulation of plaque, a mixture of necrotic food particles, saliva and bacteria. Plaque can cause progressive erosion of the gingiva, gingivitis, periodontal disease, tooth loss and oral infections. Plaque can eventually accumulate to form dental calculus (commonly referred to as dental tartar), which also contains the minerals calcium and phosphorus.

Dental Equipment

Several instruments are used for dental prophylaxis. Manual instruments include the dental probe, tartar-breaking forceps, and various types of dental scalers. The dental probe is used to evaluate the integrity of the periodontium, probing the gingival sulcus

Table 1. Dental formulae of dogs and cats.

Deciduous Teeth		Permanent Teeth
$2\left(I\frac{3}{3}\,C\frac{1}{1}\,PM\frac{3}{3}\right)=28$	Dog	$2\left(I\frac{3}{3}\,C\frac{1}{1}\,PM\frac{4}{4}\,M\frac{2}{3}\right)=42$
$2\left(I\frac{3}{3}\,C\frac{1}{1}\,M\frac{3}{2}\right)=26$	Cat	$2\left(I\frac{3}{3}\,C\frac{1}{1}\,PM\frac{3}{2}\,M\frac{1}{1}\right)=30$

I = incisor teeth PM = premolars

C = canine teeth M = molars

The numbers beside each letter represent the number of teeth $\left(\frac{\text{maxillary}}{\text{mandibular}}\right)$ on *one* side of the head.

around each tooth (Fig 32). Loose teeth are also identified with the probe. Tartar-breaking forceps are used for removing large blocks of dental calculus before scaling the teeth. The dental scaler is used to remove plaque and calculus from the teeth (Fig 33). Table 2 provides additional information about the dental probe and some of the more commonly used dental scalers. Dental elevators and extractors are primarily used for tooth extraction, not tooth cleaning.

Use of ultrasonic scalers has the advantage of being much faster and less labor intensive than manually scaling the teeth. However, these machines are expensive and, if used incorrectly, can permanently damage the tooth and surrounding gingiva. Ultrasonic

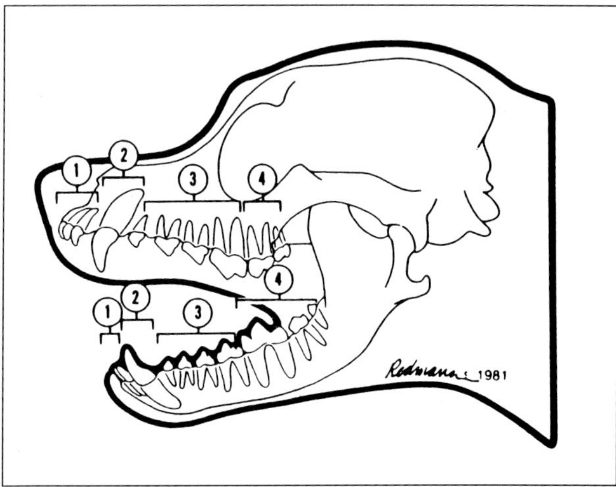

Figure 29. Dentition of the adult dog: (1) incisors; (2) canine teeth; (3) premolars; (4) molars. (Courtesy of Jane Redmann)

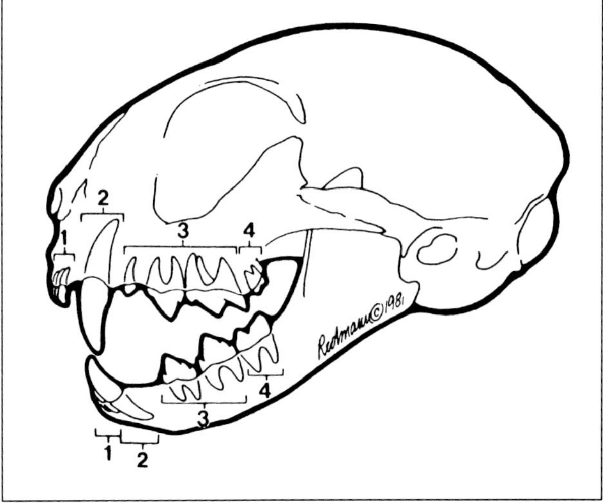

Figure 30. Dentition of the adult cat: (1) incisors; (2) canine teeth; (3) premolars; (4) molars. (Courtesy of Jane Redmann)

waves, consisting of high-frequency vibrations, are used to remove plaque and calculus from the tooth surface.

After the teeth are scaled, polishing the teeth smoothes the surface of the enamel. Pits and crevices favor proliferation of microorganisms. Polishing helps decrease growth of bacteria by eliminating surface irregularities. Dental polishers are usually low-speed, rotary hand held devices (Fig 34).

Prophylaxis Technique

Dental prophylaxis consists of several steps: thorough examination of the oral cavity, including the gums and teeth; manual removal of large amounts of calculus and debris; ultrasonic removal of plaque and calculus; manual removal of sub-gingival plaque and calculus; polishing of the tooth enamel; rinsing the oral cavity of blood and debris; and, when indicated, fluoridation of the teeth. Tooth extraction may also be part of the dental treatment, but is a therapeutic, not prophylactic, measure.

Figure 31. Anatomy of the tooth. (Modified from Bell, *J Sm Anim Pract* 6 (1967), courtesy of Lea & Febiger.)

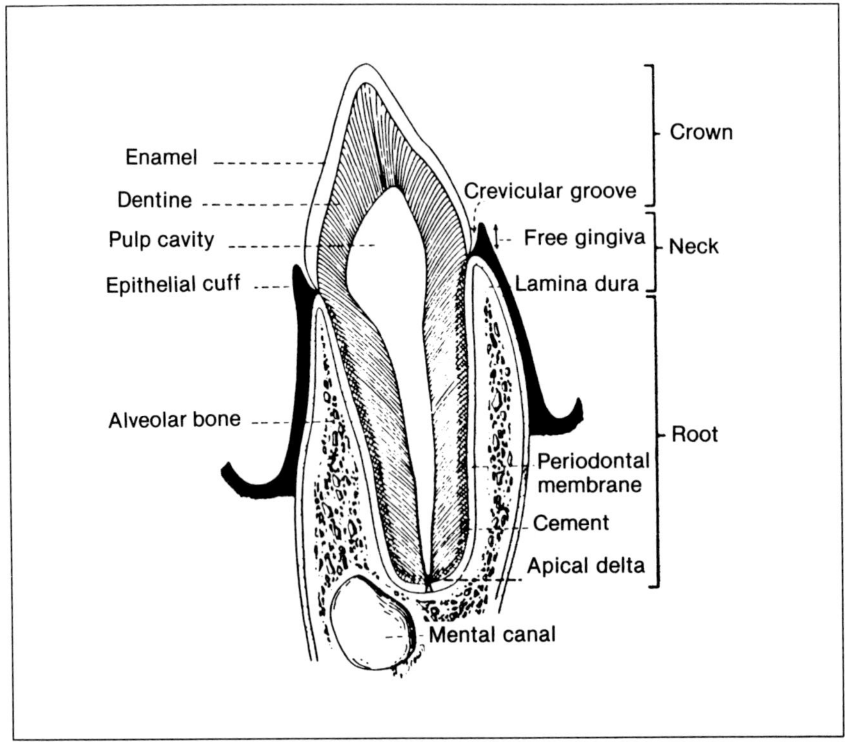

Animals with severe periodontal disease are usually pretreated with oral antibiotics before dental prophylaxis, as dental treatment may release bacteria into the blood, setting the stage for potential septicemia and bacterial endocarditis. If significant dental disease is present, oral antibiotics for several days before and after dental treatment may be indicated. Occasionally, parenteral antibiotics at the time of the procedure are required.

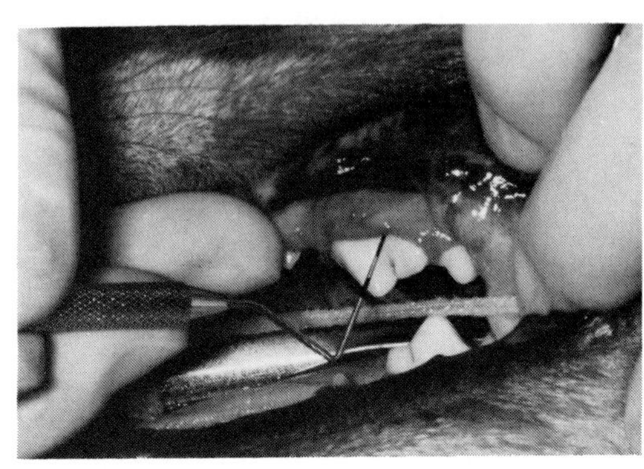

Figure 32. Periodontal probe. The depth of the gingival sulcus can be measured using the 3-mm markings on the probe.

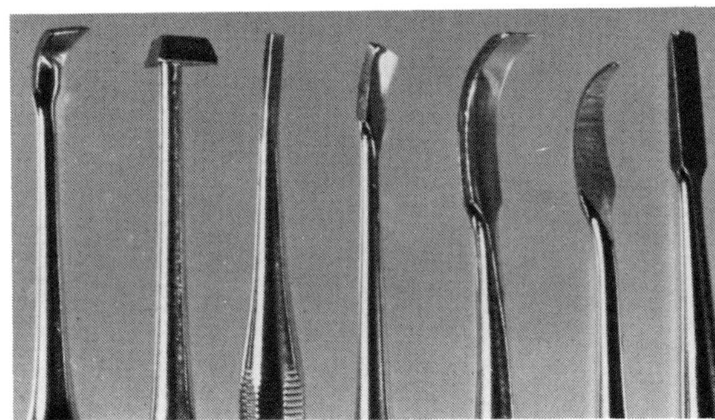

Figure 33. Manual scalers used for routine dental prophylaxis.

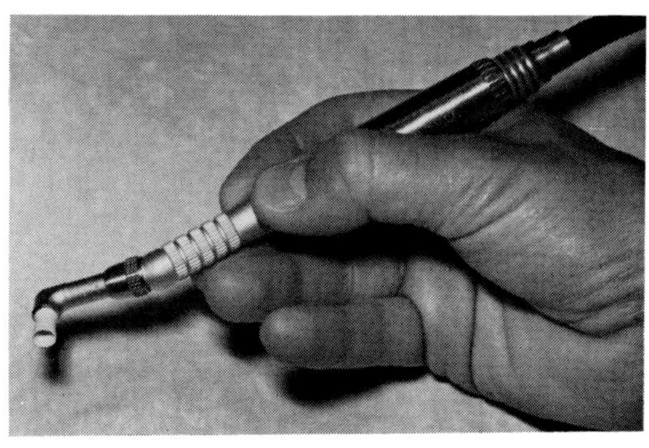

Figure 34. Low-speed rotary handpiece used to polish enamel.

Table 2. Description and use of dental instruments for oral prophylaxis.

Instrument	Description	Purpose	Placement/Movement
Explorer/Probe	The narrow shaft of the probe is marked in easy-to-read increments on one end. Blunted, pointed explorer tip on the opposite end. (*eg,* ST-4: Henry Schein)	Aids detection of decay and assessment of the perodontium.	Explorer is placed perpendicular to the tooth surface and lightly passed over the tooth to detect surface irregularities. Probe is placed parallel to the tooth and passed gently into the gingival sulcus.
Scaler	Curved blade with 3 cutting edges. Is the most versatile dental instrument for scaling. (*eg,* ST-2 and ST-3: Henry Schein)	Debridement of sub- and supragingival plaque/calculus	Short, powerful strokes from the gingival margin toward the cusp tips. Blade must remain against the enamel surface.
Curet	Elongated curved blade with 2 cutting edges. Blade terminates in a round end. The outer edge is the working (scaling) edge. (*eg,* Gracey curets 11-12 and 13-14)	Subgingival scaling. 11-12 Gracey for incisors, canine premolars. 13-14 Gracey for premolars, molars.	Gentle retraction of the free gingival epothelium with the curet. Blade is placed against the tooth surface and stroked toward the cusp tip.
Hoe	Single, right-angle cutting edge. (*eg,* ST-1: Henry Schein)	Gross debridement of supragingival calculus on the flat tooth surface.	Blade is positioned perpendicular to the tooth and pulled away from the gingival margin.

General anesthesia is always required for thorough dental prophylaxis. Because many dental patients are geriatric, a blood chemistry profile may be indicated before anesthesia. An endotracheal tube, with an inflated cuff, should be used at all times to prevent the inadvertent aspiration of debris into the lungs.

The patient is positioned in lateral recumbency on an inclined surface with the head lower than the rest of the body. This helps keep water from leaking around the endotracheal cuff and into the lungs. A mouth gag is placed on the canine teeth to keep the mouth open.

The operator should wear examination gloves, a surgical mask, a surgical cap and a smock. This is especially important when using the ultrasonic scaler because of the potential for infection from bacterial aerosol created by this instrument.

Oral Examination: The first step of dental prophylaxis is a complete oral examination, including inspection of the oral cavity. In addition to the teeth and periodontium, the tongue and oral mucosa should be evaluated for lesions (*eg*, masses, ulcerations, abscesses). The dental probe is used to assess the health of the dental sulcus, probing for deep pockets and loose teeth. Not all loose teeth must be extracted. Some may be salvaged with prophylactic therapy. However, extremely loose teeth should be removed.

Manual Removal of Calculus: The second step of dental prophylaxis is the removal of large particles of calculus, usually with tartar-breaking forceps. This facilitates the scaling process. When removing dental calculus with tartar-breaking forceps, care should be taken not to damage the gingiva.

Ultrasonic Removal of Plaque and Calculus: The third step of dental prophylaxis is mechanical removal of plaque and tartar, usually with an ultrasonic scaler. As previously mentioned, an ultrasonic scaler is more efficient at removing debris than a manual scaler. The major disadvantage of the ultrasonic scaler is the potential damage to the tooth enamel or gingiva when improper technique is used or when the tip is allowed to overheat. While cleaning the teeth, the scaler tip is moved lightly and continuously in a circular motion across the tooth's surface, keeping the tip parallel to the gingival margin. The tip must never be left on any one site for more than a few seconds, as permanent damage to the pulp may occur. When in operation, the tip of the scaler must emit water to prevent overheating the tip from the high frequency vibrations. The water flow may require some adjusting until 1-2 drops per second are emitted from the tip. The frequency is initially set on zero and then adjusted until all the water drops are aerosolized.

Manual Removal of Plaque: The fourth step of dental prophylaxis is the manual removal of any remaining plaque or calculus.

Areas that are difficult to clean effectively with the ultrasonic scaler, such as crowded teeth, sub-gingival regions and deep periodontal pockets, require hand scaling with manual dental instruments. Several types of dental scalers are available. Each type is shaped to reach a different surface of the tooth.

Polishing the Teeth: The fifth step of dental prophylaxis is polishing the tooth. Polishing paste is applied to the end of a rotary polisher. Each tooth is individually polished for 10 to 15 seconds. As with the ultrasonic scaler, the dental polisher should never be used too long at any one site, as this could result in damage to the pulp.

Rinsing the Oral Cavity: The sixth step of dental prophylaxis is rinsing the oral cavity free of blood and debris. Sterile saline, dilute povidone-iodine or an oral chlorhexidine solution can be used. If fluoride treatment is included in the dental prophylaxis, it is done under general anesthesia as the final step. Fluoride phosphate gel is applied to the dental sulci with cotton-tipped applicators and allowed to remain for 4 minutes. Excess gel is then wiped away.

Client Education

Routine dental prophylaxis may be recommended for cats and dogs with relatively healthy teeth. This involves a dental cleaning every 1-2 years. Animals with severe dental disease may benefit from more frequent cleaning, 2-4 times a year.

To maximize the effectiveness of dental prophylaxis, clients should be shown how to clean their pet's teeth at home. Dental care is best begun when animals are still young, as cats and dogs are usually more receptive to training at a young age. Additionally, if dental care is begun before the onset of gingival disease, the teeth are likely to stay healthier.

Ideally, brushing the teeth should be performed daily. However, even brushing once to twice weekly may significantly delay dental disease. A human toothbrush or specialized animal toothbrush can be used. Human toothpaste is not recommended because it can irritate the animal's stomach if swallowed. Numerous veterinary dental products are available, including gels, sprays, solutions and powders (*eg*, Nolvadent: Fort Dodge). Dental sprays may be easier to apply to patients that resist having their teeth brushed.

Diets can also play a role in prevention of dental disease in dogs and cats. Dry foods tend to be better for the teeth than semi-moist or canned products because they are more abrasive and less likely to become impacted in gingival crevices. However, if teeth have been removed during a dental treatment, a soft diet of canned food is recommended for the following 2-3 days to minimize irritation to the gingiva.

Recommended Reading

Routes of Drug Administration

McGuire BH, in McCurnin DM and Poffenbarger EM: *Small Animal Physical Diagnosis and Clinical Procedures.* Saunders, Philadelphia, 1991.

Otto CM *et al:* Intraosseous infusion of fluids and therapeutics. *Compend Cont Ed Pract Vet* 11:421-430, 1989.

Tube Feeding

Abood SK and Buffington CA: Improved nasogastric intubation technique for administration of nutritional support in dogs. *JAVMA* 199:577-579, 1991.

Bright RM *et al:* Percutaneous tube gastrostomy for enteral alimentation in small animals. *Compend Cont Ed Pract Vet* 13:15-23, 1991.

Crowe DT: Nutritional support for the hospitalized patient: an introduction to tube feeding. *Compend Cont Ed Pract Vet* 12:1711-1721, 1990.

Fox SM: Placing a pharyngostomy tube for enteral feeding. *Vet Med* 82:903-906, 1987.

Lewis LD *et al,* in: *Small Animal Clinical Nutrition III.* Mark Morris Associates, Topeka, KS, 1987.

Urine Collection

McGuire BH, in McCurnin DM and Poffenbarger EM: *Small Animal Physical Diagnosis and Clinical Procedures.* Saunders, Philadelphia, 1991.

Grooming

McGuire BH, in McCurnin DM and Poffenbarger EM: *Small Animal Physical Diagnosis and Clinical Procedures.* Saunders, Philadelphia, 1991.

Ear Care

McGuire BH, in McCurnin DM and Poffenbarger EM: *Small Animal Physical Diagnosis and Clinical Procedures.* Saunders, Philadelphia, 1991.

Eye Care

McGuire BH, in McCurnin DM and Poffenbarger EM: *Small Animal Physical Diagnosis and Clinical Procedures.* Saunders, Philadelphia, 1991.

Enemas

McGuire BH, in McCurnin DM and Poffenbarger EM: *Small Animal Physical Diagnosis and Clinical Procedures.* Saunders, Philadelphia, 1991.

Dental Prophylaxis

Aller S: Basic prophylaxis and home care. *Compend Cont Ed Pract Vet* 11:1447-1458, 1989.

Eisner ER: The instruments required for dental prophylaxis. *Vet Med* 84:1048-1054, 1989.

Eisner ER: Conducting a methodical dental prophylaxis. *Vet Med* 84:1056-1066, 1989.

Eisner ER: Helping clients care for their pet's teeth at home. *Vet Med* 84:1070-1074, 1989.

Hawkins BJ: Dental instruments and the use of dental materials. *Compend Cont Ed Pract Vet* 11:1465-1472, 1989.

Seim HB, in McCurnin DM and Poffenbarger EM: *Small Animal Physical Diagnosis and Clinical Procedures.* Saunders, Philadelphia, 1991.

Physical Therapy for Dogs and Cats

C.H. Tangner

Physical therapy is the treatment of disease or injuries by physical agents, such as light, heat, cold, water, electricity, massage and exercise. When properly applied, physical therapy can expedite healing of injured tissue, prevent disability and help restore normal function. Physical therapy can be used to rehabilitate animals with diseases of bones, muscles, joints, nerves and skin, as well as dislocations, fractures, arthritis, paresis, paralysis, infections and decubital ulcers. Physical therapy can relax muscle spasm, relieve pain, promote early resorption of swelling, increase blood and lymphatic circulation, and maintain or build muscle tone and flexibility.

Indications for physical therapy include pain, swelling, muscle spasm, and altered function of traumatized tissues, including surgical wounds. Physical therapy is also indicated to minimize muscle atrophy and joint stiffness resulting from disuse or neurologic dysfunction.

Physical therapy techniques must be performed correctly and only when indicated because physical therapy, like any other form of medical treatment, can cause harm if improperly administered.

Specific physical therapy should be designed to meet the needs of an individual patient. Once it is determined that the patient can tolerate the treatment, therapy can be continued by the pet owner at home. The client should be present at the last in-hospital physical therapy treatment just before release of the patient so the client can be shown exactly how to proceed. Patients should be reexamined regularly to assess the need for continuation or change in the prescribed protocol.

The modes of physical therapy range from simple to complex. The most important factor determining the quality of the therapy is the person administering it. A good therapist must have an optimistic attitude, a general interest in the welfare of each animal, and a great deal of patience.

Local Cold Therapy

Cold therapy (cryotherapy), administered with cold packs, cold water or ice, decreases tissue temperature, reducing pain and muscle spasms. Cold is also thought to decrease nerve conduction and create mild analgesia at the application site. Cryotherapy also causes local vasoconstriction and decreased capillary blood flow, thereby decreasing edema. Applied within 24 hours after an injury, cryotherapy can greatly reduce hemorrhage into tissue spaces. Animals with acute swelling, pain and muscle spasm can be aided by cold therapy in the first 12-48 hours after traumatic injury. Any cold pack or cold wrap can be used, provided excessive pressure, weight or cold is not applied to damaged tissue. Open wounds in the area to be cooled should be protected with sterile, impermeable dressings during treatment to avoid contamination.

Cold Packs: Commercial cold packs are manufactured for use in human medicine but can also be used in veterinary medicine. They are available in various sizes and forms (Fig 35). A disposable instant cold pack is activated by squeezing, which breaks an inner bag, mixing the contents and causing an immediate drop in temperature. The pack provides a temperature of 20 F for about 45 minutes.

Reusable cold packs contain a liquid that does not harden, even when frozen (Fig 35). This type of pack can be bulky and heavy, so it should not be applied to a fracture site. Both instant and reusable packs should be covered with a towel before application so as to prevent frostbite. Application time is generally 5-20 minutes, 2-4 times daily for up to 2 days.

The most commonly used cold packs are those used by drug companies for shipping drugs. These packs stay frozen longer than ice and are reuseable. If commercial packs are not available, apply ice to the affected site. The ice should be in a plastic, leakproof bag,

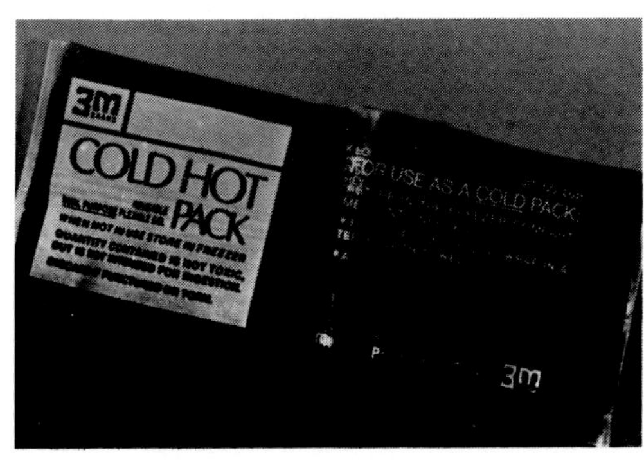

Figure 35. A reusable hot and cold pack.

wrapped in a towel. A washcloth or towel soaked in ice water can be used on injuries in body areas to which ice cannot conform, such as joints and bony prominences.

Cold-Water Immersion: Immersion of an injured limb in cold water (18 C, 65 F) is another effective cryotherapeutic method. Only the affected areas should be immersed. Cold water immersion is used specifically to rehabilitate muscles, ligaments, tendons and joints, combat high fevers, and treat burns and traumatic inflammatory conditions. Cold-water immersion is also indicated in cases in which heat therapy has been unsuccessful. An injured limb can be immersed in cold water for 5-10 minutes 2-4 times daily. A limb should not be immersed for more than 20 minutes at a time.

Cold packs or wraps are preferred to immersion if open wounds are present. A disinfectant should be added to the water if a small wound is to be immersed. Large wounds should not be immersed, as this can delay healing.

Local Heat Therapy

Heat therapy (thermotherapy) involves use of radiant, conductive or converted heat to treat disease. The purpose of heat therapy generally is to increase tissue temperature, causing analgesia (pain relief) in affected tissues and some sedation. The resulting vasodilation and increased circulation in the injured site enhance movement of phagocytes, oxygen, antibiotics and nutrients to the area. Heat relieves pain, relaxes muscle spasms and promotes wound healing. It usually relaxes the patient, increasing its sense of well-being.

Animals with contusions and sprains benefit from heat applied 48-72 hours after injury. Animals with bursitis, tendinitis, impaired circulation or noninflammatory edema have a decreased tolerance to heat and should not be subjected to heat therapy.

Freshly epithelialized wound and scar tissue are especially susceptible to thermal damage, so application of heat to these tissues should be avoided. Heat therapy should be modifed or abandoned if it causes pain or worsens clinical signs. Heat treatments should last from 10 minutes to a maximum of 20 minutes, repeated 2-3 times daily.

Heat is often combined with other forms of physical therapy. For example, heat can be followed by massage or exercise to reduce swelling. In patients that can walk, mild exercise is indicated within one hour after heat treatment to aid muscle relaxation and increase arterial flow to and venous return from the injured area.

Radiant Heat: Radiant heat transmits energy to the skin and superficial tissues, which absorb the rays and convert them to heat. Long- wave rays are emitted by all heated bodies and by such items as heating pads and hot-water bottles. Because long-wave rays only penetrate about 2 mm into tissue, being absorbed mostly in the upper skin layers, they are not recommended for therapy.

Short-wave rays emitted by generators or lamps, are the most effective rays used in physical therapy. These rays can penetrate up to 5-10 mm into tissues, influencing blood vessels, lymph flow, nerve endings and subcutaneous tissues. Infrared radiation is a powerful form of radiant heat. Animals can be severely burned by ultraviolet light (sunlamps). Infrared radiation should be used cautiously, particularly over healing skin and scar tissue and on animals with impaired circulation. It should not be used in very old or very young patients.

Conductive Heat: Conductive heat is heat transferred from an object with a higher temperature to one with a lower temperature. Hot packs are the most common method of applying conductive heat.

A protective layer of toweling should be placed between any hot pack and the skin surface. The skin should be checked every few minutes. If it feels hot or appears red, an additional layer of toweling should be added. Hot packs should never be applied over newly healed skin or scar tissue.

Hot packs are commercially available. One type is a reusable pack filled with silica gel. When heated to 170 F, the pack retains heat for 20-30 minutes, which is the usual maximum application time. The pack should be covered with a towel to delay cooling and must be kept constantly wet or it becomes unusable. Units are available for heating the water and storing the packs. These packs last for years if used with care.

Instant, nonreusable packs are also available. These are activated by breaking an inner bag and shaking the pack to mix the contents. A chemical reaction of the enclosed chemicals generates moderate heat.

Warm (about 100 F) whirlpool baths are another form of conductive heat therapy (see below). The moist heat is more effective in relieving pain and muscle spasms than is dry heat.

Converted Heat: Converted heat results from conversion of one energy form to heat in the body tissues. Ultrasound, a mode of converted or deep-heat therapy that provides deeper heat than radiation therapy, consists of mechanical vibrations that are identical to acoustic or sound vibrations except in their frequency and mode of emission. The frequency of ultrasound waves (over 20,000 cycles per second) makes them inaudible to the human ear.

Ultrasound waves are transferred from the machine producing them to the affected body area through a hand-held transducer. To eliminate air pockets between the transducer and skin, a coupling medium, such as mineral oil or lubricating gel, is used. For best results, the animal's hair should be clipped from the area to be treated.

Ultrasound therapy is applied in 3 ways. The most common is the contact technique, which is used on smooth, muscular surfaces and involves a coupling medium. The weight of the transducer or the light pressure applied usually does not cause pain.

A second method is underwater ultrasound therapy. This technique is used to treat very uneven surfaces, such as the olecranon (elbow) or stifle (knee), where good transducer-body contact is impossible. Only the area of treatment need be immersed in water.

The cushion technique, the third method of ultrasound administration, is used over bony prominences or curvatures that prevent good transducer contact and cannot be submerged in water. For this type of ultrasound treatment, a plastic bag filled with tepid water is placed between the transducer and the gel-coated skin.

Ultrasound is used for a variety of neuromuscular and musculoskeletal conditions to soften scar tissue, reduce pain of neuromas and degenerative joint disease, and treat arthritis and bursitis. The chief danger in using ultrasound is a burn. The patient should never feel any pain or discomfort during the treatment; excessive movement or other signs of pain during treatment indicate inappropriate application of ultrasound. Ultrasound should not be used over the eyes, spinal cord, brain, growing bones, heart, anesthetized areas, ischemic areas, tumors, reproductive organs, acutely infected areas, or areas previously exposed to radiation.

Massage

The simplest form of physical therapy is massage, in which the hands and fingers are used to manipulate soft tissues of the body. The primary objective of massage is to increase blood flow through the massaged tissues. Massage also enhances the flow of lymph from tissue spaces, providing quicker elimination of wastes and flow of nutrients into the site. Massage can decrease the likelihood of fibrosis, which is an abnormal formation of adhesions between connective tissue layers.

A massage medium may be used to reduce friction and soften the skin or scar tissue. Some commonly used media are mineral oil, cold cream, olive oil and petroleum jelly. Powders, such as talc or baby powder, are used more frequently in veterinary medicine in place of lubricants because they provide the same effect and are easier to remove. The medium should be placed on the hands and then massaged into the patient's skin instead of being applied directly to the skin, and never be applied to open wounds or fresh incisions. At the conclusion of therapy, the lubricant can be removed with isopropyl alcohol.

Factors that must be considered when administering massage include direction, pressure, rate and rhythm of the stroke, and duration (usually 15 minutes is enough) and frequency of massage. These factors vary, depending on the size of the area treated, and the animal's size, condition, response to and progress with treatment.

Specific conditions that massage can benefit include tight and contracted tendons, ligaments and muscles, subacute and chronic traumatic and inflammatory conditions, peripheral nerve injuries, scar tissue, and subacute and chronic edema. Specific conditions for which massage is contraindicated include acute or inflammatory processes of soft tissues, bone and joints, fractures, sprains, foreign bodies under the skin, hemorrhage or lymphangitis, and advanced skin diseases.

The 4 basic types of massage are effleurage, foulage, friction and whirlpool massage.

Effleurage: Effleurage, or stroking, is a gentle massage that accustoms the animal to the touch of the therapist, allowing it to relax before a deeper form of massage is applied. The patient is massaged from the periphery of the limb or affected area toward the center.

Effleurage can be done with a light or heavy stroke, but uniform pressure is required. A light stroke, at a rate of 15 strokes/minute, should be applied for a sedative effect. A heavy stroke, at 5 strokes/minute, should be applied to enhance drainage in veins and lymph channels. A 10-minute session should generally prepare the patient for more extensive therapy.

Foulage: Foulage, also called kneading, compression or pétrissage, is used primarily on muscle groups, individual muscles or a part of a muscle to enhance circulation and stretch muscles, tendons and adhesions. The muscle should be compressed from side to side as the hand moves up it, always in the direction of venous return (toward the heart).

Kneading massage is commonly used to assist venous and lymphatic circulation. With kneading massage, one or both hands or the fingers are used to grasp the skin and muscles, lift them away from the bones and gently roll, compress or wring them. Then the hands are repositioned 8-10 cm away from the massaged area, and the procedure is repeated.

The muscles should be compressed if they cannot be grasped. Muscles are grasped between the thumb and fingers of each hand and elevated. The tissues are then compressed alternately between the fingers of one hand and the heel of the other hand.

Massage should be firm enough to cause muscle contraction, but gentle enough to avoid causing pain. It should be performed slowly and rhythmically to avoid creating patient objection and should be done for 5-10 minutes twice daily. If the intent of the massage is to reduce limb swelling, it should be performed in a distal-to-proximal direction with the involved limb elevated. Swollen limbs should be bandaged after massage.

Friction Massage: Friction massage is used to aid absorption of local effusions and loosen superficial scar tissue and adhesions. In friction massage, the skin is moved over underlying tissue in small, circular, rhythmic motions, with the greatest pressure applied at the lowest part of the circle. The frequency and duration of friction massage vary with the animal's condition and size.

Whirlpool Massage: Whirlpool massage can be used for small animal patients (the turbulence of the whirlpool acts like manual masasge). Time can be saved by combining other treatment modalities with whirlpool treatment. Hypothermia is induced simultaneously with whirlpool massage by maintaining the water temperature at 12-22 C (55-70 F). Hyperthermia is produced if the water temperature is 36-38 C (96-104 F). Patients can be stimulated to swim in the whirlpool if they are suspended in the water and not allowed to support their weight on the bottom or sides of the tub (see below).

Exercise

Exercise is purposeful motion that involves many body systems. The goals of exercise are to increase arterial, venous and lymph flow, and to improve sensory awareness and voluntary movement. Exercise increases muscle strength, endurance and coordination of movements while preventing or reducing joint stiffness and muscle atrophy.

Immobilization of a healthy joint causes fibrous contracture, which limits movement of the joint. Immobilized muscles also lose their ability to increase in length. Prolonged immobilization or disuse of an extremity is likely to result in muscle atrophy and inelasticity, with limited joint mobility.

The 2 types of exercise used in physical therapy of small animals are passive and active.

Passive Exercise: Passive exercise is used on patients that are paralyzed or very weak, or with fractures. Passive exercise is accomplished by a therapist, with no activity on the part of the patient. This type of exercise helps prevent joint ankylosis ("freezing") and disuse atrophy. Passive exercise can also be used after certain types of surgery, such as that for intervertebral disk disease. These patients should have their hind limbs flexed and extended for 10-minute sessions several times daily.

When an animal cannot or will not exercise, each joint of the injured extremity should be moved passively at varying speeds through a full range of motion unless the movement causes pain. Painful joints should only be moved through a range of motion that is tolerable to the patient. Passive exercise should be done for 5-10 minutes twice daily, whether it is the sole treatment or is combined with other physical therapy.

Active Exercise: The most beneficial form of exercise is active exercise, which entails voluntary muscle contraction by the patient and includes many types of exercise, from walking to swimming (see below). Some patients may be willing to exercise on their own, but reluctant patients may require some stimulation and support.

Many devices can provide added support and assistance for nonambulatory (unable to walk) animals. One such device is an exercise cart, which is available commercially or can be constructed from inexpensive aluminum rods and lawn mower wheels (Figs 36, 37). The cart supports the animal's torso, allowing limb movement and exercise for patients unable to support their own weight. Carts are especially useful in rehabilitation of patients with caudal paralysis.

If an exercise cart is not available or is not well tolerated by the patient, a sling can be made with a bath towel (Fig 38). The towel

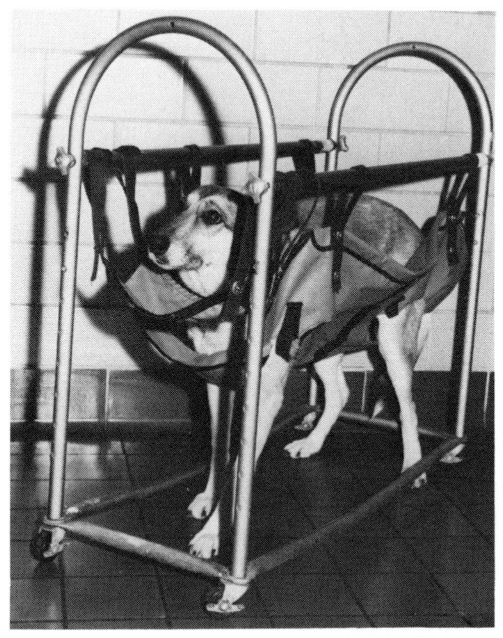

Figure 36. A full-support, wheeled exercise cart.

should not be allowed to pull against the top of the thigh because this impedes leg motion. "Tailing" exercise, which includes using the tail to support the rear quarters of the animal, can also be used intermittently with the exercise cart to prevent dependency on the cart (Fig 39). Care must be taken to grasp the tail at its base to prevent injury.

Animals that can walk and that are not experiencing pain can be walked or trotted for 10-20 minutes daily. Care should be taken to avoid overexercising the animal because overwork may cause ex-

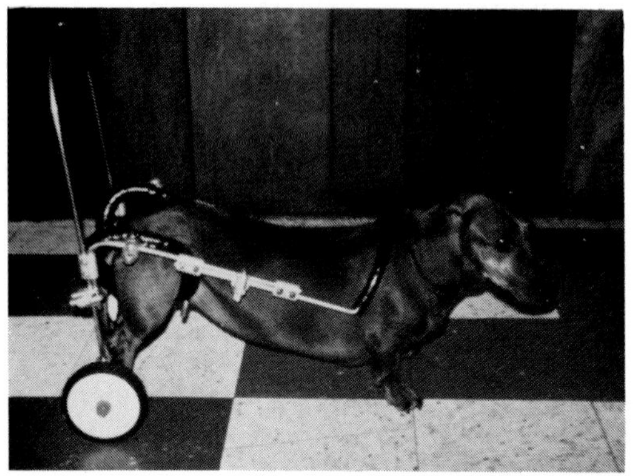

Figure 37. A commercially available exercise cart used for dogs with caudal paralysis.

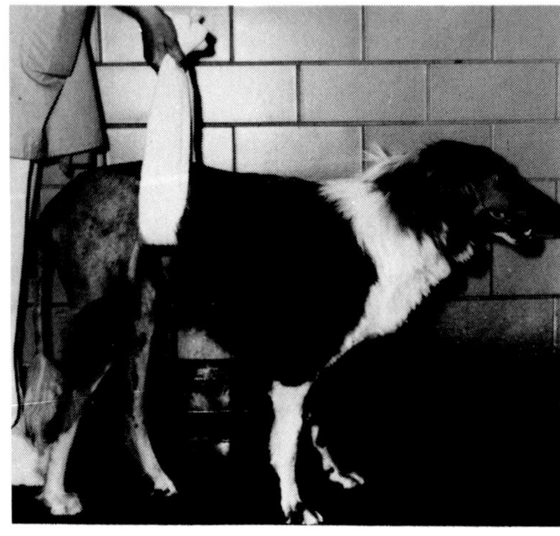

Figure 38. A bath towel can be used to support the hindquarters during active exercise of dogs with caudal paresis.

cessive muscle protein breakdown and retard return of muscle function.

Hydrotherapy: Underwater exercise is another method of providing support for an animal with locomotor difficulties. The physical properties of water provide the animal with support. Water movement or turbulence, as in a whirlpool bath, can be added to create a massage effect. Buoyancy provides a lifting effect, allowing voluntary exercise that would otherwise be impossible in animals unable to stand or walk.

The temperature of the water should be 18-24 C (65-75 F) for active exercise and 36-40 C (96-105 F) for inactive patients. With warm-water therapy, the animal gains and produces heat during exercise. These 2 combined factors increase the peripheral blood supply by dilation of superficial blood vessels, which causes increased heart and metabolic rates.

Animals undergoing hydrotherapy must never be left unattended; the possibility of drowning should always be kept in mind. If the patient has a disorder of the neck or an extremity, a sling arrangement should be used for support. Another patient safety consideration is fear. If the patient is afraid of water, the first few therapy sessions should concentrate on acclimating it to the water. Febrile patients should not be treated with warm-water therapy until their rectal temperature has been normal for at least 72 hours.

A povidone-iodine concentrate can be added to the water (1/4 oz povidone-iodine for each 1 gal water) to decrease the possibility of transmitting infections from one patient to another. The concentration can also help prevent urine scald, infection of decubital ulcers, and superficial pyoderma.

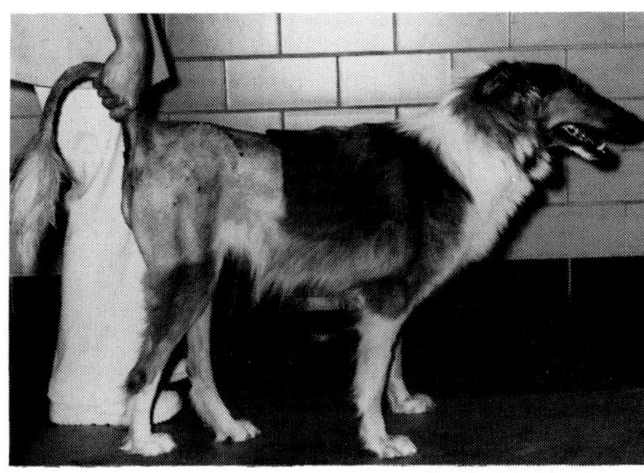

Figure 39. The tail can be used to support the hindquarters during active exercise therapy of dogs with caudal paresis. Note that the tail is grasped at the base so as to avoid tail injury.

Whirlpool Baths: The whirlpool bath, an important mode of hydrotherapy, achieves its therapeutic effects through turbulence or movement of water, accomplished with an electric turbine ejector and aerator that circulates an air-water mixture. Portable agitators are adaptable for use in almost any tank, bathtub or pool (Fig 40).

A non-skid surface should be placed on the bottom of the tub for weight-bearing patients to aid traction. The water temperature should be 41-43 C (105-110 F). The turbine must be electrically grounded and not started until the water is in the tank and the patient is safely positioned in the tub.

Contrary to common belief, the turbine should be directed so the water is emitted *away* from the affected body part. Treatments should be given after the animal has urinated and defecated so as to avoid contaminating the whirlpool bath. The length of whirlpool treatment should be about 20 minutes and should not exceed 30 minutes.

The effects of whirlpool baths are the same as those of underwater exercise. In addition, whirlpools combine the effects of gentle massage and superficial heat. The swirling action of the water helps clean and debride damaged tissues, thereby combating infection. Scar tissue is softened and metabolism, respiration and mobility of extremities are increased.

Whirlpool baths are indicated for patients with fractures in the late stage of healing, arthritis, stiff joints, adhesions, dislocations, amputations, subacute and chronic inflammatory disease, diseases associated with decubital ulcers, and skin diseases.

In treating animals with dermatologic disorders, the water aids healing by removing exudates, crusts, scales, bacteria and debris

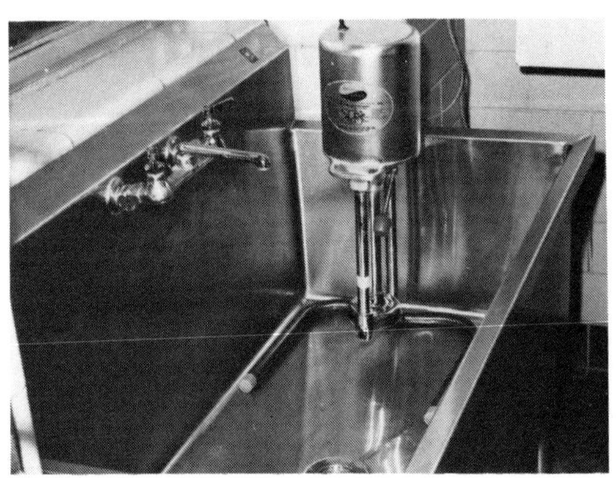

Figure 40. A portable water agitator used in hydrotherapy.

from lesions, wounds and fistulas. The whirlpool also helps alleviate pain and pruritus associated with skin disorders. The water softens the keratin of the skin and promotes epithelialization.

Whirlpool therapy is contraindicated for animals with peripheral vascular disease, acute injuries, acute inflammation, recent surgery, acute edema, fever and cardiac or respiratory disorders.

Swimming: Swimming is good exercise for animals that require more extensive exercise for rehabilitation or that are in the last phase of rehabilitation. Swimming animals are forced to move continuously, while the water's buoyancy allows an increased range of motion of their limbs.

Swimming exercise is indicated for many patients because it allows non-weight-bearing movement of weakened limbs, which is not possible otherwise without manual support. Swimming has added benefits for small animal patients with intervertebral disk disease because it removes urine and feces from the skin, thereby decreasing the likelihood of urine burns.

Swimming for 20 minutes once a day in warm water is adequate treatment for most patients. As a rule, patients with skin incisions present less than 10-14 days should not be immersed unless the incision can be completely protected from water. Small dogs can swim in a bathtub at the veterinary hospital and, after discharge, at the owner's home. Larger dogs can swim in the shallow area of a swimming pool, with a person nearby in the pool.

Rehabilitation and recovery of a patient depend on the care it receives. The importance of conscientious nursing care, with generous amounts of affection, cannot be overemphasized. Many patients have special needs for rehabilitation. It is the technician's responsibility to recognize and attend to these needs. It is also vital that the patient have a desire to recover. The technician should interact with the patient as a friend by talking in a pleasant tone and addressing the patient by name.

Hospitalized animals should be discharged as soon as possible because their familiar surroundings at home tend to improve the animal's sense of security and speed recovery. Most clients are willing to participate in the rehabilitation program at home. Physical therapy methods should be demonstrated to the client so they can be applied properly at home.

The importance of maintaining the prescribed treatment schedule should be stressed, as failure to treat the animal properly may result in relapse. Complete, written home-care instructions concerning diet, medication, exercise and treatment should be provided. Frequent communication with the client is necessary to monitor the patient's condition at home. Many animals must be returned to the hospital for additional checkups and treatment.

BLOOD COLLECTION AND TRANSFUSIONS

C.S. Intravartolo

Canine and Feline Blood Groups

One of the major concerns of transfusion therapy is whether the blood of a potential donor animal is compatible with that of the patient. Transfusion reactions are caused by an adverse antigen antibody response between the donor's red blood cells and the patient's plasma.

There are 8 blood groups in dogs, classified according to specific antigens found on the red blood cells that are sometimes responsible for transfusion reactions (Table 3). DEA 1.1, 1.2 and 7 are the most reactive antigens within the blood groups and therefore are most often associated with transfusion reactions. More than half of the canine population has those antigens on their red blood cells. These dogs should not be used as blood donors because of the potential risk of a transfusion reaction.

There are 3 blood groups in cats, classified as A, B and AB. In the past, little information was available about blood groups in cats. It was common to transfuse cats with blood that was neither typed nor crossmatched. Few transfusion reactions were noted, especially if only a single transfusion was given.

Type A is the most common feline blood type. Most type-A cats are domestic shorthairs and longhairs. Type-B blood is not as common and occurs in such breeds as the British Shorthair, Persian and Devon Rex. Type-AB blood is extremely rare.

Cats with type-A or type-B blood have naturally occurring antibodies that destroy red cells containing antigens of the other type. Depending on the donor/patient combination, reactions range from mild to severe. For example, if type-B cats are transfused with type-A blood, severe clinical signs develop. Reactions of type-A cats to type-B blood are less serious, but the transfusion is not beneficial to the patient. For this reason, the blood of the donor and the

Table 3. Blood groups of dogs. DEA = dog erythrocyte antigen.

DEA 1.1	DEA 5
DEA 1.2	DEA 6
DEA 3	DEA 7
DEA 4	DEA 8

patient should be typed or crossmatched before a blood transfusion.

Blood typing is not a routine procedure in most veterinary practices because reagents required for testing are difficult to obtain; however, some universities and clinical laboratories have facilities for animal blood typing. The laboratory should be contacted for proper instructions regarding collection and handling of the sample. In addition, 2 commercial blood banks offer various canine blood products for transfusion (Hemopet, Irvine, CA; Animal Blood Bank, Dixon, CA).

Crossmatching

Crossmatching determines donor and patient blood compatibility before blood transfusion and is easily performed in the veterinary hospital. It is not a substitute for blood typing; however, it is the best alternative when typing has not been done or when a suitable donor is not available.

Major and minor crossmatches can be performed. A *major crossmatch* involves mixing the patient's serum with the donor's red blood cells. A *minor crossmatch* combines the donor's serum with the patient's red blood cells. Significant hemolysis or agglutination indicates incompatibility between the donor and patient. Transfusion with crossmatched blood decreases the possibility of a transfusion reaction; however, it does not eliminate the possibility of sensitizing a patient, which may result in a reaction to future transfusions.

Donor Compatibility

Patients should not be transfused with blood from an incompatible donor. Transfusion of incompatible blood on the first transfusion is unlikely to cause an immediate reaction. Rather, the patient develops antibodies that may destroy constituents of the transfused blood within 7-10 days. Such antibody formation does not cause illness but sensitizes the patient to future transfusions. If the patient were to receive a second transfusion with the same donor's blood, red cell destruction could begin much sooner. Subsequent transfusions with incompatible blood increase the likelihood of a serious or fatal transfusion reaction. Cross-species transfusions (*eg,* dog to cat) are always contraindicated.

Blood Donors

There are certain advantages to maintaining donor animals with blood of known type in a veterinary hospital. Blood-typed donors reduce the possibility of giving incompatible blood. The animals are of adequate size and disposition to allow blood collection with minimal difficulty. Blood counts can be performed routinely to ensure adequate levels in the donor. The animal is maintained in good physical condition and can be fed a diet known to support blood production. Finally, the veterinarian has a readily available source of whole blood.

Animals selected as resident blood donors should be healthy young adults, 1-5 years old, that have never received a blood transfusion. Dogs should weigh at least 25 kg and should not be obese. The animals should be free of intestinal parasites and blood disorders. Dogs should be negative for *Dirofilaria immitis, Brucella canis* and other blood-borne parasites.

Donor cats should be shorthaired and easy to handle, and weigh at least 5 kg. Cats should be tested for feline leukemia virus, feline infectious peritonitis virus and *Hemobartonella felis.*

The technician should maintain accurate records for each donor animal. Records must be kept of each donation and of routine preventive care, such as immunizations and fecal and heartworm examinations. The technician may wish to develop a medical record sheet for each donor animal (Fig 41).

Blood Collection

Blood can be collected and stored for future use or collected at the time it is needed. The interval between transfusions given in a hospital determine how often blood is collected. Because most transfusions are given as part of emergency treatment, fresh blood is usually collected when it is needed.

Collection Materials

Drugs for Sedation or Anesthesia: Blood can usually be collected from most hospital donor dogs without chemical restraint. Cats often require mild sedation or anesthesia for ease of collection. Tranquilizers and anesthetics should be available when needed.

Clippers and Preparation Materials: Strict asepsis must be maintained during collection, storage and administration of blood. The blood collection site is clipped with a #40 blade and prepared with a suitable antiseptic, such as povidone-iodine, to prevent infection in the donor animal.

Blood Collection and Administration Equipment: Blood collected for transfusion in dogs is collected in commercially available plastic bags or vacuum bottles. The most commonly used anticoagulants are *citrate phosphate dextrose (CPD), acid citrate dextrose (ACD)* and *heparin.*

Plastic collection bags are available with ACD or CPD (Fig 42). The blood collection set is incorporated into the bag, eliminating the need for a separate donor set. The bags are available in a variety of styles for human use. Two styles that are useful in veterinary hospitals are the CPD Single Blood-Pack Unit (Fenwal Division, Baxter Health Care, Deerfield, IL) with a 15- or 16-ga needle for whole blood collection, and the CPD Double Blood-Pack Unit (Fenwal) with an attached 300-ml transfer pack suitable for harvesting plasma.

Vacuum bottles contain ACD and are available in 250-ml and 500-ml sizes (Fig 42). The bottles require a separate blood collection set, also called a *donor set*, when the blood is withdrawn.

In many instances, plastic bags are preferred over bottles for blood collection. Collection in glass bottles is usually quicker because of the built-in vacuum. A disadvantage of using bottles is the difficulty in maintaining sterility because the bottles must be

Figure 41. This record sheet for blood donors provides a convenient record of vaccinations, diagnostic test results and blood donations. (Courtesy of Veterinary Learning Systems)

Name ______________________ Species ______________________

Breed ______________________ Birth ______________________ Sex ______

Blood type ______________________

Vaccination History

Date												
Rabies												
DHLP												
Parvovirus												
FVRC-P												

Preventive Care Checklist

Date												
Fecal												
CBC												
Platelets												
Heartworm												
Weight												
Other												

Donation Record

Date	Amount	Next Use	Date	Amount	Next Use

vented during blood administration. The advantages of using plastic bags include: minimal loss of platelets, convenient attachment of collection tubing and needle, no possibility of breakage, less storage space required, gravity flow eliminates the foaming and mechanical trauma caused by vacuum bottle collection, and plasma can be harvested from outdated blood units.

To collect blood from donor cats, a 60-ml heparinized syringe and a 21-ga butterfly catheter (Abbott Labs, North Chicago, IL) work well (Fig 43). The syringe is flushed with heparin before venipuncture, using 0.25 ml of sodium heparin for every 50 ml of blood collected. Avoid using too much heparin, as this may cause clotting disorders in the patient.

Blood Collection from Donor Cats

The jugular vein is the preferred site for blood collection from cats. The average adult cat can safely donate 50 ml of blood every 2 weeks.

Donor cats are usually sedated or anesthetized for blood collection. The jugular site is clipped and surgically prepared. The but-

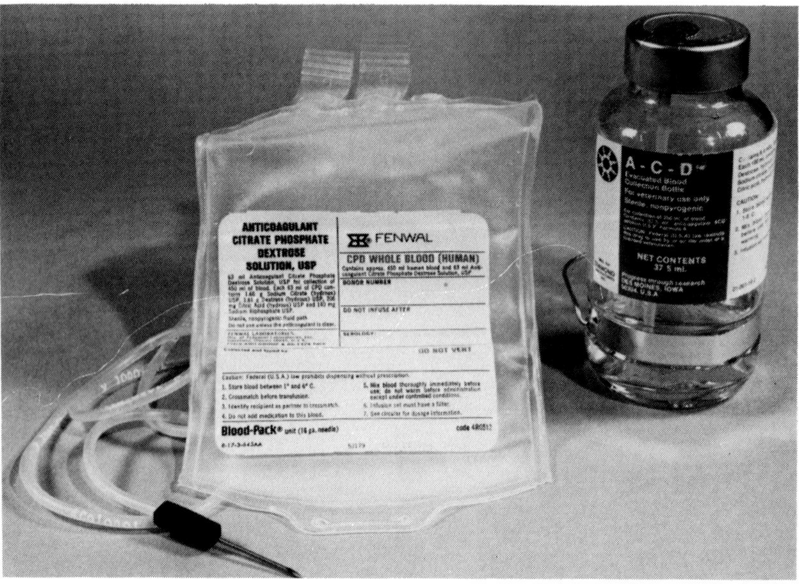

Figure 42. The CPD Single Blood-Pack Unit and the ACD collection bottle are suitable for blood collection and short-term storage of whole blood. (Courtesy of Veterinary Learning Systems)

terfly catheter is inserted cranially into the vein and the required amount of blood is withdrawn into the heparinized syringe. After the cat has been anesthetized, the entire procedure can be completed in 10 minutes with relative safety and minimal stress to the cat.

Blood Collection from Donor Dogs

The most common sites for blood collection from dogs are the jugular vein and femoral artery. Collection from the femoral artery causes less trauma to red blood cells and platelets than collection from any other site. Though this method is quick, it requires tranquilization and sometimes general anesthesia. Dogs can safely donate 22 ml/kg every 10-14 days.

Sedation or anesthesia is rarely necessary when collecting blood from donor dogs, unless the femoral artery is used. Most resident blood donor dogs become accustomed to the procedure and are easily handled. The jugular area is prepared as in cats, the collecting needle is inserted cranially into the vein, and blood is collected in a bag or bottle. Because the collection bottle or bag contains a specific amount of anticoagulant, it is important to completely fill the container with blood.

Donor Care After Collection

Following blood collection, the technician should place a bandage over the venipuncture site to prevent infection and hematoma formation. If the donor animal has been anesthetized, it should be monitored during recovery. If only plasma was needed, the red

Figure 43. Blood can be collected from donor cats using a 21-ga butterfly catheter attached to a 60-ml syringe. (Courtesy of Veterinary Learning Systems)

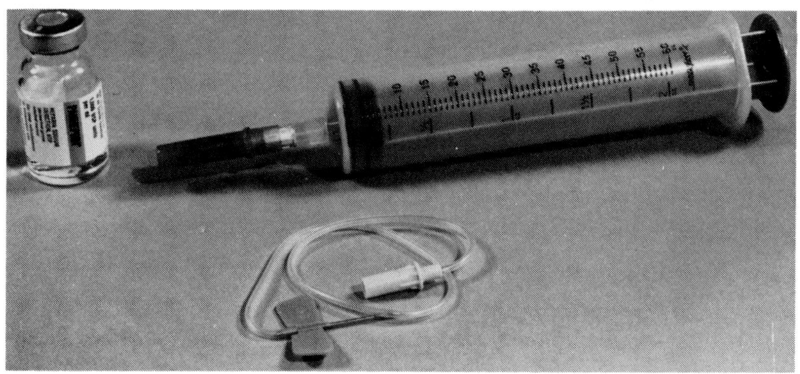

blood cells may be infused back into the donor. Cats may be given 100 ml of saline solution IV to replace lost fluid volume.

Blood Storage

Whole Blood

If blood is not to be used immediately, the container should be labeled, dated and stored at 4 C (39 F). It can be stored in a standard refrigerator for at least 21-28 days.

The dextrose in the anticoagulant helps to preserve the red blood cells. Heparinized blood contains no preservative and should be used immediately or stored in the refrigerator and used within 48 hours. Blood collected into syringes should be used within 4 hours to avoid bacterial contamination.

Plasma

Plasma is the liquid portion of the blood. It differs from serum in that *serum* is plasma from which the fibrinogen has been separated during collection. Plasma may be harvested from blood simply by allowing the red blood cells to settle and then aspirating the plasma from the top of the container. Plasma may be stored frozen for as long as 1 year.

Preparing Stored Blood and Plasma for Use

Blood that has been stored in a refrigerator should be slowly warmed to room temperature before administration. Before it is transfused, the bottle or bag should be *gently* inverted several times until the red blood cells are in suspension. Discard any previously stored and rewarmed blood that is not used. Do not refrigerate it again, as bacteria are found in blood that has been warmed. A dark brown to black color of the plasma indicates bacterial growth.

Blood Administration

Handling the Patient

It is important to remember that the patient in need of a transfusion is usually in poor physical condition. Most such animals are depressed and weak. Stress of any kind may result in sudden collapse and possibly death. For these reasons, the patient must be handled as gently as possible.

Routes of Administration

Whole blood is most effective when given IV. The most common sites are the jugular, cephalic and lateral saphenous veins. One method combines use of commercially available blood administration sets and indwelling IV catheters (Sovereign Catheter, Sherwood Medical, St. Louis, MO). Standard fluid administration sets are not designed for blood administration.

Blood administration sets differ from fluid administration sets in that they contain a special filter chamber that prevents large blood clots from entering the patient. Improperly filtered blood may cause pulmonary microembolization and respiratory distress. The blood should be given through a 20-ga or larger indwelling catheter placed aseptically into the vein. Using a smaller needle or catheter may cause hemolysis of the transfused blood.

No other drugs should be mixed with blood or plasma during transfusions, as incompatibility between the drug and blood or anticoagulant may cause complications. Certain drugs and fluids (*eg,* Ringer's solution) can cause coagulation of the blood. Sterile physiologic (0.9%) saline is the only safe fluid for diluting blood for transfusion.

Sometimes IV administration of blood is difficult. Occasionally an animal's blood pressure is so low that a vein cannot be catheterized. In small puppies and kittens, it is sometimes difficult to catheterize a vein. Blood and other fluids can be given directly through a needle placed into the intramedullary canal of a bone, such as the femur or tibial crest. A standard 18- or 20-ga needle usually can be placed into the bone without problems. If the needle becomes obstructed with bone particles, a 20-ga needle with a stylet may be used. When the needle is securely placed, blood or other fluids may be dripped in by gravity or injected through a syringe. One disadvantage of this method is the risk of osteomyelitis.

Blood should not be given SC because most of the red blood cells are destroyed in the tissues, resulting in no benefit to the patient. Intraperitoneal infusion is also not recommended because of poor absorption of the blood.

Amount and Rate of Administation

The amount of blood transfused depends upon the reason for the transfusion. Blood may be given either to effect or in amounts to replace known losses.

The average cat can usually accept about 50 ml of blood over a 30-minute period. An equation has been developed to determine blood replacement requirements based on the patient's weight and

PCV, the PCV of donated blood, the desired posttransfusion PCV in the patient, and the blood volume of dogs and cats:

$$\text{Volume of blood required} = \text{patient weight (kg)} \times 90 \text{ (dog) or } 70 \text{ (cat)} \times \frac{\text{desired PCV} - \text{patient PCV}}{\text{donor PCV}}$$

The rate for IV administration of blood should not exceed 22 ml/kg/day. Patients with heart disease may not be able to tolerate more than 5 ml/kg/day. Most blood administration sets are designed to deliver 10 drops/ml (always refer to package inserts for exact directions); therefore, the administration rate in drops per minute can be calculated.

A slow IV drip is safer and more desirable for the patient than a large, rapidly administered bolus dose. During the first 30 minutes of a slow transfusion, the patient must be closely observed for any signs of a transfusion reaction. Signs include dyspnea, shivering, vomiting, fever, coughing and urticaria (hives). If these signs occur, the transfusion should be immediately discontinued and the patient reevaluated by the veterinarian.

If no problems develop, the infusion rate can be increased to standard recommendations. When possible, the entire required volume of whole blood should be given within a 4- to 6-hour period to avoid bacterial contamination.

BANDAGES AND DRESSINGS

K. Kazmierczak

Uses

A bandage is a piece of gauze or other material applied to a limb or other portion of the body. If the animal is confined to a cage, a bandage can prevent contamination from urine, feces, dander and other contaminants. It can also prevent the animal from chewing and licking the affected area.

A bandage can maintain the proper environment for healing of an open wound by keeping the area clean and free of contaminants that could cause an infection and delay healing. A bandage can also provide support to weakened tissues or control edema associated with fractures or blunt trauma. Bandages can be used to limit or prevent use of a limb with a fracture or after joint surgery to aid healing.

A bandage can be applied to secure a catheter for IV fluid administration. Neck bandages are commonly used to secure a jugular catheter and limb bandages for a cephalic vein catheter. When large areas of skin have been undermined or large areas of tissue removed, a bandage can be applied to prevent seromas by compressing dead space.

Bandage Materials

The most commonly used bandage materials are gauze sponges, gauze, elastic gauze, roll cotton, adhesive tape, elastic tape, roll padding, nonadherent sponges, and nonadherent elastic wrap (Table 4). The type and purpose of a bandage determine the combination of materials used. For example, to prevent a seroma postoperatively, the bandage may consist of gauze sponges placed along the incision line for absorption, elastic gauze to hold them in place, and elastic tape or elastic wrap to apply slight compression. The same materials can be used for a granulating wound. However, nonadherent gauze sponges (*eg*, Telfa Pads: Colgate-Palmolive) can be used in place of gauze sponges. Nonadherent sponges cause less disturbance of a granulating tissue bed each time the bandage is changed than do other types of sponges.

Bandage Application

Application and care of the bandage are important if it is to achieve the desired results.

When bandaging a limb, the most important rule is to apply the bandage material in a spiral fashion to prevent development of pressure rings on the skin. A pressure ring occurs when bandage materials have been applied in a circular fashion or a bandage has slipped from its original position. A constrictive, encircling bandage can cause severe edema within 24 hours.

To ensure a bandage is not applied too tightly, it should be possible to easily slip 2 fingers under the edge of the bandage (Fig 40). This also applies when securing an IV catheter; if too tight, the bandage impairs flow if fluids. When the limbs have been bandaged, the toes should be checked at least twice a day for signs of edema or coldness.If this occurs, the bandage should be removed immediately to restore proper blood circulation.

Elastic tape should be pulled off the roll and then laid onto the animal without any tension, unless mild compression is desired. If stretched and applied with too much tension, it can lead to edema of bandaged limbs, dyspnea from a bandaged thorax, head or neck, or choking when applied to the head and neck region.

Chafing caused by bandages occurs most often in the axillary and groin areas. Talcum powder, medicated powder, or baking soda

Table 4. Materials used in bandages.

Materials	Trade Name	Manufacturer
Adhesive tape	Zonas	Johnson & Johnson
	Orthalectic-Porous	Parke-Davis
	Curity Standard Porous	Kendall
Elastic gauze	Kling	Johnson & Johnson
	Stretch Gauze	Parke-Davis
	Kerlix Rolls	Kendall
Elastic tape	Elastikon	Johnson & Johnson
	Conform	Kendall
Gauze	Absorbent Gauze Roll	Parke-Daivis
	Gauze Roll	Kendall
	Nu-Gauze	Johnson & Johnson
Adhesive elastic wrap	Vet-Wrap	3-M
	Coban	3-M
Nonadherent sponges	Curity Telfa Pads	Colgate-Palmolive
	Release	Johnson & Johnson
	Micro Pad	3-M
	Telfa "Ouchless"	Kendall
	Non-Stick Sterile Pads	Johnson & Johnson
Roll cotton	Absorbent Cotton	Parke-Davis
	Red Cross Cotton	Johnson & Johnson
	Curity Cotton Roll	Kendall
Roll padding	Sof-Rol	Johnson & Johnson
	Specialist Cast Padding	Johnson & Johnson
	New Webril Orthopedic	Kendall
Sponges	Topper	Johnson & Johnson
	Gauze Sponge	Parke-Davis
	Unisorb	Parke-Davis
	Kerlix	Kendall
	Sof-Wick	Johnson & Johnson
Stretch bandage	Ace	Becton-Dickinson
	Dyna-Flex	Johnson & Johnson
	Rediflex	Parke-Davis
	Tensor Elastci Bandage	Kendall

can be applied to relieve the irritation. Chafing may be prevented if the powder or baking soda is applied to the dry skin in these areas when the bandage is first applied.

The animal should be prevented from chewing, licking or scratching the bandage. Application of an Elizabethan collar (Fig 45) or side brace (Fig 46) may be necessary. Hobbles can be used to prevent scratching at a thoracic, abdominal, head or neck bandage (Fig 47). It should be noted that scratching may be a signal that the bandage is causing some discomfort.

Head and Neck

The head and neck region may be bandaged after ocular surgery, repair of an aural hematoma or cervical spinal surgery, or to secure a pharyngostomy tube or jugular catheter. Care must be taken not to restrict respiration, swallowing, eating or vision (this may be unavoidable under certain circumstances).

It should be easy to slip 2 fingers under each end of the bandage (Fig 44). If the bandage is too tight, the animal will show signs of dyspnea or difficulty swallowing, or may scratch at the bandage. To remedy this, the bandage can be cut to relieve the tension. Tape

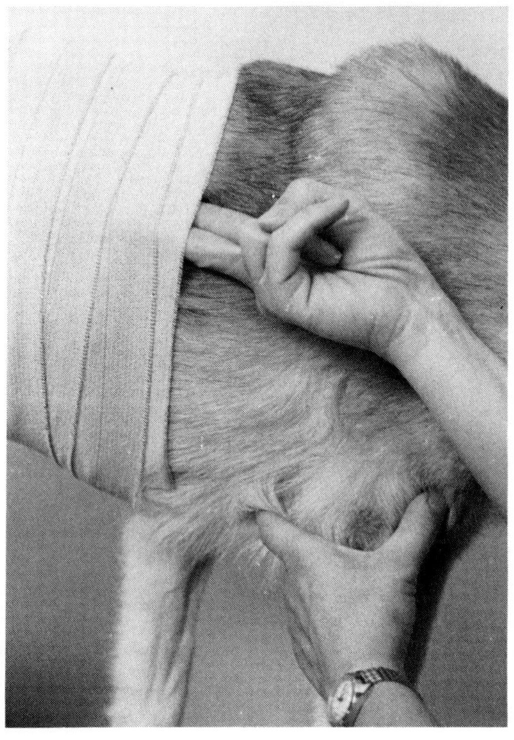

Figure 44. Testing bandage tension by inserting 2 fingers beneath the bandage.

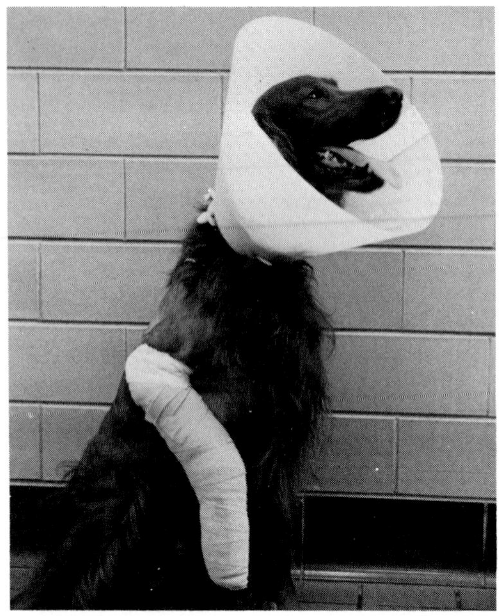

Figure 45. Use of an Elizabethan collar to prevent bandage removal by the animal.

Figure 46. A side brace can be used to prevent self-mutilation.

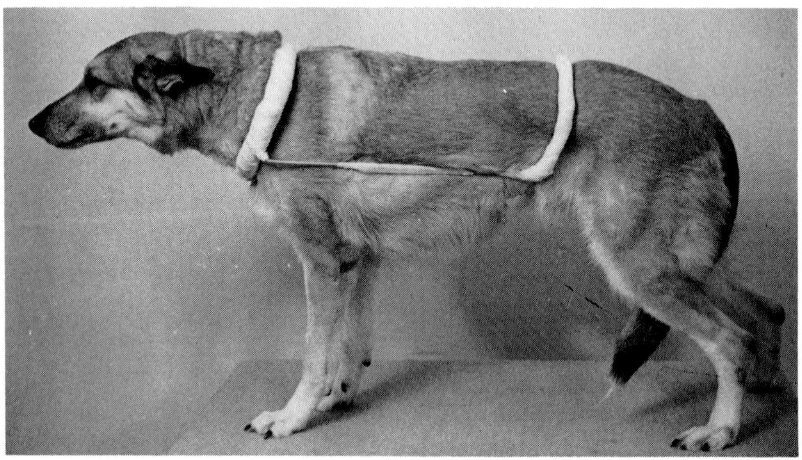

can then be laid over the cut bandage without any tension. This prevents having to replace the entire bandage.

If the bandage loosens, it most frequently slips caudad. If this occurs, the bandage should be removed immediately, as it can restrict respiration.

Occasionally an animal scratches at the bandage in an attempt to remove it. In such cases, it may be necessary to put hobbles or an Elizabethan collar on the animal.

Thorax

The thorax is most routinely bandaged when securing a chest drain, stabilizing fractured ribs, or protecting large thoracic wounds. The major concern when bandaging the thorax is not to impair respiratory movement. The tightness of the bandage can be checked by easily slipping 2 fingers under either end of the bandage (Fig 44). Tape, especially elastic tape, should be pulled off the roll and laid onto the animal without any tension. If the animal shows signs of dyspnea, remove the bandage immediately, as it may be too tight.

A common failure is slippage of a thoracic bandage. To help prevent this, be sure the tape is adhered to 1-1.5 inches of hair at the cranial and caudal edges of the bandage.

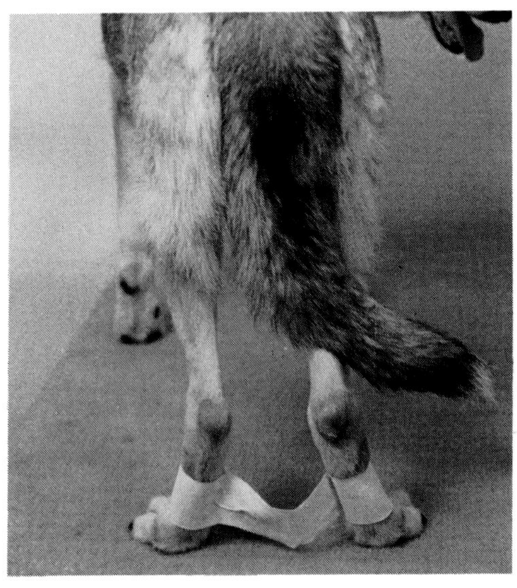

Figure 47. Hobbles made from bandaging material can be used to prevent injuries caused by excessive scratching.

If the animal scratches at the bandage in an attempt to remove it, hobbles will be necessary.

Abdomen

Indications for bandaging the abdomen are radical mastectomy or other extensive dissection of the abdominal region, hernia repair, placement of a drain, or securing a gastrostomy tube (a tube placed into the stomach through the abdominal wall).

To prevent the bandage from slipping caudad, it must be taped securely to the hair at the cranial end or even up on the chest.

It should be easy to insert 2 fingers at either end of the bandage to check that the bandage has not been applied too tightly. If the bandage is too tight, it can impair respiration or cause discomfort.

When an animal is confined to a cage and recumbent, the bandage becomes contaminated with urine and feces. This can be avoided by using a special rack to elevate the animal off the cage floor and allow for drainage of urine and feces (Fig 48).

The prepuce must not be included in the bandage on the abdomen of a male dog, as it can interfere with urination (Fig 49).

Limbs

Indications for bandaging a limb include postoperative immobilization of fracture repairs, protection of granulating wounds and stabilization of a limb for fluid therapy.

Figure 48. Use of a cage rack to elevate a patient from the cage floor and prevent bandage contamination.

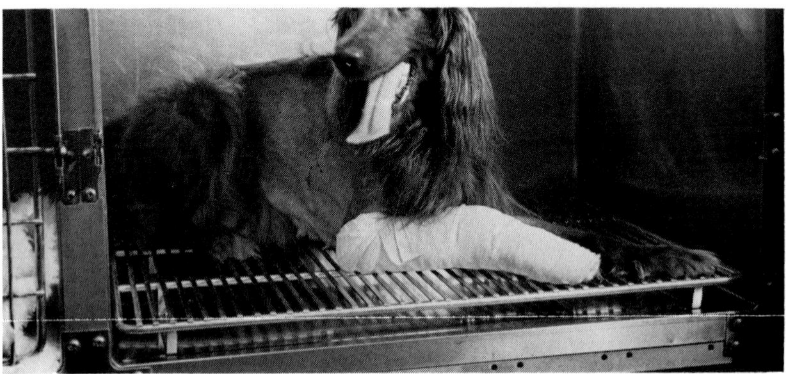

A Robert Jones bandage is commonly applied to temporarily stabilize fractures before definitive treatment. This bandage consists of several layers of roll cotton compressed tightly with elastic gauze and elastic tape. Note that this is the only type of bandage in which elastic gauze and tape are applied tightly. The underlying layers of cotton prevent constriction of the limb.

When bandaging the thigh, knee, proximal (upper) forelimb or elbow, the entire limb should be included. Application of the bandage should begin at the paw and continue proximad in a spiral fashion (Fig 50). This allows even distribution of pressure along the limb and maintains venous return from the paw.

To ensure the bandage has not been applied too tightly, it should be possible to slip 2 fingers under the proximal end of the bandage. The toes should be checked twice a day for edema, coldness or an abnormal odor, which are signs of decreased venous return.

If the bandage has slipped from its original position due to the animal's movement or chewing, the bandage may cause a pressure ring. Remove the bandage immediately if it has slipped or the toes become edematous.

Keeping a limb bandage dry and clean presents special problems in regard to exercising an animal. A wet, soiled bandage presents a perfect environment for proliferation of microorganisms, which could lead to infection or moist dermatitis. This can be avoided by taping a plastic bag around the limb when the animal is exercised outside and then removing it when the animal is returned inside. It is not advisable to use a rubber band to secure the bag, as it can slip off and constrict blood flow. If the bandage becomes wet, it should be removed immediately and a dry dressing applied.

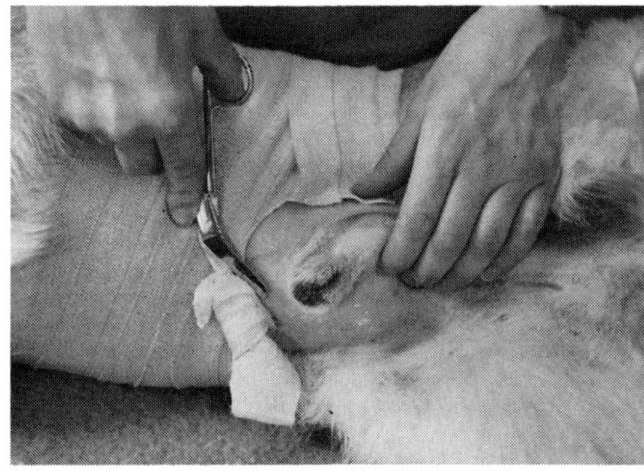

Figure 49. Modification of an abdominal bandage may be necessary in male dogs to prevent urine contamination.

Paw

The paw is normally bandaged after declawing cats, dewclaw removal in dogs, and repair of lacerations to the toes or foot pads.

To ensure adequate venous return from the paw, 2 fingers should easily slip under the proximal end of the bandage. The tape should be applied in a spiral fashion to prevent pressure rings.

When bandaging the paw, the accessory pad should always be included in the bandage. A small piece of cotton under the pad helps prevent irritation (Fig 50). Chafing could occur if the bandage were applied just under the accessory pad. To keep the bandage dry when the animal is exercised outside, a plastic bag may be applied around the bandage and secured with tape. The bag should be removed immediately when the animal is returned inside. If the bandage becomes wet, it should be removed immediately to prevent possible infection and a dry bandage applied.

Pelvis and Groin

Mastectomy, repair of perineal hernias, abscesses, wounds with drains and pelvic surgery are a few situations requiring bandaging in this area. This is perhaps the most difficult area to bandage.

The bandage should not be applied tightly. Check by slipping 2 fingers under the cranial edge of the bandage and where it encircles the legs. The legs, vulva or scrotum may become endomatous if the bandage is too tight.

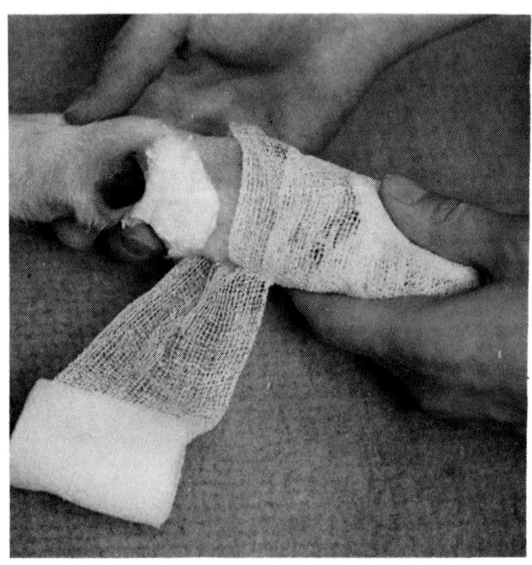

Figure 50. Starting a limb bandage at the distal end of the leg.

The bandage must not include the vulva, prepuce, scrotum or anus so as not to impair the animal's ability to urinate or defecate (Figs 51, 52). The bandage should be checked at least twice a day for dryness. If the bandage becomes soiled with urine or feces, it must be changed. Placing the animal on a rack may aid in keeping the bandage dry (Fig 48).

To prevent the bandage from slipping caudad, apply tape to 1-1.5 inches of hair around the cranial edge of the bandage.

Tail

Occasionally there may be a need to bandage the tail, as in partial tail amputation, granulating wounds or tumor removal. The major problem is securing the bandage.

In animals with a long tail, it may be necessary to apply the bandage 1 inch on either side of the lesion, or over the entire tail. In animals with a docked tail, tape should be applied loosely around the tail head.

Figure 51. Proper placement of a pelvic bandage in a female dog.

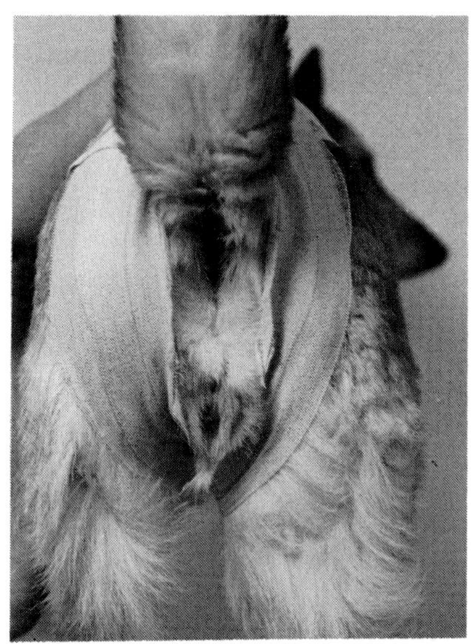

Figure 52. Proper placement of a pelvic bandage in a male dog.

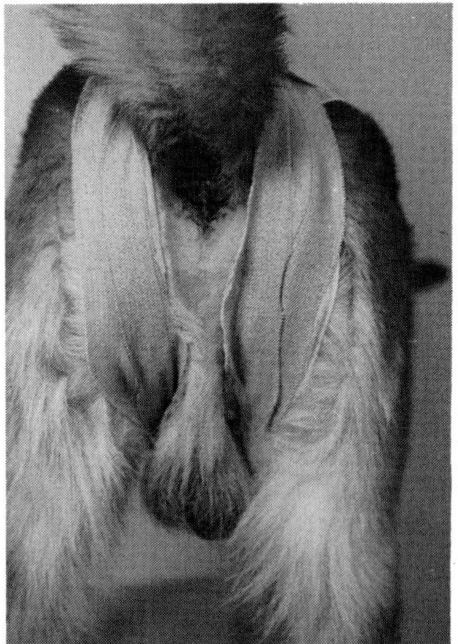

An Elizabethan collar or side brace may be necessary to prevent the animal from chewing the bandage off (Figs 45, 46).

Home Care of Bandages

When an animal is discharged, the owner must be instructed on how to maintain the bandage. The bandage should be kept clean and dry. A plastic bag can be taped over the bandage when the animal is outside and removed when indoors, so the bandage may "breathe." The animal should be relatively confined, with exercise only on a leash.

Self-mutilation must be prevented and the animal observed twice daily for edema or coldness of the toes, or an odor from the bandage. If the bandage becomes wet or loose, the toes become edematous, or the animal removes the bandage, the client should be instructed to notify the veterinarian immediately. It may be necessary to have the animal examined to evaluate the wound and possibly replace the bandage.

These home care instructions can be printed with the name of the clinic and veterinarian, and the telephone number and given to the client upon the animal's discharge. The technician should review this information with the client at the time the animal is discharged.

Recommended Reading

Giger U and Bücheler J: Transfusion of type-A and type-B blood to cats. *JAVMA* 198:411-418, 1991.

Giger U *et al:* Geographical variation of the feline blood type frequencies in the United States. *Feline Pract* 19(6):21-27, 1991.

Greene RT: Blood banking and transfusion therapy. *Vet Technician* 6:134-140, 1985.

Knecht *et al: Fundamental Techniques in Veterinary Surgery.* 2nd ed. WB Saunders, Philadelphia, 1981.

Oakley DA and Shaffran N: Blood transfusions. Part II. Collection, storage and administration. *Vet Technician* 8:189-193, 1987.

O'Neill S: Blood transfusions. Part I. The blood donor colony. *Vet Technician* 8:87-89, 1987.

Pichler ME and Turnwald GH: Blood transfusion in the dog and cat. Part I. Physiology, collection, storage and indications for whole blood therapy. *Compend Cont Ed* 7:64-71, 1985.

Poundstone M: Intraosseous infusion of fluids in small animals. *Vet Technician* 13:407-412, 1992.

Turnwald GH: Blood transfusions in dogs and cats. Part II. Administration, adverse effects and component therapy. *Compend Cont Ed* 7:115-124, 1985.

5

Treatment Techniques For Birds and Small Exotic Animals

L.A. Downey

Treatment of Birds

Restraint and Handling

Avian patients require special considerations regarding restraint and handling. First, birds are generally very susceptible to the stress of handling and examination. Efficiency and organization are critical to minimizing stress, so the veterinary team should anticipate and arrange any needed equipment and suppies before the patient is restrained. Second, restriction of the patient's chest movement interferes with respiration. The bird should not be held tightly around the chest, which would immobilize the sternum. Because cartilaginous rings completely encircle the trachea of birds, however, it is very difficult to disturb flow through this structure. Therefore, applying slight pressure on the neck to position a bird for venipuncture or examination is acceptable to faciliate the procedure. Finally, large psitticine birds are sometimes very noisy and you may want to wear protective ear coverings.

The amount of restraint necessary depends on both the temperament of the patient and the precedure being done. In general, the least amount of restraint required for the situation should be employed. All perches, dishes and toys should first be removed from the bird's enclosure to avoid injury during capture. Some tame patients readily step onto your finger or arm to be removed from the cage.

Small and medium-sized birds (*eg,* finches, budgies, cockatiels) can be grasped from behind using your bare hand or using a paper towel or small cloth. The towel or cloth acts as a visual barrier and gives the handler an opportunity to properly position the patient. The towel is placed in the palm of one hand while that hand is maneuvered behind the bird's head. Gently, but swiftly, grasp the patient's head with the thumb and forefinger on each side just ventral to the eyes. Wrap the palm of the hand and remaining 3 fingers around the bird's back and wings, folding the ends of the last 3 fingers under to avoid restricting the sternal movements (Fig 1).

For larger birds, a large towel of medium thickness should be used with the same technique. After the head is restrained, however, wrap the towel around the bird's body to control the legs, feet and wings (Fig 2). Hold the bird with one hand firmly on the head and use the other hand to cradle the bird's body next to you. The end of the towel can then be manipulated to expose the outside

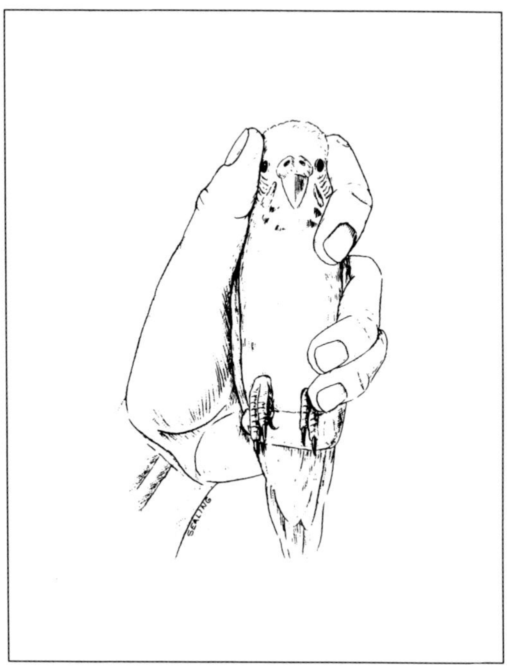

Figure 1. Grasp the bird with the thumb and forefinger on each side of the head, just ventral to the eyes. Wrap the palm of the hand and remaining 3 fingers around the bird's back and wings.

wing or leg, or to tuck the feet in and expose the sternum or abdomen.

When it is necessary to examine the opposite side of the bird, transfer the patient to the other hand. With the bird still wrapped in the towel and grasped firmly by the head, position the patient with its ventral side up. Then transfer the bird's head to the opposite hand using the same technique as previously. Finally, cradle the bird against your body (Fig 3).

Large birds can be dangerous when frightened and leather gloves are sometimes used to protect the handler. Leather gloves make handling and restraint more difficult for the handler and more stressful for the patient, however, and they are not recommended for most pet birds. Use of nets is not advised for most avian patients because of the possibility of injury to the bird.

A very nervous or antagonistic patient may first be distracted by allowing it to bite a towel, nylon bone or other object. This gives you the opportunity to capture the bird as previously described.

Once the patient has been restrained, a thorough examination may be done, along with grooming, blood collection, medication administration and other procedures.

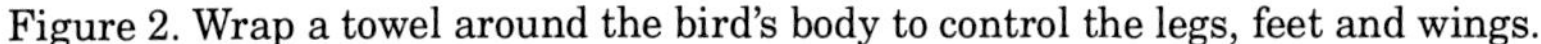

Figure 2. Wrap a towel around the bird's body to control the legs, feet and wings.

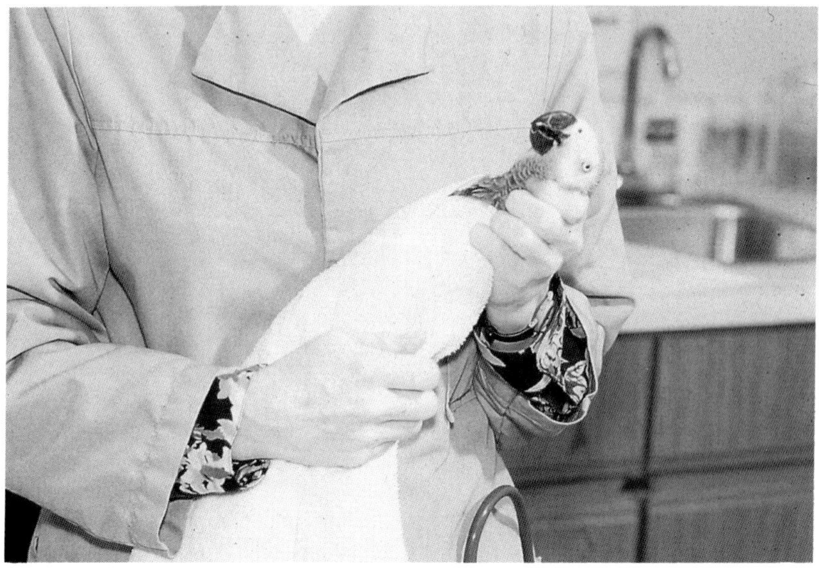

Figure 3 (A-D, left to right)). Transfer of a large bird to the opposite hand after initial restraint.

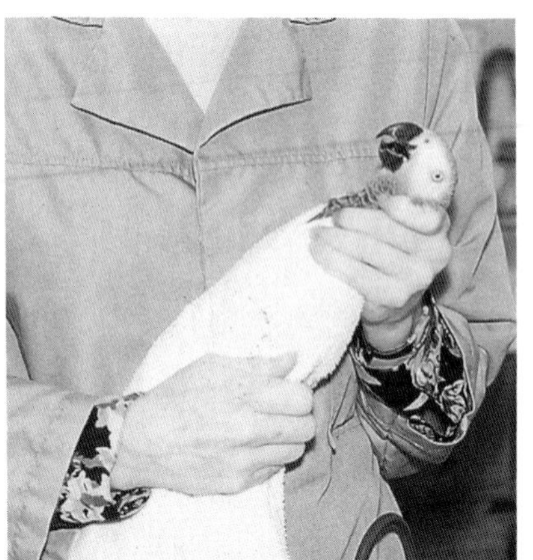

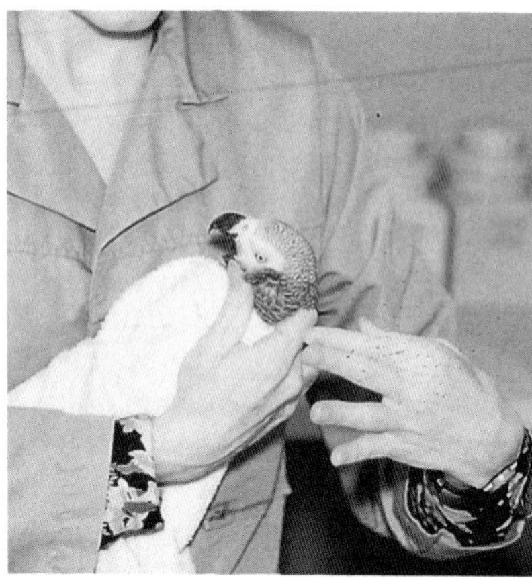

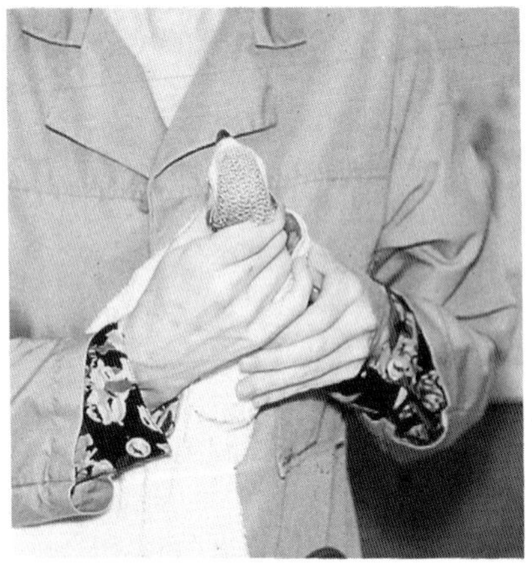

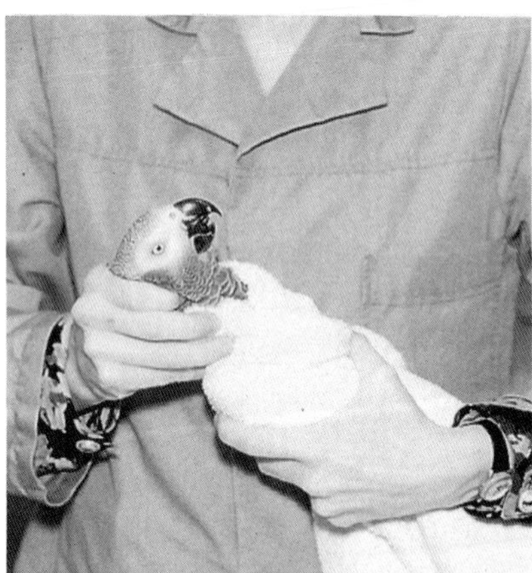

Grooming

Beak and Nail Trimming: Many pet birds have long and sharp nails and beaks, and their owners prefer to have these blunted or shortened for ease of handling. Some bird's beaks also grow overly long because of abnormal beak conformation or improper diet.

Nails of smaller avian species can be cut with suture scissors or small toenail clippers used for dogs or cats. Nails can usually be clipped just distal to the point that the nail becomes thin and claw-like. However, if the nails are extremely long, the quick may have grown past this point. If you inadvertently cut the nail a bit too short and it begins to bleed, simply grasp the toe to form a tourniquet, and apply a hemostatic powder or silver nitrate with some firm pressure on the tip of the nail to stop the bleeding. The quick of all nails is usually about the same relative length, so adjust the amount clipped from the remaining toenails accordingly.

With larger birds, many veterinarians prefer to use an electric hand-held grinding instrument to trim the nails. This often allows more control over the degree of trimming and also generates a small amount of heat to cauterize small blood vessels in the nail. Therefore a little shorter nail trim may be possible. Practice is necessary to achieve good control of the grinding instrument and the bird's toe, and it is advisable to have another handler restrain the bird in a towel as previously described. The opposite foot should be tucked into the towel used to restrain the bird, so it will not be inadvertently injured by the grinding instrument or will not latch on to a handler (Fig 4).

Similarly, most psittacine birds have very sharp and pointed beaks. A grinding instrument can also be used to blunt these for easier handling and training. Knowledge of the normal length and shape of the beak for each avian species is important. Generally, the tip and sharp edges of the upper beak can be rounded off. While holding the bird's head in one hand, place the thumb on the lower beak and the index finger on the upper beak. Hold the upper and lower beak together firmly to restrain the bird's head while grinding the upper beak (Fig 5). The tip of the lower beak can also be blunted and shaped. To expose the lower beak, push the bird's upper beak behind the tip of the lower beak with the index finger and hold it firmly in place (Fig 6). This will also prevent the bird from injuring its tongue on the grinding instrument.

Wing Trimming: Pet birds often benefit from clipped wings for purposes of training, confinement or prevention of escape or injury. This procedure limits the bird's ability to fly up and for significant distances. The goal is to limit flight but not to render the bird flightless, as it will need some control to land safely without injuring itself.

The wings of small species can sometimes be clipped by one person, but it is generally easier if an assistant restrains the bird. Larger species should be restrained in a towel, exposing one wing at a time.

After the wing is fully extended (grasp the wing bone close to the body so as to prevent injury during a struggle), first look for any blood feathers (immature feathers containing a blood vessel) and avoid cutting these. Cut the most distal 6-10 feathers closest to the tip of the wing at the level of the second row of feathers (coverts) (Fig 7). The cosmetic result can be improved if the covert feathers are not cut; however, no loss of function will occur if they are cut. It is usually advisable to clip both wings equally to allow the bird to retain its balance in flight.

When the wing clip is complete, test the bird by encouraging it to fly from a short height in a padded area, such as a carpeted room. The bird should be able to fly a short distance and land softly. If the bird can still fly in an upward direction, clip 1-2 more feathers on each wing. If the bird lands too heavily on its sternum, clip 1-2 fewer feathers on each wing at the next trim. Wing clips should be repeated as often as the feathers regrow, usually after each molt.

Figure 4. A hand-held rotary tool can be used to grind down the nails of large birds.

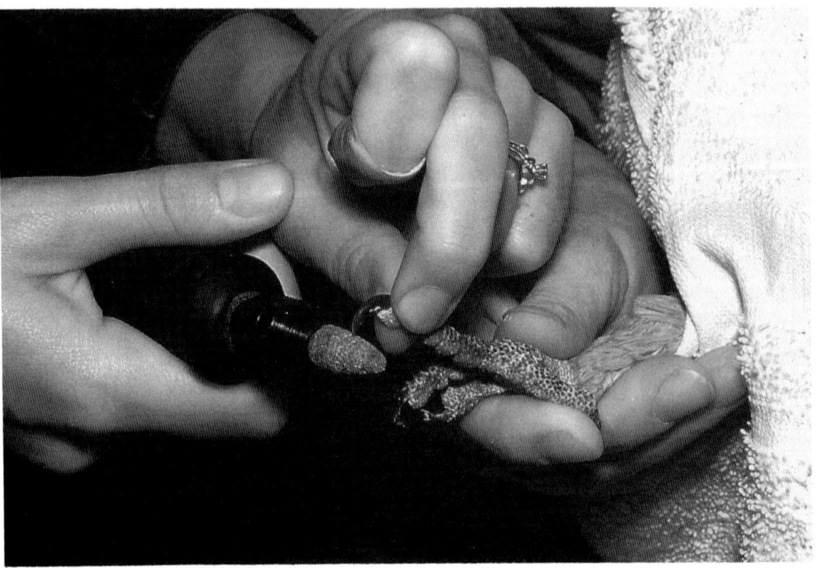

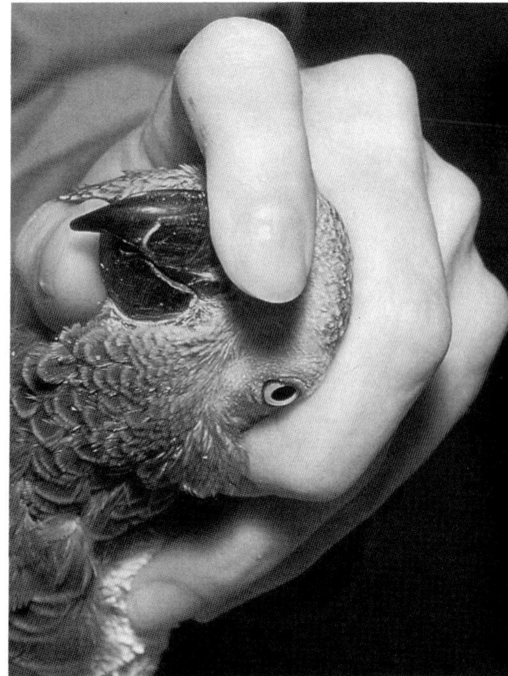

Figure 5. Restraint for grooming of the upper beak.

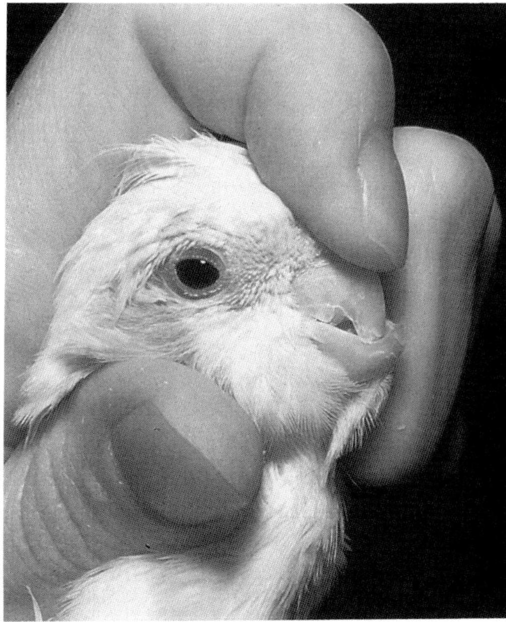

Figure 6. Restraint for grooming of the lower beak.

Blood Collection

Blood samples are commonly used for diagnostic tests. The amount of blood collected should be tailored to the size and condition of the bird. Generally, it is safe to take a sample in milliliters of 0.5-1% of the bird's body weight in grams. For example, a 100-g bird could safely give 0.5-1 ml of blood. Severely compromised patients should have a bit less blood collected, however. This sample is usually sufficient to run most hematology and serum chemistry tests.

The most efficient site of blood collection in birds is the jugular vein. The right jugular should always be used in birds because the left jugular is usually very small or absent. Restrain the bird as described previously; however, the head should be tilted away from the body by placing the index finger under the lower beak. The neck may be extended slightly dorsally or sideways to control the head for collection. At the same time, occlude the jugular vein with the thumb of the same hand. Application of alcohol to the skin of the neck allows the feathers to be parted over the vein and makes the vein more visible. Then use the opposite hand to withdraw the sample (Fig 8). A tuberculin or 3-ml syringe with a 25-ga needle is best for medium-sized to large birds; a smaller syringe and needle are often necessary for small patients.

Other sites for blood collection include the medial metatarsal vein, located superficially just distal to the tarsus (Fig 9), and the

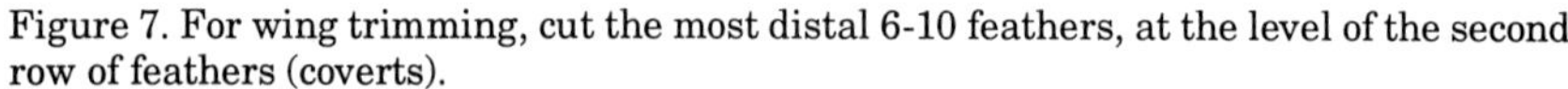

Figure 7. For wing trimming, cut the most distal 6-10 feathers, at the level of the second row of feathers (coverts).

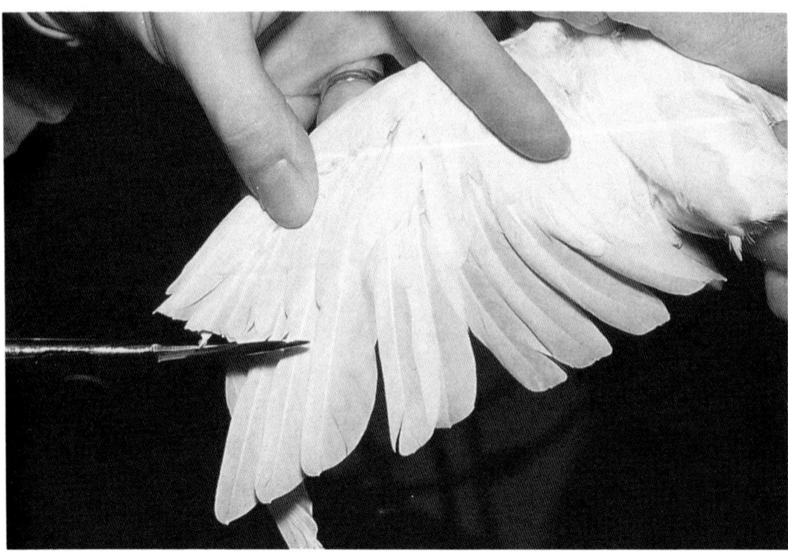

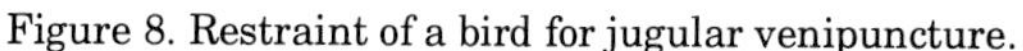
Figure 8. Restraint of a bird for jugular venipuncture.

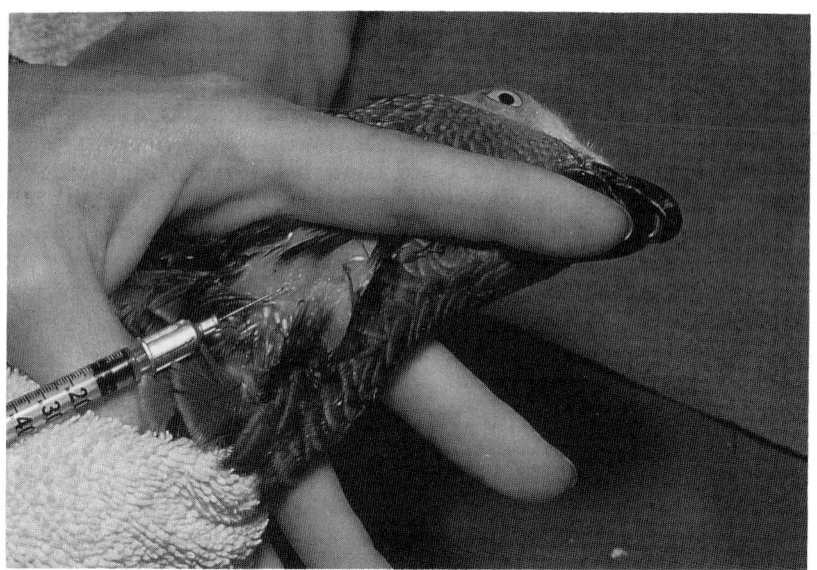

cutaneous ulnar or wing vein, located on the medial side of the wing near the body (Fig 10). The medial metatarsal vein is easily visualized and accessible, especially in larger birds. Wing veins are notorious for developing hematomas but are easy to visualize with a little alcohol applied to the skin. Hematoma formation can be minimized by sliding the overlying skin to one side during collection and letting the skin return to a normal position after sampling, thereby covering the venipuncture site. Because of the small size and low blood flow of these veins, collection can be easier by inserting a needle (unattached to a syringe) into the vein and collecting the blood into a series of capillary tubes as blood flows out of the needle.

Finally, a clipped toenail is sometimes an acceptable sample site. This method is somewhat painful for the patient, however, and is often more time consuming and therefore more stressful. Carefully clean the toe before clipping so as to avoid contamination of the blood sample with urates or other surface particles. Other blood collection methods are preferable in most birds.

Administration of Drugs and Nutrients

Oral Administration: Medication and food are often administered orally to avian patients. It must be remembered that any orally administered substance can be aspirated into the lungs if given too fast or improperly. Food or medication can be given per os (PO) by several methods. First, an eye dropper or similar device may be used to administer small amounts of food or medication to a bird. Hold the bird as described previously, but be sure to keep the bird's beak elevated above a horizontal plane. Administer the medication slowly, allowing the bird to swallow it as it is administered. Many birds try to shake their head or allow the substance to pool in their mouth without swallowing, making it difficult to give an accurate dose. Some pediatric preparations are very palatable, however, and therefore acceptable to birds.

A better way to administer oral substances is by *gavage*. This method involves delivering the substance directly into the bird's crop using a metal gavage tube attached to a syringe (Fig 11). Gavage can also be done with a rubber feeding tube or other device that can be passed directly into the crop.

To pass the tube, restrain the patient as described and pass the tube over the tongue from the bird's left to right (the esophagus is located to the right of the trachea) caudally to the level of the crop near the thoracic inlet. By palpating the patient's neck, 2 tubes should be evident if the gavage tube is in the esophagus (gavage

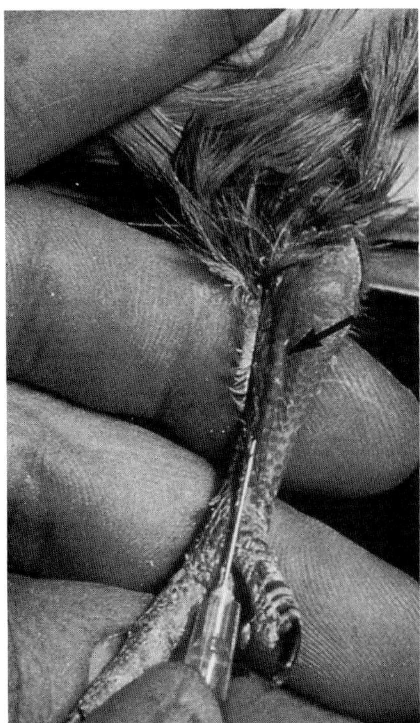

Figure 9. Venipuncture of the medial metatarsal vein of a bird.[11] (Courtesy of WB Saunders)

tube and trachea). After determining proper tube placement, slowly inject the food or medication into the crop. Filling of the crop may be evident as the substance is administered. If a soft rubber tube is used for gavage, a mouth speculum may be necessary to prevent the bird from biting off the tube. A plastic syringe case, a paper clip, or a commercial speculum can be used to protect the

Figure 10. Venipuncture of the wing vein.

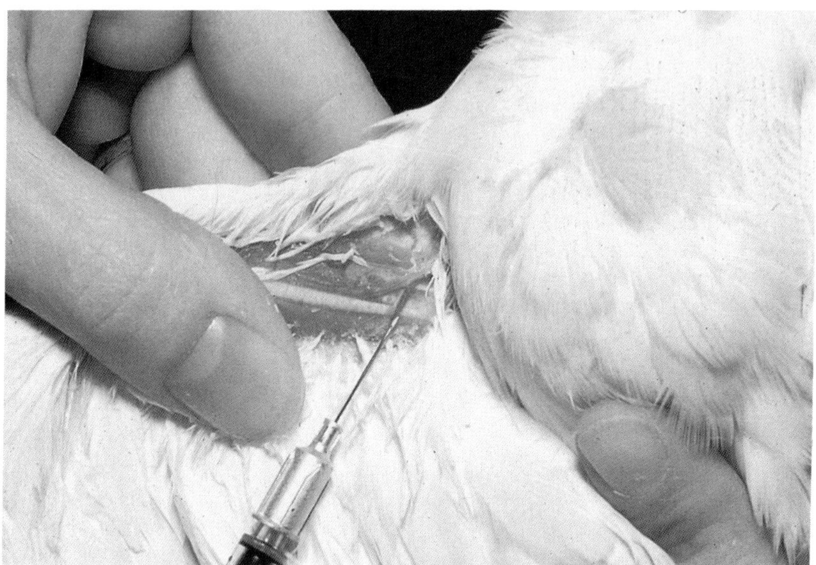

Figure 11. Curved metal gavage tubes are available in various sizes.

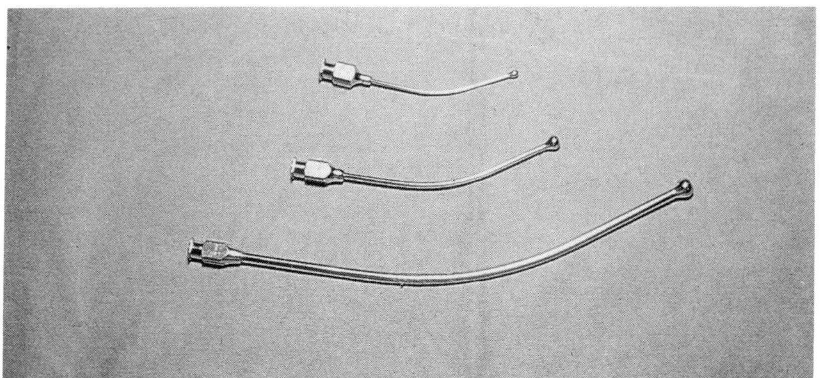

tube or prop open the bird's beak, depending on the size of the patient.

Parenteral Administration: Parenteral injection is the preferred route of drug administration because it is the most exact and effective means of dosing avian patients. The most accessible site of injection is *intramuscularly* (IM) in the pectoral (breast) muscles or, in large birds, the leg muscles.

To locate the pectoral muscles, first palpate the keel, or breast bone, on the ventral side of the patient, just caudal to the thoracic inlet. The large pectoral muscle mass is located on either side of the keel (Fig 12). It is often helpful to first wet the feathers on the ventral chest with alcohol and part them to visualize the keel and adjacent pectoral muscles. Because of the small volumes usually administered to birds, a 25-ga or smaller needle should be used, along with an appropriately sized syringe for the amount injected. Also because of the small volumes and the unlikely possibility of hitting a vein, it is usually not necessary to aspirate the syringe before injection. This omission reduces the amount of time needed to administer the substance, thereby reducing stress on the patient.

Muscle irritation or even necrosis may occur if repeated injections are given in the same muscle or if irritating substances are administered. Alternate sides of the pectoral muscles or alternate legs should be used for a series of injections. Also, because birds

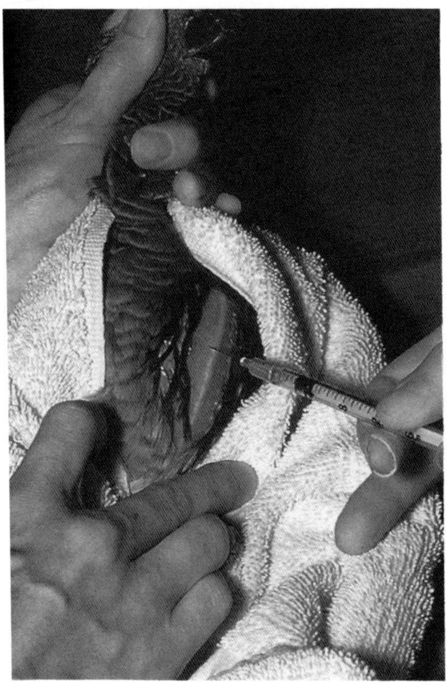

Figure 12. Injection into the pectoral muscles located on either side of the keel bone.

have a renal portal system, nephrotoxic drugs should not be given in the caudal pectoral muscles or legs.

Intravenous (IV) administration of medication is somewhat difficult in avian patients because of the fragility of the veins and the uncooperative nature of most birds. However, bolus IV injection of small amounts of fluid and medication into the jugular vein is very helpful in emergency cases and debilitated patients. The total fluid volume needed for the animal should be calculated and then divided into 3 or 4 bolus injections given over the first 24 hours of treatment.

IV catheter placement is also possible in birds weighing over 100 g. The patient must first be anesthetized (preferably with isoflurane). A small cat-sized rigid or flexible catheter can then be placed in the right jugular vein and taped into place. Most birds tolerate an IV catheter very well, but hospitalization is necessary to monitor the patient.

Subcutaneous (SC) drug and fluid administration is also possible. Because birds have a minimal amount of dermis, however, substances given SC may be poorly absorbed. Small amounts of fluids and medications can be administered SC in the interscapular (Fig 13), axillary or inguinal areas.

Intraosseous fluid administration using the proximal tibial bone is another good method to administer fluids and some medications. The technique is similar to that used in kittens.

Figure 13. Subcutaneous injection in the interscapular area.[11] (Courtesy of WB Saunders)

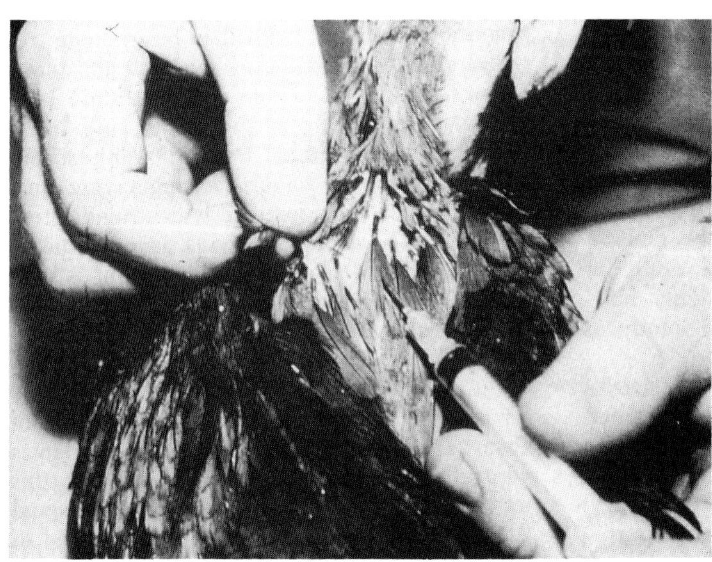

Treatment of Reptiles

Restraint and Handling

Pet reptiles are generally very docile creatures. Though often afraid, they are not usually difficult to handle. An exception is venomous snakes, which should only be handled by experienced reptile handlers with appropriate equipment.

Snakes: Nonvenomous snakes are usually presented to the veterinary clinic in some type of bag or carrier. Owners should be advised to bring their animals in some type of protective container for the safety and health of the snake, as well as the comfort of other clients and pets in the waiting area.

Restraint of snakes involves little more than supporting their head and body. Snakes have only one occipital condyle that supports the skull on the cervical spine. Rough handling or handling the snake, such that most of the body weight is borne by this structure, can occasionally dislocate the skull from the body, causing irreparable damage. Always support snakes gently by the head and neck, with adequate support also given to the body of large snakes (Fig 14).

Lizards: Lizards should be handled with similar concerns as with snakes. However, most lizards can be lifted by holding them caudal to the front legs, and supporting the trunk. A threatened or insecure iguana usually tightens its grip on the surface on which it is resting by latching on with its claws. Carefully detach each foot if this should happen. Also, many lizards try to scamper upward when handled, in an attempt to escape, so be prepared for an active

Figure 14. The head and neck of snakes must be gently supported, with adequate support given to the body of large snakes.

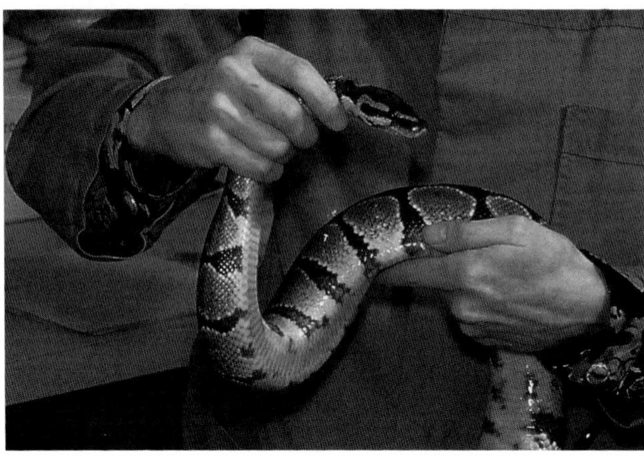

retreat. However, do not drop the animal, but firmly hold the lizard with its legs pinioned until it becomes calm (Fig 15).

Because most lizards have long, sharp toenails, it is wise to either clip these before handling, or wrap the lizard in a towel for protection of the handler. The same care concerning the head and neck must be given to lizards as to snakes.

Some large lizards can also be immobilized by employing the vago-vagal response. This technique produces relaxation for a few minutes without ill effect, though the heart rate and blood pressure are briefly reduced. Place gentle digital pressure on the patient's closed eyes for 15-30 seconds. The calming effect is abolished by loud noises, but can be reinstituted if necessary. Radiography and other short, noninvasive procedures can be done with this technique.

Turtles: Turtles can usually be restrained by holding them gently by the shell. To examine the head, it is often possible to coax them out of the shell by gently squeezing the caudal halves of the shell together. If the turtle's neck must be extended, this can be done using straight ovoid delivery forceps placed gently around the head (avoiding the eyes), with steady gentle traction just enough to overcome the neck's resistance to extension (Fig 16).

Turtles can be prevented from moving around freely by placing them on a pedestal, which prevents their legs from touching the

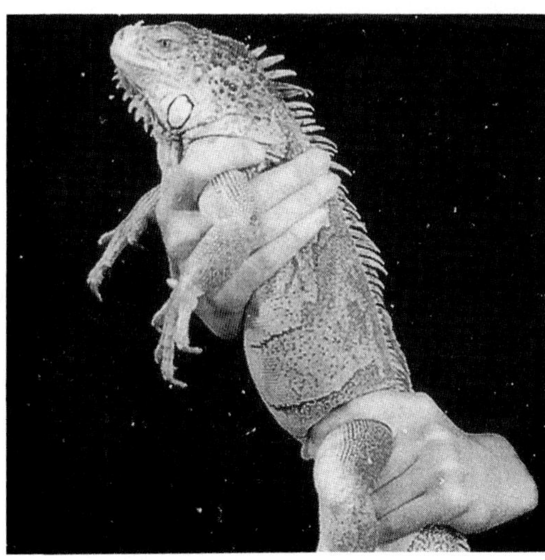

Figure 15. Lizards should be firmly held, with the legs pinioned, until they become calm.[9] (Courtesy of Krieger Publishing)

Figure 16. Extension of a turtle's head with ovoid delivery forceps.[8] (Courtesy of Krieger Publishing)

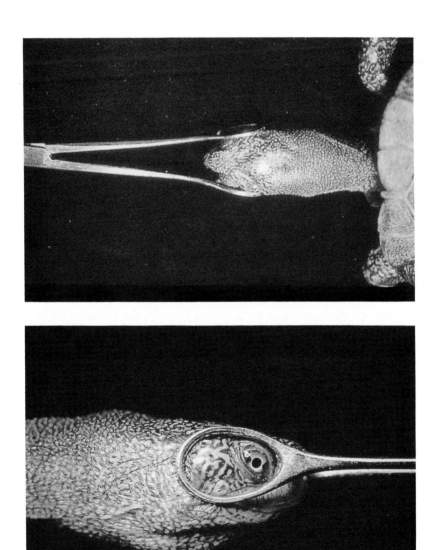

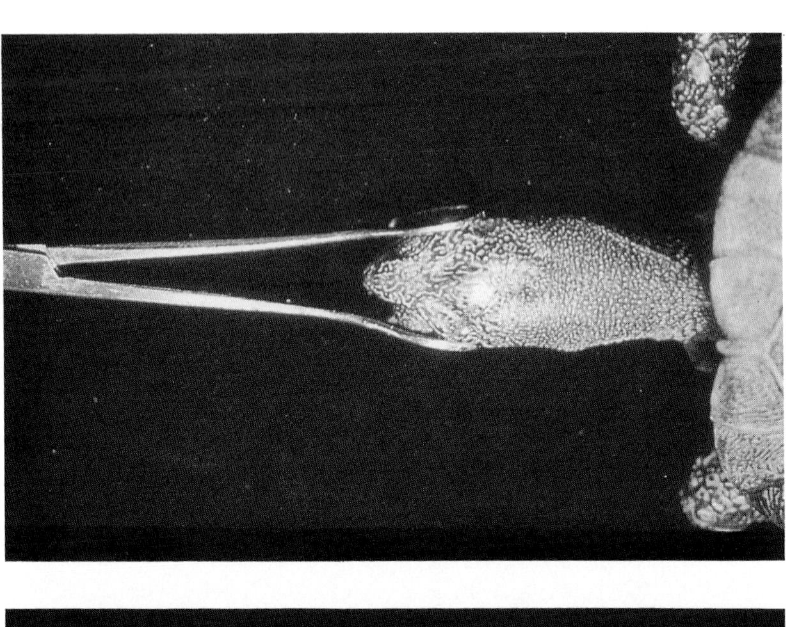

table surface (Fig 17). An inverted flower pot or coffee can may serve this purpose well. The legs can be immobilized by wrapping the entire shell in elastic bandage material.

Blood Collection

Blood can be collected for blood tests from most reptiles, even small patients. The easiest and perhaps safest method of blood collection in snakes and lizards is by direct cardiocentesis (heart puncture) into the large single ventricle.

The apical heartbeat can usually be visualized by placing the patient on its back and shining a light from the side of the body. In snakes, the heart is found one-quarter to one-third of the body length caudal to the head. After aseptic skin preparation, puncture should be done either directly over the apical beat and directed dorsally in a vertical plane, or 1-2 scales caudal to the apical beat and directed craniodorsally at an angle (Fig 18). Enter the body wall between the ventral scales to minimize discomfort to the patient. The same technique can be employed in lizards after visualizing the apical heartbeat. The size of the sample must correspond to the size and condition of the patient as well as the volume blood required for the test; the smallest sample necessary should be taken. It is generally safe to collect up to 1% of a reptile's body weight in grams. For example, 1 ml could be collected from a 100-g snake.

Figure 17. Restraint of a turtle on a pedestal.[8] (Courtesy of Krieger Publishing)

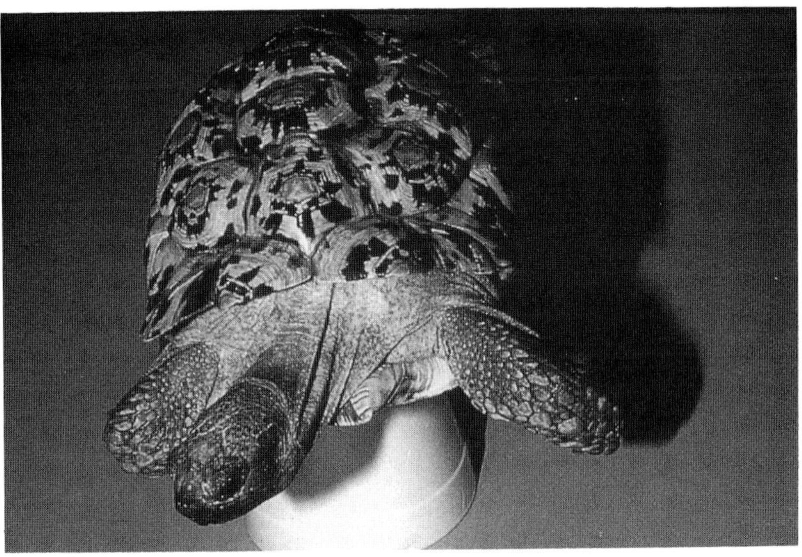

Many reptiles can give larger samples with no ill effect. A smaller volume should be collected from debilitated patients.

The ventral caudal vein may also be a useful venipuncture site in medium-sized to large snakes and lizards. With the patient on its back, direct an appropriately sized needle dorsally in a vertical plane on the midline of the tail. Gently insert the needle until it hits the vertebrae. While applying gentle suction with the syringe barrel, slowly withdraw the needle until blood is visualized in the hub and hold the needle in that position until a sufficient sample is obtained (Fig 19).

Larger turtles can often be sampled from the jugular vein (Fig 20), brachial vein (forelimbs) or popliteal vein (hind limbs). Toenail clipping can also be employed in turtles and lizards. However, nail clipping may not produce a sufficient sample in small patients, and hemostasis after sample collection may be difficult in large patients.

Other blood collection sites in reptiles include the pterygo-palatine-pharyngeal veins in snakes, the occipital sinuses in turtles, and the peribulbar and retrobulbar venous plexi in lizards. The techniques for these sites have been published.[8]

Administration of Drugs and Fluids

Oral Administration: Reptiles can be dosed orally by any of 3 methods. The first involves mixing the medication in the animal's food or, with snakes, injecting it into the prey before the snake eats

Figure 18. Cardiocentesis in a snake. The puncture site is 1-2 scales caudal to the area of the apical beat, with the needle directed craniodorsally at a slight angle.

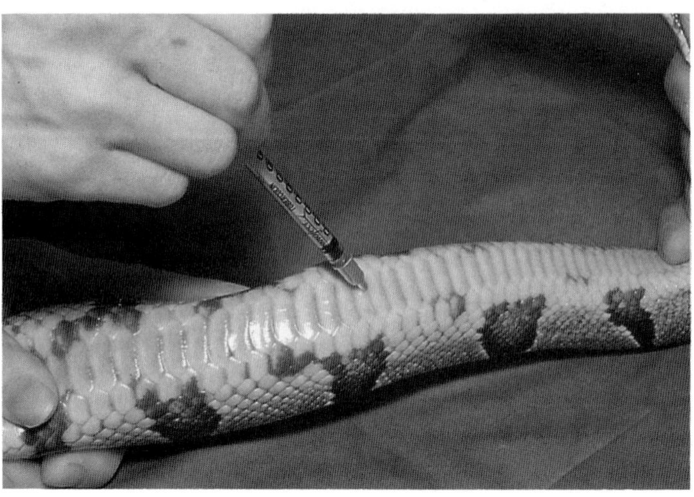

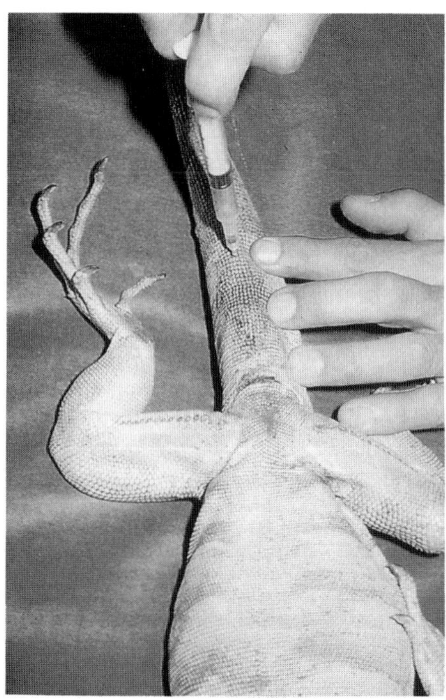

Figure 19. Venipuncture of the ventral caudal vein of a lizard.[8] (Courtesy of Krieger Publishing)

Figure 20. Venipuncture in a turtle.

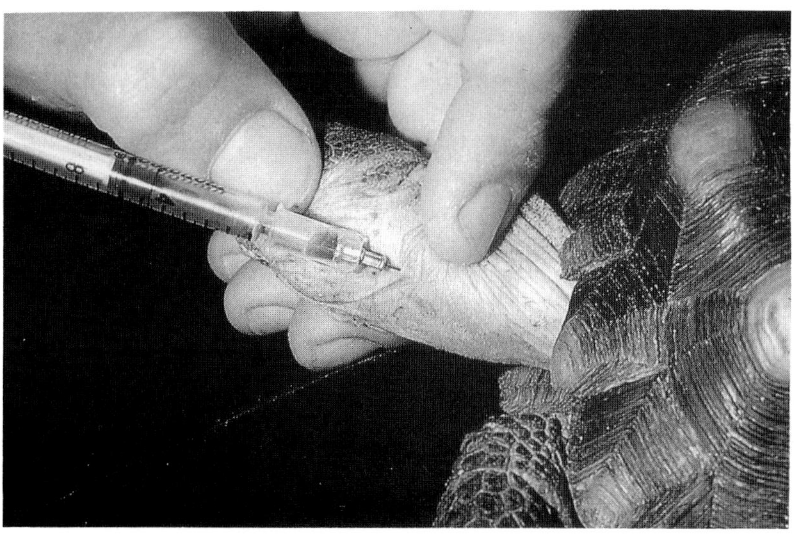

it. Some patients will not eat this altered food in sufficient quantities to obtain therapeutic levels of medication, however.

The second method is dosing by stomach tube. A red rubber feeding tube can be used for this purpose. However, cooperation of the patient and the resulting stress may limit the usefulness of this technique. Finally, topical application of certain antibiotics directly to the oral mucosa is occasionally used to treat lesions in the oral cavity.

Parenteral Administration: Veins are often difficult to access in reptiles, so parenteral therapy is usually accomplished by either intramuscular or subcutaneous injection. Intramuscular injections can be given into the epaxial muscles adjacent to the spine, or in the muscles of the forelimbs in larger lizards and most turtles. Subcutaneous injections can also be given in reptiles as in mammals. Reptiles often have less loose skin than mammals, however, so smaller volumes must be used. Subcutaneous injections of physiologic fluids may be administered into the lateral sinus of snakes, located at the junction of the epaxial muscles and the ribs. The lateral sinus is located along the entire length of the body (Fig 21). It is important to avoid injections of nephrotoxic drugs in the caudal limbs or caudal half of the body of reptiles because of their renal portal vascular system.

Figure 21. Injection into the lateral sinus of a snake.[8] The lateral sinus is located at the junction of the epaxial muscles and the ribs, and courses along the entire length of the snake. (Courtesy of Krieger Publishing)

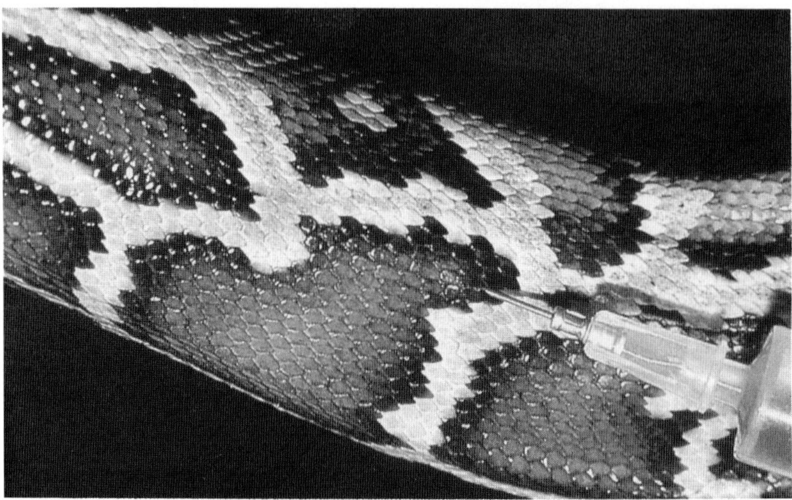

Treatment of Small Mammals

Rabbits

Rabbits are generally easily handled. They rarely bite, but their long toenails can scratch an unwary handler. Rabbits also have powerful rear legs, which they often kick forcefully when frightened while restrained. It is even possible for a rabbit to fracture its back as a consequence of these kicks. Therefore, it is important to support a rabbit's rear legs during restraint.

To lift a rabbit, grasp the skin over the dorsal neck (similar to scruffing a cat) while supporting the hindquarters with the other hand (Fig 22). Always point the rabbit's feet away from yourself to avoid being scratched. Rabbits can be carried short distances by supporting them sternally on your forearm, with the rabbit's head in the bend of your elbow (Fig 23). For transport over longer distances, the rabbit should be placed in some type of carrier, such as a cat carrier.

Rabbits can be restrained for examination by manipulating the rabbit on a mat or towel while supporting both the neck and hindquarters. Rabbits may become very nervous on a smooth surface, such as an exam table, and struggle to find stable footing. It may even be helpful to wrap the rabbit in the towel or place it in a cat bag to calm the rabbit and minimize struggling.

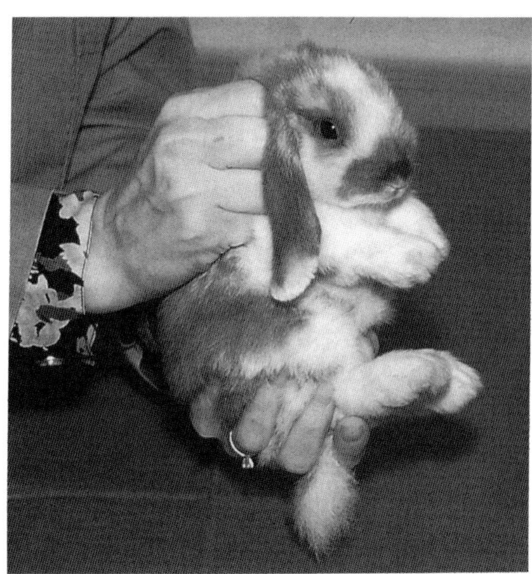

Figure 22. To lift a rabbit, grasp the skin over the dorsal aspect of the neck while supporting the hindquarters with the other hand.

When releasing a rabbit, always place the hind legs down first while retaining a grip on its neck. The rabbit may try to jump away when its rear feet are placed on a surface, so you must maintain control until the rabbit has calmed.

Blood is usually collected from rabbits via the prominent vessels in the pinna (Fig 24). The artery in the center of the dorsal pinna or the vein at the margin of the pinna can be used for this purpose. Simply wet the area with alcohol and occlude the vessel with digital pressure applied near the base of the pinna for the vein, or near the distal tip of the pinna for the artery. Some hair can aso be plucked or shaved over the puncture site to more easily visualize the vessel. If the vessel is difficult to visualize, anesthetizing the rabbit with isoflurane given by mask often causes the vein to become more prominent.

The vessels of the pinna can also be used for catheterization to provide a route for IV administration of medications or fluids. IV injection without a catheter can sometimes lead to sloughing of the skin of the pinna.

Rabbits can be force fed by one of several methods. First, a curve-tipped syringe can be used to inject food into the interdental space (the cheek pouches can hold a large amount of food). Cut the syringe tip to half its original size and then aim it toward the back of the mouth and deposit the food slowly.

The second method involves using a flexible feeding tube passed into the stomach. It is a good idea to use a mouth speculum of some kind to prevent the tube from being severed by the patient. A syringe casing with a hole drilled through it works well. Also, be

Figure 23. Rabbits can be carried short distances by supporting them on your forearm, with the rabbit's head nestled in the bend of your elbow.

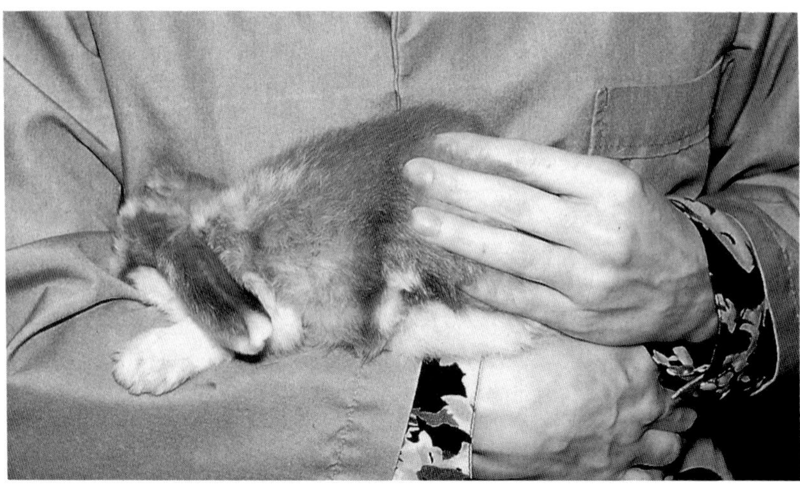

Figure 24. Puncture of the central artery of a rabbit's pinna.

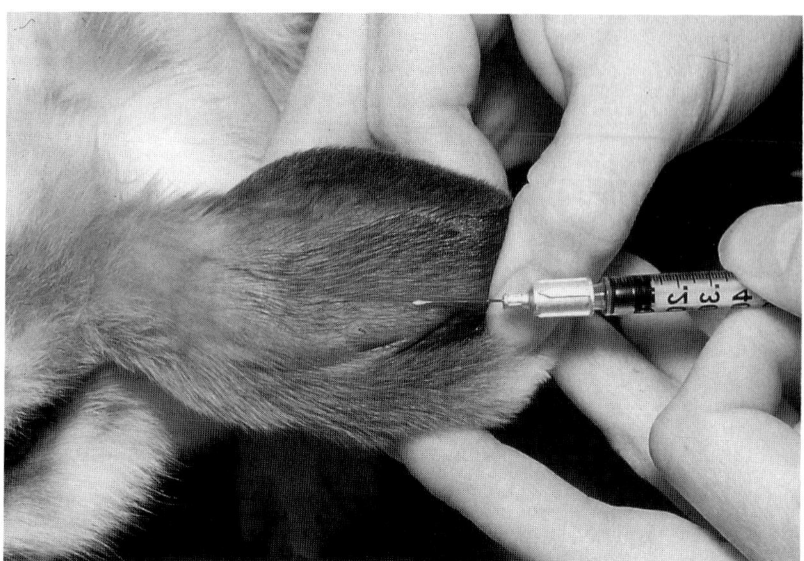

aware that the stomach wall of rabbits is thin and can be penetrated easily. Pediatric-sized nasogastric tubes can also be used in rabbits.

Injections and medications may also be given by other routes (SC, IM, PO) as in cats and dogs.

Ferrets

Ferrets are usually gentle animals, but they occasionally bite. Young ferrets can be a bit more prone to this, so a firmer hand may be indicated when restraining them. A spray bottle containing a bitter substance is often enough to induce a ferret to detach its mouth if a bite does occur.

In most respects, ferrets can be restrained much like cats. Grasping the scruff of the neck is often very effective to control movement. Additionally, if a ferret is grasped by the scruff and suspended over the exam table, some gentle stroking of the abdomen may help to relax the patient for routine examination, injections and grooming procedures. (Fig 25). Some young ferrets may resist this method of restraint and require another restraint technique.

Additional restraint techniques involve holding the patient on its back, with the back of the ferret's head in the palm of one hand and the body tucked under your arm and along your side. This restraint is useful for examining the patient's mouth or giving oral medications. Holding the ferret on its side, with one hand around the neck and the other hand around the caudal abdomen just cranial to the rear legs, serves to immobilize an uncooperative patient during injections.

Blood collection sites are generally similar to those of other mammals, and include the cephalic vein, the jugular vein, and the tail artery. Inexperienced ferret handlers should first sedate or anesthetize the patient before attempting blood collection. This not only makes blood collection easier by eliminating struggling, but it also causes less stress to the patient. Anesthesia also makes visualization of these veins easier. Isoflurane by mask is the agent of choice for short procedures.

Manual restraint may be augmented by wrapping the ferret's body in a towel. This also helps to protect the handler's clothes, as ferrets will often eliminate when restrained tightly. Many ferrets struggle fiercely for a short time when first restrained, and then become very calm. A good distraction technique is to offer the patient a little Nutrical on a tongue depressor during the restraint procedure.

Except for jugular venipuncture, a 25-ga needle attached to a 1-ml syringe should be the largest sizes used so as to avoid collapsing the vein. The needle can also be positioned in the vein without a sy-

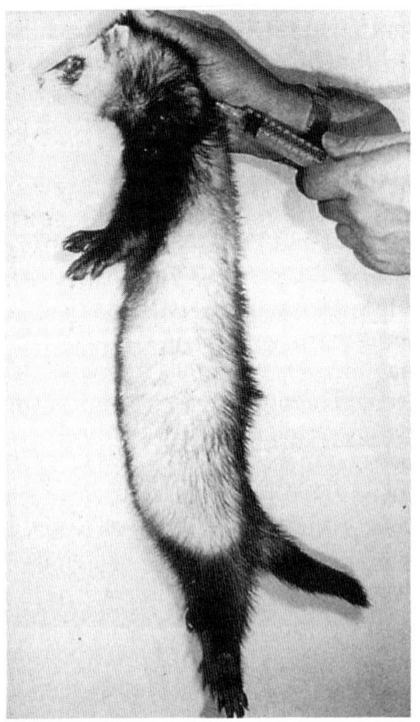

Figure 25. Ferret restrained by suspending it by the scruff.[7] (Courtesy of Lea & Febiger)

ringe. The blood sample is then allowed to drip directly into a collection tube or can be caught in microhematocrit tubes.

The technique for cephalic and jugular venipuncture is identical to that used in cats, with the added challenge of more difficult restraint on an unsedated animal. Because a ferret's front leg is very short, once blood is aspirated into the syringe from the cephalic vein, the tourniquet should be released to allow for adequate sample collection. If properly done, up to 1 ml of blood can be collected from this site, while larger amounts can be obtained from the jugular.

Intravenous catheter placement is possible in ferrets. The jugular, cephalic or lateral saphenous veins may accommodate short small-gauge catheters. Ferret skin is fairly thick, so it is sometimes necessary to first "nick" the skin with a sharp needle. Also, flushing the catheter while threading it into the vein may facilitate correct placement. Intraosseous catheter placement in the femur is also useful in some ferrets. The technique is similar to that used in kittens.

Medication and injections are given as for larger mammals. Ferrets often willingly accept pills and capsules if these are first coated with Nutrical, Laxatone or butter.

Hamsters, Gerbils, Mice, Rats and Guinea Pigs

Rodents, or so-called "pocket pets," are usually easily handled if restrained gently but firmly. Hamsters are nocturnal in nature and often bite if disturbed from sleep; however, the other species are generally quite tame.

Gerbils, rats and mice can be lifted by the base of the tail (Fig 26). This grip should only be maintained for enough time to grasp the animal in a better hold. If the tail is grasped too far caudally or for long periods, the skin may strip off the tail.

After lifting a gerbil by the base of the tail, cradle the animal in the palm of your hand with the index and middle finger around the neck (Fig 27). The haircoat of gerbils is slick and they often try to jump out of the handler's grasp, so be ready for quick movements.

Mice can be restrained by grasping the skin over the neck and back while keeping a gentle grasp on the tail base. It is sometimes helpful to place the mouse on a nonskid surface after grasping the tail to facilitate scruffing. Then the mouse can be inverted and the tail released to allow for examination or treatment of the patient (Figs 28, 29).

Rats may be restrained by grasping them gently but firmly around the back and ribs, just caudal to the forelegs. At the same time, wrapping the thumb and index finger around the neck provides additional restraint of the head (Fig 30). Rats also should be handled by the tail only for short periods and only at the base so as to prevent the skin from tearing away. Caution should be used when lifting a rat out of a wire-bottom cage by the tail, as they

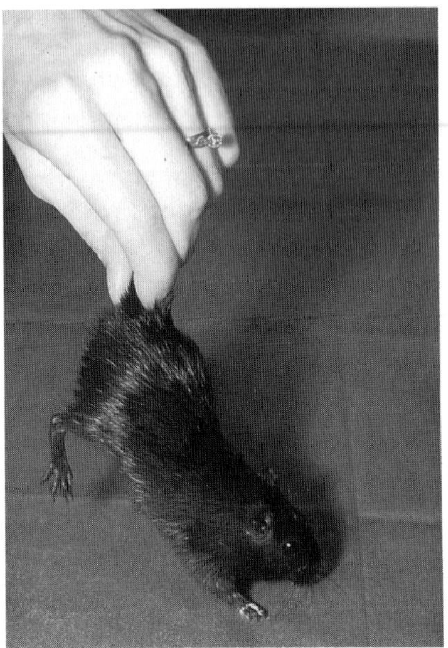

Figure 26. Gerbils, rats and mice can be lifted by the base of the tail.

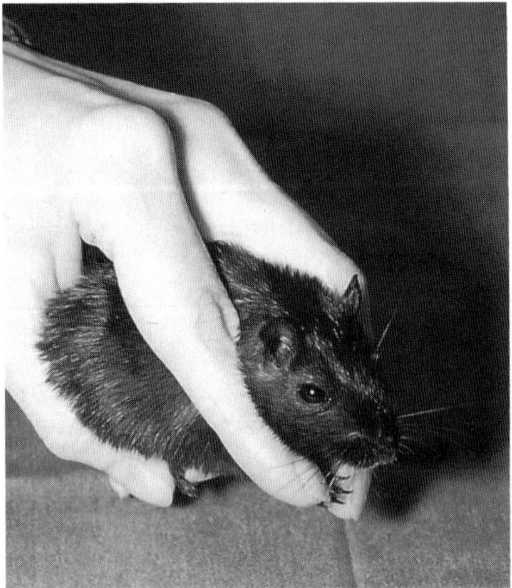

Figure 27. Restraint of a gerbil.

often grasp the wire and you can inadvertently injure its foot or tear the tail skin. Instead, lift the rat from beneath its body.

Hamsters should be first wakened from sleep before handling so as to prevent startling them and decreasing the chance of a bite.

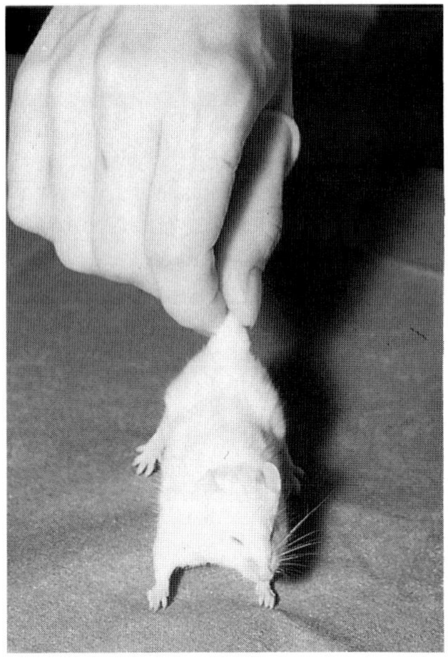

Figure 28. A mouse's tail is gently grasped as it clings to a nonskid surface.

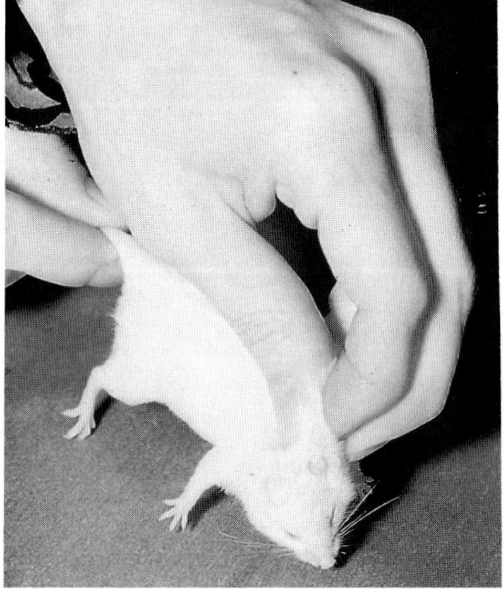

Figure 29. The mouse is grasped by the scruff as the tail is held.

They are also more likely to bite if handled roughly, frightened or injured. Use caution when dealing with hamsters under these conditions. To lift a hamster, grasp the scruff of the neck as with a cat. Grasp as much skin as possible to prevent the patient from turning its head to bite. It is more difficult to scruff a hamster with full cheek pouches. In such cases, try to coax the rodent into a small can or empty syringe case to lift it out of the cage. Tame hamsters can be cupped in the palm of both hands for restraint (Figs 31, 32).

Guinea pigs should be lifted by sliding one hand under the torso near the front legs and supporting the hindquarters with the other hand (Figs 33, 34). This hind-end support is especially important for large adult and pregnant females. The pig may be held ventral side up (dorsal recumbency) for examination if cradled in 2 hands, with one hand supporting the rear end to prevent struggling.

Blood collection can be challenging in small rodents. Blood samples of sufficient volume to run laboratory tests are difficult to obtain from mice, hamsters and gerbils. The most common sample sites include the retroorbital venous plexus and the tail vein or artery. The retroorbital sinus of rodents has a venous plexus that can be punctured for blood collection. Inexperienced handlers should first anesthetize the patient. Then insert a capillary tube at the medial canthus of the eye in a caudomedial direction. Rotation of the capillary tube within the sinus breaks the capillaries and blood flows into the tube (Fig 35). Though complications may include eye trauma, harderian-gland lesions and nasal hemorrhage, the procedure is minimally traumatic to most patients.

Figure 30. Rats can be restrained by grasping them gently but firmly around the back and chest, just caudal to the forelegs.

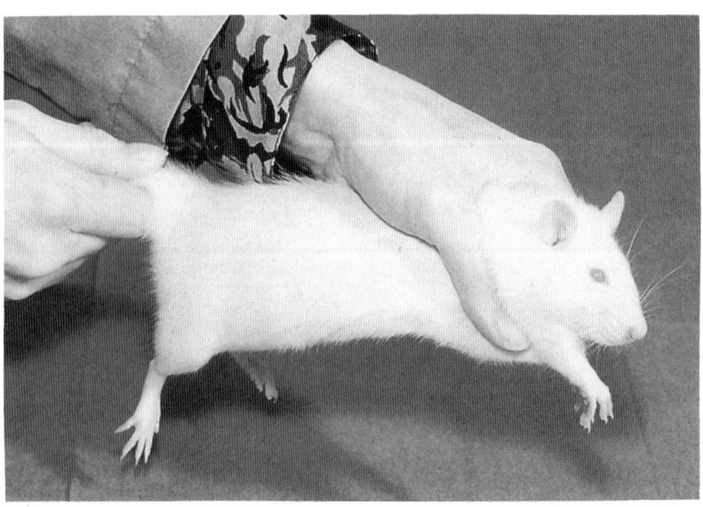

The ventral tail artery is located on the ventral midline of the tail. Two tail veins can be visualized on the lateral surfaces. All of

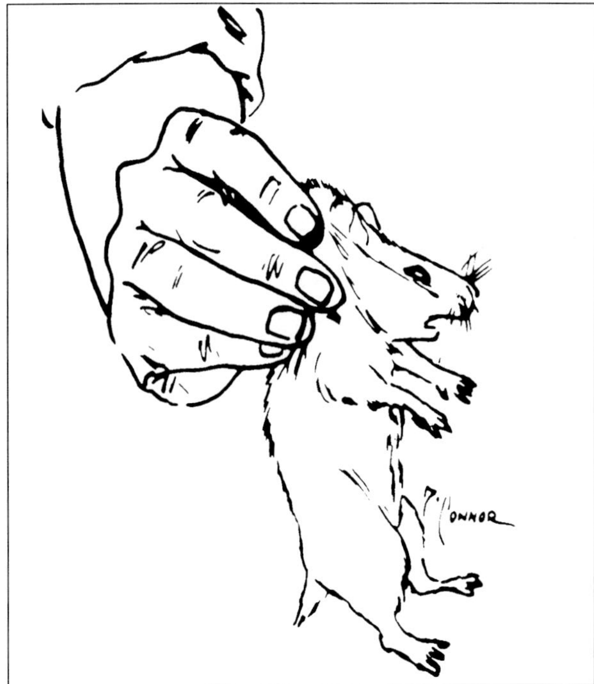

Figure 31. Restraint of a hamster.[10] (Courtesy of Iowa State University Press)

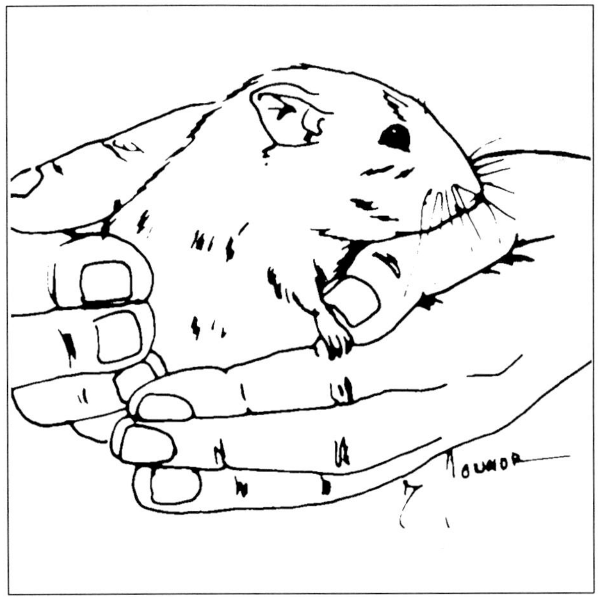

Figure 32. Restraint of a hamster.[10] (Courtesy of Iowa State University Press)

these vessels run the entire length of the tail and may be used for blood collection (Fig 36). The patient must either be placed in a restraint chamber or given anesthesia as necessary. To access the vessel, a 25-ga needle attached to a small syringe can be used,

33. Restraint of a guinea pig.

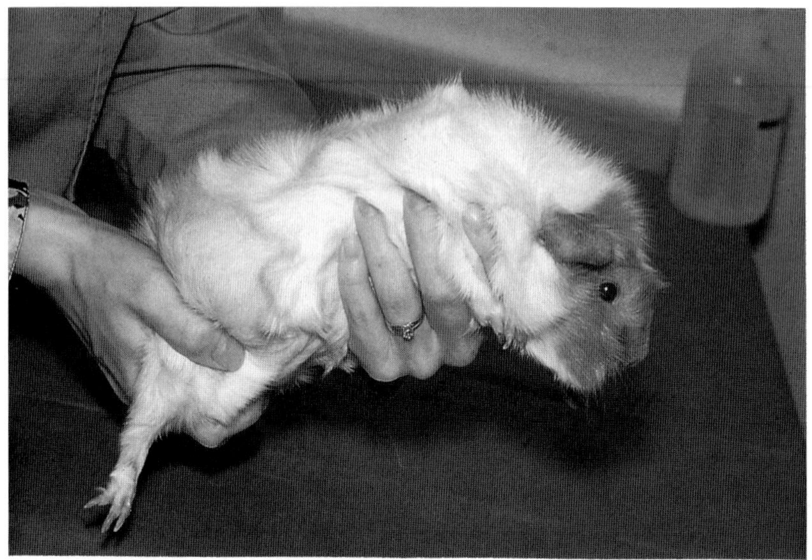

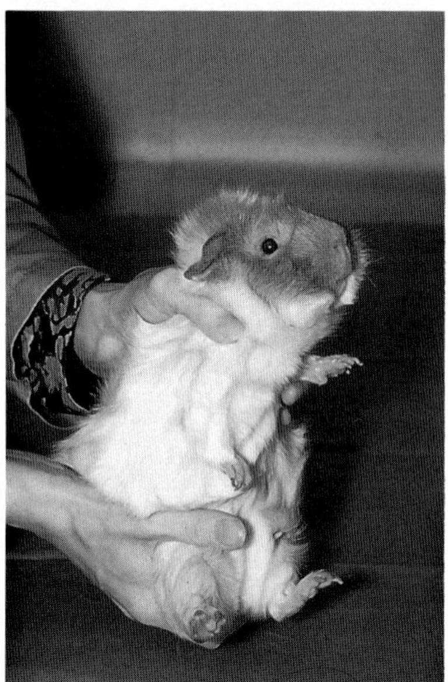

Figure 34. Restraint of a guinea pig.

though a 26- or 28-ga needle may be more effective in the smaller species.

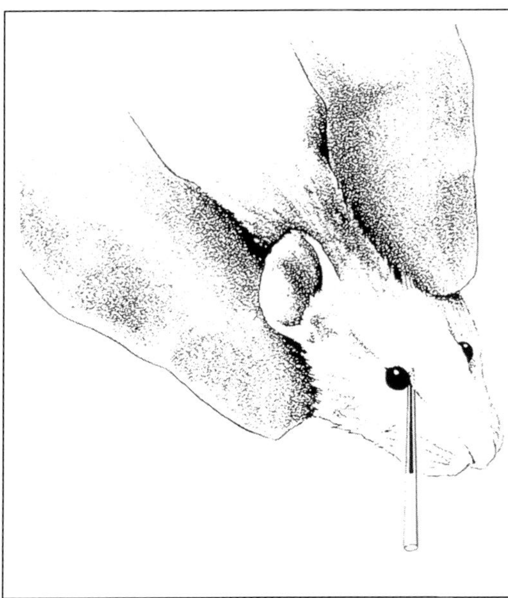

Figure 35. Blood collection from the retroorbital sinus of an anesthetized rodent.[1] With the head secured between the thumb and forefinger, insert a capillary tube at the medial edge of the globe and direct the tip of the tube toward the back of the eye socket. Carefully rotate the tube to puncture the blood sinus. Blood fills the tube by capillary action. (Courtesy of American Association for Laboratory Animal Science)

Figure 36. Blood collection from the tail vessels of rodents.

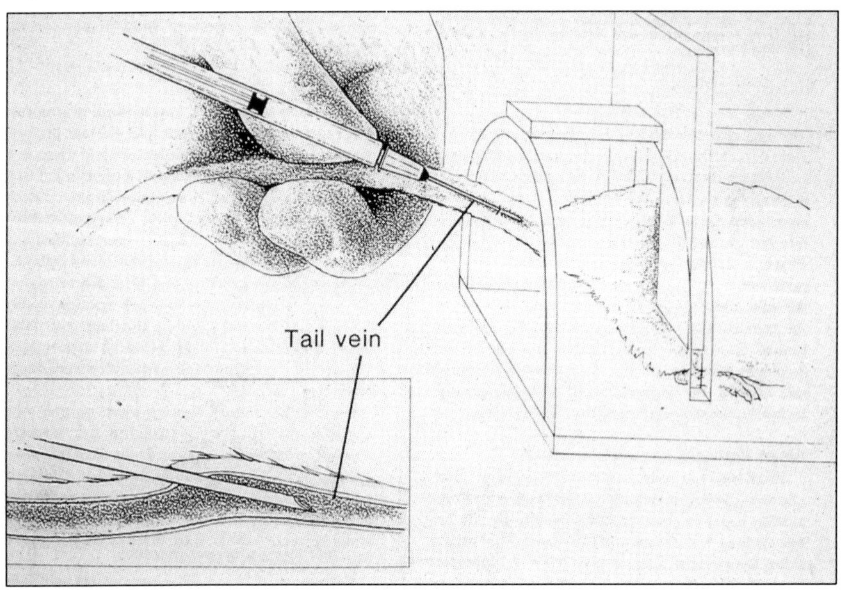

When using the ventral tail artery, the plunger of the syringe can be removed before puncture and blood pressure alone will often fill the syringe. The tail vessels can also be nicked with a needle and the blood collected directly into a capillary tube or other collection device. First immersing the tail in warm water may enhance blood flow.

To locate the ventral artery, direct the needle, bevel up, at about a 30-degree angle into the tail on the ventral midline until the needle strikes a coccygeal vertebra. Apply some gentle suction on the plunger and very slowly retract the needle until blood flows into the syringe.

References

1. *AALAS Training Manual Series.* Am Assn Lab Anim Sci, Cordova, TN, 1990.

2. Brown S: Husbandry, handling, diagnostic procedures for rabbits and rodents. *Proc Ann Mtg AAHA,* 1993. pp 52-54.

3. Brown S: Ferret practice tips. *Proc Eastern States Vet Conf,* 1989. pp 255-256.

4. Campbell TW: *Vet Clin No Am* (Small Anim Pract) 14:223-226, 1984.

5. Erdman SE: Venipuncture in the ferret. *Proc North Am Vet Conf,* 1993. p 733.

6. Fowler ME: *Restraint and Handling of Wild and Domestic Animals.* Iowa State Univ Press, Ames, 1978.

7. Fox JG: *Biology and Diseases of the Ferret.* Lea & Febiger, Philadelphia, 1988.

8. Frye F: *Biomedical and Surgical Aspects of Captive Reptile Husbandry.* 2nd ed. Krieger Publishing, Malabar, FL, 1991.

9. Frye F: *Iguanas: A Guide to Their Biology and Captive Care.* Krieger Publishing, Malabar, FL, 1993.

10. Harkness JE and Wagner JE: *The Biology and Medicine of Rabbits and Rodents.* Lea & Febiger, Philadelphia, 1989.

11. Harrison GJ and Harrison LR: *Clinical Avian Medicine and Surgery.* Saunders, Philadelphia, 1986.

12. Jenkins J: Treating rabbits and rodents: there is an easier way. *Proc Eastern States Vet Conf,* 1990. pp 276-277.

13. Sonsthagen T: *Restraint of Domestic Animals.* American Veterinary Publications, Goleta, CA, 1991.

Notes

6

Treatment Techniques for Horses

A.M. Lamar

The continuing development of new drugs and drug vehicles has changed and will continue to change the methods by which horses are treated. But even with these changes, basic treatment techniques remain essentially the same. This chapter describes several methods to give oral, parenteral and topical medication, to collect blood and urine specimens, and to apply many types of bandages.

Giving Medication

Oral Administration

Per os (PO) and oral are terms used to indicate administration of medication via the mouth. This is the most convenient and least painful method of giving medication. However, it has some disadvantages.

The effectiveness of oral medication depends on how well the drug is absorbed from the stomach or intestines. Absorption is much slower than with parenteral use (injection). It is also difficult to ensure that all of the medication has been swallowed, even when the most adept person administers the treatment. Despite these drawbacks, the oral route is used frequently by veterinary personnel and horse owners.

Several types of medication can be given PO. Anthelmintics (deworming medication) are available in various forms, such as powder, granules, liquid and paste, and are approved for use in feed or as a drench. Antiinflammatory drugs, such as phenylbutazone and flunixin meglumine (Banamine: Schering) can be given as powder or granules in the feed, tablets by bolus, crushed tablets in a palatable medium, or pastes. Antibiotics are marketed in tablet, capsule, liquid and paste forms. Oral tranquilizers may be given with grain. Electrolytes may be given as an additive to drinking water. Animals that do not tolerate injections or gastric intubation (stomach tubing) or those treated by their owners can be medicated PO.

Oral medications may be given in several ways. The least reliable method is addition of the medication to the grain or drinking water. Many horses taste the additives and totally refuse to eat or drink or, if the medication is in the grain, may pick out the grain and leave the drug, particularly if the grain and drug do not mix well.

Years ago, the balling gun was commonly used (Fig 1). It is still used for administering tablets or boluses but can cause problems. If the tablet or bolus is dry, it may become lodged in the esophagus. If the drug in the bolus is irritating, it may erode through the pharyngeal or esophageal mucosa. Tablets or boluses given by balling gun should be lubricated well and placed as far back in the mouth as possible. The patient must be watched carefully after adminis-

Figure 1. Oral medication devices. *Top:* 12-oz dose syringe with an 8-inch tip. *Middle:* 2-oz plastic catheter-tipped syringe. *Bottom:* balling gun.

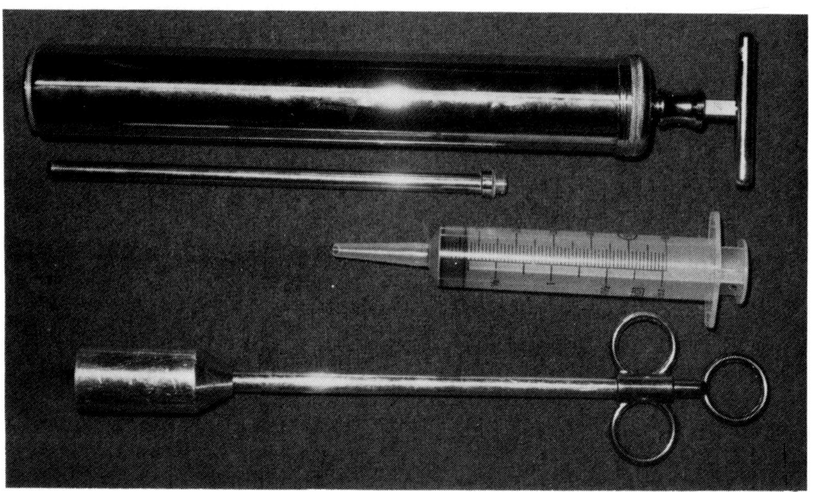

tration, as the medication may be dropped from the mouth if it is not deposited near the back of the tongue. The swallowing reflex can be stimulated by gently rubbing the roof of the mouth with the balling gun or allowing the horse to eat a small amount of grain after the tablet has been given.

Dose syringes are another common means of giving oral medication (Fig 1). They may be obtained as stainless-steel syringes in various sizes (2-, 6- and 12-oz), with tips of different lengths (4- and 8-inch), or as catheter-tipped, plastic syringes (2-oz). Care must be taken when using the plastic variety, as they can be easily crushed by the horse's teeth. Premixed liquid medication and powders or crushed tablets mixed with molasses or syrup may be given by dose syringe. Water should not be used to dissolve oral medication because the resultant solution is too thin; a gruel or paste-like consistency is best.

To properly use a dose syringe, stand at the horse's head, holding the halter with one hand, and introduce the syringe at the buccal commissure (corner of the mouth) with the opposite hand (Fig 2). Advance the syringe as far back on the tongue as possible, avoiding the cheek teeth. Discharge the medication slowly, allowing the horse to swallow while the drug is being given. If the horse does not swallow on its own, rubbing the tongue or the roof of the mouth with the tip of the syringe often stimulates swallowing. Elevating

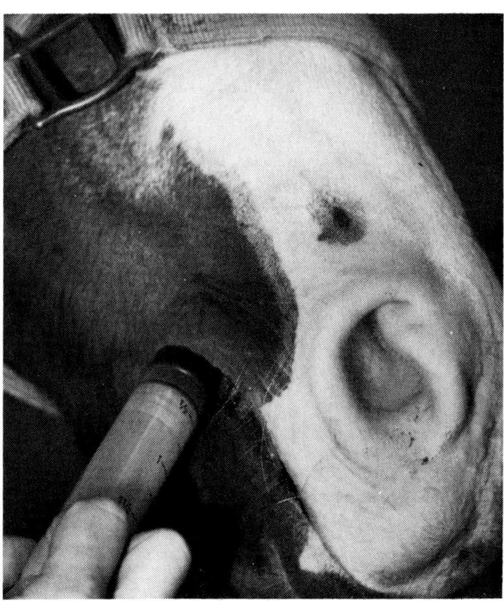

Figure 2. Use of dose syringe. Introduce the syringe at the buccal commissure, avoiding the check teeth. Inject slowly, allowing the horse to swallow frequently during administration.

the horse's head slightly also helps prevent the medication from trickling out of the mouth. If the head is held too high, however, some of the medication may be aspirated into the trachea, which could result in pneumonitis. Using drugs in paste form has helped resolve this problem. By thickening the consistency of the medication, the chance of aspiration is reduced and more of the drug is retained and swallowed.

Most horses do not object to this method, but some form of restraint may be necessary on those that do.

Nasogastric Intubation

Nasogastric intubation ("tubing") is used to deposit medication, fluids or nutrients directly into the stomach. It is more effective than the balling gun or dose syringe. Many horses object to this method of treatment; however, with proper restraint, medication can be given without difficulty. Though "tubing" horses requires extensive practice and entails the danger of nasal, pharyngeal and esophageal trauma and inadvertent tracheal intubation, nasogastric intubation is commonly used to give anthelmintics, lubricants, astringents, fluids and nutrients to horses.

Selection of a tube of proper diameter is the first step in nasogastric intubation. Tubes of varying diameter are available, from very small-diameter tubes for foals to very large-diameter tubes for draft horses. The length is generally the same despite the tube's diameter. If the tube is too small, it passes too easily, making it difficult to determine its location. If it is too large, it traumatizes the nasal turbinates and may cause epistaxis (nosebleed). An average 1000-lb horse requires a medium-sized tube (5/8-inch outside diameter).

Restraint is extremely important during nasogastric intubation. It is very difficult to pass a nasogastric tube if the horse is continually moving about. The nasal turbinates may also be damaged if the horse tosses its head while the tube is in the nasal cavity. If the horse is to be "tubed" in a stall, both restraint and intubation should be applied from the same side to decrease the possibility of injury to everyone involved. When using treatment stocks, restraint may be applied from either side during intubation. Generally, a lip twitch is sufficient restraint. If this is inadequate, tranquilization may be indicated.

Before intubation, the tube should be warmed in a bucket of clean, warm water to make it pliable. A water-soluble lubricant, such as water or K-Y Jelly (Johnson & Johnson), should be applied to facilitate tube passage. The tube may be inserted into either nostril; technicians should be able to pass the tube from both sides. If standing on the left side of the horse, loop the tube over the left arm and place the palm of the right hand over the bridge of the horse's nose, with the thumb inserted into the nostril (left hand if standing on the right side), making certain the fingers do not occlude the opposite nostril (Fig 3). When holding the horse in this manner, lateral movement of the head can be controlled, the neck can be flexed, and the tube can be easily directed into the ventral meatus of the nasal cavity.

Insert the tube into the nostril with the left hand and advance it slowly and gently, at the same time pushing down on the tube with the thumb of the right hand. In an average horse, the tube should proceed about 12 inches caudad before it stops at the dorsal pharyngeal wall. If the tube stops before this, it may be in the middle meatus. If this is the case, the procedure should be repeated and the tube directed ventrad into the ventral meatus. When the tube stops at the pharynx, gentle movement back and forth should stimulate the swallowing reflex. If this does not occur, slowly rotating or blowing into the tube may cause the animal to swallow. Throughout this portion of the procedure, the throat region should be observed. When the horse swallows, the tube should be advanced 4-6 inches. Once the tube is in the esophagus, passage of

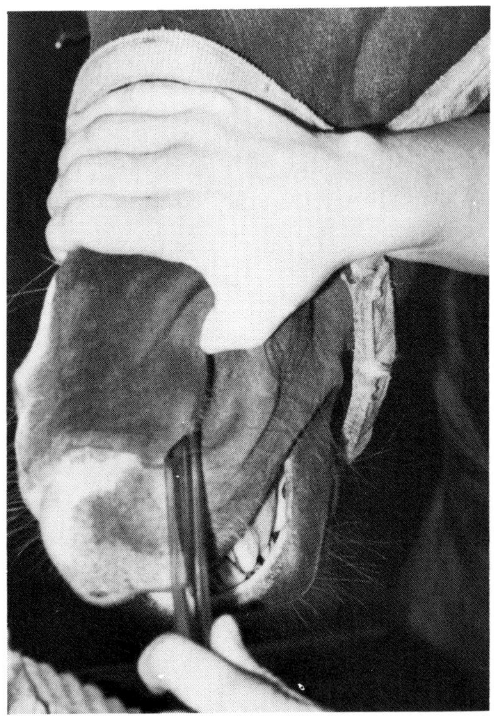

Figure 3. Passing a nasogastric tube. Place the palm of the hand over the bridge of the horse's nose, insert the thumb into the animal's nostril, and advance the tube under the thumb with the opposite hand.

the tube may be enhanced by gently blowing into the tube to dilate the muscular wall of the esophagus as the tube passes caudad.

Throughout this procedure there are numerous ways to ensure that the tube is in the correct location. As mentioned previously, if caudal progression of the tube ceases before it is inserted to about 12 inches, it is more than likely in the middle meatus. Force applied at this point often produces epistaxis.

When the tube reaches the pharynx, it can enter either the esophagus or the trachea. If it enters the trachea, most horses cough; however, this is not a reliable indicator as to the location of the tube because horses with pharyngitis may cough even if the tube is in the esophagus. Also, if the tube is in the trachea instead of the esophagus, it advances very easily because of the open structure of the trachea as compared with the collapsed state of the esophagus. (Overly small tubes also pass easily in the esophagus.) Occasionally, the tube may rattle against the sides of the trachea, which indicates its location. This is determined by shaking the trachea at the ventral aspect of the neck with one hand. If respiration can be heard or felt through the nasogastric tube, it is definitely in the trachea and should be withdrawn and the procedure repeated.

If the tube passes into the esophagus as desired, the first thing observed is the amount of pressure required to advance the tube. The esophagus is a muscular structure that remains closed, except when an object is moving through it. For this reason, the tube is much easier to advance when air is gently blown ahead of the advancing tube. Another sign of correct tube placement is visualization of the tube passing through the esophagus. This may be observed in most horses over the left side of the neck, near the jugular furrow. In some horses, however, the esophagus may be located on the right side of the neck.

It is important not to confuse passage of the tube with the jugular pulse, which is present in many horses. By slowly advancing and withdrawing the tube while applying manual pressure over the area, the tube may be felt and its presence in the esophagus confirmed. In horses with a very thick neck, the tube may not be seen at all. Two distinct tubular structures, *ie,* the esophagus with the tube in place and the trachea, may be felt in horses with a very thin neck. These cannot be discerned in most horses, however.

The final sign observed when passing a nasogastric tube occurs when it enters the stomach. Gurgling sounds are heard in most horses and are often accompanied by a distinct gastric odor. Administration of medication must not proceed until the tube is, without a doubt, in the stomach.

When the tube is in the stomach, the liquid medication may be administered with a stomach pump, dose syringe or funnel. After the medication has been given, give 12 oz of water, then gently blow through the tube to force most of this fluid into the stomach. Before withdrawing the tube, cap the end with your thumb or kink it to prevent material remaining in the tube from leaking out as the tube is pulled out past the trachea. Such leakage may cause aspiration, with subsequent pneumonitis. The head should be held very still as the tube is removed so as to prevent the end of the tube from striking the turbinates and causing hemorrhage.

One complication that may result from nasogastric intubation, no matter how carefully performed, is epistaxis. If this occurs, the patient should be kept quiet until the hemorrhage ceases (usually in 10-20 minutes). Towels held over the nostril absorb the blood, but some horses may resist this and hemorrhage even more. Because only a very small amount of blood is usually lost through intubation-related epistaxis, there is no great cause for alarm.

Intradermal Injection

The intradermal (ID) route of administration involves injection of a small quantity of medication into the dermis, the skin layer underlying the epidermis. Medication given this way is absorbed much more slowly than with SC, IM or IV injection. This route is used most often for allergy testing, though some vaccines may be given ID as well.

An ID injection may be given anywhere on the body, most commonly on the lateral aspect of the neck. Before injection, the skin should be cleansed with 70% alcohol and allowed to dry. A small area of skin may then be picked up by thumb and forefinger to isolate the area for injection.

Select a small needle (25-ga, 5/8-inch) and introduce it into the dermis by pressing it against the skin at a slight angle, pushing it forward at the same time. Once inside the dermal tissue, aspirate (withdraw the plunger of the syringe slightly) to make certain a vessel has not been entered and then inject it slowly. Resistance should be felt as the solution is injected. A prominent bleb (raised area) rises shortly after the injection has begun. If this bleb is not seen immediately, withdraw the needle and repeat the procedure.

Subcutaneous Administration

Medication given by the subcutaneous (SC) route (beneath or deep to the skin) is absorbed faster than with the oral and ID routes but slower than with the IM and IV routes. Drugs commonly given SC include some vaccines, local anesthetics and any other drug for which slow absorption is required.

Subcutaneous injections are most frequently given on the lateral aspect of the neck. The injection site is cleansed with 70% alcohol and allowed to dry. This area of skin is then firmly grasped between the thumb and index finger, forming a tent of skin into which the needle is introduced (Fig 4). A 20- to 25-ga, 5/8- to 1-inch needle is selected, inserted under the skin and advanced to the hub. Once the needle is in place, aspirate to make certain a vessel has not been penetrated; then inject slowly. The solution should flow easily and a bleb may be evident directly under the skin. Gentle massaging of the area after injection may increase circulation to that area and consequently increase the absorption rate.

Local anesthetics are given SC as diagnostic nerve blocks on the limbs, around lesions before potentially painful treatment or in areas on which surgery is to be performed under local anesthesia. These areas are usually cleansed thoroughly with a surgical scrub before injection of the anesthetic. If the anesthetic is to be deposited over the legs, abdomen or face, it is almost impossible to pick up a fold of skin. However, introducing the needle at an angle nearly parallel to the skin should result in proper needle placement. Sluggish flow of solution may indicate ID needle placement, necessitating repositioning of the needle slightly deeper. If a bleb does not appear while injecting, the needle may be placed too deeply. If the injection is made into edematous tissues, however, a bleb is rarely seen.

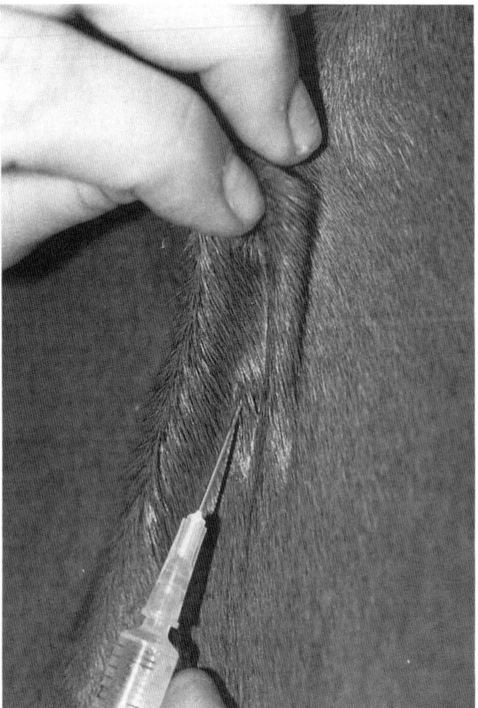

Figure 4. Subcutaneous injection. A "tent" is formed, into which the injection is given, when the skin on the lateral aspect of the neck is pinched.

Intramuscular Injection

Intramuscular (IM) injection, or injection of medication directly into a muscle, is commonly used in horses. Drugs given IM are absorbed relatively quickly. Intramuscular injection is usually easier for owners than ID, SC or IV injection. Care must be taken to make certain the drug is not inadvertently injected into a blood vessel, as severe reactions can occur if such drugs as procaine penicillin G enters the systemic circulation. This is more likely to happen using the IM route than with ID or SC injection.

Several sites can be used for IM injections in horses. A series of injection sites should be used, to minimize muscle damage and pain, if large amounts of medication are to be given over a long period. The largest muscle masses are located in the hindquarters. The gluteal muscle is located high on the rear limb, lateral to the vertebral column and caudal to the point of the hip (Fig 5). The disadvantage to using this muscle is that it is difficult to detect inflammation caused by the injection; also any injection abscesses are difficult to drain from this location. It is a large muscle mass, however, and can be used when necessary.

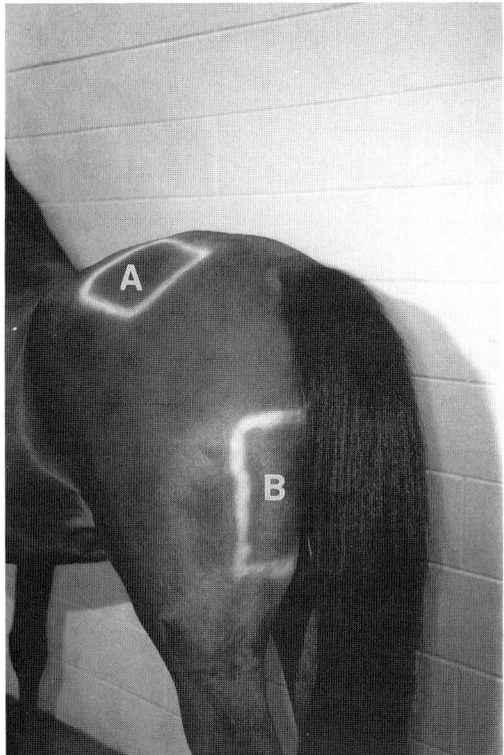

Figure 5. Intramuscular injection sites. A. Gluteal muscles. B. Semimembranosus and semitendinosus muscle groups.

The semimembranosus and semitendinosus muscle groups, located on the caudal aspect of the rear limb between the point of the buttock and the hock, may also be used (Fig 5). This large muscular area can be used often, with minimal complications. It is the choice location for IM injections in foals because of its large size. Though repeated IM injections in the rear legs may cause some degree of lameness, this usually subsides over several days after the last injection.

Another location for IM injection is the group of muscles on the lateral aspect of the neck. This area is bordered dorsad by the ligamentum nuchae, ventrad by the cervical vertebrae and caudad by the scapula (Fig 6). Large volumes of medication should not be injected in this area, however, because of the small muscle mass. Foals should not be injected in their neck muscles because the resultant soreness may inhibit nursing.

Other muscle masses that may be used are the pectoral and triceps muscles (Fig 6). However, these muscles are relatively small, even in well-developed horses, and are therefore used infrequently. Frequent IM injections in the pectoral and triceps groups may re-

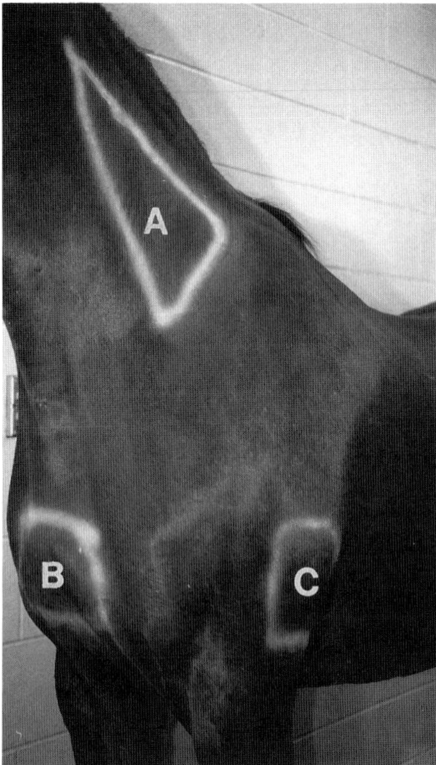

Figure 6. Intramuscular injection sites. A. Lateral muscles of the neck. B. Pectoral muscles. C. Triceps muscle.

sult in edema and pain. Nor should large amounts of medication be given in these muscles.

For an IM injection in a rear muscle mass, the animal should be properly restrained, according to its temperament, and the required materials should be readily available. An 18- to 20-ga, 1- to 1.5-inch needle is usually adequate. When injecting the gluteal muscle, the safest place to stand is very close beside the horse's hindquarters, facing caudad. If the horse attempts to kick while the operator is standing in this position, its movements can be felt and one can move aside before the kick.

The central area of the muscle is identified and the skin cleansed with 70% alcohol solution. The needle should be removed from the syringe for insertion because it is less awkward to place the needle into the muscle without the syringe attached. Also, if the horse reacts adversely to needle insertion, the needle usually remains in the muscle, should the horse move, if the added weight of the syringe is not present.

When inserting the needle in a rear muscle mass, hold it firmly between the thumb and index finger at the hub, with the point directed ventrad (downward). Immediately before introducing the needle into the muscle, tap the area firmly with the edge of the fist. This stimulates the nerve endings in the area, thereby decreasing the initial pain of needle penetration. After 2 quick, rhythmic taps, thrust the needle through the skin and into the muscle on the third tap. Very few horses react adversely to this method.

After insertion, sink the needle to the hub and attach the syringe. Before injecting the medication, aspirate (slightly withdraw syringe barrel) to make certain a vessel has not been penetrated. If blood is withdrawn into the syringe, remove the needle and repeat the procedure 2-3 inches from the original site or select a different muscle group altogether. Inject the drug slowly after the needle is properly placed. Do not inject more than 10-15 ml into one site, as excessive tissue distention by large volumes of injected liquid can result in tissue necrosis. If more than 15 ml is given, divide the dose and use 2 or more sites 2-3 inches apart. These divided doses should be given as separate injections rather than withdrawing the needle slightly and redirecting it. Moving the needle around once it is in the muscle causes excessive tissue trauma. Once the injection has been completed, withdraw the needle and properly dispose of it.

The technique used for injecting into the semimembranosus and semitendinosus muscles is similar to that described for the gluteals. The recommended injection site is about halfway between the gastrocnemius tendon and the point of the buttock, in the thickest portion of the muscle. Introduce the needle in the manner previously described. To safely inject an unruly horse, reach across the horse and inject into the opposite leg; most horses that kick will use the leg being injected. The same technique can be used when injecting into the gluteal muscle of a kicking horse, provided the animal is short enough that the opposite side can be seen.

Though the restraint techniques are similar, the method for injections into the lateral muscles of the neck differs significantly from that used in the hindquarters. The best injection site is located by drawing an imaginary triangle on the neck, with the ligamentum nuchae, cervical spine and scapula as the borders (Fig 7).

Clean a small area within this triangle with 70% alcohol and allow to dry. Grasp a portion of the skin immediately adjacent to the selected injection site between thumb and index finger (Fig 8). This acts as a form of restraint, transferring painful sensations elsewhere while the needle is inserted. Also, after the injection has been given and the skin is released, the needle holes in the skin and muscles are several inches apart, preventing leakage of the drug to the exterior, as so often occurs in the hindquarters. The slapping technique used for IM injections in other muscle groups may cause some skittish horses to become head shy after repeated

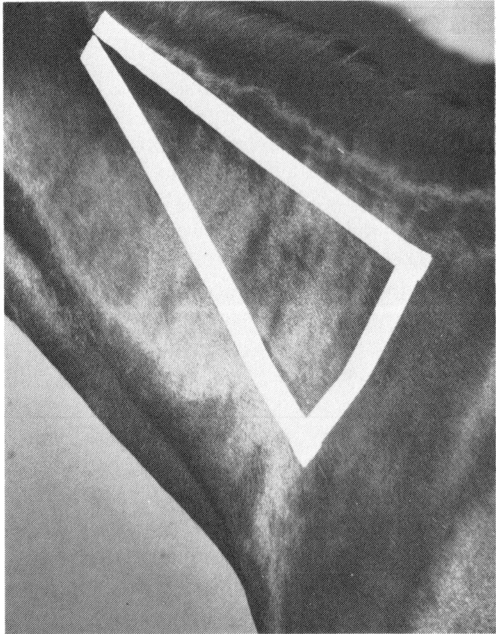

Figure 7. The muscular area of the neck is bordered dorsally by the ligamentum nuchae, caudally by the scapula, and ventrally by the cervical vertebral column.

injections into cervical muscles. For this reason, many technicians and veterinarians avoid "slapping" a needle into this area.

After the skin has been elevated, insert the needle gently to the hub, with or without the syringe attached (Fig 8). After aspiration to avoid inadvertently injecting into a vessel, slowly inject the medication. After the injection, withdraw the needle and release the skin. Premature release of the skin may bend the needle, traumatizing surrounding tissues.

Other muscle groups that may be used for IM injections are the triceps and the pectoral muscle (Fig 6). The technique used in these areas is identical to that used in the hindquarters.

Intravenous Injection

Intravenous (IV) injection allows the drug to bypass the absorption process and enter the bloodstream directly, rapidly providing high blood levels of the drug given.

Several veins are used for IV injections in horses. The most common vein used is the jugular vein, a large vein located on the ventrolateral aspect of the neck in what is termed the "jugular furrow" (Fig 10). In most horses this can be recognized as a depression, 1-2 inches wide, extending bilaterally along the entire length of the neck from the angle of the jaw to the shoulder.

Other vessels that may be used include the cephalic and saphenous veins. The cephalic vein is located on the medial aspect of the forearm, proximal to the carpus (Fig 9A). The saphenous vein is on

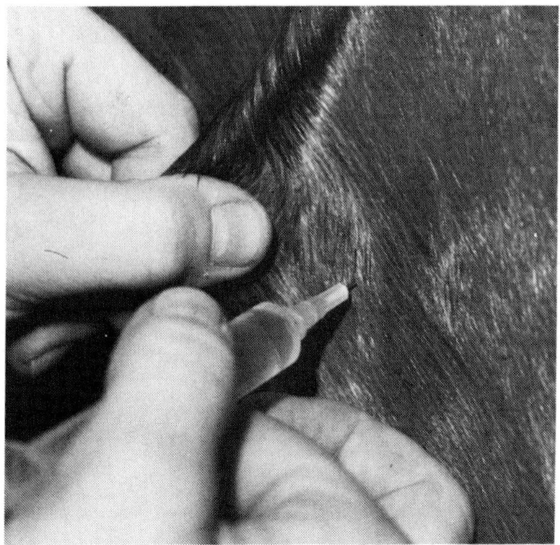

Figure 8. Injection into the lateral muscles of the neck. Grasp a fold of skin, introduce the needle perpendicular to the muscle, aspirate, inject, remove the needle and release the skin.

the medial aspect of each rear limb, extending from the inguinal region to the distal tarsus (Fig 9B). Though they are both rather prominent vessels, it takes skill to penetrate them because they move freely under the skin and most horses resent being injected in these areas.

The size of the needle used for IV injections should be proportional to the size of the vein. In the cephalic and saphenous veins, a 20- to 22-ga, 1- inch needle is used, while an 18- to 20-ga, 1- to 1.5-inch needle is used in the jugular veins. Smaller needles may be required when working on ponies and foals. If repeated injections are to be given, a smaller needle should be used to minimize the tissue trauma associated with venipuncture.

The technique used for venipuncture is essentially the same for all veins. To locate (raise) the jugular vein, digital pressure is applied with a thumb over the jugular furrow about two-thirds of the way down (caudal on) the neck. With blood flow obstructed, the distended vein is seen immediately above (cranial to) the thumb (Fig 10). If the vein is not readily identified, alternate application and release of pressure over the jugular furrow to detect filling of the vein with blood. "Strumming" or lightly tapping the vein cranial to the thumb with the opposite index finger may cause waves in the jugular vein, which assist in identifying the vessel. Because the ce-

Figure 9. A. The cephalic vein (arrows) on the equine forelimb. B. The saphenous vein (arrows) on the equine hind limb. In both of these photos, the horse's head is to the left.

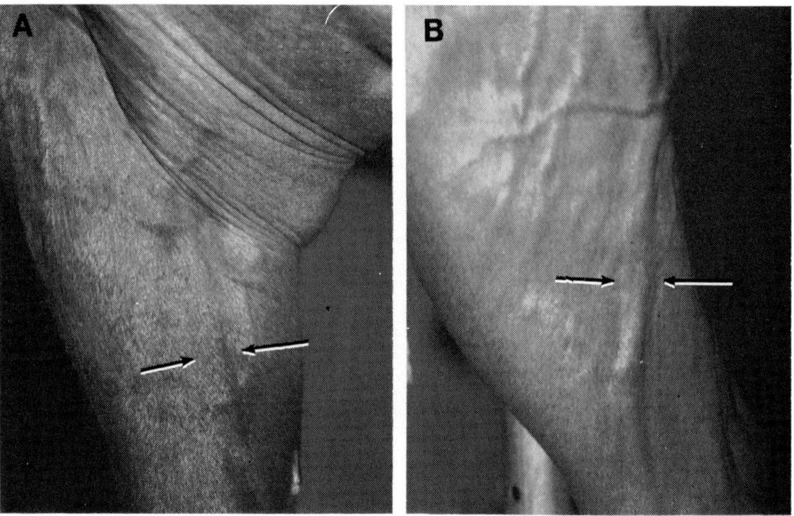

phalic and saphenous veins are very superficial in most horses, raising of these veins is usually unnecessary.

In horses with a very thick neck, it may be very difficult or nearly impossible to see the jugular vein. Palpating the muscles on either side of the jugular furrow may be the only means of locating the vein in such horses. Once the vein is identified, cleanse the overlying skin thoroughly with 70% alcohol. This not only cleans the skin but also smoothes the hair, making the vein more visible. Insert the needle, bevel up, at a 30-degree angle to the vein. It may be inserted toward the heart or toward the head, depending on personal preference.

Whether or not the syringe should remain attached during venipuncture is open to discussion. When the syringe is in place during the procedure, very little manipulation of the needle is required to complete the injection; however, it is more difficult to determine if the blood aspirated into the syringe is venous or arterial. This problem may be remedied by inserting the needle alone and observing the character of the blood exiting the needle. If, however, a very small-bore needle is used, the characteristic "arterial spurt" may not occur, which may lead to an intraarterial injection that could have serious side effects. The technique used is based on personal preference.

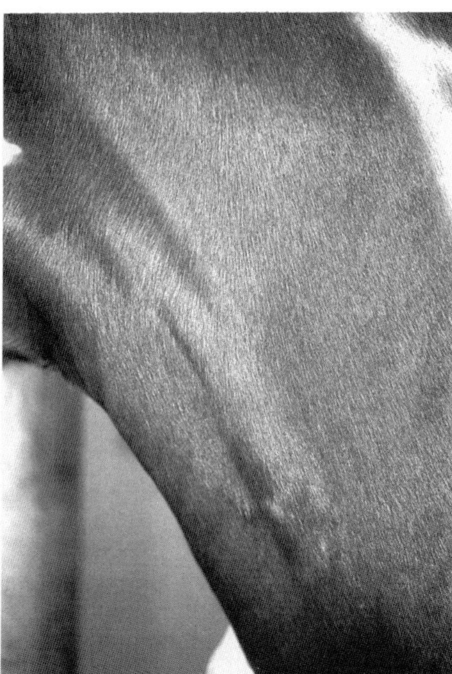

Figure 10. Occlusion of the jugular vein midway down the jugular furrow allows the vein to fill. A distinct distention of the vein is evident cranial to the thumb.

The venipuncture method selected depends on the patient's behavior. One successful method involves pressing firmly, with the needle, on the skin over the vessel while slowly sliding the needle forward and into the vein. This eliminates the possibility of surprising the animal, thereby dislodging the needle. The needle is more accurately placed and trauma to surrounding tissues is minimized. If the patient reacts adversely to this approach, a quick thrust with the needle through the skin may be required for venipuncture. With the quick-thrust method, the needle may not properly enter the vein, and may require redirection once it is through the skin and the patient quiets down.

When the needle is believed to be in the vein, aspirate to ensure a good backflow of blood. If this is not observed, slightly advancing, withdrawing or rotating the needle may position it so it is directed into the vessel's lumen. Once the needle is properly placed, release the vessel and inject slowly and evenly. Aspirate frequently throughout the injection, especially after any movement of the animal, to ensure that all of the medication is given IV. After the injection, remove the needle and apply digital pressure (with fingers) to the injection site until all hemorrhage has ceased.

Complications: The most common mistake made during IV injections is injecting medication into the perivascular tissues (around, rather than in, the vein). Severe irritation by such drugs as phenylbutazone or sodium pentothal may lead to sloughing of the overlying skin. If a caustic drug is injected outside a vein, infiltrate the SC tissues at the site with saline and lidocaine. This dilutes the drug and relieves the pain an irritating drug may cause.

Another complication of improper IV injection is phlebitis, which may result from perivascular injection but is also associated with undue trauma to the vessel during venipuncture. Dull or barbed needles can extensively damage the vessel wall, as can repeated attempts to enter the vessel. Progression of this condition to thrombophlebitis may result in complete occlusion of the vessel. If this occurs bilaterally, the head may swell because of poor venous return.

A very serious complication of improper IV injection is intraarterial injection. Medication given in this way may produce disorientation, convulsions and possibly death within a few seconds after beginning the injection. If the animal does recover, it may take only a few minutes or several days. Intraarterial injections are best avoided by working in a well-lit area, applying adequate restraint, using an appropriately sized needle, observing the character of the blood aspirated, and recognizing the early signs of intraarterial injection so that immediate steps can be taken to treat the patient.

Intravenous Catheterization

Intravenous catheterization is commonly used in horses requiring extensive fluid therapy. If properly maintained, indwelling catheters may remain functional for several days. However, when IV catheters are improperly placed or poorly maintained, several complications may result. These may range from local infections at the catheter exit site, to thrombophlebitis and embolus formation, which could eventually lead to death. Therefore, proper aseptic technique is required for this avenue of therapy.

The jugular veins are most frequently used for IV catheterization. The cephalic and saphenous veins may also be catheterized, but limb movement often results in excessive movement of the catheter, which may lead to thrombosis of these vessels. The lateral external thoracic vein is used occasionally but only when the previously mentioned veins are no longer patent (open or clear). This vein is located on the lateral thorax, immediately caudal to the elbow; it is not easily discerned, making a "cut down" (incision and retraction of overlying skin) necessary before catheterization.

Many types of catheters are available for use in horses (Fig 11). The selection of catheter size is based on vessel size and the rate at which the fluids must be given. Over-the-needle catheters are most often used in adult horses because of the large diameter and durable construction of these catheters. Through-the-needle catheters are available in smaller sizes that are ideal for ponies and foals. These smaller catheters are less rigid, however, and caution is required to prevent bending upon insertion.

Commercially prepared sterile catheter units are most often used. Catheters may also be prepared from polyethylene or Silastic

Figure 11. Intravenous catheters. *Top:* Over-the-needle catheter. *Bottom:* Through-the-needle catheter.

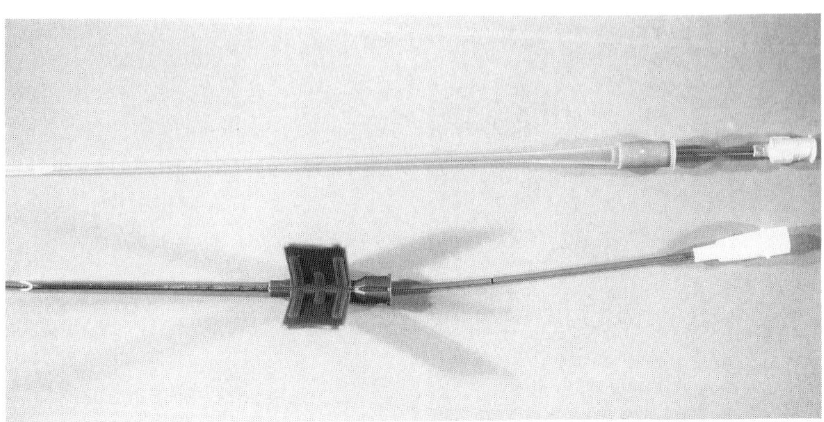

tubing, and fitted with a needle adaptor. These pieces of tubing are sterilized and inserted through a large-bore needle.

The area chosen for catheterization should be clipped and surgically scrubbed, with local anesthetic injected if desired. Wearing sterile gloves, locate the vein and insert the needle through the skin and into the vein, toward the heart. Before removing the needle from the catheter and threading the catheter down the vein, aspirate with a syringe or hold off the vein securely to ensure a backflow of blood, signifying proper placement. Advance the catheter off the needle and down the vein gently until its entire length is in the vein. Catheter placement must again be verified before continuing (Fig 12).

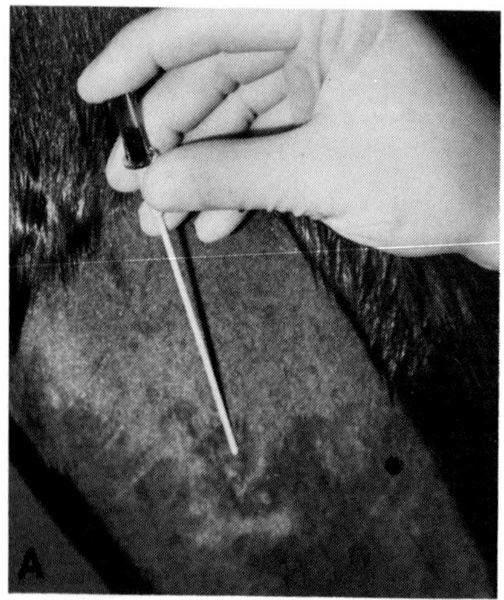

Figure 12. Intravenous catheterization. A. After surgical preparation of the skin over the jugular vein, the catheter is introduced through the skin and into the vein, directing it toward the heart. B. When blood is observed exiting the catheter, the stylet is held securely and the catheter is threaded into the vein. C. The position of the catheter must be verified before proceeding.

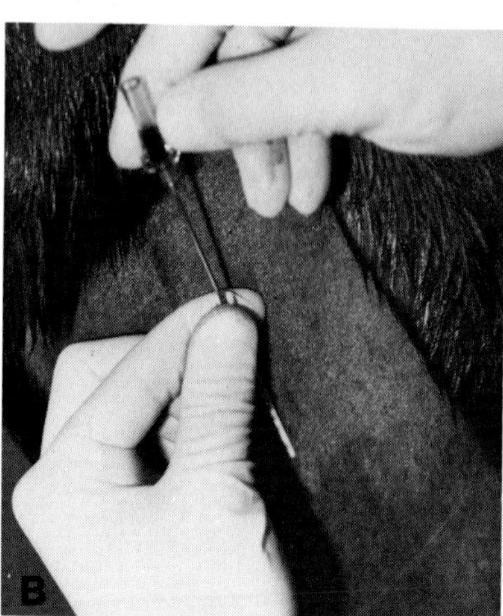

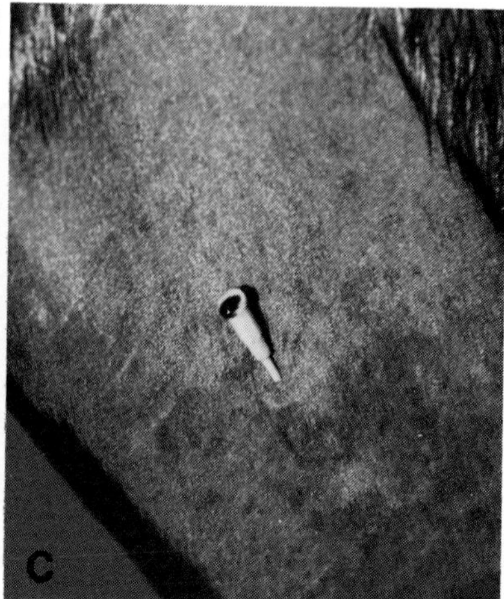

Once the catheter is in its proper position, cap it and then flush it with heparinized saline. To prevent the catheter from moving about within the vessel, the catheter's end should be sutured to the underlying skin. Securing the catheter by bandaging is inadequate if it is to be left in place for an extended period. Catheters may be secured by various methods. Using a tape "butterfly" is one method (Fig 13). There are some disadvantages with this technique, however. The tape is not sterile and may increase the possibility of infection at the catheter's exit from the skin. Also, if the catheter becomes wet, the tape may loosen, which reduces its holding power. It is a relatively easy procedure, however, and works well under most circumstances.

Another method that may be used to secure the catheter involves placing a suture immediately above any outcropping on the

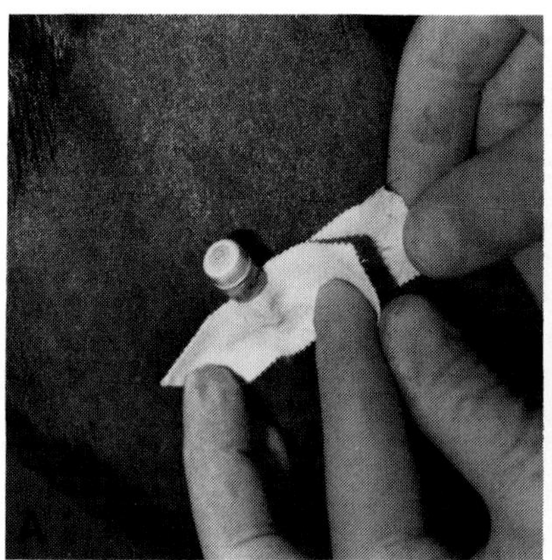

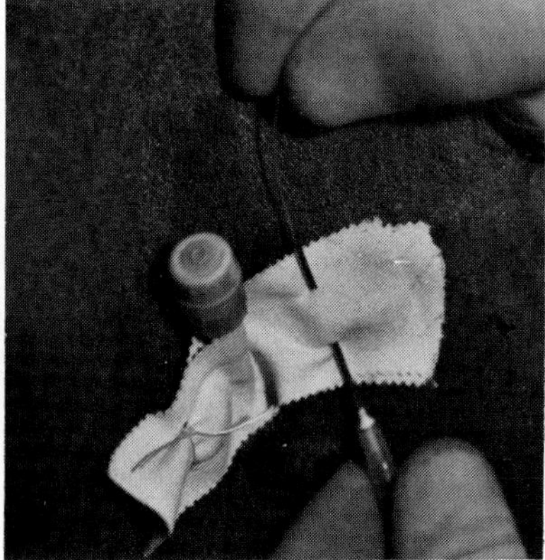

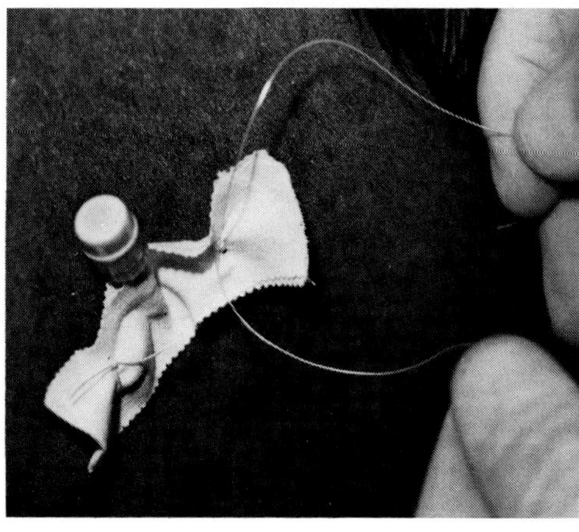

Figure 13. Securing the IV catheter with a tape butterfly. A. A 4-inch section of adhesive tape is folded in half and secured to itself around the catheter. B. A piece of suture material is placed through the tape and skin, using a hypodermic needle as a guide. C. The sutures are tied over the tape.

extension line (Fig 14). This prevents the catheter from backing out of the vein by seating the hub at the catheter exit.

When using the more flexible catheters, a few drops of surgical glue (Nexaband: Tri Point Medical) applied at the catheter exit helps keep the catheter in place.

Once the catheter is secured, place antibacterial ointment at the catheter's exit from the skin, using a piece of sterile gauze and adhesive bandage material (*eg,* Elastikon: Johnson & Johnson) looped into or on top of the bandage and held in place with adhesive tape (Fig 15). Looping the extension line prevents direct traction on the catheter when the animal moves.

Complications: Complications can be minimized by using aseptic technique during catheterization, and by frequent examination and appropriate maintenance of the catheter and associated equipment. All supplies required must be sterile before use, and needles and catheters must be free of barbs and frays that could damage the vessel wall. Because the likelihood of thrombophlebitis increases the longer a catheter is left in place, the catheter should be changed at least every 72 hours. All associated IV tubing should be changed every 24-48 hours and the dressing replaced every 24 hours to decrease the possibility of contamination and resultant infection.

Figure 14. Placement of a suture through the skin above any outcropping on the extension line helps prevent the catheter from backing out of the vein.

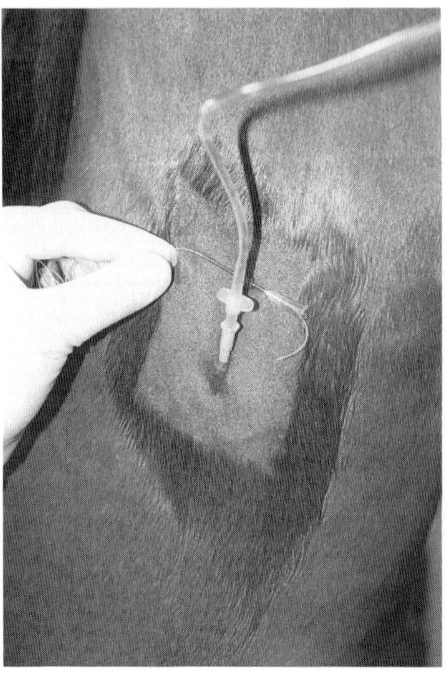

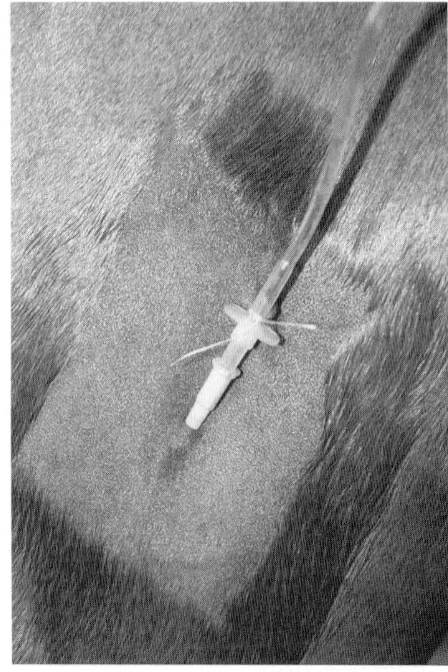

Intrauterine Infusion

Intrauterine infusions involve injection of liquid medication through an infusion pipette or catheter passed through the vulva, vagina and cervix, into the uterus (Fig 16). Indications for this procedure include treatment of intrauterine infections, and prophylactic medication after diagnostic procedures or artifical insemination. Because technicians are not permitted to give intrauterine infusions in some states, the clinician should be consulted before such treatment is given.

Proper preparation of the mare is important to avoid introducing microorganisms into the reproductive tract during the procedures. The tail should be wrapped with gauze or a clean bandage, after which it is held or tied up out of the way. The vulva must be scrubbed and rinsed thoroughly to remove contaminants, after which a small piece of wet cotton is used to swab the inner surface of the dorsal labial commissure (dorsal, internal aspect of the vulva) to remove fecal material that often collects there, particularly after rectal palpation.

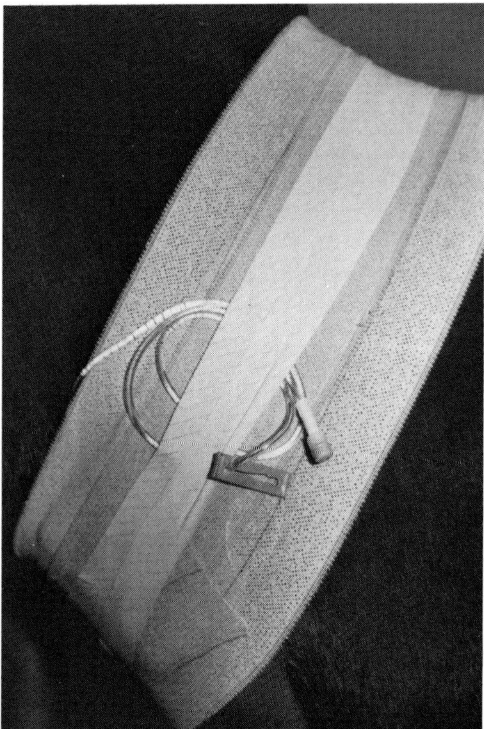

Figure 15. Apply a sterile dressing and gauze over the catheter's exit from the skin and bandage with an adhesive bandage. Loop the extension lines and secure with adhesive tape.

Use of sterile equipment is essential. Disposable obstetric (OB) sleeves may be gas sterilized or a sterile surgeon's glove may be placed over a nonsterile OB sleeve. Place an infusion pipette or Chambers intrauterine catheter (Wellcome) in the palm of the hand, with index finger covering the opening. Apply a sterile, water-soluble lubricant, such as K-Y Jelly (Johnson & Johnson) or Ster-L-Jel (McCullough Cartwright), to the dorsal surface of the hand and arm, which are then inserted through the vulva. Rotation of the hand and arm during insertion distributes the lubricant evenly and minimizes reproductive tract irritation. If the mare strains when the arm is inserted, wait until the animal relaxes and then proceed.

At the cranial wall of the vagina lies the cervix. In an estrual mare (in estrus), the cervix is relaxed and lies near the vaginal floor. Diestrual mares have a firm cervix located near the center of the cranial aspect of the vagina. During diestrus, digital (finger) manipulation may be required to enter the cervix because of its increased muscular tone. Postpartum mares (after foaling) have a dilated cervix that may allow passage of the entire hand.

Once the cervix is located, advance the index finger through the os (opening) and slide the pipette under (ventral to) the finger until the pipette is 3-4 inches inside (cranial to) the cervix, near the uterine body. Then infuse the medication through the pipette. If resistance is met during fluid infusion, withdraw or advance the pipette

Figure 16. Intrauterine infusion. After thoroughly cleansing the perineal area, insert a sterile-gloved, lubricated hand through the vulva into the vagina, guarding the tip of the catheter with the index finger. Insert the finger into the cervix and advance the catheter under the finger and into the uterus.

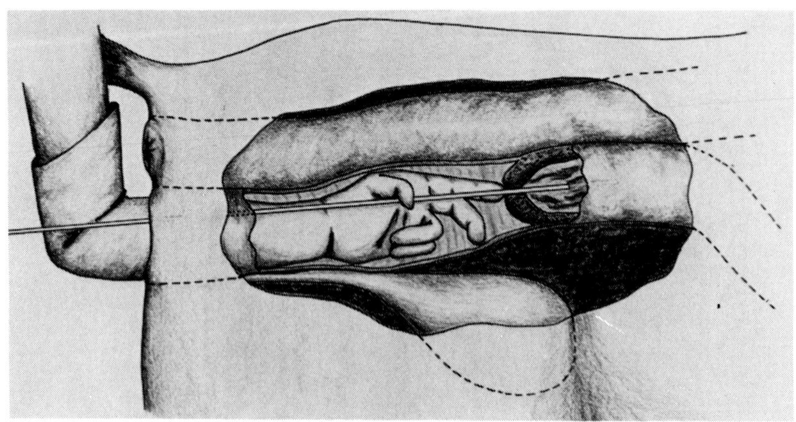

slightly, as its opening may be against the uterine wall. After the infusion, withdraw the pipette and cleanse the mare's vulva to remove excess lubricant.

Medicating the Eye

Diseases of the eye, such as keratitis, corneal ulcers, corneal abrasions and lacerations, and conjunctivitis are often treated by topical application of ointments or solutions. A horse's cornea may be exposed by placing the index finger immediately dorsal to the margin of the upper eyelid and pushing it dorsomediad until it contacts the supraorbital process. The lower lid is everted by rolling it into position with the thumb of the same hand (Fig 17). A thin "ribbon" of ointment or a few drops of solution is then applied to the ventral conjunctival fornix. If ointment and solution must be used together, the solution should be applied first to prevent it from running over the ointment and out of the eye, wasting the solution and reducing its efficacy. Ophthalmic solutions must be instilled often to maintain an effective concentration of the drug; ointments can be applied less often because of their prolonged contact item. The veterinarian should be consulted on which form to use.

Subpalpebral catheters are often used in uncooperative patients that require ocular therapy for extended periods. Most horses tolerate placement of these catheters under local or regional anesthesia; however, extremely fractious animals may require general anesthesia. Polyethylene tubing (PE 160 or 200) is prepared by applying heat to one end to create a flange (flared end) at the open-

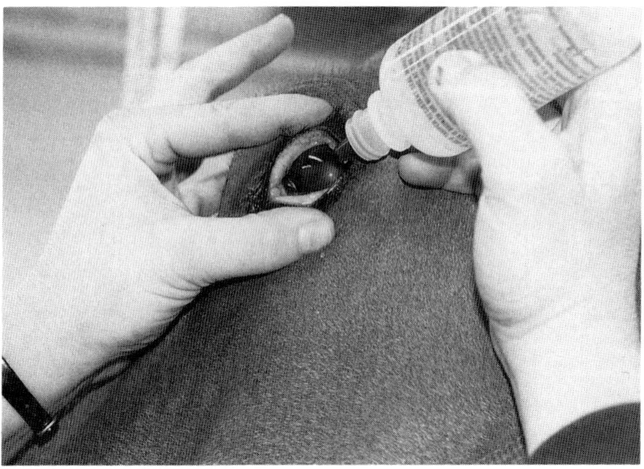

Figure 17. Topical application of ocular medication. Place the index finger dorsal to the margin of the upper eyelid and direct it dorsomedially, ventral to the supraorbital process. Evert the lower lid with the thumb of the same hand.

ing. The tubing should be long enough to reach from the eye to the withers.

Introduce a large (12-ga), hubless needle into the dorsal conjunctival fornix at the dorsolateral aspect of the upper eyelid. Thread the plain (unflared) end of the catheter through the needle until the flange is fitted snugly into the conjunctival space (Fig 18), after which the needle is removed. Suture the catheter to the skin dorsal to the eyelid with the aid of a tape butterfly (Fig 18). Fit the free end of the catheter with a needle adaptor and injection cap (Becton-Dickinson), through which the medication is injected, and then secure it to the mane at the withers with adhesive tape. After injecting solutions through the system, it is important to then inject air so that the medication is flushed out of the catheter and over the eye.

Nasolacrimal Duct Irrigation

Obstruction of the lacrimal apparatus (tear ducts) of the horse is usually unilateral (only on one side) and may be identified by epiphora (constant tearing) on the affected side. Retrograde (nose to eye) irrigation of the nasolacrimal duct is the most common means used to open obstructed ducts. A smooth-tipped catheter, such as a 5-Fr polyethylene catheter, is most commonly used for this procedure.

Figure 18. Subpalpebral catheter. A. The catheter sutured in place. B. Lateral section of the eye shows the flared end of of the catheter fitted into the conjunctival fornix.

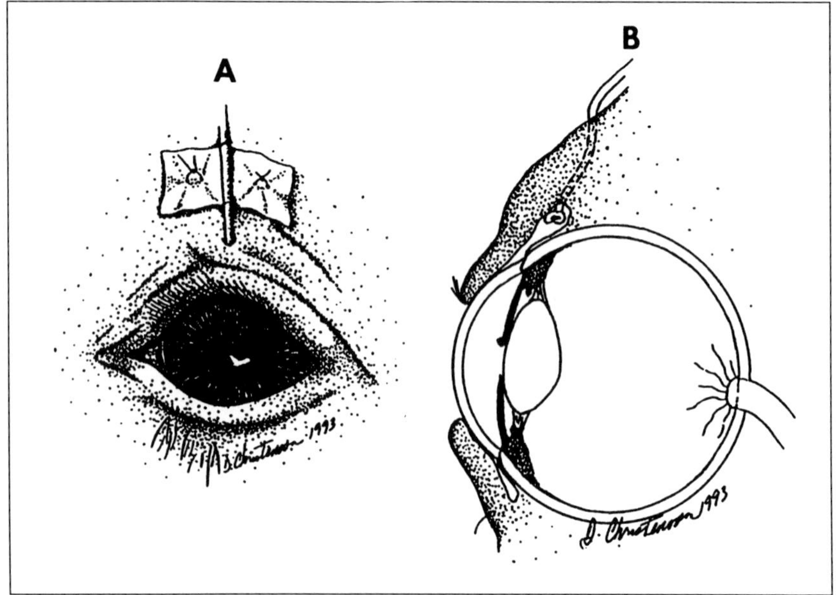

With the horse properly restrained, identify the nasolacrimal duct opening in the nostril on the floor of the nasal cavity near the junction of the skin and mucous membrane. Gently thread a smooth-tipped, 5-Fr polyethylene catheter 2-3 inches into the duct (Fig 19). Seal the opening of the nasolacrimal duct around the catheter by applying digital pressure over the area to prevent backflow of the irrigating solution. The duct is considered patent (open) when irrigation fluid flows easily and exits readily at the medial canthus (inner corner) of the eye.

The ventral palpebral punctum at the medial canthus of the eye may be catheterized in cooperative horses. Because this opening is significantly smaller than the opening in the nostril, a smaller-gauge catheter is required than for retrograde flushing. The catheter is introduced through the punctum and into the nasolacrimal duct, after which irrigating solution is injected slowly and gently. The duct is considered patent when the solution flows easily from the opening in the nostril.

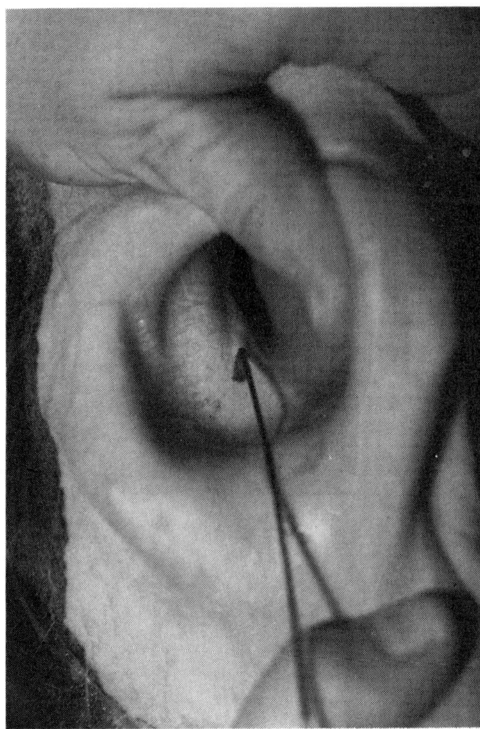

Figure 19. Retrograde catheterization of the nasolacrimal duct. The duct opening is located on the floor of the nasal cavity, near the junction of the skin and mucous membrane. Insert a smooth-tipped catheter into the duct, occlude the surrounding duct opening and gently inject the irrigating solution.

Blood Collection and Administration

Collecting Blood Samples for Diagnostic Tests

Blood samples are required for various diagnostic tests, such as complete blood count (CBC), packed cell volume (PCV), blood chemistry analyses, blood gas studies, coagulation profiles, equine infectious anemia tests and many others. The amount of blood needed for these tests varies from less than 1 ml to 10 ml. The type of sample collected (coagulated or anticoagulated) depends on the requirements of the test. These samples may be collected with a needle and syringe or with vacuum tubes and their needles (*eg,* Vacutainer: Becton-Dickinson).

The jugular vein is most commonly used to obtain venous blood samples, though the cephalic and saphenous veins may be used if necessary. An arterial sample may be obtained from the carotid artery, located dorsomedial to the jugular vein in the jugular furrow, or from the great metatarsal artery, found along the cranial aspect of the fourth metatarsal bone. The skin overlying the vessel should be prepared as for IV injections.

A 20- to 22-ga, 1- to 1.5-inch needle is used for venous samples. The needle is introduced into the vein as for IV injections. If the Vacutainer system is used, the needle must be threaded into the vein and advanced to its hub. Failure to do so may result in penetration of the opposite wall by the needle or withdrawal of the needle from the vein when the tube is attached. When a backflow of blood is observed, release digital pressure on the vein. Hold the needle firmly between the thumb and index finger and force the external end of the needle through the center of the rubber stopper and into the tube (Fig 20). Use of the Vacutainer needle holder provides more accurate placement of the needle into the tube, with minimal manipulation (Fig 20).

If blood is not flowing adequately once the tube and needle are connected, withdraw, advance or rotate the entire unit slightly. The tube quickly fills with blood until the vacuum is depleted. Because the amount of anticoagulant present in each vacuum tube corresponds to the volume of blood the tube accommodates, it is important to allow these tubes to fill until the vacuum is depleted or the sample will be incorrectly diluted.

When the tube has filled, remove the needle from the vein, gently invert the tube to mix the blood with the anticoagulant (if any is present in the tube), and apply digital pressure over the venipuncture site to prevent hemorrhage.

If Vacutainer needles are not used, blood may be collected with a needle and syringe and immediately transferred to an appropriate tube. Hemolysis (rupturing of RBCs) may occur if the blood is rapidly injected into the tube through the needle. Hemolysis may be

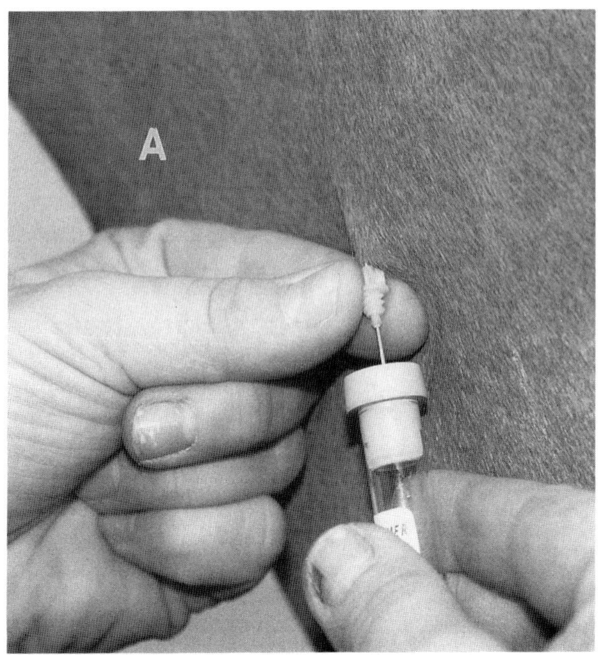

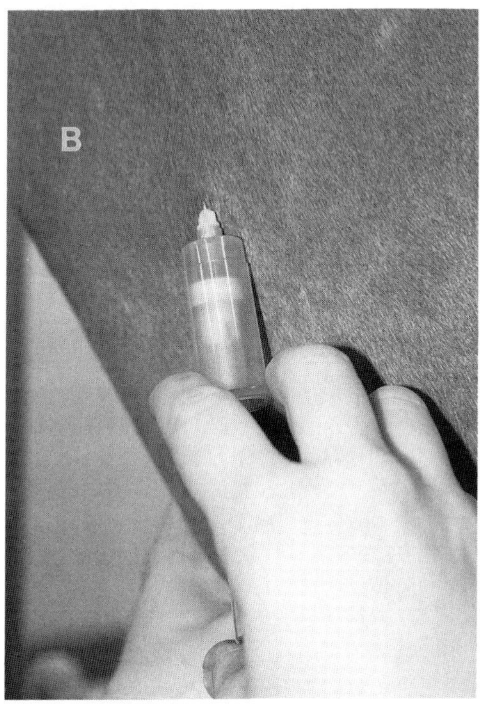

Figure 20. Blood collection. A. Using the Vacutainer system to collect blood, hold the hub of the needle securely, while advancing the tube onto the needle so that the other end of the needle remains in the vein's lumen. B. Use of a Vacutainer needle holder allows the tube to be attached to the needle with very little manipulation.

prevented by detaching the needle and depositing the blood directly from the syringe into the open tube.

When collecting small amounts (0.5-2 ml) of blood for such tests as a PCV or blood gas analysis, use of a needle and small syringe is adequate. Before collecting blood, flush the syringe with a small amount of heparin to prevent coagulation of the sample. When collecting a sample for blood gas evaluation, expel all air from the syringe after the blood is obtained so the values obtained are accurate. Insertion of the needle end into a rubber stopper prevents air from entering the blood-filled syringe during transport.

Palpation of an arterial pulse is the only indication as to the location of an artery. When attempting to obtain blood from the carotid artery, an 18- to 20-ga, 1.5-inch needle attached to a heparinized syringe is used, as previously described. The arterial pulse may be detected by palpating the distal third of the jugular furrow. The carotid artery is more superficial in this area than at any other point along its course. It is located dorsal to the jugular vein and trachea.

Once the pulse is identified, the needle is inserted at a 90-degree angle (perpendicular) to the skin and advanced slowly toward the artery. Because the carotid artery moves rather freely in this location, several attempts may be required before the sample is collected. A bright-red spurt of blood exits the needle once the arterial lumen has been entered. After withdrawal of the needle, digital pressure must be applied over the site for as long as 5 minutes to prevent hematoma formation, a common event after arterial puncture.

The great metatarsal artery is much smaller than the carotid artery; therefore, a smaller (22- to 25-ga, 1-inch) needle is required for collection of blood from this artery. The artery is used frequently to obtain samples for blood gas analysis on foals; however, because of its location, it is rarely used on adult horses because few will stand quietly for this procedure. The arterial pulse may be detected along the cranial aspect of the fourth metatarsal bone. Introduce the needle at a 15- to 30-degree angle and collect the blood in a heparinized syringe. Digital pressure must be applied to the area after collection, as in carotid artery puncture, to avoid hematoma formation.

Another artery that may be used is the facial artery. This artery is located immediately rostral to the facial crest. Again, because of the vessel's size, a very small needle (25-ga, 5/8-inch) is required.

Blood Transfusions

Severe blood loss, anemia, hypoproteinemia, hypogammaglobulinemia and neonatal isoerythrolysis are some conditions for which transfusions may be indicated in horses. Transfusions may consist of only blood cells, whole blood or plasma, depending on which deficiencies are present. Before blood is transfused, it should be crossmatched to assess the compatibility of the donor's and recipient's blood. Failure to do so may result in administration of incompatible blood, with a subsequent transfusion reaction. If whole blood is to be given, it must be compatible in both major and minor phases; that is, agglutination must not be observed when the donor's cells are added to the recipient's plasma (major) or when the recipient's cells are added to the donor's plasma (minor). When only plasma is to be given, compatibility is necessary only in the minor phase.

Blood Collection for Transfusion

After selecting a healthy, compatible blood donor, prepare the equipment used to collect large volumes of blood. Plastic bags are available as single or multiple Blood-Pack units (Fenwal), which have a detachable collection set containing citrate-phosphate-dextrose-adenine (CPDA-1), with or without an attached empty bag (transfer pack) (Abbott) that receives the cells or plasma from the original container. These plastic bags typically hold 500 ml of blood. Larger quantities of blood can be collected using a Whole Blood/Plasma Collection Kit (Veterinary Dynamics). This kit contains a 2-liter collection bag with a collection needle, a 1-liter bag into which to transfer the plasma, a bag of sodium citrate anticoagulant, a blood administration set and a complete set of instructions on how to use the system.

The donor horse's jugular vein should be thoroughly scrubbed, after which a large (10- to 12-ga, 2- to 3-inch) needle is inserted into the vein, toward the heart. Attach the collection tube to the needle. The jugular vein must be occluded (held off) continually throughout the procedure to enhance flow of blood into the container. During collection, rock the collection container gently back and forth to mix the blood with the anticoagulant. Hemolysis may result if this is not done carefully. After the blood is collected, remove the needle and apply digital pressure to the site until all hemorrhage has ceased. Immediately label the container of blood with donor identification and the date and time of collection.

Whole blood may be given immediately after collection, but plasma may be given only after centrifugation or sedimentation to remove blood cells. The cells usually settle to the bottom of the container within 2 hours at room temperature. If plasma is not to be immediately transfused, the whole blood may be refrigerated for 12 hours, after which the blood cells may be separated. After the blood cells are separated, plasma may be siphoned off or aspirated into a vacuum container.

The transfusion recipient must have an IV catheter inserted before the transfusion. The transfusion should be given through an administration set containing an in-line filter to prevent infusion of fibrin and blood clots. The first 100-200 ml should be given very slowly and the patient watched closely for signs of a transfusion reaction. The first sign of such a reaction is uneasiness, followed by dyspnea, tremors, and a fast, weak pulse. Collapse and apnea may result if the condition is not treated immediately. The transfusion should be immediately discontinued after the first signs of a reaction. Epinephrine and antihistamines may be required to treat horses with a transfusion reaction; therefore, these emergency drugs should always be immediately available when transfusions are given. Monitor the patient throughout the transfusion; if no abnormalities are initially evident, slowly increase the flow rate and complete the transfusion.

Urine Collection

Urine may have to be collected from a horse for several reasons. A urinalysis may be part of a routine physical examination. Such conditions as myositis, azoturia and urolithiasis may be diagnosed and monitored by urinalysis. The response to treatment of such conditions as cystitis may also be monitored by urinalysis. Finally, testing of the urine for the presence of certain drugs is now required at many race tracks and competitive horse shows.

Urine specimens may be obtained by catching a mid-stream sample during urination or by catheterizing the bladder. Catheterization provides an uncontaminated sample, more suitable for microbial analysis than “free catch” samples.

Collecting Urine from Male Horses

A urine sample may be obtained easily from some male horses by placing the animal in a stall with fresh straw bedding. If the horse does not urinate within a short time, urination can occasionally be hastened by kicking the straw about. If a urine sample is required in a short period, an injection of furosemide (a diuretic) promotes urination. When collecting a voided sample, allow the horse to urinate a small amount before collection, as the initial flow of urine often contains urethral debris, which may alter the results of the urinalysis or drug test. Collect the mid-stream sample in a clean, labeled container and refrigerate it until the analysis can be performed.

Male horses usually must be tranquilized for bladder catheterization. Acepromazine maleate relaxes the retractor penis muscle, allowing the penis to protrude from the prepuce. Once this has occurred, grasp the penis caudal to the glans penis and wash it with a mild soap and rinse it thoroughly. Direct your attention while washing the penis to the glans penis, urethral process and urethral diverticulum. The diverticulum is a blind pouch, dorsal to the urethral process, that collects smegma. This collection of smegma has been referred to as a "bean" because of its shape.

Using sterile gloves, introduce a lubricated, sterile plastic or rubber stallion catheter into the urethra, and advance it slowly and gently to avoid traumatizing the urethra (Fig 21). As the catheter reaches the ischial arch, just ventral to the anus, slight force may be required to pass the catheter through the curvature of the urethra in this area. As the catheter passes over the ischial arch, the horse usually raises its tail, indicating the catheter is near the bladder. Gentle aspiration with a sterile syringe may be required to start the flow of urine unless the bladder is full. Collect a midstream sample of urine passively exiting the catheter in a labeled, sterile container and refrigerate it until it is analyzed.

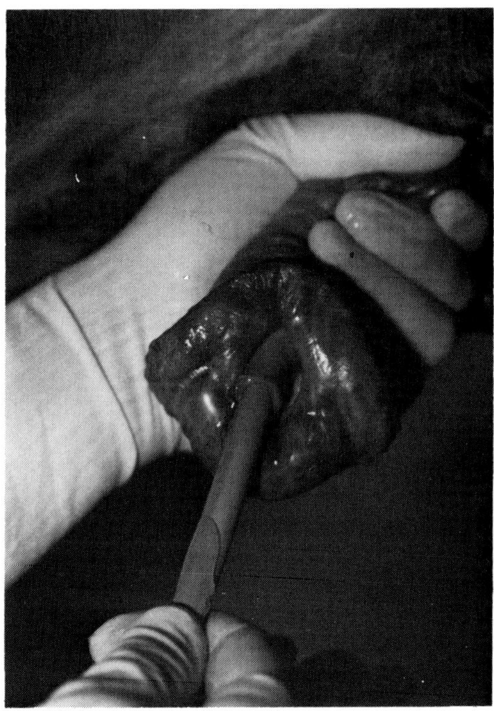

Figure 21. Urethral catheterization of the male horse. After thorough cleansing of the glans penis, a sterile, lubricating plastic or rubber catheter is introduced into the urethra and advanced into the urinary bladder.

Collecting Urine from Female Horses

Urine collection is comparatively difficult in mares. Mares generally do not react in the same manner as geldings or stallions when placed in a freshly bedded stall. A voided sample is often obtained, however, during catheterization, as manipulation of the urethral orifice often results in urination. If a sample is not collected during catheterization, most mares attempt to urinate when taken back to their stall. Collect a mid-stream sample in a labeled, sterile container and refrigerate it until it is analyzed.

Catheterization of a mare's bladder does not generally require tranquilization. Sterile equipment must be used to obtain a sterile sample and avoid contamination of the urinary tract. The perineum should be thoroughly cleansed before catheterization (see Intrauterine Infusion).

Several types of catheters are available for use in mares; the one selected is determined by personal preference (Fig 22). The metal mare urinary catheter (Wellcome, Kansas City, MO) is used most frequently. A rubber stallion catheter may be used, though greater manipulation of the catheter may be required to complete the procedure. Uterine pipettes or Chambers catheters (Wellcome) may be used in fillies and small mares when a smaller-diameter catheter is required.

Sterile surgeon's gloves should be used to manually guide the catheter, if necessary. Apply sterile water-soluble lubricant and insert the hand through the vulva and into the vaginal vestibule. The urethral orifice may be palpated on the floor of the vestibule 4-6 inches from the ventral vulvar commissure (ventral aspect of the vulva). To enter the urethral orifice, pass the catheter ventral to the hand and guide it into the urethra by the index finger. Gentle

Figure 22. Urinary catheters. *Top:* Rubber stallion catheter. *Middle:* Chambers catheter. *Bottom:* Metal mare urinary catheter.

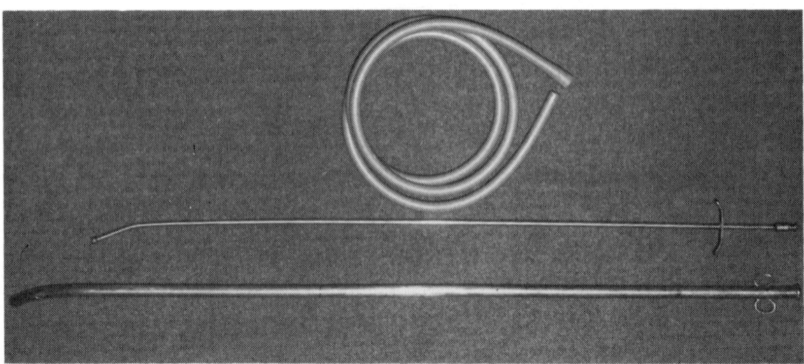

aspiration with an attached sterile syringe may be required to obtain the urine. If this is unsuccessful, gently manipulate the catheter craniad and caudad, making certain the catheter does not leave the urethra. Such stimulation of the urethra often causes the mare to urinate. Once urine is obtained, remove the catheter and rinse the mare's vulva with clean water to remove excess lubricant.

The mare urinary catheter may be passed into the bladder without manual guidance. The mare is prepared in the same manner as above. Insert the catheter through the vulva and into the vaginal vestibule, with the tip remaining in contact with the floor of the vagina. A small amount of resistance is felt when it reaches the urethral orifice. At this point, turn the tip of the catheter slightly to one side and advance it slowly. The catheter should slide directly into the bladder. The procedure used to obtain the urine is the same as above.

Enemas

Enemas are used to facilitate passage of feces from the terminal colon and rectum. Constipation that is not corrected by oral administration of lubricants often requires use of an enema. The fluid volume and equipment used differ significantly between mature horses and foals.

Enemas in Foals

In foals, enemas are most often used to relieve meconium (fetal feces) impactions. Meconium is normally passed 3-12 hours after birth. Foals that experience difficulty in expelling this firm, tenacious material show abdominal straining, anal protrusion and frequent tail raising when attempting to defecate. Many breeding farms routinely give enemas to all newborn foals to prevent meconium retention.

Fleet enemas (Fleet, Lynchburg, VA), available in most drug stores, may be used safely in foals (Fig 23). These squeeze bottles have a flexible tip and contain a premixed liquid (mineral oil or phosphate solution). Insert the tip into the foal's rectum and slowly infuse the contents of the bottle, then discard the container.

Warm water may also be used in enemas. The fluid may be delivered through a plastic or rubber catheter or IV line attached to a bottle or dose syringe. Enema buckets (Haver-Lockhart, Shawnee, KS), manufactured with an outlet valve, to which rubber tubing may be connected, are ideal for warm-water enemas (Fig 23). Insert the lubricated tubing into the rectum and advance it slowly and gently while the fluid is infused. The foal's fragile rectum can be torn or punctured if undue force is used during the procedure. Only a small amount (2-4 oz) of fluid should be infused so as to prevent overdistention of the rectum. After infusion, wait until the foal expels most of the fluid and repeat the procedure, if necessary.

Enemas in Adult Horses

Adult horses rarely need enemas, but enemas can be used to soften and remove feces in mares with perineal laceration repairs. Fecal material often collects cranial to the repair because of the discomfort during attempts to defecate. Warm water is infused through a medium-sized nasogastric tube, using a funnel or stomach pump for delivery. Large quantities (1-3 gal) of fluid can be infused, but administration should be intermittently interrupted to allow evacuation of feces. It may be necessary to repeat these enemas for several days until the discomfort subsides and the mare defecates unassisted.

Application of Limb Bandages

Bandages are commonly applied to the legs of horses to protect wounds and surgical incisions, and to prevent self-inflicted injury during training, racing, working or trailering. They provide support to the tendinous structures of the opposite weight-bearing limb when an injured leg cannot bear full weight. In emergency situations, bandages are used to control hemorrhage and support fractures until definitive treatment can be initiated. Certain types of bandages, in conjunction with sweats and poultices, help control limb edema. Because of their extensive use, it is important to be able to select appropriate materials and properly apply different types of bandages.

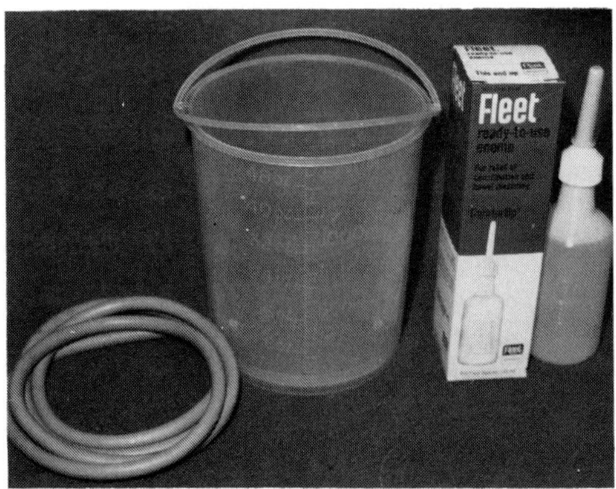

Figure 23. Enema units for use in foals. *Left:* Enema bucket with attached rubber tube. *Right:* Fleet enema.

Bandage Materials

The foundation of every leg bandage consists of good padding material. Failure to apply adequate padding under a bandage could result in injury from excessive pressure. Roll cotton is ideal as a bandage foundation. It is very soft and absorbent, and conforms well to the limb. It is available in 1-lb rolls and is relatively inexpensive. Sheet cotton is also used extensively. These broad, thin sheets of cotton may be layered to produce the amount of padding desired. Quilted pads may be purchased or prepared from mattress pads and used as shipping bandages. This type of padding is washable and may be reused numerous times.

The form of wrapping material used is based on the type of injury, cost of bandage materials, frequency of bandage changes, and personal preference. Roll gauze, available in several widths, does not stretch, and is relatively inexpensive. Elastic bandages (*eg,* Ace Bandage), also available in various widths, stretch and are washable, and conform well to the limb. "Derby" bandages, commonly used as shipping bandages, are made of cotton-knit material that stretches and is washable, and are available with ties or Velcro closures. Disposable elastic bandages (*eg,* Vetrap: 3M, Elastikon: Johnson & Johnson) are commonly used on equine limbs. Vetrap is made of crepe material that adheres to itself, while Elastikon adheres to nearly any surface. Kling (Johnson & Johnson) is a disposable, double-layered stretch gauze that conforms well to the limb and clings to itself.

Flannel is an inelastic, reusable material available in large sheets that can be cut to any size desired. Stockinette (Johnson & Johnson), a knit material manufactured as a tube bandage, is available in many sizes. It is often used under casts and is excellent for bandaging the head and neck. Adhesive tape is used primarily to secure the ends of bandages. It should not be used as the primary bandage material because of its tendency to tighten around the limb if the bandage shifts in position.

Bandaging Principles

The principles of bandaging should be followed closely so as to prevent injuries, strictures, or loosening of the bandage. As previously mentioned, failure to use adequate padding could produce tendinitis, particularly if the wrap is applied tightly. Pressure sores may occur, for the same reason, over bony prominences, such as the accessory carpal bone or tuber calcis. Even if the proper amount of padding is used, irritation may develop if wrinkles or folds are formed during bandage application. This may be prevented by applying both padding and wrapping material smoothly, snugly and in one (the same) direction. About an inch of padding must be left at the top and bottom of the bandage to avoid impairing blood circulation, which may occur if the wrapping material binds around the limb.

Derby bandages should be tied on the lateral aspect of the limb to prevent excessive tension over the extensor and flexor tendons. When knots are tied on the medial aspect of the limb, the horse may accidentally step on the ties and loosen the bandage. The ends of the bandage should be secured by taping them to the bandage. Adhesive tape should be applied, without tension, in a spiral around the bandage. If the tape is wrapped around the leg and reattached to itself, it could tighten and bind if the bandage slips, resulting in severe tendinitis. It is advisable to make a tab at the end of the tape by folding the end on itself so it may be easily located to facilitate bandage removal.

Bandage Types

Standing Bandage: A standing or support bandage is applied to the distal limb, from the distal carpus or tarsus to the hoof. Many trailering injuries occur at the level of the coronary band; therefore, it is imperative that this area be protected. The padding material should be wrapped securely around the limb and any wrinkles smoothed out to prevent irritation to underlying tissues (Fig 24A). The wrapping material is started at the level of the fetlock. It is wrapped snugly around the limb, working distad (toward the hoof) (Fig 24B). Including the bulbs of the heel in the bandage holds it more securely in place. The wrap is then worked proximad (upward), toward the carpus or tarsus, relaxing the tension somewhat over the tendons. The bandage is completed with adhesive tape applied in a spiral around the bandage (Fig 24C). The standing bandage is often used as a base, upon which other bandages are built; therefore, application of this bandage must be mastered before attempting to apply other types.

Carpal / Tarsal Bandages: Extensive practice is required to properly apply bandages over the carpal and tarsal joints so that they remain secure, without producing pressure sores over the bony prominences in these areas. To prevent slippage of these bandages, a standing bandage is applied as previously described. A "stovepipe" bandage, which overlaps the standing bandage by several inches, is then applied.

Another method of bandaging the carpus/tarsus uses roll cotton and gauze (or elastic bandages) in the standing bandage, with a similar bandage applied proximad (Fig 25A). The 2 bandages are then "tied in" by placing a sheet cotton bandage over the junction of the original 2 bandages and wrapping the entire leg with a third gauze roll (Figs 25B, 25C). Excessive pressure over the accessory carpal bone and tuber calcis can be avoided by creating a slit through the bandage in this area (Fig 25C).

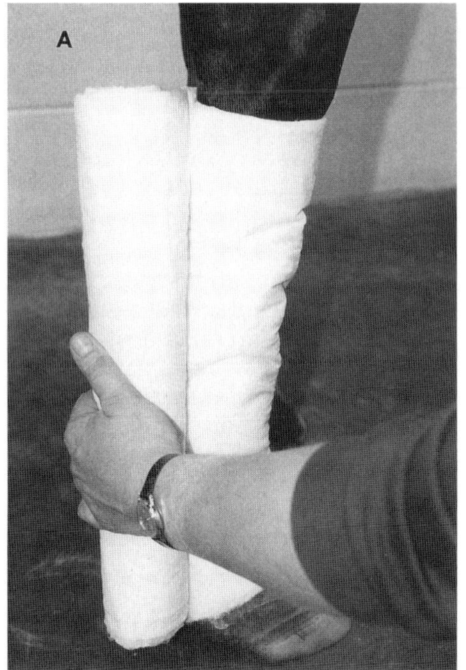

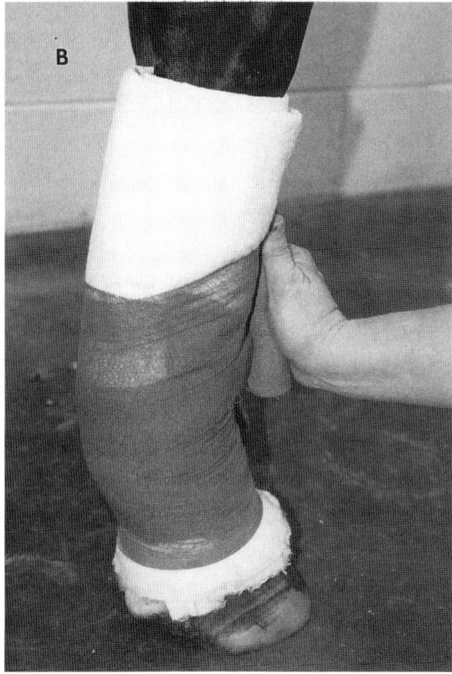

Figure 24. The standing bandage. A. Padding material is wrapped smoothly and snugly around the limb, from the proximal metacarpus/metatarsus, distally to the ground. B. The wrapping material is started at the level of the fetlock and progresses toward the hoof, leaving at least 1 inch of cotton uncovered. C. The wrap is applied proximally toward the carpus/tarsus, somewhat relaxing the tension over the tendons. Adhesive tape is then applied over the gauze in a spiral fashion, ending with a tab on the lateral aspect of the bandage.

Use of arthroscopic surgery in horses has resulted in a shortened recovery period and minimal postsurgical wound care. For this reason, a much lighter bandage can be applied after arthroscopy. These postsurgical bandages consist of a nonadhesive dressing, followed by gauze and adhesive bandage material. When bandaging the carpus or tarsus, apply each layer of the bandage in a figure-8 pattern to allow more flexibility and reduce the possibility of excessive tension in any one area that could result in pressure sores (Fig 26).

Foot Bandage: The primary reason a bandage is applied to a foot is to keep it clean. In cases where a subsolar abscess has been diagnosed, the foot is pared out, producing an open area on the bottom of the foot. The abscess is treated, after which a medication boot or bandage must be applied. The bandage material used may be an adhesive wrap, such as Elastikon (Johnson & Johnson), or household duct tape. When applying this bandage, avoid placing excessive pressure around the coronary band. Apply enough material on the bottom of the foot and around the edges of the hoof so the bandage does not wear through before the next treatment (Fig 27).

Support Bandages: The prognosis of a fractured leg may be affected by the type of support bandage applied before transport of the patient; therefore, knowledge of emergency bandage application is important. With a compound fracture (bone exits the skin), the wound should be covered with a very clean or, preferably, a

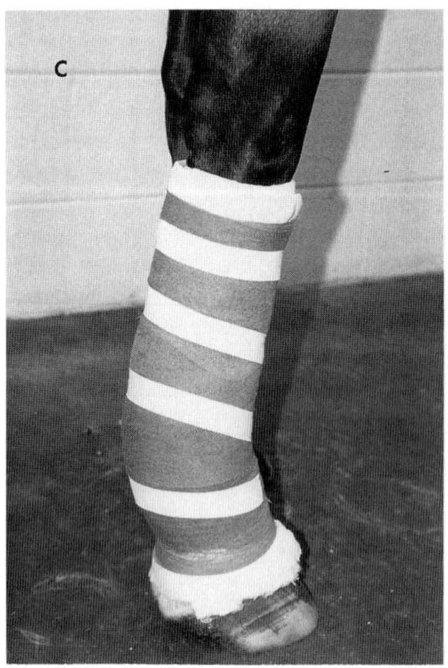

Figure 24, continued.

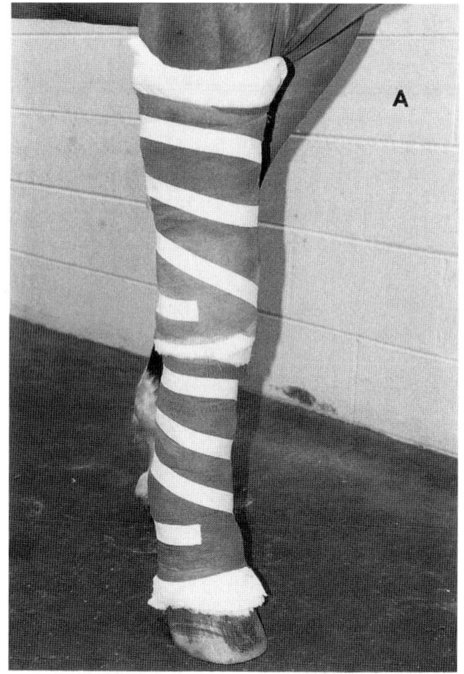

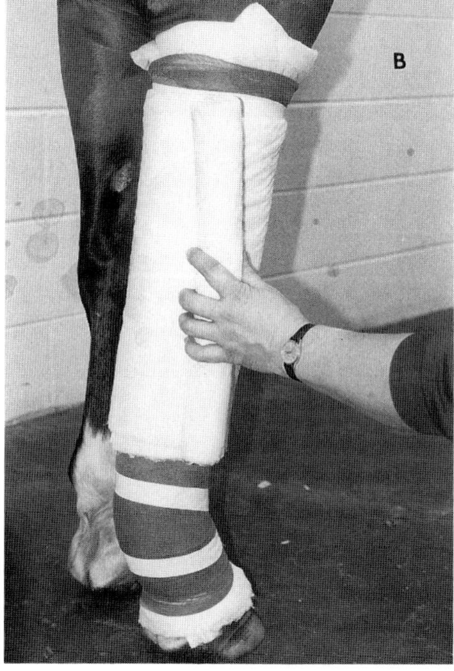

Figure 25. Carpal bandage. A. A standing bandage of cotton and gauze is applied to the distal limb and a similar bandage applied proximal to it. B. These 2 bandages are "tied in" by applying sheet cotton over the junction of the underlying bandage. C. The bandage is completed by wrapping another roll of gauze over the bandage. A slit in the bandage over the accessory carpal bone helps prevent pressure wounds in this area.

sterile wrap. Soaps or detergents should not be used to clean such wounds, nor should ointments be applied if surgical intervention is being considered.

When a fractured limb is bandaged, the joints proximal and distal to (above and below) the fracture site must be immobilized by application of large amounts of padding and tightly wrapped bandages. Up to 12 1-lb rolls of cotton may be used in these bandages. If the usual bandage materials are not available, several large pillows and 4- to 6-inch strips of a bed sheet may be used. The leg may be further stabilized by incorporating broom sticks or small boards into the bandage. This type of emergency bandage is referred to as a Robert Jones bandage.

Ointments, powders, dressings or sterile wound dressings may be applied beneath the previously mentioned bandages. A leg sweat may be applied to the skin beneath the bandage to "sweat out" fluid that may accumulate in interstitial tissues. Such sweats often contain equal parts of alcohol and glycerin. After this substance is massaged into the leg, an impermeable wrap, such as Saran Wrap or a plastic OB sleeve, is applied smoothly and evenly, followed by a standing bandage. This sweat bandage is left in place for 12-24 hours, after which it may be removed or reapplied.

Poultices: Poultices are also used to remove excessive fluid from inflamed tissues. Poultice application involves applying a thick

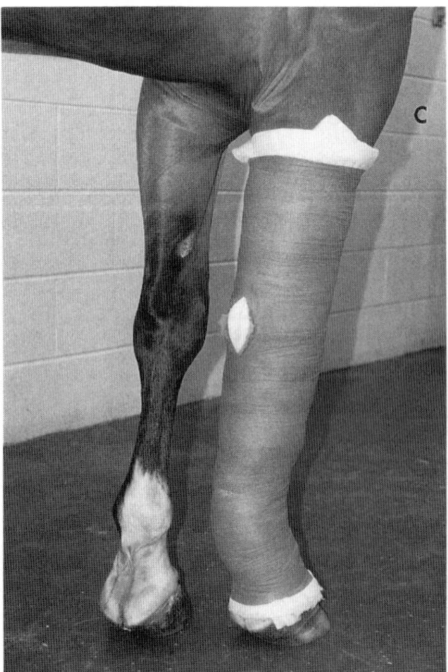

Figure 25, continued.

layer of the poultice material over the affected area, smoothing it on gently with damp hands and covering it with a plastic wrap and then an appropriate bandage. The poultice is left in place for 12-24 hours, after which it is rinsed off and reapplied if necessary.

Casts: Casts are sometimes used instead of bandages. They are most frequently used to stabilize fractures following fracture reduction (manipulative realignment) and/or surgical fixation. Foals with angular limb deformities may have casts applied. Because most foals adjust to casts very well, this form of stabilization may be superior to bandages, especially when pressure sores develop from bandaging these young patients. Casts may also be used on horses with chronic, slow-healing wounds, for which repeated bandage changes could be very expensive.

Before cast application, the leg is cleaned and covered with a double layer of stockinette, and orthopedic felt is fastened around the coronary band and the point at which the cast will terminate. Many types of cast material are available; selection is based on the desired weight of the completed cast, frequency of cast changes and personal preference. Though the veterinarian usually applies the cast, the technician should be able to prepare the limb and the materials required for completion of the procedure.

Splints: Splints may be applied over bandages to further reduce limb flexion or extension. It is very important to apply adequate

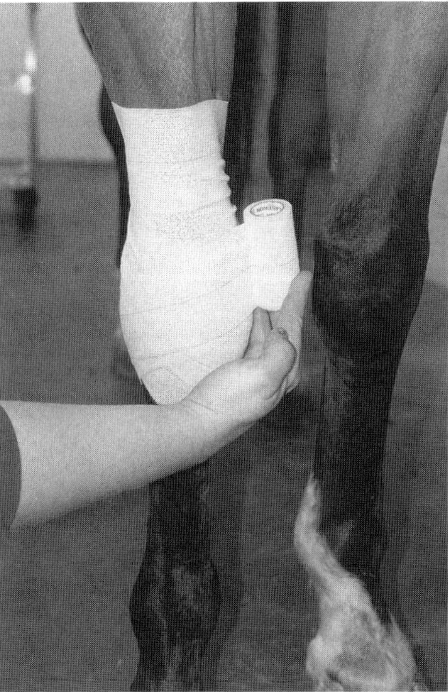

Figure 26. Applying a light, protective bandage in a figure 8 around a joint allows more flexibility and reduces excessive pressure over any one area of the limb.

Figure 27. To prevent the bandage on a foot from wearing through, apply several layers of material over the weight-bearing edges of the hoof.

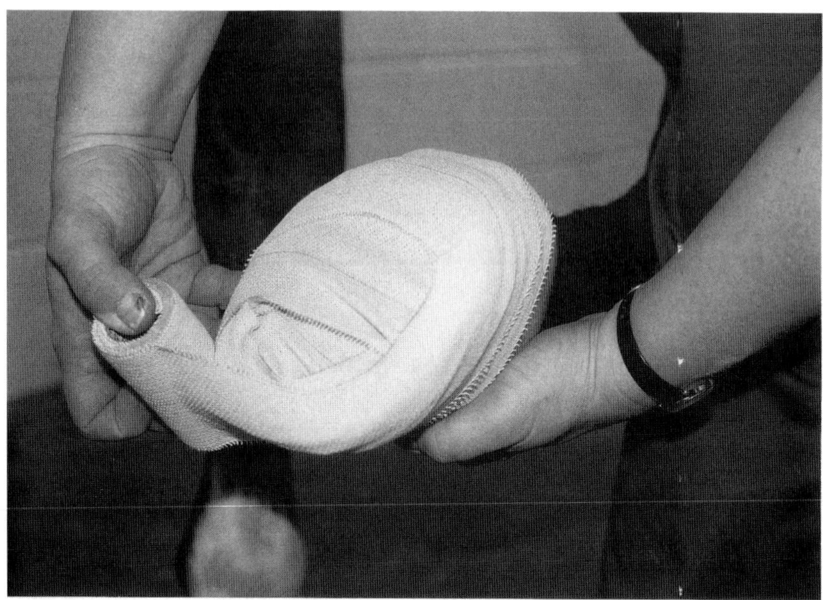

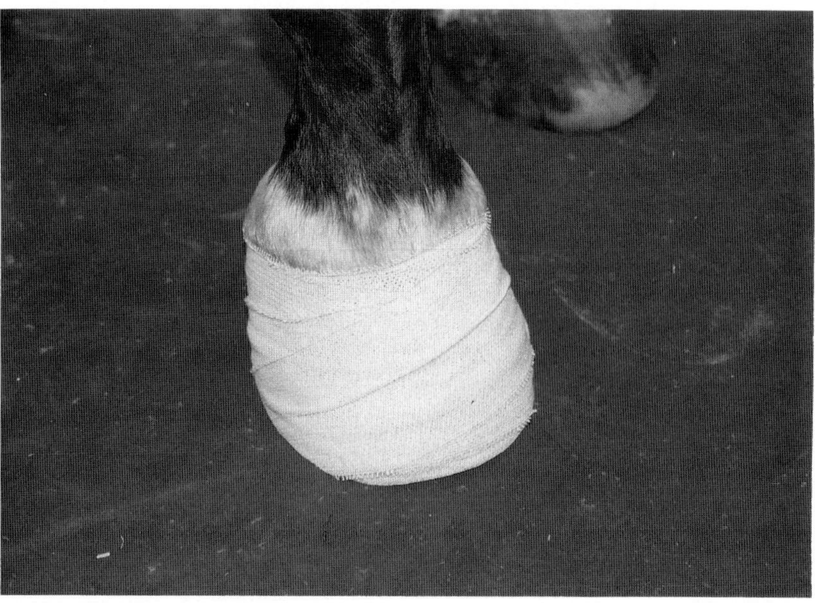

padding beneath the splint to prevent severe pressure sores. Splints may be prepared from broom handles, boards or longitudinal halves of PVC (plastic) drain pipe. The PVC pipe is available in many sizes at most plumbing or hardware stores and may be cut to an appropriate length and width with a cast-cutting saw. The selected splint material is then applied over the well-padded bandage with adhesive bandage or tape.

Application of Abdominal Bandages

Abdominal bandages are most frequently applied to support and protect incisions after abdominal surgery. These bandages usually consist of a sterile bandage applied over the incision, and gauze wrapped around the abdomen, followed by an adhesive bandage material. The bandage should be applied tightly to support the abdomen during healing.

Because these large bandages are comparatively expensive, they are changed only when necessary. Many horses resent having their hair pulled upon removal of an adhesive bandage. For this reason, nonadhesive gauze is applied beneath an adhesive bandage, except at the cranial and caudal ends to facilitate removal. If the patient continues to object, application of ether to the sticky underside of the adhesive bandage during removal helps loosen it with little discomfort to the horse.

Application of Tail Bandages

Tail wraps may be applied to prevent the hair from being soiled with loose feces and to retract the tail during breeding, genitourinary tract or rectal examinations or when working on the hind limbs. Using gauze or elastic bandage material, the wrap is started at the tailhead and continued caudad to the last coccygeal vertebra. The bandage may be completed at this point or the tail may be folded craniad and included in the bandage (Fig 28). If the bandages must stay in place for several hours or days, it may be further secured by including a few tail hairs in the first few wraps of the bandage.

Tail bandages must not be applied too tightly, especially if they are to be left in place for several hours, as the circulation may be impaired, resulting in ischemic necrosis and sloughing of the tail.

Preventing Self-Mutilation

Complications may result from improper bandaging, as previously mentioned, but self-mutilation may also occur when the patient attempts to remove its own bandage. This may be prevented by the use of bibs, cradles and cross-ties (see Chapter 2). Bibs allow free movement while preventing the animal from reaching the bandage with its teeth. Cradles restrict flexion of the neck, preventing the horse from reaching its limbs. Cross-ties, attached to the stall walls, hold the horse's head in a central location so that lateral movement is nearly eliminated and flexion is severely restricted. Some horses may work their way around these obstacles, however. In these instances, application of a red-pepper paste or tabasco sauce to the external surface of the bandage often prevents chewing on it.

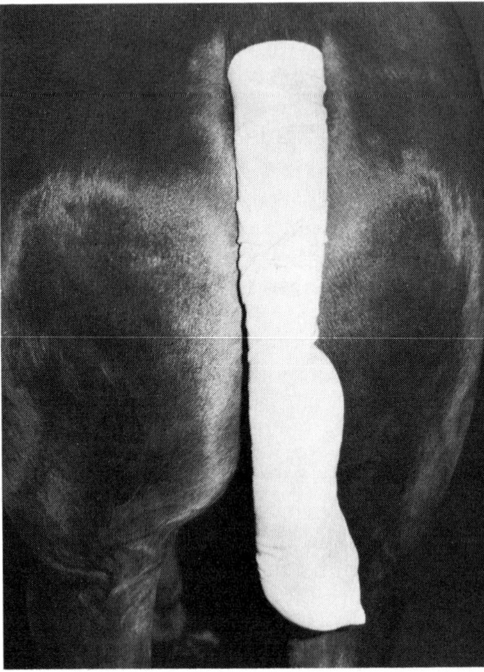

Figure 28. Tail wrap. This bandage incorporates the folded distal ends of the tail hairs.

Recommended Reading

Anon: *Giving Medication: A Nursing Photobook.* Intermediate Communications, Horsham, PA.

Bayly WM and Vale BH: Intravenous catheterization and associated problems in the horse. *Compend Cont Ed* 4: S227-S237, 1982.

PHYSICAL THERAPY

M. Porter

Physical therapy, as applied to horses, is used to prevent injury or disease and to aid in recovery from injury or disease. Methods or modalities include use of cold, heat, electricity, light, sound, water, magnetic fields, massage and exercise. Modalities are applied to reduce or eliminate the sensation of pain, to enhance tissue healing, and to improve the ability of a body part to move through its normal range of motion.

The techniques and tools of physical therapy have the potential for doing harm. No modality that can create a biological change is innocuous. One must thoroughly understand the tool and thoroughly evaluate the injury to create the desired effects. Also, knowledge of the physiology of tissue repair and an understanding of the pain response are important.

Veterinarians have only recently begun to include physical therapy in treatment of injuries to horses. The promise of increased performance potential, rapid recovery from injury, and prevention of reinjury has drawn attention to physical therapy techniques for horses. Decreasing turnout space and the desire to avoid extensive drug use have also prompted interest in these techniques.

Hundreds of articles in athletic training and physical therapy journals describe the effects of ultrasound, electrical stimulation, and other modalities. An increasing number of studies are appearing in veterinary journals. Anyone attempting to use physical therapy should acquaint himself with the current scientific literature. The references listed at the end of this chapter offer an entry to the literature.

The Role of the Equine Therapist

Physical therapy fits comfortably in the equine health care scheme. The role of the equine therapist can be compared with that of the athletic trainer or sports therapist in human sports medicine. The athletic trainer works cooperatively with the physician and the coach, implementing conditioning and rehabilitation programs for the athletes. The athletic trainer or sports therapist applies therapeutic modalities to ease the discomfort of injury and facilitate exercise following the physician's evaluation of injury. As more people, of varying backgrounds, become interested in equine therapy as a career, it becomes necessary to delineate the requirements of an equine therapist. The knowledge and personal qualities of the therapist determine the success of treatment to some extent.

Qualities of the Equine Therapist

The equine therapist must have good horsemanship skills. An equine therapist must be able to detect subtle lameness and discomfort in the horse. One must be aware of hazardous situations around the barn and help correct them. One must give full attention to each equine patient during the work day.

The equine therapist must recognize that the horse is an athlete. Personal experience as an athlete or involvement in fitness activities gives the equine therapist insight into such concepts as overuse injury and the process of rehabilitation. An equine therapist must have curiosity about the rehabilitation process and be willing to devote time and energy to study in this field.

An equine therapist must have knowledge of equine anatomy and physiology, pharmacology and nutrition, sports medicine and modality use. College-level courses in physical therapy or athletic training, coupled with certain veterinary courses, provide educational basics. One must be dedicated enough to read scientific journals and books in several fields to gain knowledge about therapy. Finally, one must be experienced in use of therapeutic modalities and know their indications and contraindications.

The Modalities

The tools and techniques of equine physical therapy should be applied as part of complete management of the condition. Therapeutic modalities are useful in the relief of clinical signs and in improving function of the affected area. Pain-free function is important in avoiding secondary complications related to connective tissue adhesions.

Massage and Stretching

Massage involves use of the fingers, hands and elbows to manipulate soft tissues. Manual stroking, pressing, tapping, kneading and knuckling increase local circulation and lymphatic drainage. Massage stretches superficial muscles and tendon fibers and can help maintain mobility as these tissues remodel in response to training.

Deep tissue massage is the preferred technique when massaging a horse (Fig 29). Equine musculature has considerable depth and muscle tension is deep seated. Deep tissue massage requires strength and accuracy of finger placement. Tissue is moved at right angles to the long axis of the fibers to reduce adhesion formation between the fibers.

Stretching exercises should follow deep tissue massage. Manual or controlled active exercises can be used. When one thinks of controlled exercises for the horse, work on the lunge line, hand walking, and controlling speed under saddle come to mind. These exercises develop or maintain the horse's muscle strength or cardiovascular endurance. Addition of manual stretching may be necessary to increase flexibility (Fig 30).

Optimal flexibility is an aspect of fitness often overlooked in equine athletics. Flexibility, or the ability of a body part to move

Figure 29. Deep tissue massage.

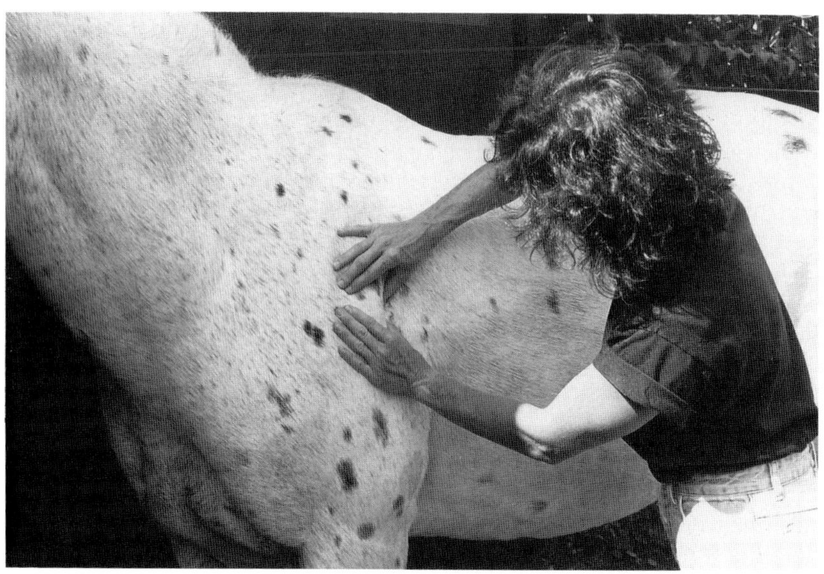

Figure 30. Gentle manual stretching increases joint range of motion.

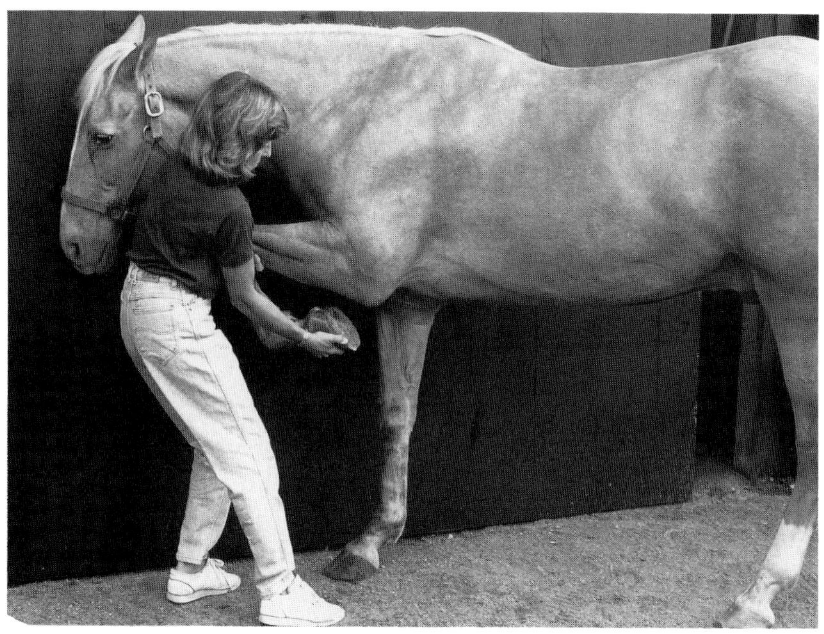

through a complete range of motion, is an important component of injury rehabilitation. Limited range of motion can be a result of muscle splinting or bracing to protect an injured part, or from scar tissue formation within the muscle after injury. Adhesions within the connective tissues interfere with joint mobility, straining related joints and muscles and compromising their function.

Stretching exercises can be used to detect muscle soreness or weight-bearing problems. Before lameness develops, a horse may exhibit an imbalance in joint and muscle flexibility that could be detected with manual stretching.

A combination of massage and stretching helps increase the range of motion and inhibits adhesion formation in muscle tissue. Rapid restoration of function is more important in athletic rehabilitation than pain-free rest. Correct use of these techniques can promote a shorter rehabilitation period and an earlier return to exercise.

Therapeutic Ultrasound

Therapeutic ultrasound is used to elevate the temperature of deep tissue. Because of its large energy output, ultrasound has the potential to benefit or harm the horse. Ultrasound produces heat, so a complete veterinary evaluation is necessary to determine the status of healing and to identify the tissues involved in the injury.

Therapeutic ultrasound is not to be confused with *diagnostic* ultrasound. Diagnostic ultrasound uses a lower level of power and produces no heating effects. At up to 20 watts of power output, therapeutic ultrasound can raise intramuscular temperature 3 degrees centigrade and bone cortex 3.9 degrees centigrade using 1 watt/cm^2 for 1 minute.

The sonic wave frequency from diagnostic units ranges from 1 mHz (1 million cycles per second) to 10 mHz. Therapeutic units manufactured in America today operate at a frequency of 1 mHz, an appropriate frequency for absorption of energy by the tissues. (There is an inverse relationship between beam absorption and hertz level. When the hertz level is high, there is greater scattering of the sound beam in the tissues. At 1 mHz, the beam's energy is readily absorbed.)

Ultrasound generates high-frequency sound waves by converting electrical energy to mechanical energy. This mechanical energy flows through the tissues in compression waves that are absorbed or reflected. The molecular concussion of the wave produces heat. Applying a high-frequency, low-voltage alternating electrical current to a crystal with piezo-electrical properties creates ultrasound waves. This crystal is cemented to a thin layer of metal on the inside surface of the applicator, called a *sound head.* The crystal expands and contracts in time with the cycles of electrical current.

Pressure waves caused by these vibrations pass from the sound head into the body tissues. These pressure waves move in a straight line from the source. This differs from audible sounds in that the sounds we hear are vibrations that are propagated in all directions from the source.

Tissues of high collagen content readily absorb therapeutic ultrasound waves (Fig 31). Because of its affinity for collagenous structures, ultrasound can be used to selectively heat certain tissues, such as superficial cortical bone, periosteum and joint structures (ligaments, menisci, synovium, capsule).

Of soft tissues, muscle absorbs the most heat, allowing heating of myofascial interfaces, tendons and nerves. Because tissues of the dermis absorb little energy, skin surface temperature does not increase. This may lead the novice operator to increase the intensity beyond proper therapeutic levels. Heat on the skin surface indicates inadequate transmission gel or inconsistent contact of the sound head and skin surface.

Ultrasound waves are reflected when they encounter an interface of 2 tissues that absorb sound differently. Reflected waves add to the intensity of the sound beam at that point. "Hot spots" can cause endothelial damage.

As a rule, bone reflects about 70% of sound waves reaching it. As 30% of this energy is absorbed by the bone, the periosteum is sub-

Figure 31. Ultrasound application.

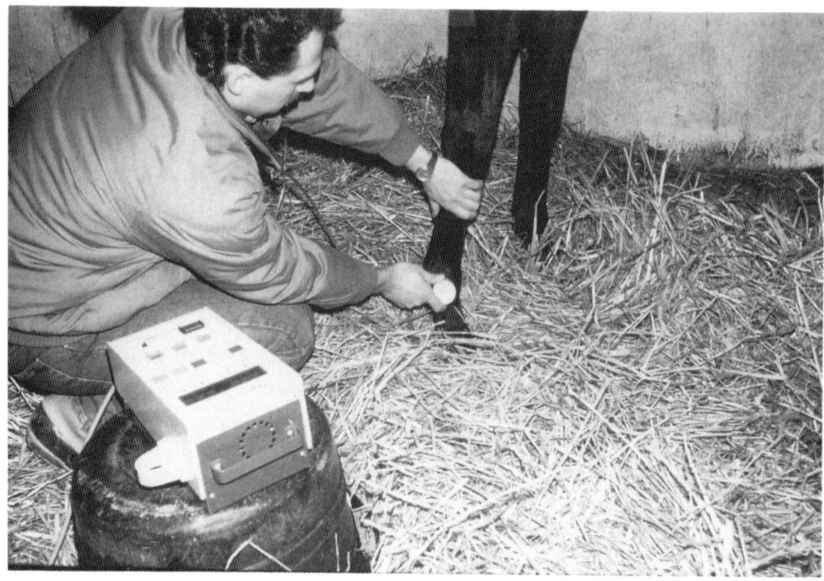

ject to energy entering and leaving it. The reflected wave passing through the periosteum can cause overheating and may create a dull aching pain.[1] Horses and people do not react immediately to this type of pain, and tissue burning may occur before the operator becomes aware. Maintaining proper treatment levels and remaining attentive during treatment sessions are important when applying ultrasound. When used correctly, ultrasound produces no sensation.

Heating Effects of Ultrasound: The thermal effects of ultrasound are comparable to other forms of heat. Ultrasound is unique in that its effects reach much more deeply than those of hot packs, massage or whirlpools. The principal physiologic effects of heat are increased cellular metabolic rate, vasodilation, increased extensibility in collagen, increased membrane permeability, and an increased pain threshold.

Mechanical Effects of Ultrasound: In addition to increasing tissue temperature, mechanical activity of the sound wave stimulates other cell processes. In the ultrasonic field the tissue components oscillate and flow as the compression wave moves into the tissue. This flowing movement, driven by the sound wave, impacts the membrane of cells and membranes of organelles within the cells, causing them to become more permeable. Diffusion across cell membranes is accelerated. No other heating modality can create this effect. By stimulating the diffusion process, ultrasound can help remove the debris of injury and enhance tissue repair.

Restoring Joint Range of Motion: Early restoration of full joint range of motion is of primary importance in recovery from surgery or injury. The heating and mechanical effects of ultrasound render newly formed scar more susceptible to remodeling by stretching forces.

Phonophoresis: An ultrasound beam can force substances through the skin and into the underlying tissue. *Phonophoresis* is the use of ultrasound to enhance the dispersion of topical or injected medications throughout the underlying soft tissues. The major medications used in phonophoresis are antiinflammatory agents and anesthetics. Hydrocortisone is used in most phonophoresis treatments.[2]

Contraindications: Ultrasound applications just above the therapeutic dosage cause a variety of problems. Overheating bone causes pain. Using an excessively high intensity level or holding the sound head stationary causes this to occur. Excessive use does not speed healing.[3]

Ultrasound is not dangerous if the operator carefully follows the treatment rules and understands the capabilities of ultrasound.

Therapeutic Electricity

The essentially electric nature of the body must be appreciated when using therapeutic modalities, whether on horses or people. No modality more clearly illustrates this than therapeutic electricity.

Therapeutic electricity is used to create muscle contractions, to stimulate sensory nerves for pain inhibition, to increase local blood flow, and to stimulate wound healing. Therapeutic gains from electrically stimulating muscle contractions include muscle re-education, retardation of atrophy, and muscle strengthening (Fig 32).

Muscle Stimulation: Immobilization is widely used in horses and people. Muscle tissue atrophies and has reduced contraction force following prolonged disuse or restricted joint mobility, as when a limb is placed in a cast or bandage. Electrical muscle stimulation is used to retard atrophy and to maintain muscle integrity following an injury or surgery. For example, after knee surgery in people, profound inhibition occurs in the quadriceps muscle. Often the patient cannot lift his leg for several days after surgery. Patients receiving electrical stimulation have increased muscle function and less atrophy than those doing exercise alone.[4]

Stall rest is often used following injury to horses. During stall confinement, disuse atrophy and adhesions occur in unused muscles. Electrical stimulation induces rhythmic muscle contraction

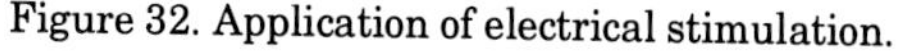

Figure 32. Application of electrical stimulation.

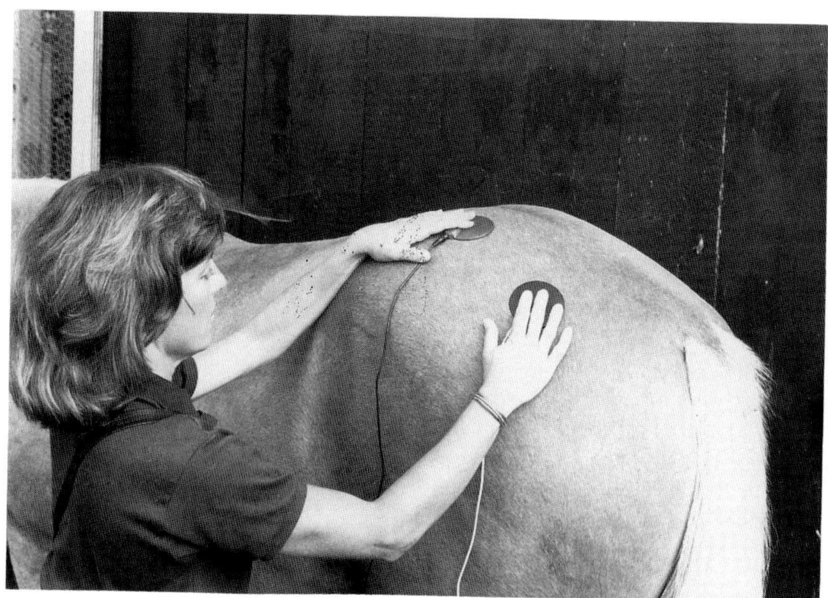

and relaxation and maintains muscle fiber volume, muscle blood volume, and contractile enzyme volume. A combination of electrical stimulation and controlled exercise is superior to stall rest.

Pain Control: Electrical stimulation may help manage degenerative joint disease in horses. Signs include pain and swelling around the joint. Electrical stimulation relieves many types of pain, including that of rheumatoid arthritis and osteoarthritis. Stimulation of nerves in the joint capsule suppresses pain. Electrical stimulation also has a direct effect on synovial fluid volume and reduces leukocyte count in the joint.[5] A histologic section from an unstimulated arthritic synovial membrane shows massive leukocytic infiltration and congested capillaries.

Electrical stimulation is useful in locating muscle soreness in horses. The horse's body language and facial gestures indicate when active trigger points or acupuncture points have been stimulated. These can be used as indicators of areas of soreness. Treating the affected trigger points reduces the pain response considerably.

Increased Local Circulation: Circulation can be stimulated through the pumping action created by rhythmic muscle contractions. Blood flow is increased through a rhythmically contracting muscle, whether it is voluntarily or electrically stimulated. Edema fluid resulting from damage to the vascular structures or loss of normal muscular activity is absorbed.

Swelling around a joint limits the joint's range of movement. Swelling can be caused by excessive intraarticular synovial fluid, excessive fluid in the bursae surrounding the joint, and fluid around the tendon inside the tendon sheath. Standard first-aid practice to control swelling uses ice, compression and elevation. Because one cannot practically elevate a horse's distal extremities, electrical stimulation can be of great help in augmenting the effects of cooling and compression. Following the acute phase of injury, electrostimulation can be used to dilate local blood vessels. This accelerates delivery of nutrients and resorption of blood plasma and interstitial fluid into the venous blood.

Wound Healing: Wounds of soft tissue are repaired by a dynamic process of epithelialization, cell regeneration, scar formation and tissue contraction. Successful repair depends on the animal's general state of health and nutrition. Other factors include an adequate blood supply to the wound, and an absence of infection and physical barriers, such as foreign particles or dead tissue. Passage of electrical current through a wound stimulates protein synthesis, transport of free amino acids, and generation of ATP.[6]

Contraindications: There are few contraindications or cautions associated with use of therapeutic electrical current. Do not apply electrodes over abraded or lacerated skin, as the current produces an uncomfortable sensation because of lowered skin impedance.

Also, the wound may become contaminated. When treating injuries, the operator should avoid thinking that "more is better" and should not increase the current until the horse is uncomfortable.

Therapeutic Laser

The laser is a somewhat new tool, developed in the 1960s. Because of lack of FDA approval, the laser is considered an experimental tool in human physical therapy.

Lasers used for therapy are called *cold* or *low-power lasers*. The energy level is so low that temperature in treated tissue does not rise above normal body temperature. They produce a form of radiant energy that falls in the near-infrared portion of the electromagnetic spectrum.

A laser alters light to increase its speed and its energy so that it can penetrate skin. Two types of low-power lasers are commonly used. The infrared *gallium arsonide* type has a wavelength of 904 nanometers (nm). The *helium neon* type has a visible red beam in the wavelength of 632 nm.

Gallium arsonide crystals are a synthetic substance that emits light when stimulated by electricity. Manufacturers advertise the peak power of gallium arsonide lasers as 2 watts. Because of the pulsing of the beam and the brevity of the pulses (200 nanoseconds), the average power used is only 0.2 milliwatts or less.

Helium neon lasers amplify light by passing it through a gas-filled tube with multiple silver resonator mirrors. The altered light is transmitted through a flexible monofilament fiberoptic system to the tip of the hand-held wand.

Laser therapy is used to treat superficial wounds and injuries near the skin surface (Fig 33). Laser energy is absorbed to a greater extent in dark or pigmented tissue. Infrared modalities, which include hot and cold packs or hot and cold whirlpools, penetrate 1 cm or less. Laser light penetrates 1-3 mm. Longer wavelengths of laser light have deeper penetration. Denser tissues allow less penetration. Skin cells are stimulated by absorption of laser light.

Pain Relief: A primary use of laser is pain relief. Laser is used for direct stimulation of a painful site or to stimulate related nerves and acupuncture and trigger points. One study showed that a helium neon laser slowed nerve conduction, similar to the effect of cooling, suggesting the possible mechanism of pain relief often reported with this modality.[7]

Laser is used as a noninvasive form of acupuncture. In a study using horses, laser-stimulated acupuncture points produced the same results as needle acupuncture.[8] Laser stimulation raised the skin resistance to electricity and stimulated release of endogenous opiates.[9] For this technique the operator must be precise in point location and knowledgeable of acupuncture theory.

Wound Healing: Laser can be used to stimulate the repair of nonhealing ulcers and to accelerate healing of skin wounds. (Nonhealing wounds are those that do not respond to conventional therapies.) Patients with wounds that had not healed for many years healed completely with a few months of laser therapy.[10] Increased strength of healed tissue, accelerated healing of burns, increased phagocytic activity of leukocytes, and increased collagen synthesis have been reported.[11,12]

When injury occurs, current flows between the injury site and the local lymph and blood vessels. This current signals the body to bring in the chemicals and cells needed for healing. Application of electrons from an external source can trigger this effect.

Contraindications: There are few contraindications to use of cold lasers. The cold laser, with less than 1 milliwatt of power, is an insignificant risk to people unless held close to the cornea of the eye. Research describing damage to the cornea used higher-intensity lasers than those available for use in horses; nonetheless, the eye should be avoided during laser therapy.

Many laser manufacturers place a warning in their operating manuals advising the operator to avoid using the laser in patients treated with certain drugs. Such drugs as cortisone, furacin and iodine are light sensitive and their effects on tissue may be altered

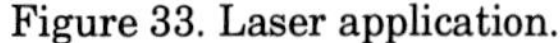

Figure 33. Laser application.

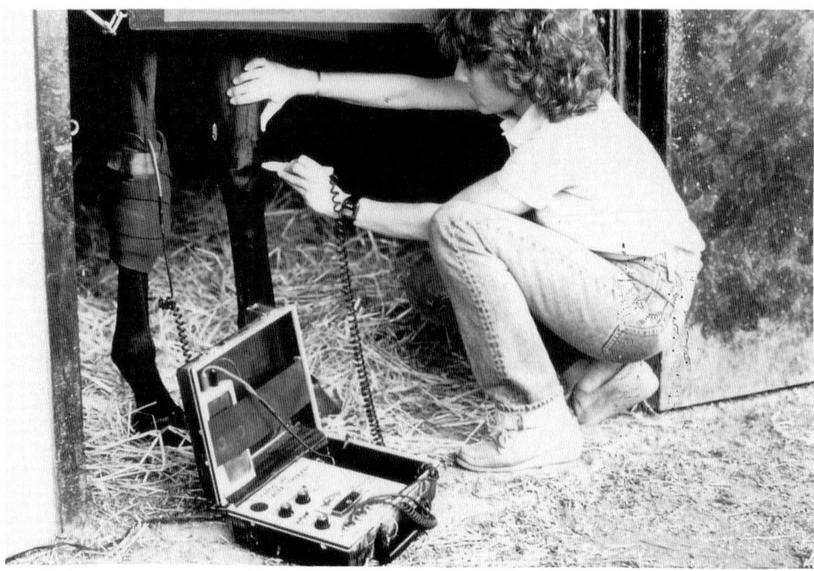

when exposed to laser light. This effect is undocumented in the scientific literature, but avoiding the interaction is a reasonable precaution.

Lasers can be misused if applied without a complete veterinary examination. Pain is nature's signal of a problem. If the signal is ignored or covered up through pain-reduction techniques, the problem may become untreatable or more difficult to treat successfully.

Magnetic Therapy

Magnets were used in ancient cultures, such as the Egyptian and the Chinese, for thousands of years. The therapeutic effects of magnets were described in this country as early as 1938, by a researcher who applied an electromagnet over a painful area. In this study, the pain subsided or disappeared after magnet treatment, documenting the value of magnets for pain relief.[13]

Instruments that make use of permanent magnets (*static magnets*) or magnetic fields with a superimposed electric field (*electromagnets*) are applied for pain relief. Changes in nerve membrane permeability and decreases in sodium pump activity have been documented.[14] Clinical findings include pain relief and reduction in posttraumatic edema. Edema reduction results from increased circulation in the vessels within the magnetic field. Charged particles in the blood flowing through the magnetic field deflect at right angles to the field, causing turbulence of the blood within the vessel. This turbulence increases flow velocity across the diameter of the vessel. A recent unpublished scintigraphic study showed increased circulation and metabolic activity in soft tissue and bone within a magnetic field.[15]

Highly specific pulsing electromagnetic fields have been of great scientific interest in orthopedics for the past 15 years. Research centers on osteogenesis, particularly of non-union fractures and pseudoarthrosis. In 1979, the FDA approved use of magnetic fields in treating recalcitrant fractures, but this is the only approved use in human medicine to date.

Examples of Application

Painful conditions that diminish performance and limit but do not completely incapacitate the horse are commonly seen wherever horses are in use. In human athletes, physical therapy techniques are used to help control painful conditions and promote rapid return of function. These same techniques can also be useful in rehabilitation of equine injuries.

An example of a typical case referred from the veterinarian to the equine therapist could include the following findings:

During a recent event a 12-yr-old gelding failed to clear a jump. Though the horse did not fall and was unhurt from the incident, initial examination revealed back muscle soreness and soreness in the right hock. Radiographs of the hocks revealed no fractures. The rider complains that the horse has not been performing up to his former ability, but no specific injury is diagnosed.

The therapist first becomes acquainted with the horse through palpation of the musculature to detect muscle splinting and to look for a twitch response in a tight band of muscle. An electrical stimulator could be used to seek out areas of muscle soreness by moving the electrodes slowly over the body surface, and watching the horse's facial expressions and "body language." Electrically induced contraction of a sore muscle elicits a change in the horse's facial expression or body language. Where soreness is noted, therapeutic electricity can be used to reduce the pain and spasm. In this particular horse, pain and spasm were detected along the muscles of the back and hip, especially on the right side.

Electrical currents are especially useful for reducing the muscle splinting that occurs as the horse tries to guard a sore area of the body. In this horse, reluctance to use the right rear leg through its full range of motion has caused splinting along the right side. Splinting of the back and hip muscles prevented muscle contractions powerful enough to propel the horse over the jump. A program designed to increase range of motion in the right rear leg and reduce back muscle soreness would include daily electrical stimulation to the trigger points found in the large muscle groups of the hip and back, followed by gentle stretching.

The equine therapist should spend time watching the horse at work to see how the injury affects the animal's ability to function optimally. In this horse, slight dragging of the right rear leg was noted at the trot. Further questioning of the owner provided information that the horse had been cast in his stall a year ago; this had resulted in a very swollen right hock. It was concluded that the wear and tear of steady training had caused some joint surface degeneration in this previously traumatized joint. The discomfort involved in moving this joint through its full range of motion had resulted in atrophy in the right gluteus muscle. The joint condition could be addressed with ultrasound applications to the hock joint and application of a magnetic hock wrap. Electrical stimulation would aid in restoring gluteal muscle volume.

Another interesting observation is asymmetry in the biceps muscles of the front legs, with the left leg hypertrophied as compared with the right. The left radial artery is enlarged compared with the right, indicating overuse of the left limb. The subtle muscle imbalances indicate how effectively the horse is able to compensate for areas of weakness or discomfort. Through use of physical therapy, these areas can be made less painful, while function is restored through range-of-motion exercises and carefully balanced riding.

The equine therapist could contribute significantly to the comfort of a horse suffering from laminitis. A typical example is a broodmare with laminitis and abscesses in the front feet. Constant weight shifting to the rear legs has resulted in soreness in the rear musculature. Electrical stimulation to these muscles can reduce discomfort temporarily, but the therapist must also consider providing pain relief to the feet. Abscesses can be resolved more quickly with application of ultrasound to the coronary band twice daily. Ultrasound can also be applied underwater if the feet are being soaked in warm water. Electrical stimulation to the coronary band reduces hoof pain and increases blood flow to the foot. Laser application could be used to stimulate acupuncture points to increase blood flow to the feet, as well as to acupuncture points related to hip and back soreness.

Physical therapy treatments are usually carried out on a daily basis. For optimum effectiveness, physical therapy should follow a careful veterinary diagnosis and be applied with specific goals in mind. It is beyond the scope of this chapter to teach the application of physical therapy techniques. Until a college-level course in equine therapy is established, the equine therapist must pursue human physical therapy studies to gain an understanding of the array of instruments and techniques that could be applied to horses.

References

1. Gersten JW: Effect of metallic objects on temperature rises produced in tissue by ultrasound. *Am J Phys Med* 37:75-82, 1958.
2. Quillen WS: Phonophoresis: A review of the literature and technique. *Athletic Training* Summer:109-110, 1980.
3. Oakley EM: Dangers and contraindications of therapeutic ultrasound. *Physiotherap* 64:171-174, 1978.
4. Eriksson E and Haggmark T: Comparison of isometric muscle training and electrical stimulation supplementing isometric muscle training in the recovery after major knee ligament surgery. *Am J Sports Med* 7:169-171, 1979.
5. Abelson K *et al:* Transcutaneous electrical nerve stimulation in rheumatoid arthritis. *N Zeal Med J* 96:156-158, 1983.
6. Cheng N *et al:* The effects of electric currents on ATP generation, protein synthesis, and membrane transport in rats. *Clin Ortho Rel Res* 171:264-272, 1982.
7. Snyder-Mackler AL and Bork CE: Effect of helium-neon laser irradiation on peripheral sensory nerve latency. *Physical Therap* 68:223- 225, 1988.
8. Martin BB and Klide AM: Treatment of chronic back pain in horses. *Vet Surgery* 16:106-110, 1987.
9. Shoen AM: *Veterinary Acupuncture.* American Veterinary Publications, Goleta, CA, 1994.
10. Mester E: *Lasers in Medicine.* John Wiley & Sons, New York, 1980. pp 83-95.

11. Mester E *et al:* The stimulating effects of low-power laser rays on biological systems. *Laser Review* 1, 1968.

12. Mester E and Jaszsagi-Nagy E: The effects of laser radiation on wound healing and collagen synthesis. *Studia Biophysical* 35:227-230, 1973.

13. Hansen KM: Some observations with view to possible influence of magnetism upon human organisms. *Acta Med Scand* 97:339-364, 1938.

14. Hong CZ *et al:* Magnetic necklace: Its therapeutic effectiveness on neck and shoulder pain. *Arch Phys Med Rehab* 63a:462-466, 1982.

15. Kobluk C *et al:* Summary of the effects of magnetic field therapy on the equine third metacarpal bone. Coll Vet Med, Univ Missouri, Columbia, MO, unpublished data, 1993.

Notes

7

Treatment Techniques for Food Animals

L.R. Krcatovich

There are many routes for administering the various forms of medication used to treat food animals. Technicians must become proficient in all forms of treatment so they may medicate animals in the most efficient, humane and safe method. It is important, especially when treating large herds, for the veterinary team to choose the least expensive and most effective route to medicate the animals.

INTRAVENOUS INJECTIONS

Intravenous (IV) administration of medication results in high blood levels of the drug in a short time. Though farm personnel may learn to give IV injections, most veterinarians prefer that laymen use the intramuscular (IM) or oral route to avoid possible phlebitis and thrombosis caused by poor venipuncture technique.

Cattle

The veins most often used for IV injections in cattle are the jugular veins, coccygeal (tail) vein and the subcutaneous abdominal (milk) veins. The jugular veins are most often used for large-volume IV injections. In addition to their accessibility, there is less chance of being kicked when using these veins. The jugular vein is always used for IV injections in calves because it is the largest accessible vessel.

The coccygeal (tail) vein is used for IV injection of small volumes (3-5 ml) of drugs. Though most cows are more tolerant of tail venipuncture than jugular injections, there is a greater chance of being kicked. This can be minimized with proper restraint.

The subcutaneous abdominal vein, also called the "mammary" or "milk" vein, is used mainly when the jugular veins are thrombosed (occluded) or cannot be located. There are several disadvantages to milk vein injections. The technician has an increased risk of being kicked. A second person may be required to provide additional restraint. The milk vein rolls easily under the skin, making it hard to puncture the vein and thread the needle. Finally, hematomas are easily formed and may result in thrombosis of the vein.

Preparation for venipuncture is similar for all 3 veins. A disinfectant, such as 70% alcohol, should be applied to the injection site to remove gross contamination, provide antibacterial activity, and increase visibility of the vein. Venipunctures should not be made through dirt or fecal material, as phlebitis, septicemia and/or contamination of medication and samples may result.

Jugular Venipuncture

Restraint: Good restraint is necessary when attempting any venipuncture. Ideally, the animal should be restrained in a head gate or stanchion. Injecting medication into the jugular vein of an animal that is not properly restrained is difficult and dangerous. Therefore, never attempt venipuncture on a free, moving large animal. A halter should be applied and the head raised and pulled to one side (Fig 1). A quick-release knot should be used when tying an animal to a stationary object. If the animal should fall during infusion of medication, the head can be released immediately to prevent injury to the animal. If a recumbent cow must be treated, its head can be secured by tying the free end of the halter back above the hock with a quick-release knot (see Chapter 2). Tying the head to one side secures it, making the vein accessible, but it may also make it more difficult to distend the vein. Nose tongs (nose lead) may be applied to help quiet fractious cattle.

A standing calf may be restrained by pulling it close to your body, immobilizing its head. Older calves can be restrained like adult cattle, but application of nose tongs is usually not necessary. A recumbent calf should have its head firmly held with the neck extended. If the calf moves excessively, a second person should aid in restraint.

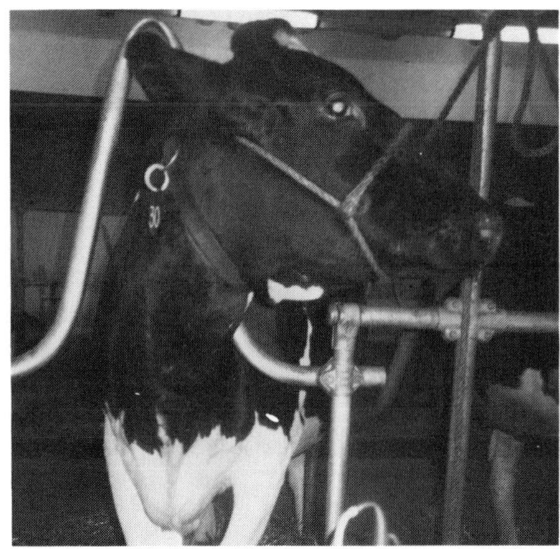

Figure 1. Correct restraint of the head for jugular venipuncture in cows.

Materials: All required materials should be assembled before attempting venipuncture. The needle selected for IV injection of large volumes of fluids varies according to personal preference and the flow rate desired. A 12- to 14-ga, 2- to 3-inch needle is best for giving large volumes to adult cattle. Needles less than 2 inches long should not be used. A correctly threaded 3-inch needle is not likely to slip from the vein if the cow thrashes around, decreasing the chances of perivascular infiltration of irritants and the chances of perivascular infiltration of irritants and hypertonic solutions. For injections of small volumes into the jugular vein, use of a 16-, 18- or 20-ga, 1.5-inch needle is recommended for cows and calves. These small-gauge, disposable needles are easier to insert than the reusable, large-bore needles, as disposable are used only once and are very sharp, whereas reusable needles tend to become dull.

A rubber IV line, referred to as a simplex, is used for IV infusions. This is commonly referred to as "jugging." A syringe may also be used to inject medication. Its size depends on the volume of medication to be injected.

Technique: One should never kneel or stand directly in front of the animal during jugular venipuncture. To distend the jugular vein, apply pressure at the jugular furrow, about two-thirds of the way caudad on (down) the neck. Allow time for the vein to fill. Briskly stroking the vein with a finger in a downward motion (toward the heart) helps raise it for easy visualization. Unless the animal is in shock or is severely dehydrated, jugular venipuncture should not be attempted without sufficiently raising the vein. Though the jugular vein is quite large when raised, it is easily missed by the inexperienced technician.

Bovine skin is thick and difficult to penetrate with a large-gauge needle; therefore, the needle must be inserted with considerable force. Grasp the needle by the hub, using the thumb and first knuckle of the forefinger (Fig 2). Warn the cow of the impending needle insertion by repeated taps on the neck, near but not over the injection site, using the back of the hand holding the needle. These warning strokes may upset the animal more than the insertion of the needle. Gradually increasing the intensity of the strokes often prevents this. After 2-3 warning strokes, flip the hand over and thrust the needle through the skin at a 45- to 90-degree angle to the vessel, with the needle directed toward the heart. Keep the jugular vein occluded to observe for blood flow from the needle, indicating proper placement.

If the vein was entered on the initial attempt and a steady flow of blood exits the needle, lay the needle parallel to the skin and advance it further caudad into the vein. The needle may be directed toward the head for administration of small volumes, but larger volumes should be given with the needle directed toward the heart. If the needle slips out of the vein during insertion, retract it until blood steadily flows from it; then attempt to rethread it.

Occasionally, the needle does not enter the vein, but only penetrates the skin. When this occurs, relocate the vein and thrust the needle into it without withdrawing it from the skin. Redirection of

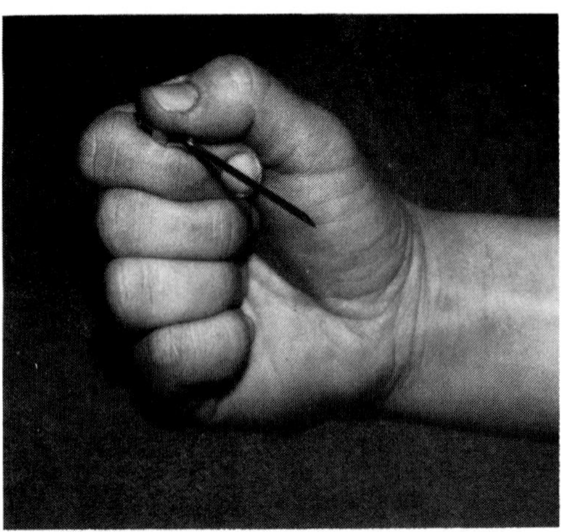

Figure 2. Correct positioning of the needle for jugular venipuncture.

the needle may be necessary to find the vein. Once a steady flow of blood is present, the needle should be threaded to its hub. If the needle has been inserted too deeply and has penetrated entirely through the vessel, pull the needle back slowly until the blood flows freely from the hub; at this point the needle can be threaded. Apposition of the bevel of the needle against the vessel wall may also occlude it. This may be corrected by slightly rotating the needle. Care must be taken when redirecting the needle to prevent laceration of the vein and consequent hematoma formation.

Small-gauge, disposable hypodermic needles may be inserted as are large-bore needles. However, it is not necessary to use as much force to insert these needles or to strike the animal before insertion, as they are very sharp and easily penetrate the skin. The needle is introduced into the vein at a 30- to 45-degree angle, with or without a syringe attached. The needle may be correctly positioned by attaching a syringe and aspirating blood.

When the needle is correctly threaded, the syringe or simplex is attached. Aspirate (slightly withdraw the syringe barrel) and then inject the medication. If a bottle is used, it should be held in an inverted position. A steady bubbling in the bottle indicates that the medication is flowing into the vein and is being replaced by air in the bottle. If the bubbling becomes irregular or stops, the needle may be occluded or out of the vein. In such cases, lower the bottle, check the needle for correct positioning and make the appropriate adjustments. When the inverted bottle is lowered, blood flows into the IV line. This can be used to check correct positioning of the needle.

Whether using a simplex or a syringe to administer fluid, observe the jugular furrow for gradual swelling around the needle. This may indicate that medication is flowing into the perivascular space (outside the vein). Correct the needle's position and continue. After IV injection is complete, remove the needle and apply digital (finger) pressure for 15-20 seconds over the venipuncture site to prevent a hematoma.

Correct and sanitary venipuncture technique must be used to prevent formation of hematomas and thrombi. If phlebitis or thrombosis develops, the routes for IV administration become severely limited. Perivascular injection of caustic or hypertonic solutions may produce tissue damage. Perivascular injection of a hypertonic solution, such as 50% dextrose, results in localized edema. This not only provides a medium for growth of bacteria and may develop into an abscess, but it also looks unprofessional.

Coccygeal Venipuncture

For smaller volumes of medication, the coccygeal (tail) vein is often used rather than the jugular vein. Cattle usually become less agitated when the tail is used for venipuncture. This method also usually requires less restraint than when the jugular vein is used.

Restraint: Limited restraint is needed for coccygeal venipuncture. Dairy cattle require a halter or stanchion and a "tail jack" (Fig 3). Beef cattle generally are more fractious and may require restraint in a chute. A tail jack must be used for coccygeal venipuncture, as it is impossible if the tail is not held in a vertical position. Holding the tail in this manner also simultaneously serves as restraint.

Materials: An 18- or 20-ga, 1.5-inch needle attached to a 3-, 5- or 10-ml syringe is appropriate for coccygeal venipuncture. A needle larger than 18 ga is too large for the coccygeal vein. A 20-ga needle is most commonly used.

Technique: To locate the correct sites for injection, one must know the position of the coccygeal vein in the tail (Fig 4). The middle coccygeal vein and artery run together along the ventral midline of the tail between the hemal arches of the coccygeal vertebrae. As the vein and artery course caudad along the tail, their size de-

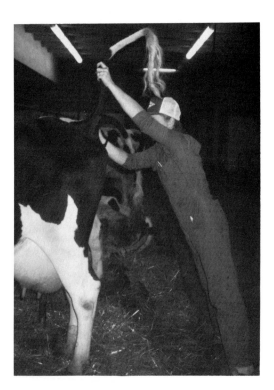

Figure 3. A proper "tail jack" is required for coccygeal venipuncture in cattle.

creases; therefore, the first 3 coccygeal vertebrae (near the tail base) are the best sites for the coccygeal venipuncture.

To locate the correct site, apply a tail jack and clean the ventral surface of the tail to remove gross contamination (Fig 5). Palpate the tail for the bony protrustions (hemal arches) of the vertebrae while gently aspirating, directly on the midline at a 45-degree angle to the tail. If the blood is not withdrawn into the syringe, check the needle for the correct angle and position. It may be necessary to advance or retract the needle to locate the vein. Remove the needle and redirect it if necessary. Inject the medication when the needle is correctly positioned. Periodically aspirate blood into the syringe and reinject this to clear the needle of residual medication. Either the coccygeal artery or vein may be used for injection. After the injection is completed, remove the needle, lower the tail and apply digital pressure for 10-15 seconds. Hematoma formation is usually not a problem, though digital pressure should be applied if the artery was punctured.

Subcutaneous Abdominal Venipuncture

The milk veins are used when the jugular veins cannot be raised or are inaccessible for other reasons. These veins should be used for administration of large volumes of medication only. It is too dangerous to obtain routine blood samples from them.

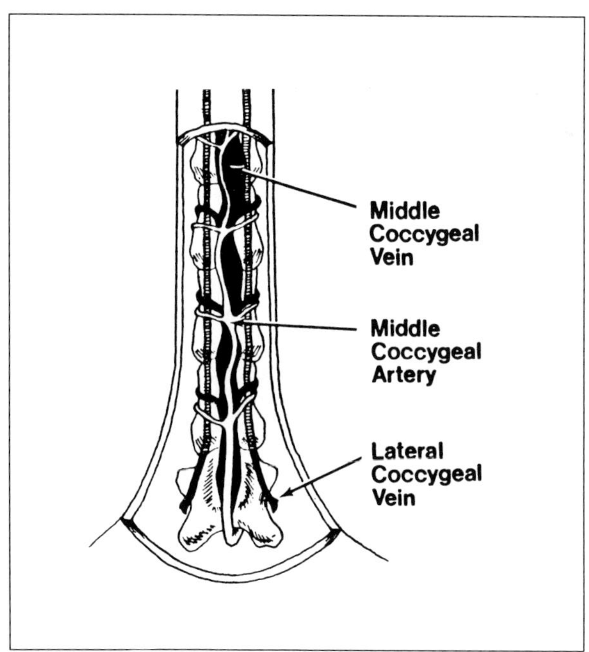

Figure 4. Ventral view of coccygeal vessels at the base of the bovine tail.

Restraint: The animal should be tied securely or restrained in a stanchion. Stand close to the cow's flank, facing the same direction as the cow (Fig 6). One should not face the cow's rear, as the cow may kick.

Materials: A 14-ga, 2- to 3-inch needle is used for venipuncture. A syringe may be used to inject medication; however, a simplex system is frequently used. Because blood flows slowly in this vein, administration through a simplex may require more time than anticipated.

Technique: It is not necessary to occlude the milk vein before puncturing it, as it is normally distended (Fig 7). The preferred venipuncture site is immediately caudal to the point where the vessel enters the abdomen; this section of the vein is the most stable (Fig 7). As with jugular veinpuncture, it takes some force to introduce the needle through the skin. The needle should be inserted caudad and threaded into the vein. If blood does not flow freely from the needle, check the position of the needle and redirect it. Exercise caution when redirecting the needle, for it is easy to create hematomas in this area. Observe the area for perivascular infiltra-

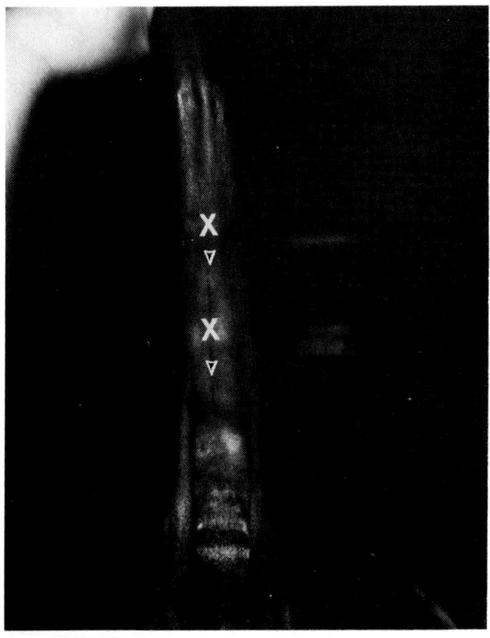

Figure 5. Location of the hemal arches (X) and venipuncture sites (arrowheads) on the ventral aspect of the bovine tail.

tion during administration. When the injection has been completed, remove the needle and apply digital pressure for several minutes. Even with digital pressure, hematomas form easily.

Swine

The vein used in pigs for IV injections is the caudal auricular vein (ear vein). The jugular veins are too deep to be used. A surgical cutdown may be performed if necessary, but this is rarely done for routine injections. The volume injected into the ear vein is limited

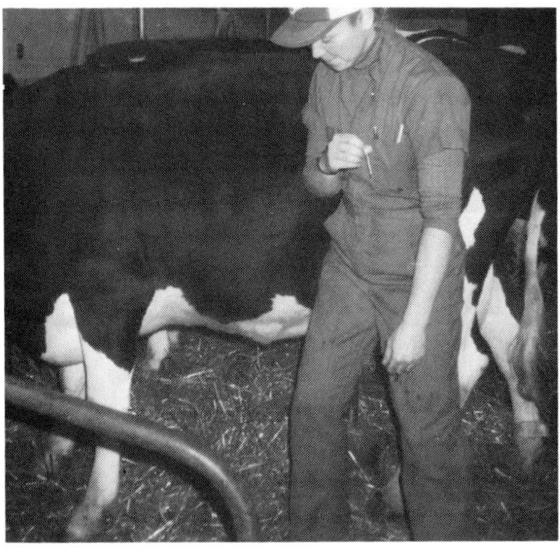

Figure 6. The correct and safest position for subcutaneous abdominal venipuncture in cows.

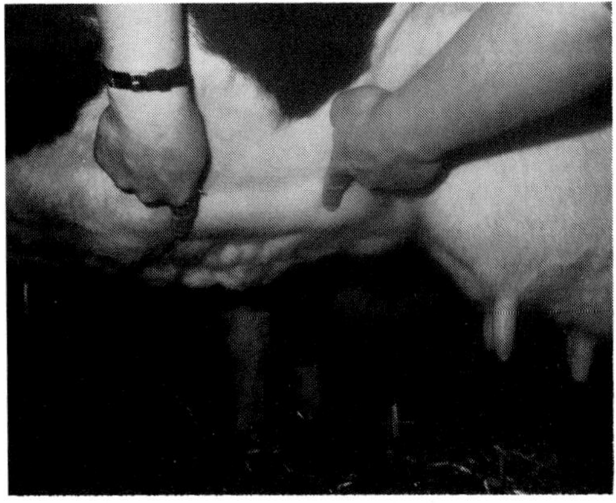

Figure 7. Segment of the subcutaneous abdominal vein most commonly used for venipuncture in cattle.

because of the vein's small size. Catheterization of the vein is possible, but this is difficult unless tranquilization is used. Fortunately, most injections in swine are given by other routes.

Restraint: If not tranquilized, pigs are restrained with a hog snare or noose (see Chapter 2). They may be backed into a corner or pinned against a wall.

Materials: A 20- to 22-ga, 1.5-inch needle and a 3- to 5-ml syringe are appropriate. A rubber band placed around the base of the ear or rubber tubing pulled tightly around the ear and clamped with hemostats distends the vein for venipuncture.

Technique: Venous distention can be hastened by clapping or rubbing the ear. Clean the injection site with an antiseptic. The thumb may be placed beside the vein to prevent the vein from rolling. The needle should be inserted, bevel up, into the distal portion of the vein (near the ear tip) and threaded into the vein to the hub. Aspirate to check for correct needle placement. Aspirate gently, for even a little negative pressure may collapse the vein. Before injecting the medication, release the rubber band. Observe the vein for perivascular infiltration as the medication is injected. If the medication is injected perivascularly or a hematoma forms, remove the needle, apply pressure at the site, and attempt another venipuncture closer to the base of the ear.

Goats and Sheep

Intravenous medication is almost always given in the jugular vein of goats and sheep. The cephalic and femoral veins are used only if both jugular veins are thrombosed.

Jugular Venipuncture

Restraint: For jugular venipuncture, sheep and goats should be restrained as are calves. The head is elevated and turned slightly to one side by an assistant. Sheep may also be "thrown" into a sitting position (see Chapter 2). A single person can perform venipuncture on a sheep in this manner.

Materials: An antiseptic is applied to the jugular furrow. Sheep may require clipping in the jugular area to increase visibility of the vein in adults; a 20- or 22-ga, 1.5-inch needle is good for lambs and kids.

Technique: The vein is held off about two-thirds of the way down (caudal on) the neck at the jugular furrow, or at the thoracic inlet. Stroking the vein with a finger helps raise it. The needle is inserted at a 30- to 45-degree angle, with or without the syringe attached. The vein seems deeper in unshorn sheep because of the thickness of overlying wool. Thread the needle into the vein and aspirate to check its location. If the needle position is correct, inject the medication. Remove the needle while applying digital pressure.

Cephalic and Femoral Venipuncture

The techniques for venipuncture of these veins are similar to those used in large dogs (see Chapter 4). When choosing the type of restraint, remember that most goats and sheep are not pets and therefore are not as docile.

Llamas

The most accessible vein of llamas is the jugular vein. There are many difficulties encountered when attempting jugular veinpuncture on a llama. Many llamas have not been trained or socialized to people; therefore, they can be very difficult to handle. Also, restrained llamas have a very thick, long haircoat that increases the difficulty of venipuncture. In most cases, clipping of the hair is not acceptable to the client. Remember to always ask the client for permission to clip hair anywhere on a llama.

The skin of the neck is extremely thick and coarse. This is a measure of protection for the llama from attacks of predators. The jugular vein is most accessible cranially and caudally because of the anatomy of the llama. The jugular vein is most superficial at the cranial site and at a farther distance from the carotid artery than it is at the caudal site. The skin is not as difficult to penetrate at the caudal site and the neck is stable for injection. When performing venipuncture at the caudal site, the right side is usually used to avoid the esophagus.

Restraint: Restraint of llamas for venipuncture can be quite a task but is essential for successful venipuncture. The approach to a llama should be quiet and calm, with no quick movements. In attempting to restrain a llama, do not approach it directly from the front and reach for its halter and/or head. Llamas may object to this, usually by regurgitating rumen contents and expelling them at the handler. Calmly approach the llama and attempt to put an arm around the base of the neck, then reach for the halter. The llama can also be put into a llama chute or backed into a corner or against a wall or fence.

Depending on the llama's personality, it may take several people to assist with restraint. Because of the llama's long neck, it is hard to stabilize the head and neck for venipuncture. An ear twitch can be very helpful on difficult animals. Many llamas react to restraint or procedures by laying down or leaping straight up or forward. The person restraining the llama must be prepared for anything.

The person restraining the head should keep his or her face turned away from the animal. Placing a towel over the llama's head may help keep the animal calm.

Young crias (immature llamas) may be placed in lateral recumbency to make venipuncture easier and less stressful for the animal.

Once the llama is safely restrained, the hair can be wetted down to help increase visibility of the jugular vein.

Technique: Occlude the jugular vein approximately one-third of the way down (caudally) the neck. Frequently the jugular vein is not visible when occluded because of the thick skin and haircoat. The jugular vein can be located by strumming the vein cranial to the occlusion. Feel for movement of blood against the hand that is occluding the vein. Occasionally release the hand that is occluding the vessel and observe the area for movement when the vein collapses. Locate an area approximately 3-6 inches caudal to the mandible. The skin may be extremely thick at this location. An 18- to 20-ga, 1.5-inch needle with syringe can be used. The needle is inserted at a 45- to 90-degree angle into the vein. On male llamas, this may require some force. The technique for injection of medications is similar to that for other species.

At the caudal location, the vein is occluded at the thoracic inlet and the vein strummed with a finger. Venipuncture can be performed 6-12 inches cranial to the occlusion. Normal venous blood from llamas may appear brighter red than that of other species. Make certain there is no pulsing, as this would indicate penetration of the carotid artery.

INTRAVENOUS CATHETERIZATION

Intravenous catheterization is primarily used for prolonged fluid therapy, but is also used for administration of injectable anesthetics or repeated IV injections. The jugular vein is most often chosen for IV catheterization in cattle, sheep, goats and llamas. The caudal auricular vein can be catheterized in swine and cattle, though this vein is used mainly for injection of small volumes of medication. It is difficult to secure a catheter in the ear vein for an extended period because of its location.

Restraint: Restraint required for IV catheterization is identical to that described for IV injection. Restraint needed for catheterizing the auricular vein involves securing the head and possibly use of nose tongs. It may help to cover the animal's eyes with a towel.

Materials: A 10- to 14-ga catheter is used for adult cattle. Calves, goats, llamas and sheep require a smaller-gauge catheter (14, 15 or 18 ga). An 18- to 22-ga, 1.5-inch catheter is adequate for kids, crias and lambs. A butterfly catheter or a 22-ga, 1.5-inch catheter is used to catheterize the ear vein of pigs.

To catheterize the ear vein of cattle, one can use an 18- to 20-ga, 1.5- to 2-inch over-the-needle catheter. On large bulls, a 14-ga, 2-inch catheter may be used if the ear vein is large enough.

Technique: The site should be clipped and surgically scrubbed. Local anesthesia is not required for most food animals. An antiseptic is applied to complete skin preparation. Because of the skin's thickness, attempts to introduce a catheter through it may bend the catheter or damage the tip. To help introduce a catheter, a disposable needle of the same gauge is used to puncture the skin. This enables the catheter to pass through the skin with ease. This is necessary when placing a jugular catheter in a llama. A #15 surgical blade can be used for this purpose also.

Cattle, Sheep, Goats

Catheterization of the jugular vein in cattle, sheep and goats is similar to that used in horses (see Chapter 6).

The procedure for placing a catheter in the auricular vein of cattle is similar to that used in swine. A local anesthetic is useful to decrease ear movement. Skin glue or a suture can be used to secure the catheter. The catheter site should be bandaged. To give the ear some stability, insert a 4-inch roll of gauze into the ear before bandaging the ear.

Llamas

Clients must be informed that the llama needs to have the IV catheter site clipped and surgically prepared.

A 14- to 16-ga over-the-needle catheter may be placed. Because of the thickness of the skin, a long catheter (6 inches) may be difficult to advance into the vein. A shorter catheter (4 inches) is often used with success.

A through-the-needle type of catheter has proven quite successful in llamas. The vein is punctured with the needle and the catheter is advanced through the needle and into the jugular. Some types of through-the-needle catheters may be left in the vein for longer periods than other catheters. This is an advantage, as the catheter does not have to be changed as often, which decreases the stress on the patient.

Swine

A rubber band placed around the base of the ear distends the vein. Introduce the catheter at the distal section of the vein (near the ear's tip) at a 30- to 45-degree angle. When blood enters the catheter, advance it into the vein to the hub. Remove the stylet if using an over-the-needle catheter, attach a syringe and aspirate. Blood should flow easily through the catheter. Place an injection cap or an IV extension set onto the catheter's hub. Remove the rubber band, then flush the catheter with heparinized saline and observe the site for perivascular infiltration. Dry the ear before attempting to secure the catheter. A 0.5-inch strip of adhesive tape is placed around the catheter's hub and wrapped around the entire ear.

It is important to use aseptic technique when inserting a catheter to minimize the chances of such complications as hematomas, phlebitis, thrombosis and catheter breakage.

INTRAMUSCULAR INJECTIONS

Intramuscular (IM) injections are commonly used in cattle, llamas and swine. Other routes are preferred in sheep and goats because of their small muscle mass.

Cattle

Several large muscles masses are available for IM injections in cattle, including the gluteals, semimembranosus, semitendinosus and lateral cervical muscles. The gluteals are located on the dorsal aspect of the rear legs. The semimembranosus and semitendinosus are located in the rear limbs, between the stifle joint and ischium. The lateral cervical muscles are cranial to the scapula, dorsal to the cervical vertebrae and ventral to the ligamentum nuchae.

The needle selected for IM injection depends on the viscosity (thickness) of the medication to be administered and the size of the muscle mass selected. A 16-, 18- or 20-ga, 1.5-inch needle is commonly used for adults. A smaller-gauge needle is used for calves (18, 20 or 22 ga).

Gluteal Injection

The gluteal muscles may be injected with minimal restraint; securing the animal's head is usually adequate. The site is swabbed with an antiseptic solution and allowed to dry. One should stand close to the cow's flank, cranial to the stifle, facing the opposite direction as the cow (Fig 8). The needle can be inserted into the muscle mass nearer the technician or into the muscles of the opposite hip (Fig 9). Because an animal usually kicks on the same side where the pain is felt, the needle should be inserted into the opposite side to reduce the chances of being kicked.

The needle is removed from the syringe before insertion and held by its hub, between the thumb and forefinger. Strike the animal several times with the back of the hand holding the needle. Keeping the same rhythm, flip the hand over and insert the needle into the muscle. The preliminary strokes are used to warn the animal of the impending injection. Attach the syringe and aspirate. If blood is withdrawn into the syringe, withdraw the needle and repeat the procedure at another site. Once it is certain the needle has not entered a vessel, the medication may be injected. The site may require digital pressure after withdrawing the needle to prevent leakage of medication from the site.

Semimembranosus/Semitendinosus Injection

The restraint, equipment and site preparation for semimembranosus or semitendinosus injections are the same as for the

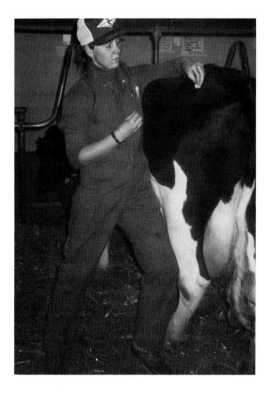

Figure 8. Correct position for IM injection into the gluteal muscle mass of a cow.

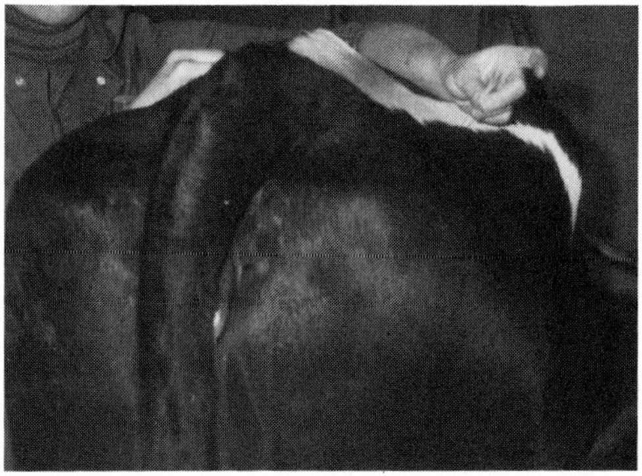

Figure 9. Insertion of the needle into the muscle mass on the cow's opposite side.

gluteals. As with the gluteals, medication can be injected into the opposite muscle mass or into that nearer the technician. The needle is inserted and medication injected in the same manner as previously described for gluteals.

Lateral Cervical Injection

The neck muscles may be used for IM injections, though the muscles of the rear legs are preferred (Fig 10). In general, cows are "head shy" and react more to injections into the neck than at other sites.

Restrain the animal and prepare the site with an antiseptic. It is best if the neck region is not struck before inserting the needle, as the animal may become "head shy." Attach the syringe, aspirate and inject the medication. Withdraw the needle and apply digital pressure to the site to prevent leakage of medication.

The maximum volume of medication that can be deposited per IM site in adult cattle is 15-20 ml. Up to 10-15 ml can be injected per site in calves, depending on their muscle mass. For numerous injections, injection sites should be rotated to prevent soreness and local inflammation in one particular muscle.

Swine

The sites for IM injections in swine are limited, as drug residue in various muscles may decrease the animal's market value. The gluteal, semimembranosus and semitendinosus muscles can be used, but must be avoided in market-bound swine. The dorsolateral muscles of the neck, directly caudal to the ear, are best for IM injections in swine.

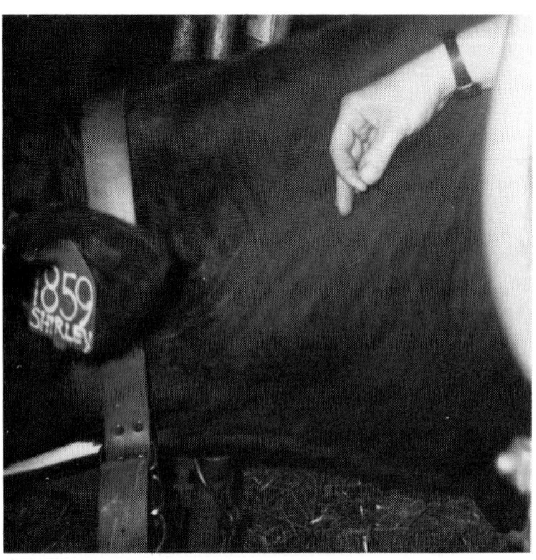

Figure 10. Correct site for IM injection into the cervical muscles of cattle.

The animal should be adequately restrained before IM injection. When a number of swine are to be injected, it helps to crowd them into a pen. Then inject each animal and walk among the pigs. Piglets may be restrained by holding them up by their rear legs.

A disposable 18- to 20-ga, 1.5-inch needle is appropriate for IM injections in adult pigs. Piglets require a smaller-gauge needle. Wipe the site with an antiseptic and remove the needle from the syringe before insertion. Striking the animal before inserting the needle is not necessary, as it may excite the animal. Insert the needle with a quick thurst and attach the syringe. If no blood is present upon aspiration, inject the medication. The needle is removed and digital pressure is applied briefly to the site. A maximum of 1-15 ml may be injected per site, depending on the size of the muscle mass.

Sheep, Goats and Llamas

The semimembranosus and semitendinosus muscles are commonly used for IM injections in sheep and goats. The gluteals and triceps may be used, but these have such a small muscle mass that only minimal amounts may be injected at these sites. Injection into the cervical muscles generally is not recommended, as the animals become too sore. This is important in young animals, as they may refuse to nurse if they become too sore to lift their head.

Sheep and goats are easily restrained by an assistant or by confinement to a small area. Restraint of a llama can vary greatly because of the llama's disposition. An assistant is usually needed to restrain the llama. An ear twitch or flank twitch may be useful if added restraint becomes necessary. Placing fractious llamas in a chute or against a wall or fence may be useful.

The injection site is prepared with an antiseptic solution. An 18- to 20-ga, 1.5-inch needle is recommended for use in adult sheep, goats and llamas. Young animals require a 20- to 22-ga needle.

When medicating a llama, stand next to the llama's rear legs, facing the opposite direction of the llama. Insert the needle at a 90-degree angle to the muscle, with or without the syringe attached. After aspirating, inject the medication. Apply digital pressure to the site after withdrawing the needle. The maximum volume that may be injected is 15 ml, with an average of 5-10 ml. Care must be taken in kids, lambs, crias (immature llamas) or thin animals to avoid hitting the sciatic nerve, running down the caudomedial aspect of the rear legs.

SUBCUTANEOUS INJECTIONS

Subcutaneous (SC) injections are given anywhere loose skin can be raised with one's fingers. In cattle and goats, this is easily done on the lateral aspect of the neck and thorax, the axillary region, the fold of the flank and the brisket. The sites chosen in sheep should be free of wool and hair, such as on the axillary region and flank folds. Sites for SC injections should be just cranial to the shoulder. Subcutaneous injecitons are not commonly used in swine because of the difficulty in raising loose skin. Possible sites for SC injections in swine are the axillary and inguinal areas. The area just caudal to the base of the ear also may be used.

Restraint: Subcutaneous injections generally require minimal restraint. Swine, sheep, llamas, goats and calves can be cornered in a small area. Small pigs can be held by the rear limbs for injections into the fold of the flank. Adult cattle should have a halter applied to be placed in a headgate or stanchion. Aggressive animals may require a chute.

Materials: An 18-, 20- or 2-ga, 1.5-inch needle is used for SC injections in goats, llamas, sheep, calves and swine. A 14-, 16- or 18-ga, 1.5-inch needle is used for cattle. The needle size selected depends on the viscosity of the drug and thickness of the skin. A syringe is used to inject small quantities. A simplex system may be used to administer larger quantities.

Technique: The site should be cleaned with an antiseptic, such as 70% alcohol. Pinch the skin and raise it to form a "tent," taking care not to penetrate the other side with the needle. After the needle is positioned, aspirate, If blood is not observed upon aspiration, inject the medication. If there is blood present in the needle, withdraw the needle and attempt the injection at a new site. when the injection is completed, withdraw the needle, release the skin fold and massage the area to enhance spread of the medication and increase its absorption rate.

The volume of medication injected at each SC site varies according to personal preference, the species involved and the animal's size. For cattle, 50-100 ml per site is the recommended maximum, through up to 250 ml may be given SC. When giving large volumes, the needle should be intermittently redirected to prevent depositing large quantities in one site. The amount that can be injected at each SC site for goats, llamas, sheep and calves varies from 2 to 30 ml, with a maximum volume of 50 ml. The maximum volume that can be injected SC in swine is about 30 ml.

INTRADERMAL INJECTIONS

Intradermal (ID) injection is directed into the dermis, the skin layer underlying the most superficial epidermis. In food animals, ID injections are used mainly to aid in diagnosis of certain diseases. Cattle and goats are tested for tuberculosis using ID injection of bovine tuberculin. Intradermal injections are also used for allergy testing, a procedure usually limited to companion animals.

Local anesthetics are injected ID to anesthetize sites for surgery or other invasive procedures.

The caudal tail fold is the site used most often for ID injections of tuberculin. They may also be given on the lateral aspect of the neck and abdomen. In swine, ID injections are given at the base of the ear.

Restraint: The restraint required depends on the site chosen, the number of injections to be given and the animal's temperament. Most animals require minimal restraint. The sites must be free of hair before ID injection is attempted. If a diagnostic test is to be performed, the site should not be cleaned with antiseptics, as they might create a skin reaction and interfere with test results. Usually removal of dirt and feces is all that is required for preparation. Antiseptics can be applied to the site if local anesthetics are being deposited before surgery.

Materials: For goats, llamas, sheep and swine, a 25- or 22-ga, 0.5- to 1-inch needle is used for ID injection. Cattle require a larger needle, such as a 20- to 22-ga, 1.5-inch needle, because of their thicker skin. A tuberculin or 3-ml syringe is adequate for injecting small volumes ID.

Technique: The needle, with the syringe attached, is placed parallel to the skin. The free hand is used to pinch the skin. This pulls the skin taut and helps stabilize it. With the bevel directed up, gently insert the needle into the dermis of the skin. Aspirate if the injection is for local anesthesia over a vessel. A raised area ("bleb") should be visualized as the drug is deposited. If a bleb does not form, the needle is too deep; retract it a small distance and inject the drug. It is not necessary to massage the site, as the object is to keep the drug localized.

INTRAPERITONEAL INJECTION

Intraperitoneal (IP) injections are not recommended for routine injection of medication. This technique is used when IV administration is impossible or in local treatment of peritonitis.

Cattle

In adult cattle, IP injections are given in the paralumbar fossa. The rumen could be punctured if the injection is given on the left side. Injections into the right paralumbar fossa could puncture loops of intestines or dilated organs, such as the cecum or a displaced abomasum.

With the animal securely restrained, the site is clipped and surgically scrubbed, and local anesthesia is administered.

A 14-ga, 2-inch needle is commonly attached to a 20- to 50-ml syringe for IP injections. A simplex system may be used to deliver large volumes. The needle is gently inserted into the peritoneum. Air may be heard escaping through the needle as the peritoneum is punctured. If the rumen or intestines have been inadvertently punctured, a distinct gas odor can be detected. A syringe can be attached and aspirated to check for gastrointestinal contents. As the medication is injected, it should run in freely if the needle is correctly placed in the abdominal cavity.

Llamas, Calves, Goats, Sheep and Swine

The caudoventral abdominal wall is best for IP injections in llamas, calves, goats, sheep and swine. The animal is restrained in dorsal recumbency, with the rear limbs elevated. The site is prepared as for IP injections in adult cattle.

A 16- or 18-ga, 1.5-inch needle and a 10-, 20- or 50-ml syringe are used. The needle is inserted and directed caudad. To avoid puncturing the bladder or to prevent penile injury in males, insert the needle slightly off midline. Aspirate and inject the medication.

Several complications may occur with IP injections. Puncturing the gastrointestinal tract or other vital organs may result in peritonitis. Inadequate site preparation and poor technique may also result in peritonitis or an abscess.

INTRAMAMMARY INFUSION

Veterinarians and dairy farmers often employ intramammary infusions to treat mastitis or to infuse udder quarters when cows are dry (not lactating). The best time to infuse the udder is after the last milking of the day, which allows the medication to remain in the udder overnight. The udder should not be infused before milking because the beneficial effect of the medication would be lost. Because intramammary antibiotic therapy affects the results of milk culture, milk samples from mastitic quarters must be obtained before treatment.

Restraint: Minimal restraint is required for intramammary infusion. Tail restraint may be necessary for fractious cows. Care must be taken with beef cows, especially if they have been separated from their calves, as they are usually very aggressive.

Technique: Crouch beside the udder to work; never sit down or kneel. This makes it easier to avoid injury from kicking. Thoroughly clean the udder before treatment, using warm water and antiseptic soap. Use a separate cloth or paper towel to wash each teat so as to decrease the spread of microorganisms among the quarters. Dry each teat with a separate towel to remove contaminated water droplets. Wipe the teat orifice with an alcohol swab and allow to air dry. If all 4 quarters are to be infused, swab the far teat before swabbing the near ones, so as to prevent contamination when reaching past the near teats.

Empty the quarter by manually "stripping" out the milk before infusing medication, as residual milk mixes with the medication and dilutes it. Collect the discarded milk in a bucket to prevent contamination of the environment by the bacteria in the milk. After the teat is prepared, grasp it near the base and insert a teat cannula or sterile, disposable mammary infusion cannula into the teat orifice. More commonly, commercially prepared, disposable syringes with an attached cannula are used. Advance the cannula just through the teat sphincter a short distance and inject the medication slowly. Do not insert the cannula to the hub, as this predisposes to mastitis. As little as 10-20 ml or as much as 250 ml may be infused into a quarter. Remove the cannula and massage the teat and quarter to disseminate the medication. When the procedure is completed, dip the teat in teat dip to prevent invasion of microbes. If the weather is extremely cold (0 C or less), do not let the cow outside until the udder is dry, so as to prevent chapping and frostbite. Mark the cows that were treated so their milk can be discarded.

Always use sanitary techniques when manipulating the udder, as mastitis can be transferred to uninfected quarters in cows with mastitis or to other cows in the barn.

The veterinarian is responsible for informing the client of withdrawal times for any drug given to a food animal. Most pharmaceutical companies furnish drug withdrawal times on the labels of their products.

Of the food animal species, only cows and goats are milked on a routine basis. Intramammary infusion techniques, as described for dairy cows, also apply to treatment of goats.

INTRANASAL INSUFFLATION

The intranasal route is the most commonly used to administer vaccines and local anesthetics. As of this writing, intranasal vaccines have been approved only for infectious bovine rhinotracheitis (IBR) and parainfluenza-3 (PI_3) infection. Vaccines not designed for intranasal use are not effective when given by this route.

Intranasal anesthetics may be given before potentially painful procedures on the nasal cavity, such as nasogastric intubation, bronchoalveolar lavage and endoscopy.

Restraint of the head is a necessity. Calves may be manually restrained, while adults should be secured with a halter and headgate.

Nasal secretions should be wiped from the nostril with moist cotton before medication administration. A 3- to 5-ml syringe is filled with the vaccine or local anesthetic, with a disposable, blunt tip attached to inject the drug, though the syringe alone may be used (Fig 11). Facing the same direction as the animal, one hand is placed over the head, pulling it close toyour body. The head must be slightly elevated to prevent the medication from running out of the nostril. The free hand is used to insert the syringe into the nostril (Fig 11). When the injection is completed, elevate the head for 10-15 seconds before releasing it.

OCULAR MEDICATION

Ocular medication techniques are used to locally treat ocular disorders with ointments and solutions. The techniques for application of ocular medication are similar for all species. Immobilization of the head is required.

Rest the hand holding the medication on the animal's head, dorsal to (above) the eye. With the free hand, separate the lids and apply the medication. Do not touch the tip of the aplicator to the eye, as this may traumatize the cornea and contaminate the applicator. When applying both solutions and ointments to the eye, administer the solution first, as the solution will run off if it is applied on top of an ointment.

INTRAUTERINE MEDICATION

Medication is placed in the uterus to locally treat metritis. Though this technique may be performed by veterinary technicians, they are not routinely instructed in this procedure. It is up to the veterinarian as to whether technicians should perform this procedure.

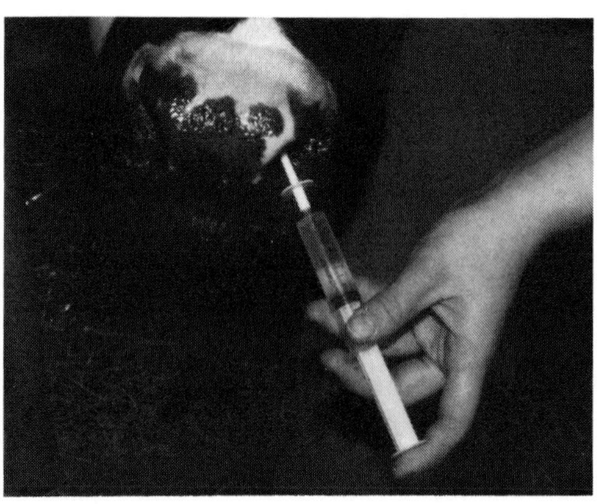

Figure 11. A syringe and a blunt-tipped cannula are often used for intranasal injection. One hand is placed over the animal's head and the other hand is used for injection.

Uterine medication is available as boluses, capsules and solutions. The form of the drug used depends on the condition of the uterus, the stage of the reproductive cycle, the types of drugs available and personal preference.

Cows require minimal restraint for this procedure. The tail should be secured away from the perianal region. Feces should be "raked" (manually removed) from the rectum before the vulva is cleaned, so as to aid in palpation and prevent contamination of the area and equipment. An antiseptic soap, warm water and cottom are used to wash the vulva and surrounding area. Wipe the vulva, starting at the dorsal commissure of the labia and progressing down to the ventral commissure. The soap should be rinsed off before treatment.

Intrauterine Infusion

A uterine pipette is used to infuse solutions into the uterus, using a syringe to inject the medication through the pipette. An equine nasogastric tube and stomach pump may be used to inject large volumes of medication into the uterus.

To aid passage of the pipette into the uterus, guide it with the opposite hand, placed into the rectum. Grasp the cervix, which lies about 3-4 inches cranial to the vulva, with the left hand (for a right-handed person) so the thumb is dorsal to the cervix and the fingers are located ventrad. Insert the pipette into the vulva, exercising care to avoid touching the pipette's tip to the labia. Advance the pipette at a 30- to 40-degree angle for 3-4 inches. This prevents the pipette from entering the urethral opening, located on the floor of the vagina. Once the tip is past the urethral orifice, advance the pipette in a horizontal position. To aid in passage of the pipette, pull the cervix craniad to straighten the folds of the vagina. As the pipette is advanced, it may become caught in a vaginal fold. If this occurs, do not force the pipette craniad, but simply withdraw and redirect it.

Introduce the pipette's tip into the cervical opening, which is usually in the center of the cervix. Gently manipulate the cervix over the pipette. Once the pipette is through the cervix, it slides craniad easily and may be palpated rectally. Beginners commonly deposite the medication in the vagina or cervix, rather than in the uterus. Always make certain the tip has passed into the uterus. Inject the medication and then flush the pipette with air to remove residual medication.

Through the entirety of this procedure, it is important never to force the pipette craniad, as this may damage vaginal or cervical tissue. Also, the vaginal and rectal walls may be penetrated if excessive force is used. This could result in such complications as peritonitis, metritis, abscesses and reproductive disorders.

Intrauterine Boluses

A sterile sleeve should be worn to insert boluses or capsules into the uterus. Advance the hand into the vulva and vagina until the cervix is located. Form your hand into a wedge, insert it into the dilated os cervix (cervical orifice) and advance it into the uterus, where the medication is deposited. There are fewer complications with this method of intrauterine medication othan with infusion. The primary complication is introduction of bacteria into the uterus by using poor sanitary techniques. Rough handling can damage vaginal and cervical tissue.

Many farmers medicate their animals with these methods. They should be carefully instructed in use of the proper techniques and informed of possible complcations. They should also be informed of drug withdrawal times so meat or milk from treated animals is not immediately sold.

ORAL MEDICATION

Oral medication is available in many forms, including liquids, pastes, powders, tablets, capsules and boluses. Instruments sued to deliver oral medication include the balling gun, Frick's speculum, dose syringe, drench bottle and stomach tube.

The different methods used for giving oral medication require similar restraint measures. The head is secured in a stanchion or headgate. Halters are not usually required. If they are used, they should not be applied too tightly over the muzzle so the animal can adequately open its mouth. Llamas, swine, sheep and goats may be restrained by backing them into a corner or against a wall.

Balling Gun

Boluses, capsules or magnets may be given *per os* (PO) with a balling gun (Fig 12). This instrument is available in various sizes for use in different species. Cattle require a gun with a large head and long handle, with a metal or flexible plastic head. The plastic head produces less trauma to the pharyngeal tissue than a metal head but is easily damaged by teeth. Small balling guns are manufactured for use in sheep, goats, swine and calves.

The methods of introducing a balling gun, dose syringe, drench bottle or Frick's speculum are similar in all species. For cattle, standing cranial to the animal's shoulder and facing the same direction as the animal, place one arm over the animal's head and caudal to the poll, with the animal's head positioned on your hip. This technique may not be possible for people with short arms. In this case, reaching across the bridge of the nose is acceptable. Insert the fingers of this hand into the mouth at the interdental space

Figure 12. Various sizes of balling guns are available.

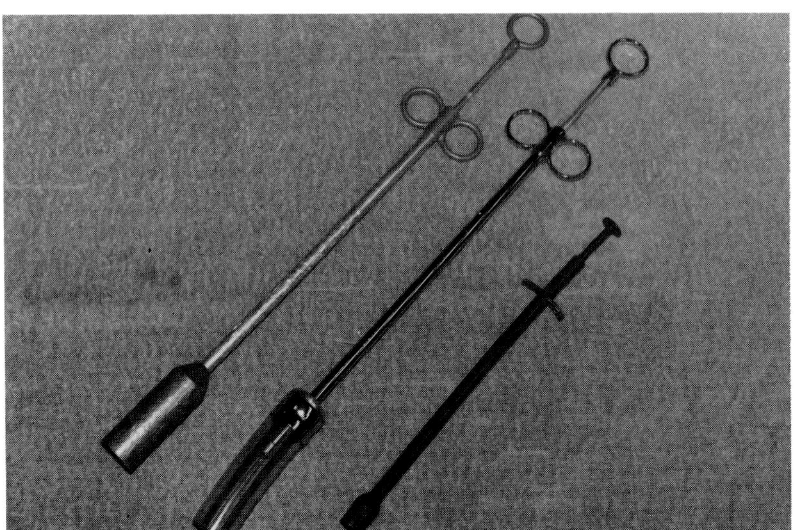

and apply pressure to the hard palate, which causes the animal to open its mouth.

Insert the balling gun or similar instrument at an upward angle at the interdental space, opposite the restraining hand. Direct the instrument caudad and advance it over the base of the tongue. Once it is over the tongue's base, advance the balling gun caudad in a horizontal position until the rings of the handle reach the buccal commissure (corner of the mouth) (Fig 13). This ensures that the gun is back far enough in the mouth to deposit the bolus, forcing the cow to swallow and preventing expulsion of the medication. Depress the plunger to eject the bolus and remove the instrument. Observe the animal to be sure the medication was swallowed. It is not necessary to elevate the head until the bolus is swallowed if the bolus was deposited correctly.

Frick's Speculum

A Frick's speculum may be used to give 2 or more boluses to cattle (Fig 14). Insert the speculum in the same manner as the balling gun. Once the speculum is placed over the base of the tongue, the boluses are inserted into the speculum. Allow the boluses to travel down the speculum and into the mouth. Remove the speculum and observe for swallowing. This method is used to save time but has the added danger of aspiration of medication.

Drenching

Giving small volumes of liquids PO is often referred to as "drenching." Drenching is done with a dose syringe or a drench bottle (Fig 15). A 60-ml catheter-tipped syringe or a bulb syringe may be used as a dose syringe in calves, sheep, swine and goats. The drench bottle, commonly a wine or a soft drink bottle, should be made of strong glass and have a long, tapered neck and smooth mouth.

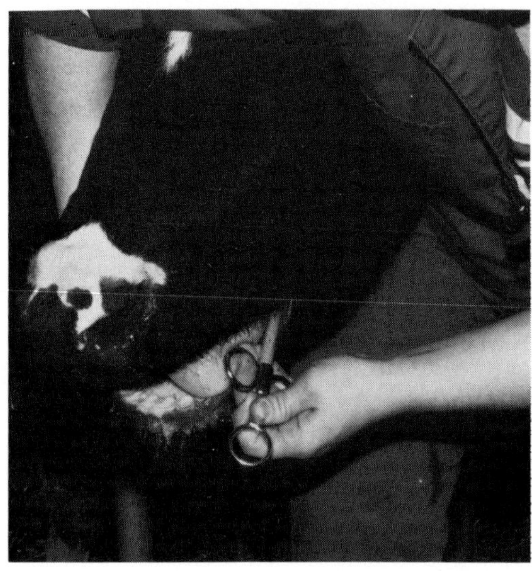

Figure 13. Correct positioning of the cow's head and insertion of the balling gun.

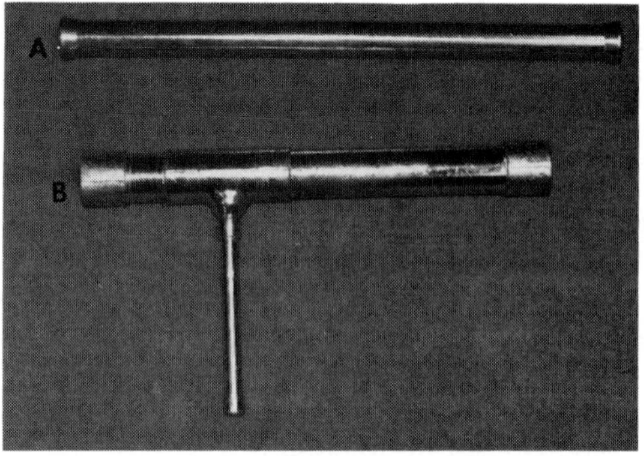

Figure 14. Regular Frick's speculum (A) and a modified Frick's speculum (B).

The technique for drenching is similar to that described for the balling gun. Be certain to insert the drench bottle at the interdental space to prevent the cow from breaking it with its molars. The head should be held slightly elevated so the nose is level with the animal's eye. If the head is raised excessively, the animal could aspirate some of the medication. Give the medication slowly, allowing the animal to swallow at its own pace.

Dose syringes are also used to give pastes. Commercially prepared syringes containing medication are available, though these are used more often in horses.

Orogastric Intubation

"Stomach tubing" is a quick and relatively painless method to deliver large quantities of liquid medication or fluids. A stomach tube may be passed through the nasal cavity, as in horses, but this method is not commonly used in food animals. Llamas do not tolerate nasal intubation well. In food animals, the stomach tube is usually passed through the oral cavity, with the aid of a metal speculum.

Cattle: An oral speculum is required to prevent damage to the soft stomach tube from the animal's teeth. Specula used in cattle are the Frick's speculum (Fig 14) and Colorado bovine speculum (Fig 16). The Frick's speculum is inserted into the mouth and held in place by an assistant. The Colorado bovine speculum, once inserted, is secured behind the poll with straps (Fig 16). Using the Colorado speculum allows one person to complete the intubation procedure, whereas use of the Frick's speculum requires 2 people.

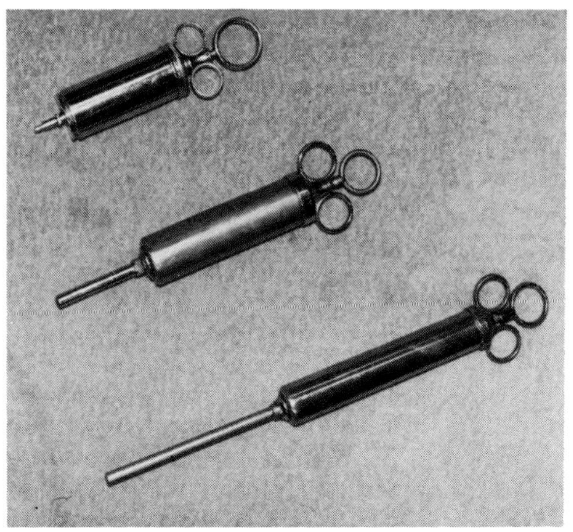

Figure 15. Various sizes of dose syringes.

Stomach tubes are available in different lengths and diameters. Choose an appropriately sized tube for the individual animal. A tube with an outside diameter of 5/8 to 1 inch is the average size used for adult cattle. A foal stomach tube is often used for "tubing" calves. A stomach pump or a funnel can be used to facilitate administration.

Measure the distance externally from the mouth to the rumen and insert the tube approximately this distance. Once this skill has been mastered, the mouth-rumen distance is easily estimated. The first 3 feet of the tube should be lubricated with water or water-soluble lubricating jelly before intubation. With an assistant holding an oral speculum in place, insert the tube into the speculum and advance it with gentle pressure (Fig 17). Some resistance may be felt when the tube reaches the esophagus. Observe for swallowing, then advance the tube into the esophagus. If passage is difficult, rotate the tube slightly and apply gentle pressure to advance the tube.

After inserting the tube the measured distance, check for correct placement in the rumen. If the stomach tube was inadvertently placed in the trachea, the animal may cough, though this should not be used alone to determine correct placement. If the tube has been inadvertently passed down the trachea, air may be felt exiting the tube upon exhalation. Remove the tube and reintubate. Another test used to check if the tube has been passed into the rumen is to have one person blow air into the end of the tube while another listens with a stethoscope at the rumen. A gurgling should

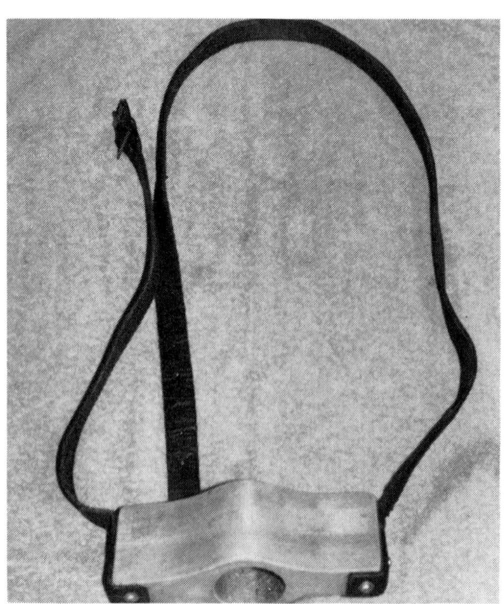

Figure 16. The Colorado bovine speculum is positioned in the animal's mouth, with the straps fastened behind the poll.

should be heard as air is blown into the tube. The smell of rumen gas may sometimes be detected exiting the tube. In some lightly muscled animals, the tube can be observed progressing caudally down the esophagus. In these animals, one may also palpate the neck for 2 tubular structures, *ie,* the trachea and the stomach tube within the esophagus.

Once the stomach tube is correctly positioned, the medication can be given. After the medication has been infused, rinse the tube with water to flush out remaining medication. Kink the tube or occlude its end and withdraw it quickly. This prevents any fluid remaining in the tube from entering the trachea upon tube removal.

Swine, Sheep, Goats and Llamas: A stomach tube with an outside diameter of 3/8-1/2 inch can be used to give liquid medication PO to swine, sheep and goats. A stallion urinary catheter or a small canine stomach tube may be used for kids, crias and lambs.

A swine mouth speculum can be used not only for swine but also for llamas, sheep, goats and calves (Fig 18). This instrument is placed into the mouth in a horizontal position (see Chapter 2) and then rotated to a vertical position at the interdental space. A hollow tube, simulating a Frick's speculum, may also be used as an oral speculum.

The technique for stomach intubation used in cattle also applies to sheep, swine, llamas and goats. Tests to confirm the tube's position are the same as for cattle. However, it is difficult to palpate a pig's neck or observe tube passage because of the fat and muscle in its neck.

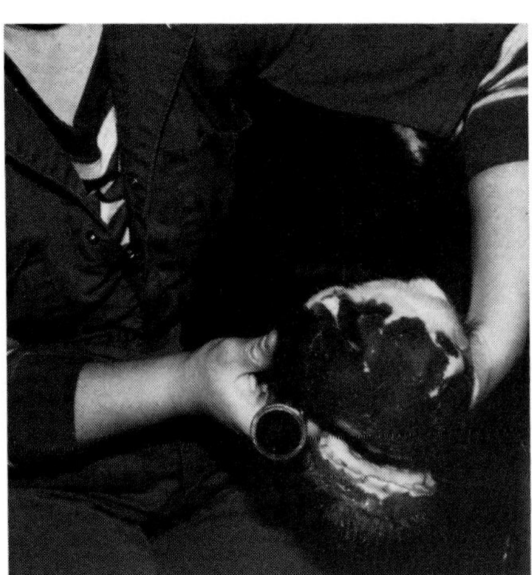

Figure 17. Correct placement of a Frick's speculum for passage of a stomach tube.

BLOOD COLLECTION AND TRANSFUSION

Small volumes (0.5-10 ml) of blood may be collected for various blood tests, such as hematologic examination and serum chemistry analysis, to aid in diagnosing a disease, or to monitor a disease's progression or an animal's recovery. Blood is also collected for transfusion of whole blood or plasma to treate anemic or hypoproteinemic animals.

Collecting Samples

Cattle

The veins more often used to obtain blood samples from cattle are the jugular and coccygeal (tail) veins. Blood can also be collected from the mammary vein, though this is rarely done. The coccygeal vein is easily accessible and blood collection is less traumatic to the cow than with use of the jugular vein. The jugular vein is used for blood collection in calves, as their coccygeal veins are difficult to puncture because of their small size.

A syringe and needle combination or a convenient vacuum tube system (Vacutainer) may be used (see Chapter 6). When a syringe is used, the blood must be immediately transferred to a vial containing an anticoagulant to prevent the sample from clotting. A syringe that has been flushed with an anticoagulant, such as heparin, can be used to obtain small volumes (3-5 ml) of blood. Vacuum tubes are available with various anticoagulant or no anticoagulant. Tubes containing an anticoagulant must be gently inverted several

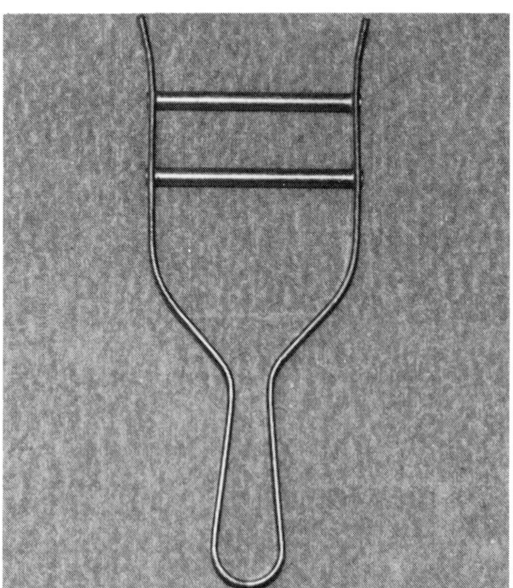

Figure 18. A swine oral speculum may be used on other species.

times immediately after blood collection to thoroughly mix the blood and anticoagulant to prevent clot formation.

Jugular Vein: A 22- or 20-ga Vacutainer needle is used to collect blood from calves. Adult cattle require a 20-ga Vacutainer needle for jugular veinpuncture. The collection tube chosen depends on the type of tests requested. A 20-ga, 1.5-inch injection needle is more suitable for adults.

With the animal properly restrained, cleanse the site with an antiseptic. Distend the vein and insert the needle at a 30- to 45-degree angle to the skin, directing it craniad (toward the head). Thread the needle into the vein, observing the hub for blood. Attach the syringe and withdraw the amount required. After removing the needle, apply digital pressure to the venipuncture site.

When using the Vacutainer system, insert the needle as previously described. Observe the needle's end for blood droplets and attach the collection tube to the needle. Blood flows into the tube until the vacuum is depleted. After the first collection tube is removed, another may be attached if necessary. A Vacutainer needle holder is available to facilitate attaching the tubes to the needle (see Chapter 6).

Coccygeal Vein: An 18- or 20-ga, 1.5-inch needle with an attached 3-, 5- or 10-ml syringe, or a 20-ga Vacutainer needle and collection tubes, can be used to obtain blood from the coccygeal vein. Use of a Vacutainer holder makes this procedure easier for beginners. The technique of coccygeal venipuncture is identical to that described for giving coccygeal vein medication.

Auricular Artery: Samples from this artery are used for blood gas analysis on anesthetized cattle or those with severe respiratory or metabolic disorders. An 18- to 22-ga, 1.5-inch needle and a 3- to 5-ml syringe flushed with an anticoagulant are used to collect the sample.

In animals that are not anesthetized, the head must be restrained for this procedure. The artery is located by palpating the ear for a pulse. The site is shaved and scrubbed with an antiseptic. Insert the needle into the artery, with the bevel directed up. Aspirate slightly to collect the sample. Withdraw the needle and apply digital pressure over the site. Remove all air bubbles from the syringe and quickly cap the end of the needle with a cork to prevent air entry into the syringe. The blood gas analysis should be done immediately after sample collection.

Sheep, Goats and Llamas

The jugular vein is most commonly used to collect blood from sheep and goats, though the cephalic or femoral veins are occasionally used. The venipuncture technique for these veins is similar to that used on dogs (see Chapter 4).

Jugular venipuncture can be accomplished with a 16- to 20-ga, 1.5-inch needle for adults and a 22- to 20-ga needle for lambs, crias and kids. Alternatively, a 22- to 20-ga Vacutainer needle and tubes may be used. The technique for jugular veinpuncture in sheep and goats is identical to that used in cattle.

Swine

Venipuncture sites are limited in swine by their lack of accessible veins. The caudal auricular (ear) vein may be used to obtain small volumes (3-5 ml) of blood. The cranial vena cava is used for collection of larger blood volumes. This vein is located deep in the thoracic cavity and requires skill and practice for venipuncture.

Cranial Vena Cava: An 18- or 20-ga, 3- to 4-inch needle should be used to collect blood from the cranial vena cava of adult pigs. Large boars may require a 5-inch needle. Small pigs (under 40-50 lb) require a shorter needle (1.5-inch needles are usually sufficient).

The cranial vena cava is located by using several landmarks. Adult pigs should be restrained in a standing position for this procedure, though small pigs may be held or placed in dorsal recumbency. The same landmarks are used for all positions.

Palpate the manubrium sterni, a bony projection located on the ventral midline, cranial to the forelegs. Move the hand to the right of the manubrium, where a slight depression should be felt. This may be difficult to feel in large pigs. Pigs are bled from their right side to avoid the phrenic nerve, which is located on the left side.

Insert the needle through the skin in the depression. Use an imaginary line drawn from this depression to the opposite shoulder to direct the needle. It may help to place your free hand on the pig's opposite shoulder and aim the needle toward that hand. Aspirate slightly to create a negative pressure in the syringe and advance the needle with short stabbing movements. When the needle punctures the cranial vena cava, blood immediately enters the syringe. Maintain the needle in this position and withdraw the desired volume of blood. If blood is not obtained at the first attempt, withdraw the needle but do not remove it entirely from the animal. Never redirect the needle when it is deep inside the pig, as laceration of the vena cava could result in death from hemorrhage. Before another attempt, check the needle's direction and repeat the procedure. Withdraw the needle once the sample is obtained and apply digital pressure to the site to control hemorrhage from skin vessels.

Caudal Auricular Vein: To collect blood from the auricular (ear) vein, a 22-ga needle attached to a 3- to 5-ml syringe, previously flushed with an anticoagulant, may be used. A rubber band or tubing, applied to the base of the ear, serves as a tourniquet.

Swab the ear with an antiseptic and place the rubber band around the ear's base. Allow time for the vein to become distended. Insert the needle into the distal portion of the vein. Aspirate slightly, as excessive vacuum collapses the vein. After the sample has been collected, place a thumb over the site and withdraw the needle. Immediately release the tourniquet and apply digital pressure.

Collecting Blood for Transfusion

Transfusions are not commonly used in most food animal practices, but are done more frequently in dogs, cats and horses (see Chapters 4, 6).

The needle size depends on the species involved. Adult cattle require a 10- , 12- or 14-ga, 2- to 3-inch needle for blood collection. A 16- or 18-ga, 1.5-inch needle is sufficient for sheep, goats, llamas and calves.

The jugular vein is almost always used for collecting large volumes of blood. The site should be clipped or shaved and cleaned with an antiseptic, and the needle inserted into the vein toward the heart (see Jugular Venipuncture). A collection line is then connected to the needle. During blood collection, gently invert the container to mix the blood and anticoagulant. To prevent hemolysis of the sample, avoid excessive or rough movement of the bottle or bag. When the desired amount is collected, remove the needle and apply digital pressure to the site.

Transfusions

Many food animal veterinarians do not cross-match donor and recipient blood before transfusion.

An IV catheter is placed in the recipient's jugular vein and a blood administration set is connected to the catheter. The transfusion is started at a low rate, while the animal is observed for possible reactions, such as increased respiration, dyspnea and tremors. Blood or plasma administration should be stopped immediately and emergency drugs administered under a veterinarian's supervision to control any adverse reaction during transfusion.

Recommended Reading

Howard JL: *Current Veterinary Therapy 3: Food Animal Practice.* Saunders, Philadelphia, 1993.

Radostits OM *et al: Herd Health: Food Animal Production Medicine.* 2nd ed. Saunders, Philadelphia, 1994.

Smith BP: *Large Animal Internal Medicine.* Mosby, St. Louis, 1990.

Veterinary Clinics of North America: Food Animal Practice. Published quarterly. Saunders, Philadelphia.

Notes

8

Anesthesia and Anesthetic Nursing

H.C. Lin, G.J. Benson, J.C. Thurmon

Anesthetized animals require the full attention of the anesthetist. A well-trained, experienced veterinary technician can contribute significantly to the patient's safety. It is important to understand that there are no safe anesthetic drugs or anesthetic techniques, only safe anesthetists. Therefore, a disciplined and skilled approach is required to safely induce and maintain anesthesia. As technician-anesthetist, your duties include preoperative patient evaluation, drug and equipment setup, induction and maintenance of anesthesia, patient monitoring and postoperative care during recovery, record keeping, stocking anesthesia supplies and maintenance of the "crash cart." Discussions in this chapter include preanesthetic considerations, pharmacology of anesthetics, anesthetic equipment, patient monitoring, fluid therapy, postoperative management and personnel safety.

PREANESTHETIC CONSIDERATIONS

History and Physical Examination

A complete history for all animals scheduled for elective surgery and/or diagnostic procedures must be obtained. A thorough physical examination must be performed before any anesthetic drugs are given. Patient history should include information on any previous illness, existing disease, reproductive status, current drug therapy, previous and potential drug reactions or allergies, previous blood transfusion and recent feeding.

The physical examination can be conducted by the technician under the direct supervision of a licensed veterinarian. The examination should include body weight and rectal temperature, temperament and activity level, auscultation of heart and lung sounds, pulse amplitude and duration, hydration, mucous membrane color, and capillary refill time. The veterinarian should be informed of any abnormal findings.

Laboratory Tests

Laboratory tests help to identify subclinical disease and provide useful information regarding the patient's ability to metabolize and excrete anesthetics and to tolerate the stress of anesthesia and surgery. Table 2 lists appropriate tests that should be conducted before anesthesia.

Nature and Duration of the Procedure

The nature and duration of the procedure should be considered before selecting the anesthetic technique. Tranquilization or sedation may be sufficient for many nonpainful procedures. Procedures that cause pain require use of an analgesic, such as an opioid, local/regional analgesia or general anesthesia. With local analgesia, pain perception is blocked by injecting a local anesthetic in the region of pain receptors or, alternatively, along the trunk of specific peripheral nerves, often while the patient remains conscious. General anesthesia induces an unconscious state as a result of the anesthetic's action on the central nervous system (CNS). Minor surgical procedures can be performed with short-acting injectable anesthetics (*eg,* a xylazine-ketamine combination or thiopental). However, inhalation anesthesia is preferred for lengthy procedures in most situations.

Physical Status of the Patient

The findings of the physical examination, the patient's history, and laboratory tests should provide information essential for determination of anesthetic risk to the patient. Table 1 presents a classification of physical status, developed by the American Society of Anesthesiologists (ASA).

Animals classified as *ASA I* or *II* are most often safely anesthetized using routine protocols. Animals classed as *ASA III* should be stabilized with fluid therapy and other drugs before inducing anesthesia. Alternative techniques may be indicated. Animals in *ASA IV* and *V* require extensive monitoring and cardiovascular and pulmonary support before and during anesthesia.

Preanesthetic Preparations

Patients scheduled for elective surgery should be admitted the day before surgery. This allows time for physical examination, laboratory analyses of health status, and acclimatization to the hospital environment. Food should be withheld for 8-12 hours before anesthesia. Water can be provided *ad libitum* until just before preanesthetic medication is given. In very young patients, prolonged fasting depletes liver glycogen reserves and decreases the animal's ability to withstand the stress of surgery and anesthesia. Therefore, a shorter fasting period is safest and preferred in young animals.

Regurgitation of rumen contents and bloat (distention of the rumen) are potential hazards that are often encountered during

Table 1. Categories of physical status of surgical patients, developed by the American Society of Anesthesiologists (ASA).

Category	Physical Status	Examples
ASA I (Minimal Risk)	Normal healthy animal	Ovariohysterectomy, castration, declaw
ASA II (Slight Risk)	Slight systemic disease, no clinical signs of disease, no functional limitation	Neonate or geriatric animals, obesity, fracture without shock, compensated heart or kidney disease
ASA III (Moderate Risk)	Moderate to severe systemic disease, slight clinical signs of disease, definite functional limitation	Anemia, low-grade heart murmur, moderate fever, anorexia, moderate dehydration
ASA IV (High Risk)	Preexisting systemic disease that is a constant threat to life	Shock, high fever, uremia, toxemia, severe dehydration, severe heart disease, severe pulmonary disease, severe kidney disease
ASA V (Grave Risk)	Moribund animal not expected to survive 24 hours with or without surgery	Severe shock, severe head injury, severe trauma, advanced major organ disease (heart, liver, lung, kidney)

Table 2. Reasonable diagnostic laboratory tests for patients scheduled for general anesthesia.

Physical Status	<5 Years Old	5-10 Years Old	>10 Years Old
ASA I and II	PCV, total protein	PCV, total protein, BUN, urinalysis	CBC, BUN, urinalysis
ASA III	CBC, BUN, urinalysis	CBC, urinalysis, serum chemistry profile	CBC, urinalysis, serum chemistry profile
ASA IV and V	CBC, urinalysis, serum chemistry profile	CBC, urinalysis, serum chemistry profile	CBC, urinalysis, serum chemistry profile

anesthesia of ruminants. For large mature ruminants, food and water should be withheld for 24-36 hours before anesthesia. For small ruminants, food should be withheld for 12-24 hours and water for 8-12 hours before anesthesia.

PHARMACOLOGY OF ANESTHETIC AGENTS

Preanesthetic Agents

Preanesthetics are given to calm the patient, to aid in restraint, to reduce pain and discomfort, to decrease salivation and vagus-mediated reflexes, to smooth anesthetic induction and recovery, and to minimize the doses of anesthetics required for induction and maintenance. It is important to remember that preanesthetics are a part of the medication used to induce and maintain anesthesia and the choice of preanesthetics varies with the veterinarian's preference and experience, the patient's general health and temperament, the type and duration of surgical procedure to be performed, and anticipated complications.

Preanesthetics include anticholinergics, tranquilizers and sedatives, opioids, and a combination of an opioid and tranquilizer, referred to as a *neuroleptanalgesic*. Dosages of preanesthetics used in domestic animals are summarized in Tables 3 and 4.

Anticholinergics

Anticholinergics are used to eliminate some of the undesirable actions of tranquilizers, opioids and general anesthetics. Of concern is increased vagal tone, often characterized by bradycardia and excessive salivation. Two commonly used anticholinergics are atropine sulfate and glycopyrrolate.

Atropine sulfate (Atropine Sulfate Injection: Vedco) decreases respiratory tract secretions but increases their viscosity. It induces bronchiolar dilation, and decreases motor and secretory properties of the gastrointestinal tract. Atropine also dilates the pupils, inhibits vagal tone and increases the heart rate (and thus, cardiac work and oxygen consumption). Clinical doses of atropine may induce an initial slowing of the heart rate (bradycardia) as a result of central vagal stimulation.

In horses, atropine decreases gastrointestinal motility, resulting in ileus and colic. Thus, it is seldom used in horses. The ocular effect (mydriasis) may impair depth perception. Horses and cats given atropine should be approached with caution because they tend to panic in response to sudden poorly visualized movements.

Glycopyrrolate (Robinul-V: Robins) reduces gastric acidity, decreasing the severity of the lung's inflammatory response to aspiration of vomited stomach contents. However, aspiration of stomach

Table 3. Intravenous dosages of preanesthetics in domestic species. Many of these drugs have not been approved for use in veterinary practice, even though they are widely used and the dosage has been established.

Drugs	**Dosage (mg/kg)**				
	Dogs	**Cats**	**Horses**	**Pigs**	**Cattle**
		Anticholinergics			
Atropine	0.02	0.02	0.01-0.02	0.02	0.03-0.1
Glycopyrrolate	0.005	0.005	0.0015-0.003	0.0015	0.005
		Tranquilizers			
Acepromazine	0.03-0.05, total ≤3 mg	0.03-0.5, total ≤3 mg	0.02-0.05	0.03-0.4	0.1
Diazepam	0.1-0.5, total 10 mg	0.1-0.5, total 10 mg	0.02-0.1	0.2-0.4	0.02-0.08
Midazolam	0.2-0.4	0.2-0.4	0.02-0.04	—	—
Azaperone	—	—	0.2-0.4	1.0-2.0	—
		Sedatives			
Xylazine	0.5-1.0	0.5-1.0	0.3-1.1	1-2	0.02-0.1
Detomidine	—	—	0.005-0.02	—	0.03-0.06
Medetomidine	0.015-0.02	0.04-0.5	—	—	—

Table 4. Intravenous dosages of commonly used opioids and neuroleptanalgesic combinations in domestic species. Many of these drugs have not been approved for use in veterinary practice, even though they are widely used and the dosage has been established.

Drugs	Dosage (mg/kg)				
	Dogs	Cats	Horses	Pigs	Cattle
Narcotics					
Morphine	0.44-1.1	0.11-0.22	0.04-0.11	0.44-0.88	—
Oxymorphone	0.11-0.22, total 4 mg	0.44	0.02-0.11	—	—
Meperidine	0.44-1.1	0.22-0.44	0.44-1.1	0.44-1.1	—
Butorphanol	0.11-0.22	0.11-0.22	0.011-0.22	—	—
Buprenorphine	0.005-0.03	0.005-0.03	0.01-0.02	—	—
Neuroleptanalgesic Combinations					
Fentanyl Droperidol (Innovar-Vet)	1 ml/10-27 kg	1 ml/20 kg	—	1 ml/20-40 kg	—
Diazepam Oxymorphone	0.44, total 10 mg 0.22, total 4 mg	0.44, total 2.5 mg 0.22, total 10 mg	—	—	—
Acepromazine Meperidine	0.1, total 3 mg 1.0-3.0	0.1, total 3 mg 0.5-3	0.04 0.6	—	—
Acepromazine Oxymorphone	0.1, total 3 mg 0.1-0.3, total 4 mg	0.1, total 3 mg 0.1-0.3, total 4 mg	0.04 0.02	—	—
Acepromazine Butorphanol	0.1, total 3 mg 0.05-0.1	0.1, total 3 mg 0.05-0.1	0.08 0.04	—	—
Xylazine Morphine	0.55-1.0 0.25-0.5	—	0.66 0.22-0.66	—	—
Xylazine Meperidine	0.06 1.1	—	0.66 1.1	—	—
Xylazine Butorphanol	0.1-0.2 0.1-0.2	0.1-0.2 0.1-0.2	0.66 0.02	—	—
Xylazine Buprenorphine	—	—	0.66 0.01	—	—

contents is not without severe consequences, even in glycopyrrolate-treated animals.

As compared with atropine, glycopyrrolate has a longer duration of action (twice as long as that of atropine) and has fewer CNS effects because it does not readily cross the blood-brain barrier. Thus, glycopyrrolate has less effect on vision than atropine and appears to be more suitable for use in horses and cats when an anticholinergic is required.

Tranquilizers and Sedatives

Premedication of healthy animals with a tranquilizer or sedative is recommended because it decreases anxiety, aids in restraint, decreases the amount of general anesthetic required and helps provide a smoother recovery from anesthesia. A number of tranquilizers are available. They are classified as *minor* and *major.*

Benzodiazepines (diazepam and midazolam) are minor tranquilizers that induce only mild tranquilization. They are commonly used for their antianxiety, anticonvulsant and central muscle relaxant actions. These drugs minimally depress cardiovascular function.

Diazepam (Valium: Roche), though not approved for use in animals, is the most widely used of the benzodiazepines. The injectable form is dissolved in a propylene glycol vehicle. Because of its water insolubility, diazepam should not be diluted with water or mixed with other drugs. Rapid intravenous injection of diazepam induces hypotension and bradycardia. These effects are probably caused by the propylene glycol vehicle rather than diazepam itself.

Midazolam (Versed: Roche) is water soluble and has greater potency and a shorter duration of action than diazepam. Like diazepam, midazolam has been used in conjunction with ketamine and opioids in small animal patients.

The *phenothiazine* (acepromazine) and *butyrophenone derivatives* (droperidol and azaperone) are major tranquilizers that induce widespread CNS depression. Therefore, major tranquilizers induce a more reliable degree of tranquilization than minor tranquilizers.

Acepromazine (PromAce: Fort Dodge) is the most commonly used tranquilizer in veterinary medicine. Additional properties include antiemetic, antihistaminic and antiarrhythmogenic actions. Acepromazine may induce hypotension because of its CNS depression and peripheral alpha-adrenergic receptor-blocking actions. In animals with hypovolemia or low cardiac output, acepromazine may cause severe hypotension, which can lead to circulatory shock during general anesthesia. Acepromazine is contraindicated in animals prone to epileptic seizures because it lowers the seizure threshold.

Butyrophenones are rarely used alone because they can induce dysphoria. *Droperidol* is available in combination with fentanyl as Innovar-Vet (see Neuroleptanalgesics below). *Azaperone* (Strensil: Pitman-Moore) is a butyrophenone derivative used in pigs. Azaperone has little effect on heart and respiratory rates but causes a slight decrease in blood pressure. When given intramuscularly, azaperone induces good sedation, but excitement may occur if the animal is disturbed during the first 20 minutes following injection. Intravenous administration of azaperone is not recommended because it often causes transient excitement.

Xylazine (Rompun: Haver/Mobay, Gemini: Butler, Anased: Lloyd), an alpha-2 agonist, is a potent sedative, analgesic and muscle relaxant used widely in most domestic species. The 2 most common side effects of xylazine are bradycardia and emesis. Unlike acepromazine, xylazine may sensitize the heart to the arrhythmogenic effects of circulating catecholamines during halothane anesthesia. Following intravenous administration of xylazine, blood pressure increases transiently and then decreases. The initial increase in blood pressure is not always evident after intramuscular injection. Despite its profound sedative effect, xylazine is not recommended for use in seriously ill animals.

Ruminants are very sensitive to xylazine, requiring only one-fifth to one-tenth the dose used in horses. Another well-known side effect of xylazine is uterine contraction, with the most pronounced effect in ruminants. Only small doses of xylazine should be used in the late stages of pregnancy. High dosages (0.1-0.2 mg/kg) may induce early calving and lead to retained placenta.

Detomidine (Dormosedan: Norden/SmithKline) and *medetomidine* (Domitor: Farmos) are newer alpha-2 agonists with greater potency than xylazine. The effects of detomidine are similar to those of xylazine but longer lasting (1 hour). It is only approved for use in horses. The major difference between xylazine and detomidine appears to be in their effect on the uterus. Detomidine does not increase uterine contraction in ruminants.

Medetomidine is more potent than either detomidine or xylazine. A medetomidine dosage of 30 µg/kg induces sedative effects comparable to those of xylazine at 2.2 mg/kg.

The effects of xylazine and detomidine can be antagonized with an alpha-2 antagonist, such as *yohimbine* (Yobine: Lloyd) at 0.125 mg/kg or *tolazoline* (Priscoline: Ciba) at 2-4 mg/kg. However, yohimbine has proven to be ineffective for this purpose in ruminants. Its effectiveness can be improved if its administration is followed by *doxapram* (Dopram: Robins) IV at 0.5-1 mg/kg. Medetomidine has a specific antagonist, *atipamezole* (Atipamezole: Farmos), which is given IV at 0.06-0.24 mg/kg.

Opioids

Opioids are commonly used in dogs to induce preanesthetic analgesia and sedation. Combinations of *morphine* (Duramorph: Elkins-Sinn, Astramorph PF: Astra) and atropine or *oxymorphone* (Numorphan: DuPont) and atropine are commonly used, not only for their profound analgesic effect but also because they minimally depress cardiovascular function. Though opioids cause minimal cardiovascular depression, they often cause significant respiratory depression. When given rapidly IV, some opioids induce excitement. Atropine should be administered to prevent opioid-induced bradycardia.

If needed, the effects of opioids can be reversed by an antagonist, such as *naloxone* (Naloxone HCl Injection: Pitman-Moore) given IV at 2.2-33 μg/kg or *nalbuphine* (Nubain: DuPont). Because naloxone is a pure antagonist, all the effects of opioids including analgesia are antagonized. Analgesia is partially reversed when the agonist-antagonist nalbuphine is used. Strict records of acquisition and administration of opioid agonists must be kept.

Agonist-antagonists, such as *butorphanol* (Torbugesic: Fort Dodge) and *buprenorphine* (Buprenex: Norwich Eaton) have gained popularity because of their mild CNS depression and profound analgesic effect. Butorphanol is 3-5 times more potent than morphine, while buprenorphine is 30-50 times more potent than morphine. In small doses, butorphanol or buprenorphine induce similar respiratory depression to that of morphine, but a "ceiling effect" is seen, in which larger doses of either drug do not induce further depression. Similar ceiling effects occur with regard to their analgesic actions.

Neuroleptanalgesics

Combinations of tranquilizers and opioids induce *neuroleptanalgesia,* which is an intense analgesic and amnesic state. The opioid is used to induce analgesia and the tranquilizer acts to sedate and counteract the side effects of the opioid, such as vomiting and excitement. These combinations induce sufficient sedation and analgesia for minor surgery, but they do not produce total unconsciousness and the animal may be aroused by a severely painful stimulus or a loud auditory stimulus.

A combination of *fentanyl* and *droperidol* (in 1:50 ratio) is available as Innovar-Vet (Pitman-Moore). Each milliliter of Innovar-Vet contains 0.4 mg of fentanyl and 20 mg of droperidol. Innovar-Vet can be used to tranquilize vicious dogs. The tranquilizing action of Innovar-Vet lasts longer than the analgesia because of droperidol's longer duration of action. This becomes significant when repeat doses are given. Other combinations, such as acepromazine and oxymorphone or diazepam and oxymorphone, can be used independently to induce neuroleptanalgesia.

Anesthetic Agents

General anesthesia can be induced in several different ways: with injectable anesthetic drugs only; with an inhalation anesthetic only; or with injectable drugs for induction and an inhalant for anesthetic maintenance. In general, inhalation anesthetic techniques are more complex and require expensive equipment, but anesthetic depth is more easily controlled and recovery does not depend on hepatic metabolism and renal excretion to the extent of injectable anesthetic drug anesthesia. Anesthesia for short surgical procedures can be safely induced and maintained with injectable anesthetics that are short-acting or reversible.

Veterinary anesthesia has become sophisticated and the anesthetist should understand the basic pharmacology of anesthetics and fully appreciate how these drugs function.

Injectable Anesthetics

Barbiturates: Barbiturates are classified into 4 groups according to duration of action: *long, intermediate, short* and *ultra-short. Long-acting* and *intermediate-acting barbiturates* are generally used as sedatives or anticonvulsants. *Short-acting* (*eg,* pentobarbital) and *ultra-short-acting* (*eg,* thiopental, thiamylal, methohexital) *barbiturates* are most commonly used to induce general anesthesia.

Because of its low lipid solubility, *pentobarbital* (Nembutal: Abbott) has a relatively slow onset (5 minutes) and a rather long duration of action. It crosses the blood-brain barrier and is redistributed away from brain tissue more slowly than is *thiopental* (Pentothal: Abbott/Ceva) and *thiamylal* (Bio-Tal: Bio-Ceutic, Surital: Parke-Davis). Pentobarbital is usually administered intravenously (or intraperitoneally in small laboratory species). It may cause excitement when given by slow intravenous infusion. For this reason, pentobarbital anesthesia should be induced by rapid (bolus) injection of half of the calculated total dose (Table 5), with the remaining dose given in increments over several minutes, allowing time to assess the full effect.

Pentobarbital induces a transient increase in heart rate (for 10-20 minutes) and a decrease in arterial blood pressure. Respiration and renal function are depressed following pentobarbital injection. Complete recovery usually requires 6-24 hours. Prolonged recovery is common with large doses or repeat dosing. Today, pentobarbital is rarely used in veterinary practice because of this undesirable effect.

Thiopental and *thiamylal* are the most popular ultra-short-acting thiobarbiturates. These drugs have a very rapid onset (60-90 seconds) and short duration of action (10-20 minutes) because of their high lipid solubility and rapid redistribution from the brain to muscle and other nonneural tissues. Complete recovery generally occurs within 1-2 hours.

Rapid intravenous injection causes a transient decrease in blood pressure and a compensatory increase in heart rate. Dose-dependent respiratory depression and a short period of apnea are characteristic responses following induction. Thiopental and thiamylal sensitize the myocardium to circulating catecholamines during halothane anesthesia. This effect can be mitigated by preanesthetic medication with acepromazine.

These 2 drugs are best used for induction or for a short period of anesthesia. Prolonged recovery is often observed when repeat doses are given to prolong anesthesia beyond a duration of 20-25 minutes. A reduced dose is indicated in patients with acidemia, anemia, hypoproteinemia, hypovolemia or hepatic disease.

Perivascular injection of thiopental and thiamylal causes tissue irritation and necrosis because of their high alkalinity. Therefore, areas of perivascular injection should be infiltrated with a dilute solution (1:9) of 2% lidocaine hydrochloride in saline. Lidocaine causes vasodilation and prevents vasospasm in the affected areas, thus increasing the rate of absorption of the thiobarbiturate. Accidental perivascular injection can be prevented by placing an indwelling catheter in the vein before drug injection.

Sighthounds, such as Greyhounds and Whippets, have less body mass for redistribution; thus, smaller doses should be used in these dogs to avoid prolonged recoveries.

The Drug Enforcement Administration (DEA) classifies thiopental and thiamylal as controlled substances, so special DEA order forms and records are required.

Methohexital (Brietal: Lilly) is an ultra-short-acting oxybarbiturate with an extremely short duration of action but twice the potency of thiopental. The onset of action is faster with methohexital (15-60 seconds) than with thiopental or thiamylal. Surgical anesthesia lasts only 5-15 minutes and full recovery is also rapid (30 minutes) because of its rapid hepatic metabolism. Consequently, this barbiturate is used primarily for induction of anesthesia.

Methohexital causes dose-dependent respiratory depression and apnea upon induction. Excitement may occur during induction or recovery if the patient is not premedicated with a tranquilizer or sedative.

Methohexital is the barbiturate of choice for induction of anesthesia in sighthounds because of its rapid metabolism.

Dissociative Drugs: Dissociative drugs induce a state of *cataleptoid* anesthesia characterized by profound analgesia, cataleptic immobility, amnesia and loss of responsiveness to external physical stimuli while preserving pharyngeal, laryngeal and eye reflexes. Occasionally, random movements of the head or limbs occur independently of surgical manipulations. It is important not to confuse these movements with insufficient depth of anesthesia.

Unlike other conventional anesthetics, dissociatives do not depress the cardiovascular system. On the contrary, they induce a stimulatory effect by direct action on the CNS and increased circulating catecholamines. Therefore, heart rate and blood pressure increase in animals anesthetized with dissociatives. Respiration is characterized by an apnestic breathing pattern (breath holding). Rapid intravenous injection and overdosage cause respiratory depression and sometimes apnea.

The most widely used dissociatives in veterinary medicine are *ketamine* (Ketaset: Aveco, Vetalar: Parke-Davis) and *tiletamine. Ketamine* is used both as a preanesthetic and general anesthetic in cats. The degree of muscle relaxation is poor when ketamine is used alone. This is generally overcome by simultaneous administration of a tranquilizer, such as acepromazine or diazepam. Salivation is common and can be reduced by premedication with atropine. If salivation is excessive, tracheal intubation is advised to prevent aspiration. Because the eyes remain open during ketamine anesthesia, an ophthalmic ointment should be applied to the corneas to prevent corneal damage.

In dogs, ketamine is used in combination with a tranquilizer to prevent excitement and clonic activity (paddling) during recovery. In horses, a sedative (*eg,* xylazine) should always be given before ketamine administration, and sufficient sedation should be evident before giving ketamine so as to prevent excitement upon induction.

In most species, ketamine is removed from the body through liver metabolism and renal excretion. Cats, however, appear to excrete ketamine largely unchanged in the urine.

Tiletamine is available in combination with *zolazepam* as Telazol (Robins) in a 1:1 ratio. The effects of tiletamine last longer than those of ketamine, and it is 2-3 times more potent than ketamine. *Zolazepam* is a benzodiazepine derivative similar to diazepam.

Combining zolazepam with tiletamine decreases the unfavorable effects of tiletamine (*eg,* poor muscle relaxation). This combination induces tachycardia accompanied by a slight increase in blood pressure and initial respiratory stimulation, followed by mild respiratory depression.

Telazol is recommended for short surgical procedures in dogs and cats. In large doses, respiratory depression and prolonged recovery are major disadvantages. In dogs, tiletamine appears to be metabolized less rapidly than zolazepam. A rough recovery, similar to that induced by ketamine alone, may occur when large doses of Telazol are given alone. Telazol has been used successfully for chemical restraint and anesthesia in a wide variety of exotic and domestic animals.

Steroid Anesthetics: Saffan (Althesin: Glaxo) is a combination of 2 steroids: *alphaxalone* and *alphadolone*. Each milliliter of saffan contains 9 mg of alphaxalone and 3 mg of alphadolone.

Saffan has been used for clinical anesthesia in cats in countries other than the United States since 1970. Saffan can be used alone for sedation or for short-term general anesthesia (10-20 minutes). Similar to thiopental, saffan decreases blood pressure and increases the heart rate, but the effect on blood pressure is not dose-dependent. The decrease in blood pressure is transient with smaller doses but is more prolonged with larger doses.

Major advantages of saffan anesthesia are a wide safety range, lack of accumulation in tissues, rapid recovery of consciousness, little respiratory depression with good muscle relaxation, and lack of tissue irritation. However, transient swelling of the ears and paws has been reported in cats. The cause of this is not clear. It may be related to histamine release. Pigs that are susceptible to malignant hyperthermia have been safely anesthetized with saffan. Use of saffan is not recommended in dogs because the vehicle in which it is dissolved induces profound histamine release.

Propofol: Propofol (Diprivan: Stuart) is a hypnotic unrelated to barbiturates or steroid anesthetics. The active ingredient of propofol, 2,6-diisopropylphenol, is suspended in an emulsion containing soybean oil, purified egg phosphatide and glycerol. Similar to thiopental, propofol induces rapid onset and short duration of hypnosis without excitatory side-effects. The cardiovascular and respiratory effects induced by propofol are similar to those of thiopental.

The major advantages of propofol over thiopental are the lack of a cumulative effect, and rapid recovery even after a long period of infusion. Because vomiting and retching have been observed in some dogs and cats upon recovery, close observation during recovery is required.

Etomidate: Etomidate (Amidate: Abbott), another non-barbiturate hypnotic, is an imidazole derivative prepared in 35% propylene glycol and water. Induction and recovery with etomidate are rapid. Excitement during induction can be prevented by premedication with diazepam or other tranquilizers. Among all the intravenous induction agents, etomidate has the least effect on the cardiovascular system. However, it does cause hemolysis in dogs and people.

Respiration is characterized by initial hyperventilation, followed by a period of respiratory depression, but the depression is less than that of other intravenous anesthetics. In people, etomidate inhibits the increase in plasma cortisol and aldosterone concentrations during surgical stress. Suppression of adrenocortical function for 2-3 hours after etomidate administration also has been reported in dogs. This suppression of adrenocortical function may decrease an animal's ability to tolerate the stress of surgery and anesthesia. Nevertheless, etomidate is often used in debilitated animals or animals with preexisting cardiac disease when maintenance of cardiovascular stability is desired.

Table 5 summarizes the recommended dosages of commonly used injectable anesthetics for induction or short-term anesthesia.

Inhalant Anesthetics

Inhalant anesthetic techniques offer several advantages over injectable anesthetics, including good control of anesthetic depth, good muscle relaxation and analgesia, rapid recovery, and minimal cumulative effects after long periods of anesthesia. As mentioned previously, a disadvantage of inhalation anesthesia is that it requires complicated anesthetic equipment and the knowledge to operate and maintain it.

The action of inhalant anesthetics is governed by the potency of the individual anesthetic, the solubility of the anesthetic in blood and different tissues, and its effects on organ systems. This section presents information on 4 commonly used anesthetics: *nitrous oxide, methoxyflurane* (Metofane: Pitman-Moore), *halothane* (Halothane: Fort Dodge) and *isoflurane* (AErrane: Anaquest).

Anesthetic Potency: Inhalant anesthetics enter the body through the lungs and the depth of anesthesia is determined by the concentration of the anesthetic in the brain. Adequate concentration of the anesthetic vapor must be achieved in the lung for an inhalant anesthetic to reach the brain. The potency of an anesthetic is determined by the alveolar concentration required to produce a given anesthetic effect.

The *minimum alveolar concentration (MAC)* of an anesthetic is defined as the lowest alveolar concentration required to prevent gross purposeful movement to a graded noxious stimulus (such as skin incision or tail clamp) in 50% of patients. Thus, the MAC value indicates the *potency* of an anesthetic. An anesthetic with a low MAC value is a more potent anesthetic than an anesthetic with a high MAC value.

Table 5. Intravenous dosages of commonly used injectable anesthetics for short-term anesthesia in domestic species. Many of these drugs have not been approved for use in veterinary practice, even though they are widely used and the dosage has been established.

Agents	Dosage (mg/kg)				
	Dogs	Cats	Horses	Pigs	Cattle
Thiopental	8.8-13.2	8.8-13.2	5-8	10-20	6-12
Thiamylal	8.8-13.2	8.8-13.2	4-6	6-18	4.4-11
Methohexital	6.6-15.4	6.6-15.4	2-5	5	5.5
Ketamine	—	2.2-6.6	—	2.2-6.6	2
Tiletamine-Zolazepam	4.4-11	2.2-11	—	4.4-11	4.4-11
Etomidate	1.1-4.4	1.1-4.4	—	1.1-4.4	—
Propofol	4.4-6.6	6.6-8.8	—	—	—
Saffan	—	3-9	—	4-6	3
Acepromazine-Ketamine	0.22 11	0.1 12	—	0.15 7	—
Xylazine-Ketamine	0.66 6.6	0.66 2.2-6.6	1.1 2.2	1.1 9	0.1 2.2
Medetomidine-Ketamine	0.02 2.5	0.035- 0.045/3	—	—	—
Diazepam Ketamine	0.2-0.4 8.8-11	0.55, total 2 mg 4.4-8.8	—	0.5-1.1 5-8	0.22 4.4-6.6
Acepromazine with Tiletamine-Zolazepam	0.1 2.2	0.05 1.1-1.5	—	—	—
Xylazine with Tiletamine-Zolazepam	0.4 6.6	0.66 2.2-6.6	1.1 1.1-2.2	0.5-1.1 0.5-1.5	0.1 4
Detomidine with Tiletamine-Zolazepam	—	—	0.02-0.04 1.1-2	—	—

Isoflurane is the least potent of the 3 most commonly used halogenated anesthetics, with halothane of intermediate potency, and methoxyflurane the most potent. Nitrous oxide (N_2O) is a weak anesthetic, with a MAC value of 150-200%. Nitrous oxide alone does not induce general anesthesia in animals. Thus, it is most commonly used as a supplement to methoxyflurane, halothane or isoflurane. The concentration of N_2O should not be greater than 60-70% when used as a supplement to other anesthetics. Oxygen (O_2) should be administered simultaneously to prevent hypoxemia.

Table 6 shows MAC values of these 4 anesthetics used alone in domestic animals. It is very important to remember that *MAC values may change with the animal's physical condition* (*eg,* disease or pregnancy), concurrent medications or body temperature (Table 7).

Solubility Coefficient: Solubility coefficient is the ratio of concentrations of an anesthetic in 2 phases at equilibrium, such as blood and gas or tissue and blood. Equilibrium concentration is based on the amounts of anesthetic contained in the 2 phases at equal partial pressure.

During induction, the anesthetic gas crosses the alveoli-capillary membranes into the blood by which it is distributed to all body tissues, including the brain. The anesthetic molecules continue moving down the pressure gradient between 2 phases (blood/gas or brain/blood) until the pressures reach an equilibrium.

The faster the alveolar anesthetic pressure rises to equal the inhaled anesthetic pressure, the faster the equilibrium is achieved between the pressure of the alveoli and pulmonary capillaries. Similarly, the faster the pressure of the alveoli and pulmonary capillaries equilibrate, the faster the pressure of the cerebral blood can rise and the faster the partial pressure of the anesthetic in the brain is achieved to induce anesthesia.

Table 6. Minimum alveolar concentration (MAC) for inhalant anesthetics. (Adopted from Booth NH and McDonald LE: *Veterinary Pharmacology and Therapeutics,* 1988.)

Anesthetics	MAC (%)				
	Dogs	Cats	Horses	Pigs	Cattle
Methoxyflurane	0.23	0.27	—	—	—
Halothane	0.87	1.19	0.88	0.91	0.76
Isoflurane	1.5	1.61	1.31	1.55	—
Nitrous Oxide	222	255	190	195[a]-277[b]	—

a–Tranquilli WJ *et al. Am J Vet Res* 46:58-60, 1985.
b–Weiskopf RB and Bogetz MS. *Anesth Analg* 63:529-532, 1984.

Table 7. Impact of physiologic and pharmacologic factors on minimum alveolar anesthetic concentration.

No Changes in MAC	Decrease in MAC	Increase in MAC
Duration of anesthesia	Hypothermia	Hyperthermia (to 42 C)
Magnitude of metabolism	Hyponatremia	Hypernatremia
$PaCO_2$ below 95 mm Hg	Pregnancy	
PaO_2 above 38 mm Hg	PaO_2 below 38 mm Hg	
Blood pressure above 40 mm Hg	$PaCO_2$ above 95 mm Hg	
Hyperkalemia or hypokalemia	Blood pressure below 40 mm Hg	
Metabolic acid-base changes	Increasing age	
	Lidocaine	
	Preanesthetics: α_2-agonists Narcotics Acepromazine Benzodiazepines	
	Injectable anesthetics	
	Other inhalation anesthetics	

The processes during recovery from anesthesia are the reverse of those during induction. When anesthetic administration is discontinued, the inspired anesthetic pressure falls and the equilibration process changes direction until the partial pressure of the anesthetic in the brain falls below the level that causes loss of consciousness, and the animal recovers.

An anesthetic with a high blood/gas solubility coefficient, such as methoxyflurane, takes longer to reach equilibrium because the anesthetic is rapidly removed from the alveoli and a concentration gradient between the alveoli and blood is established very slowly. Conversely, an anesthetic with a low blood/gas solubility coefficient, such as isoflurane, tends to remain in the alveoli and rapidly achieves a high concentration in the alveoli and increases the diffusion gradient between the alveoli and the blood. Thus, induction and recovery of anesthesia are more rapid with isoflurane than with methoxyflurane. Halothane has an intermediate blood/gas solubility coefficient; therefore, induction and recovery with halothane is slower than with isoflurane but faster than with methoxyflurane (Table 8).

Effect of Body Tissues: Body tissues are classified into 4 groups according to their blood supply: *vessel-rich* (brain, heart, liver, kidney, gastrointestinal tract, lungs), *muscle* (muscle, skin), *vessel-poor* (bone, ligaments, cartilage, tendon) and *fat.* The vessel-rich and muscle groups are the most important body tissues for uptake, distribution and elimination of inhalant anesthetics.

Vessel-rich tissues constitute 9% of the body mass and receive 75% of cardiac output. Because of their rich blood supply, anesthetic is most quickly equilibrated in vessel-rich tissues, usually in 5-20 minutes.

The *muscle group* of tissues constitutes 50% of the body mass but receives only 15-20% of cardiac output. Uptake of anesthetics by these tissues continues for a longer period before reaching equilibration (90 minutes to 4 hours).

Body fat receives approximately 5% of cardiac output and constitutes about 20% of the body mass. In general, anesthetics are more soluble in fat than in other body tissues, but the low blood flow delays anesthetic uptake. Because of this, the proportion of fat in body mass has little effect on induction of anesthesia but plays a more important role in recovery from prolonged anesthesia (over 4 hours).

Vessel-poor tissues constitute 20% of the body mass and receive only 2% of the cardiac output. Thus, these tissues have no effect on anesthetic induction and recovery.

In general, anesthetic uptake by vessel-rich tissues ceases after 20 minutes, at which time uptake by muscle and fat has just started. A state of general anesthesia does not occur until the concentration of anesthetic in the brain is great enough to induce loss of consciousness. The more soluble the anesthetic (*eg,* methoxyflurane, halothane) in the blood, the slower the induction time.

Table 8. Partition coefficient of inhalant anesthetics at 37 C. (Adapted from Miller RD: *Anesthesia,* 1990.)

Anesthetic	Blood/Gas	Brain/Blood	Muscle/Blood	Fat/Blood
Methoxyflurane	15	1.4	1.6	61
Halothane	2.4	2.0	4.0	62
Isoflurane	1.41	1.6	3.4	52
Nitrous Oxide	0.47	1.1	1.2	2.3

Increasing the inspired anesthetic concentration (*concentration effect*) above the usual maintenance level shortens the time required to induce anesthesia. Nitrous oxide can also be used concomitantly with other inhalation anesthetics to speed induction. This is known as the *second gas effect.*

Effects on the Cardiovascular System: All inhalant anesthetics depress myocardial contractility; the effect is dose-dependent and reversible. Depression of *myocardial contractility* decreases cardiac output and blood flow to vital tissues. With normal blood carbon dioxide levels and absence of surgical stimulation, halothane depresses cardiac output more than isoflurane. Methoxyflurane affects the cardiovascular system in much the same way as halothane, but to a lesser extent. Cardiac output is modestly increased by N_2O administration, which may be attributable to its sympathetic-stimulating effect.

Reduction of *blood pressure* is also dose-dependent, with isoflurane producing a somewhat greater decrease than halothane. A decrease in peripheral vascular resistance is responsible in large part for the decrease in blood pressure with isoflurane, while halothane decreases myocardial contractility and cardiac output. Blood pressure with N_2O alone remains unchanged or slightly increased.

Heart rate remains unchanged in animals during administration of halothane, N_2O or methoxyflurane. Isoflurane increases the heart rate by decreasing blood pressure and vagal activity. The effects of inhalant anesthetics on the heart rate and blood pressure may be influenced by preanesthetic drugs.

Both methoxyflurane and halothane sensitize the myocardium to epinephrine and may induce cardiac arrhythmias, while isoflurane does not. As mentioned previously, N_2O alone is not potent enough to induce anesthesia but may be used as a supplement to a more potent anesthetic. Administration of 60-70% N_2O reduces the dose of halothane or methoxyflurane required to maintain anesthesia and therefore reduces the cardiovascular depressant effects seen when halothane or methoxyflurane is used alone.

Table 9 summarizes the cardiovascular effects of various anesthetics.

Effects on the Respiratory System: Halothane and N_2O produce dose-dependent increases in the *respiratory rate.* Isoflurane produces similar increases in respiratory rate up to 1 MAC, but further increases do not occur when isoflurane concentrations above 1 MAC are given. *Tidal volume* (volume of air expired during each breathing cycle) is decreased during increased respiration.

The net effect of these changes is rapid, shallow breathing during general anesthesia. However, the increased respiratory rate is not sufficient to overcome the reduced tidal volume, resulting in decreased minute ventilation (minute ventilation = respiratory rate x tidal volume) and increased arterial partial pressure of CO_2.

Methoxyflurane, unlike other anesthetics, induces dose-dependent respiratory depression, reducing both the respiratory rate and tidal volume. Nitrous oxide use should be avoided in animals with respiratory dysfunction because it decreases the inspired O_2 tension. In these ill animals, high inspired O_2 tension is necessary to prevent hypoxemia. Use of N_2O must also be avoided in animals with pneumothorax because N_2O worsens the preexisting pneumothorax, leading to increased intrathoracic pressure and decreased lung volume. If unrecognized, these changes compromise ventilation and blood circulation, possibly leading to death.

Effects on the Liver and Kidney: Inhalant anesthetics are primarily eliminated through the lungs. Approximately 99% of isoflurane, 80% of halothane and 50% of methoxyflurane is eliminated by this route, with the remainder metabolized by the liver. The metabolites of these anesthetics are eliminated via the kidney in the urine. Isoflurane does not cause postanesthetic liver or kidney complications, probably because of its low lipid solubility and minimal metabolism. Thus, isoflurane is a preferred anesthetic for animals with preexisting hepatic or renal disease.

Postanesthetic hepatitis has been reported in people anesthetized with halothane. Liver necrosis is believed to be induced by irreversible binding of halothane to a phospholipid component of the liver cell membrane. This syndrome is exacerbated by hypoxemia. Despite the fact that this syndrome has only been suggested in goats, it still could occur in animals, though at a very low incidence. Thus, halothane should be used with some caution in animals with liver disease and the technician should ensure adequate oxygenation of patients in which it is employed.

Table 9. Effects of inhalant anesthetics on cardiovascular function. N/C = no change.

Anesthetic	Heart Rate	Cardiac Contractility	Stroke Volume	Cardiac Output	Mean Arterial Pressure	Peripheral Vascular Resistance
Methoxyflurane	↑	↓	↓	↓	↓	↓ or ↑
Halothane	N/C or ↓	↓	↓	↓	↓	↓
Isoflurane	N/C or ↓	↓	↓	↓	↓	↓
Nitrous Oxide	↑	↓	↓	N/C	N/C	↑

A nephrotoxic syndrome has been reported in people and animals anesthetized with methoxyflurane, caused by the inorganic fluoride metabolite of methoxyflurane. This nephrotoxic syndrome is characterized by nephrogenic diabetes insipidus that is unresponsive to fluid restriction or administration of antidiuretic hormone. Severity of the syndrome is proportional to the total dose of methoxyflurane administered. Concurrent administration of nephrotoxic agents, such as tetracycline and gentamicin, aggravates this syndrome. Obese animals are more susceptible to the nephrotoxic action of methoxyflurane because more drug is retained in the fat for a relatively longer period and slow release allows longer exposure to the toxic metabolite. Thus, methoxyflurane should be used cautiously in animals that are obese, that have renal disease, or that have been treated with nephrotoxic drugs.

ANESTHESIA EQUIPMENT

The basic anesthesia equipment necessary for induction and maintenance of anesthesia is listed in Table 10. Anesthesia equipment that is used routinely should be kept in a location close to the induction area and operating room.

Anesthesia Machines

There is a wide variety of types of inhalant anesthesia machines, but all of these machines have essentially the same basic compo-

Table 10. Basic anesthetic equipment for induction and maintenance of anesthesia.

- Needles (18, 20, 22 and 25 gauge) and syringes (1, 3, 5, 10 and 20 ml).
- Intravenous catheters and fluid administration sets.
- Laryngoscope with infant and adult blades, one spare set of batteries, and functional light bulbs.
- Endotracheal tubes in a wide range of different sizes, cuffed or noncuffed.
- Stylet for easy intubation.
- Topical anesthetic, either aerosol or viscous form, to anesthetize the laryngeal mucous membrane, facilitate intubation and prevent laryngeal spasm.
- Face mask for induction of anesthesia with inhalants.
- Manual ventilation apparatus, Ambu bag.
- Oxygen and inhalation anesthesia machine and accessories.
- Anesthetic, emergency drugs and balanced electrolyte solutions.

nents (Fig 1). The primary purposes of an anesthesia machine and a breathing system are delivery of O_2, delivery of the inhalant anesthetic, removal of CO_2 from exhaled gases, and provision for positive-pressure ventilation.

Inhalant anesthetics can be administered by *open* or *semi-open nonrebreathing systems,* or by *semi-closed* or *closed rebreathing (circle) systems*. These classifications are based on the degree of rebreathing of exhaled gases, use of a reservoir bag, CO_2 adsorbent or valves within the system, and the flow rate of fresh O_2. Patient size, fresh gas flow requirements, mechanism for proper direction of gas flow, method of mechanical ventilation, and elimination of CO_2 are important in selecting the appropriate system for a particular animal.

Nonrebreathing Systems

Open System: An open nonrebreathing system does not provide for rebreathing of exhaled gases; therefore, it does not have a reservoir bag or CO_2 absorber. The animal breathes only the gas(es) and anesthetic vapor presented by the anesthesia machine. *Open insufflation* is similar in that anesthetic vapor, together with air or O_2, is delivered to the mouth or trachea through a mask or

Figure 1. Basic components of an anesthesia machine. A. Small animal machine. B. Large animal machine. a. Vaporizer. b. Oxygen flowmeter. c. Nitrous oxide flowmeter. d. Ventilator. e. Carbon dioxide absorber. f. Y-piece breathing circuit. g. Rebreathing bag.

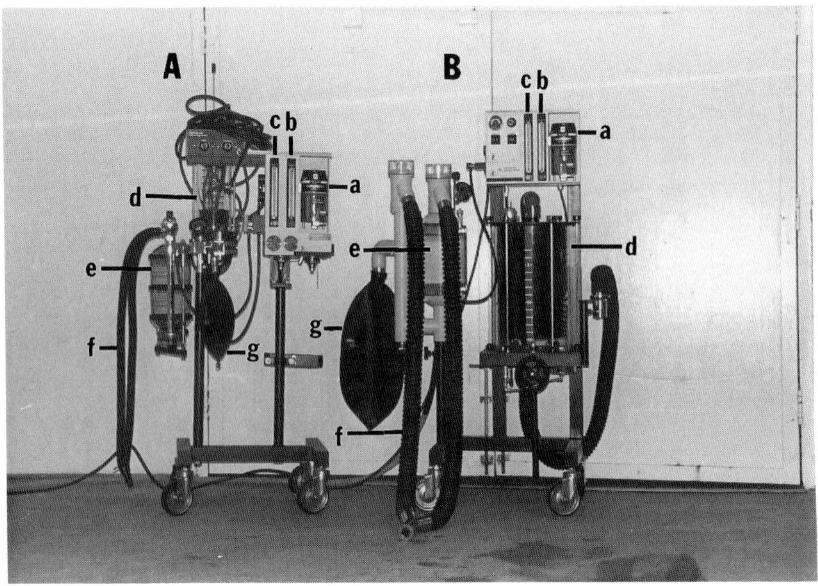

catheter. The catheter used should be small so as to avoid restriction of the airway and to allow exhaled gases to escape around the catheter.

Inhaled gases include room air as well as anesthetic gas mixtures. An O_2 flow twice the minute ventilation (440 ml/kg/minute) prevents rebreathing of exhaled gases. This technique is simple and safe, and is most frequently used for small laboratory animals in which minimal airway resistance and dead space is desirable. Major disadvantages are variable anesthetic concentration because of dilution with room air, and pollution of the environment with anesthetic gases.

Semi-Open System: Semi-open nonrebreathing systems are recommended for animals that weigh less than 7-10 kg. Thus, this system is frequently used in small animals, small exotic patients, birds and "pocket pets." Using this system, anesthesia is commonly induced with a face mask or induction chamber.

Semi-open systems do not provide significant rebreathing of exhaled gases, nor do they use a CO_2 absorbent. A reservoir bag is used to store anesthetic gases in O_2 for inhalation and for assisted or controlled ventilation.

Advantages of nonrebreathing systems include: rapid changes in anesthetic depth because the inspired anesthetic concentration is equal to the output of the vaporizer and a change of vaporizer setting immediately changes the anesthetic inspired concentration; reduced work of breathing and enhanced gas exchange because they produce less resistance to breathing than a circle system; and easy positioning because they are light-weight and compact.

The major disadvantages of nonrebreathing systems include: high gas flow required to prevent rebreathing of exhaled gases, resulting in waste of O_2 and anesthetic gas and increased cost; significant loss of body heat and humidity with high gas flow dries the respiratory tract mucosa and promotes hypothermia; and contamination of the operating room with anesthetic gases.

The most commonly used nonrebreathing systems in veterinary medicine are the *Bain coaxial system* and the *Norman mask elbow system* (Fig 2). When using these 2 systems, a fresh gas flow of 2-3 times the patient's minute ventilation (440-660 ml/kg/minute) is recommended. Some authors have proposed that a lower fresh gas flow (100-130 ml/kg/ minute) can be used safely with the Bain coaxial system in veterinary patients.

An *anesthesia chamber* is frequently used to induce anesthesia in small patients weighing less than 7 kg (Fig 3). It is particularly useful if intravenous injection is difficult. The animal is placed in the chamber and the lid is secured. The animal should first be allowed to breathe only O_2 for a few minutes. Oxygen flow is usually set at 5 L/minute, depending on chamber size. This denitrogenates the chamber and the patient's lungs.

A mixture of halothane or isoflurane in O_2 and/or N_2O is introduced into the chamber via the inspiratory limb of a regular breathing circuit or the fresh gas line. Excess gas is allowed to escape through the expiratory limb or relief valve that is connected to a scavenging system to minimize operating room pollution. The va-

Figure 2. Non-rebreathing systems. A. Norman elbow system. B. Bain coaxial system.

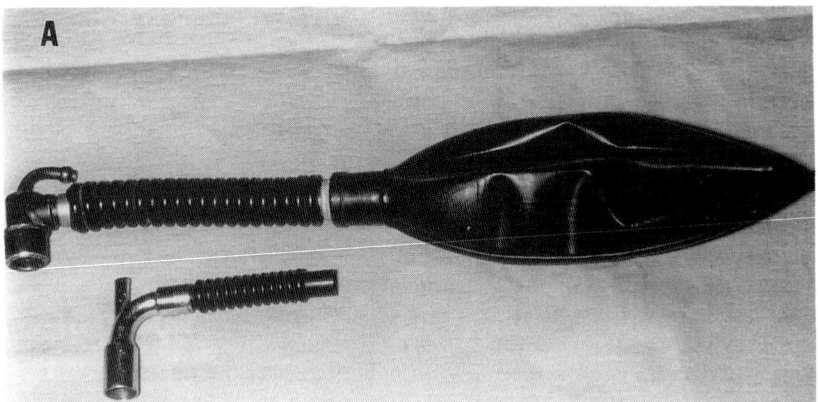

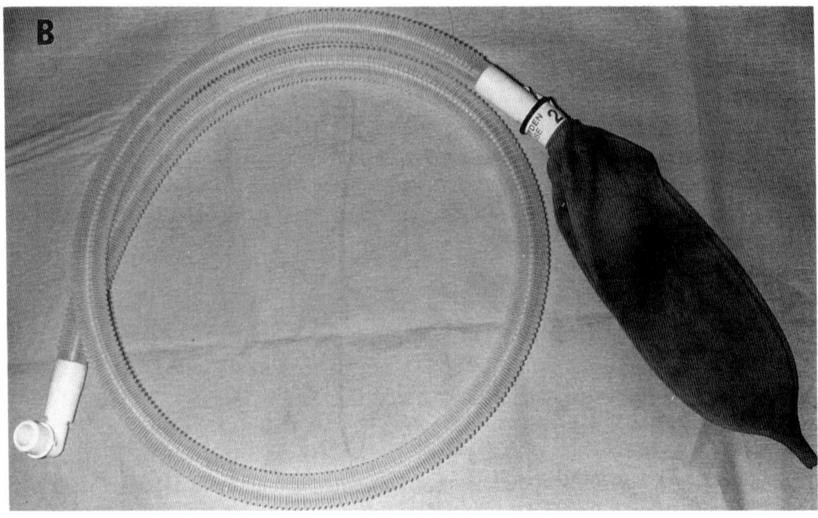

porizer is set initially at 0.5 or 1% for a short period until the animal becomes accustomed to the odor of the anesthetic. After this period, the vaporizer setting can be increased gradually to a final vaporizer setting of 4-5%.

Most patients become unconscious within 3-5 minutes. When this occurs, the patient is removed from the chamber and induction is completed by face mask and a breathing system (Fig 4).

Chamber induction is not suitable for animals with upper airway obstruction or respiratory depression, as apnea (cessation of breathing) may occur in the chamber if the patient's airway is compromised. It is also not recommended for use in animals with a full stomach, as vomiting may occur before the trachea is intubated.

Rebreathing (Circle) System

A rebreathing or circle system, by definition, allows rebreathing of exhaled gases. A rebreathing system is somewhat more complicated and expensive than a nonrebreathing system. It is composed of: a fresh-gas inlet (near the inspiratory limb of the breathing circuit); corrugated tubing; one-way valves that allow only unidirectional gas flow around the breathing circuit; a CO_2 absorber placed downstream from the gas-relief valve to ensure efficient removal of

Figure 3. Anesthesia induction chamber. This chamber can be adjusted to the size of the patient.

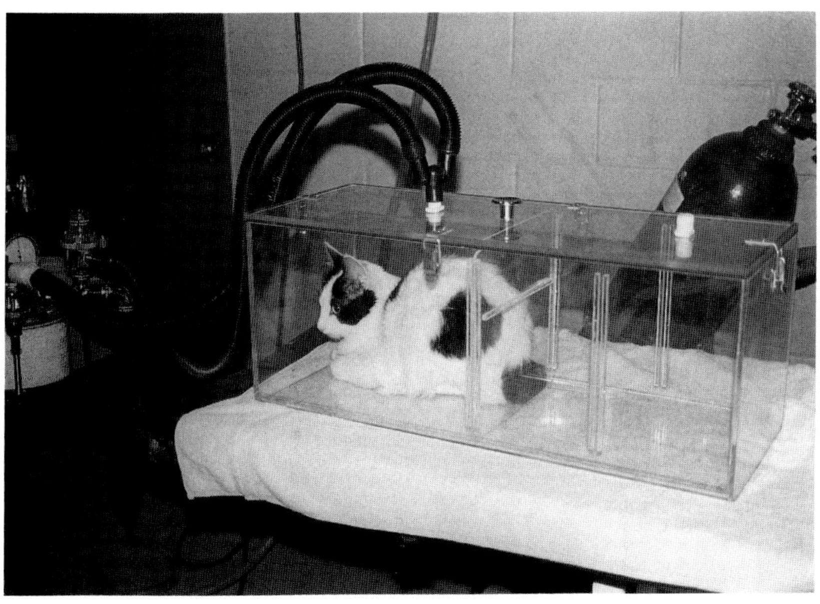

CO_2 from the rebreathed gases; a reservoir bag to accommodate changes in circuit volume during peak inspiration; and a pressure-relief ("pop off") valve to permit release of excess gases from the circuit (Fig 5).

Circle systems are subdivided into *closed* and *semi-closed systems*. There is no actual configurational difference between a semi-closed and a closed system. They use the same circle rebreathing system. Differentiation between the 2 systems is the fresh gas flow rate.

Semi-Closed Rebreathing System: With a semi-closed system, the rate of fresh gas flow is greater than the patient requires. Excess gases exit the breathing circuit through the "pop-off" valve and finally the scavenging system. Exhaled CO_2 is removed by the CO_2 absorbent. Generally, the flow rate of fresh O_2 during maintenance of anesthesia is 22-44 ml/kg/minute for small animals and 10 ml/kg/minute for large animals when a semi-closed system is used. The actual metabolic O_2 requirement is 4-7 ml/kg/minute for most small animals and 2-3 ml/kg/minute for large animals. High O_2 flow ensures adequate gas flow to the patient, decreases the time required for equilibration after adjustment of the vaporizer set-

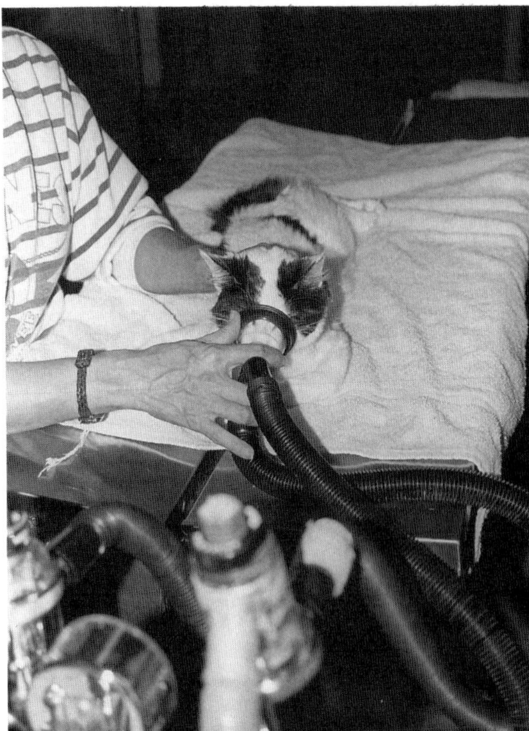

Figure 4. Face mask induction.

ting, and ensures an appropriate concentration of oxygenation when N_2O is used simultaneously.

Current recommendations are for a low-flow system using a fresh O_2 flow rate only slightly greater than the metabolic O_2 requirement (4-7 ml/kg/minute) but less than the traditional fresh O_2 flow (22-44 ml/kg/minute) used with a semi-closed system. Low-flow systems offer the advantages of conserving heat and moisture because less body energy is used to warm and humidify the dry cold gases with high fresh gas flows, decreasing anesthesia cost by decreasing the amount of O_2 and anesthetic used, and decreasing waste gas pollution in the operating room environment. The expense of CO_2 absorbent is increased with a low-flow system because proportionately more CO_2 must be removed from the system. Thus, the CO_2 absorbent is more rapidly exhausted and requires more frequent changing.

The decision to use a high or low fresh O_2 flow must accommodate the type of anesthesia equipment used, the type of vaporizer, the physical condition of the patient, and the technician's ability to identify and correct problems when they arise.

Closed Rebreathing System: A closed system exists when the O_2 flow is equal to the animal's O_2 metabolic requirement, which is 4-

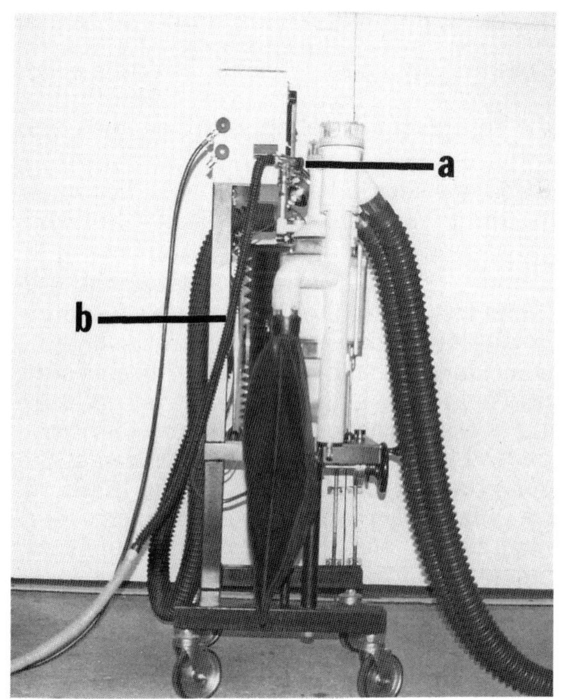

Figure 5. a. Pressure-relief (pop-off) valve. b. Disposal system.

7 ml/kg/minute for small animals and 2 ml/kg/minute for large animals. Because all of the fresh gas delivered to the breathing system is taken up by the patient, little or no gas escapes through the "pop-off" valve. The "pop-off" valve can be left closed as long as the fresh gas delivered to the system does not exceed the animal's metabolic requirement.

Similar to the low-flow system, a closed system minimizes loss of body heat, conserves energy, decreases the incidence of respiratory tract complication, and produces less environmental pollution. Of all inhalant anesthetic techniques, the closed system is the most economical.

It is extremely important to remember that *N_2O should never be used in a closed system because it decreases the inspired O_2 concentration.* Low-flow and closed systems are used for maintenance of anesthesia but not for induction or when rapid changes in anesthetic depth are required.

Maintenance of Anesthesia Equipment

With routine use, anesthesia machines and the breathing circuit become contaminated with microorganisms. When improperly maintained, they can harbor microorganisms and transfer contagious respiratory diseases from patient to patient. Further, the defense mechanism of the respiratory system against infection is depressed during general anesthesia. Thus, it is very important to ensure that all anesthesia equipment is well maintained and clean to minimize these risks.

The blade of the laryngoscope should be washed with hot water to remove oral secretions and to minimize the possibility of transferring infectious respiratory organisms from patient to patient.

Endotracheal tubes should be washed with a detergent and brushed inside and out, and then rinsed with hot water. Endotracheal tubes should then be sterilized with disinfectant solutions, such as benzalkonium chloride (Zephiran or Roccal) or by gas sterilization (ethylene oxide). Thorough rinsing before use is necessary when a liquid disinfectant is used so as to prevent injury to the tracheal mucous membrane and consequent tracheitis. When ethylene oxide is used, ambient aeration for at least 7 days or mechanical aeration for at least 8-12 hours is required to ensure removal of residual ethylene oxide to a level that is safe for personnel and animals. The cuff of the endotracheal tube should be tested for leaks before use.

Manufacturers' instructions should be carefully followed for maintenance and servicing of anesthesia machines and vaporizers. Major service should only be performed by trained, qualified personnel. Anesthesia machines and accessories should be examined before each use to ensure proper function during anesthesia. Breathing tubes, Y-pieces and rebreathing bags should be washed with hot water immediately after each use and hung to dry. The O_2 supply should be checked daily to prevent disastrous depletion of O_2 during surgery.

Many anesthesia-related incidents and accidents are the result of inexperience, poor organization, and inattention to detail (Table 11). These problems are preventable (Table 12). Proficiency is only acquired through conscientious repetition and practice. A daily check list can be used to help prevent anesthetic accidents and ensure proper equipment maintenance and an adequate stock of supplies (Table 13). By doing so, the technician can then devote full attention to anesthesia duties during surgery.

MONITORING THE PATIENT DURING ANESTHESIA

Monitoring of the patient's vital signs is essential for safe anesthesia. Monitoring equipment is helpful in assessing the animal during anesthesia. However, one should always remember that machines are subject to malfunction and should never be trusted implicitly.

For example, an apparently normal electrocardiogram (ECG) does not ensure that the patient's heart is beating because the ECG monitors only the electrical activity of the heart, which continues when the heart is not beating forcefully during electromechanical dissociation. Therefore, the ECG machine should never be a substi-

Table 11. Some factors frequently associated with anesthesia problems.

- Lack of experience.
- Inadequate familiarity with equipment.
- Failure to organize drugs and equipment.
- Inattention, carelessness.
- Haste, emergency.
- Excessive dependency on other personnel.
- Distractions by other activities.
- Supervisor frequently unavailable.
- Restriction of visual field.

tute for listening to the heart with a stethoscope and palpation of the pulse.

Safe anesthesia is more closely related to keen observations and proper use of drugs as they relate to the patient's physical condition than to a specific piece of monitoring equipment.

Table 12. Preventable anesthetic accidents.

- Breathing circuit disconnection.
- Breathing circuit misconnection.
- Loss of airway or endotracheal tube dislodged.
- Anesthetic vaporizer set at a high concentraion, resulting in anesthetic overdosage.
- Anesthetic vaporizer filled with wrong anesthetic.
- Incorrect gas flow rate.
- Intravenous line disconnection.
- Laryngoscope malfunction.
- Exhaustion of carbon dioxide absorbent.

Table 13. Daily check list for technician-anesthetist.

- ✔ Inspect and turn on electrical equipment, such as monitors, anesthesia machine.
- ✔ Inspect anesthesia work area for laryngoscope, endotracheal tubes, stylets, essential drugs and supplies.
- ✔ Inspect crash cart for emergency drugs and equipment.
- ✔ Inspect anesthesia machine: flow meters, vaporizer, gauges, supply hoses, breathing system, fresh soda lime, correct mounting of cylinder.
- ✔ Connect scavenging system.
- ✔ Verify oxygen and nitrous oxide cylinder supplies, wall and/or cylinders.
- ✔ Test anesthesia machine flow meters.
- ✔ Examine unidirectional valves for proper function.
- ✔ Test for machine and breathing system leaks; test scavenging system.

Physiologic Indicators

Physiologic indicators that allow early detection of problems must be observed continuously throughout the anesthetic period. Intraoperative monitoring should focus on the cardiovascular system, respiratory system, central nervous system and body temperature. The minimal vital signs to observe and record in relatively healthy animals are *heart rate, respiratory rate and character, pulse pressure and character, mucous membrane color, capillary refill time, and CNS signs.* Animals with preexisting disturbances, such as fluid, electrolyte and acid-base abnormalities, may require specific monitoring.

Each sign monitored may have its own specific meaning; however, body systems do not function as separate entities. Overall significance can only be fully appreciated by correlating each functional sign and value with the trends of previous values and concurrent surgical maneuvers, and by considering it with other factors, such as the patient's history, disease state and the effect of the anesthetic(s) used. Normal heart and respiratory rates in domestic animals are shown in Table 14.

Depth of Anesthesia

A well-trained technician should know how to accurately assess the level of anesthesia. Depth of anesthesia can be evaluated using the patient's involuntary reflexes; however, one should realize that individual as well as species variation and the anesthetic may influence the reliability and significance of these reflexes. Reflexes and functions commonly assessed during anesthesia are the *tactile (eyelash) reflex, palpebral reflex, corneal reflex, pupil size, oropharyngeal and laryngeal reflexes, pinna and pedal reflexes, muscle tone, respiratory rate and character, heart rate and response to surgical manipulation.*

In general, a strong palpebral reflex indicates a light plane of anesthesia. At a medium or deep level of anesthesia, palpebral reflexes are sluggish or completely disappear.

Table 14. Normal heart rates and respiratory rates of domestic species.

	Dogs	Cats	Horses	Pigs	Cattle
Heart Rate (beats/min)	70-110	90-200	30-45 (foal 50-70)	60-90	60-80
Respiratory Rate (breaths/min)	20-40	20-40	8-20 (foal 15-30)	20-40	20-40

Table 15. Guedel's classification of stages and planes of ether anesthesia.

Pulse Rate and Blood Pressure	Respiration	Pupil	Eye Movement and Position	Reflexes[a]	Muscle Relaxation
Stage I: Amnesia					
Rapid PR, elevated BP	Regular	Normal size, responsive to light	Voluntary movement	Cough + pedal + anal + palpebral + corneal +	Normal tone
Stage II: Excitement or Delirium					
Rapid PR, elevated BP	Irregular	Dilated	Involuntary movement (nystagmus, centrally fixed)	Cough + pedal + anal + palpebral + corneal + exaggerated reflexes to external stimuli	Excited movement Uncontrollable paddling of limbs
Stage III: Anesthesia Plane I: Light Anesthesia					
Normal PR, normal BP	Increased rate and depth	Constricted, responsive to light	Involuntary movement, slight nystagmus, medially fixed, prolapsed nictitans	Cough + pedal + anal + palpebral – corneal +	Slight relaxation
Plane II: Surgical Anesthesia					
Normal PR, normal BP	Regular rate and depth	Normal size	Rotated medially	Cough ± pedal ± anal + palpebral – corneal +	Moderate relaxation
Plane III: Deep Anesthesia					
Slightly decreased or rapid PR, normal BP or slow fall in BP	Decreased rate and depth	Slightly dilated, unresponsive to light	Centrally fixed	Cough – pedal ± anal ± palpebral – corneal –	Marked relaxation

Table 15, continued					
Plane IV: Overdosage					
Slow, weak pulse, then no pulse, fall in BP to zero	Abdominal breathing, followed by complete paralysis of respiratory muscles	Moderately dilated, unresponsive to light	Centrally fixed	Absence of all reflexes	Flaccid
Stage IV: Terminal					
Circulatory collapse, cardiac arrest	Respiratory arrest	Totally dilated, unresponsive to light	Centrally fixed	Absence of all reflexes	Flaccid

a: + = strong reflexes, ± = weak or absent reflexes, – = absent reflexes

Most of the time the eyeball rotates ventromedially and less frequently it may rotate ventrolaterally at a medium level of anesthesia. The pupil is centrally located during light or deep anesthesia. The pupil is difficult to visualize, the nictitans is protruded, the cornea is moist, and the eyelids are closed when the animal is in a medium plane of surgical anesthesia. Deep anesthesia is evidenced by loss of palpebral and corneal reflexes, and lack of pupillary responsiveness to light and a dry cornea.

The pedal reflex is assessed by firmly pinching the skin between the toes of the rear limb. The normal response in conscious animals is withdrawal of the limb. This reflex is sluggish or even absent during surgical anesthesia. When the hair along the lateral aspect of the external ear canal in cats is lightly touched, a flicking movement of the pinna occurs. This pinna reflex is a useful indicator in cats during anesthesia because its disappearance coincides with the onset of deep anesthesia. A similar response is seen in cattle.

Jaw muscle tone is often used to assess the depth of anesthesia in dogs and cats and small ruminants. It is useful in that it generally parallels skeletal muscle relaxation. With most anesthetics, unconsciousness and analgesia usually occur before muscle relaxation. Jaw muscle tone varies from considerable in light anesthesia to absent in deep anesthesia. Assessment of jaw tone during anesthesia provides useful information associated with the changes of the level of anesthesia. However, in cats and brachycephalic dogs (*eg,* Bulldogs), jaw tone may remain considerable even in deep anesthesia.

In horses, the heart rate usually remains constant during anesthesia, so it is a less useful indicator of anesthetic depth. Respiratory rate and depth are usually irregular during light anesthesia. Breathing pattern becomes regular when surgical anesthesia is achieved. Further deepening of anesthesia reduces the depth of respiration (shallow breaths). Low PaO_2, high $PaCO_2$ or surgical manipulation may affect the way respiratory patterns change in response to the depth of anesthesia.

Traditionally, the level of anesthesia was classified into 4 stages by Guedel (Table 15). This classification was based on the actions of diethyl ether and modified to reflect responses to methoxyflurane and halothane. This classification is still used, but modification is needed when anesthesia is induced with combinations of drugs. For example, ketamine anesthesia is characterized by increased muscle tone, persistent palpebral reflex, nonclosure of the eyelids, and sometimes spontaneous limb movement. When used in large doses, opioids may induce spontaneous or reflex movement along with increased muscle tone.

FLUID THERAPY

Animals that require anesthesia may be presented in a diseased state or, even worse, in shock. Disturbances of water distribution, electrolyte balance and/or acid-base status in these patients pose a great challenge to the technician in terms of maintaining homeostasis in the perioperative period. In addition, most anesthetics induce some degree of physiologic change in body systems, particularly the cardiovascular and pulmonary systems. Supportive therapy thus becomes a critical component of safe anesthesia and serves to improve the patient's physical status and chances for subsequent survival. Laboratory tests, such as blood counts, serum chemistry assays and blood gas analyses, aid in accurate diagnosis and help guide appropriate therapy as it relates to individual needs.

Numerous types of fluids are commercially available and the choice for a particular patient should be based on the patient's needs. When in doubt, the veterinarian in charge should be consulted.

Fluid therapy is essential to maintain homeostasis in anesthetized animals. The largest component of an animal is water. In adult animals, water constitutes 60% of the body weight vs 80% in neonates. Obese animals have less body water than do thin or muscular animals. Approximately 60% of total body water is located in the intracellular space, primarily in skeletal muscle and skin. The remaining 40% of body water is located in the extracellular space. About 25% of this water is in the plasma and the remaining 75% is in the interstitial space.

Sodium and chloride are the major electrolytes in extracellular fluid, whereas potassium and phosphorus are the major electrolytes in intracellular fluid.

Placement of a large-gauge indwelling catheter (18-20 ga for small animals and 12-14 ga for large animals) is necessary to facilitate routine infusion of intravenous fluid and to administer emergency drugs when required. In relatively healthy animals undergoing elective surgery, a balanced electrolyte solution (*eg,* lactated Ringer's solution) can be infused IV at 10 ml/kg/hour for maintenance of normal hydration and replacement of insensible water losses. Larger volumes may be needed in patients with significant dehydration.

Estimation of the degree of dehydration is shown in Table 16. Packed cell volume (PCV) and total plasma protein (TP) can be used to determine dehydration. Loss of body fluid elevates the PCV and TP. The amount of fluid to be administered depends on the amount required for rehydration, maintenance and continuing losses.

The *rehydration requirement* is the amount of fluid needed to correct the deficit. The volume of fluid (ml) needed for rehydration = % dehydration x body weight (kg) x 1000.

The *maintenance requirement* is the amount of fluid required to maintain normal hydration over a 24-hour period (50-60 ml/kg/24 hours).

A fluid therapy plan should consider the amount of *continuing losses* that result during surgery.

Serial measurement of PCV and TP should be done when a large amount of fluid is given during anesthesia so as to prevent severe hemodilution, which could result in pulmonary edema from fluid overloading. Return of capillary refill time, pulse strength and heart rate toward normal indicates the effectiveness of fluid administration.

Animals with significant blood loss may be presented for emergency surgery or blood loss may occur during surgery. Assessment of acute blood loss based on the TP and PCV may be difficult at that time because both values remain normal for some time after blood loss.

When less than 20% of the total blood volume is lost, balanced electrolyte solution or saline can be given to restore the intravascular volume. Such fluid should be infused at 3 times the volume of the estimated blood loss. Blood volume in most animals is estimated at 90 ml/kg, but in cats blood volume is less than in other species (*eg,* dogs) and is estimated at 60 ml/kg.

If greater than 20% of the total blood volume is lost, plasma or whole blood should be infused. Stored blood should be warmed

Table 16. Assessing the severity of dehydration.

Dehydration (%)	Mucous Membrane Dryness	Skin Turgor	Slowed Capillary Refill Time	Sunken Eyes	Tachycardia	Poor Pulse Quality	PCV (%)	Total Plasma Protein (g/dl)
3-5	+	0	0	0	0	0	30-45	5.5-7.0
5	+	+	0	0	0	0	40-45	7.0-8.0
6-8	+	+	+	+	+	0	50	8.0-9.0
9-12	+	+++	+	+	+	+	55	9.0-10.0
12-15	+++	+++	+++	+++	+++	+	60	12.0

0 = normal, + = slight, ++ = moderate, +++ = marked

with a water bath or an in-line heating device to at least room temperature but preferably to 37C (98.6F) before administration.

POSTOPERATIVE MANAGEMENT

After surgery, the patient should be moved to an area specifically designed for anesthetic recovery and allowed to breathe O_2 after discontinuation of the inhalant anesthetic. The cuff of the endotracheal tube should be deflated and removed after the animal regains laryngeal and pharyngeal reflexes. In ruminants, the endotracheal tube should be removed with the cuff inflated so that accumulated regurgitant and/or saliva are removed as the tube is withdrawn, minimizing the chance of aspiration of these foreign materials.

In small patients, general anesthesia often causes hypothermia. Recovery may be prolonged in cold patients. Warm-water blankets or heat lamps should be used in small patients and neonates of large species to prevent further decrease in body temperature and to assist rewarming. Horses should be allowed to recover in a small well-padded recovery stall to prevent self-injury.

When postoperative pain is expected, analgesics should be administered *before* the animal regains consciousness (Table 17). Postoperative pain can also be prevented by blocking regional nerves with a local anesthetic (*eg,* intercostal nerve block for thoracotomy or brachial plexus nerve block for forelimb amputation). Intravenous fluid administration should be continued during recovery when necessary. Patients should be monitored at regular intervals until consciousness is fully regained.

Table 17. Signs of pain and surgical procedures that often result in moderate or severe postoperative pain.

Signs of Pain	Painful Procedures
• Vocalization	• Mastectomy
• Biting at the wound site	• Limb amputation
• Salivation	• Cervical spine surgery
• Avoidance behavior	• Joint surgery
• Frequent repositioning	• Corrective orthopedic surgery
• Restlessness	• Jaw fracture
• Agitation	• Laminectomy
• Pale mucous membranes	• Thoracic surgery
• Pupillary dilatation	• Declaw
• Tachycardia	• Abdominal surgery with deep dissection and retraction
• Tachypnea	• Ovariohysterectomy
• Depression	• Joint dislocation

Agitation and excitement may occur during emergence from anesthesia and, when severe, can result in self-injury. When these reactions occur, a tranquilizer and/or analgesic should be given. However, before administering CNS depressants, one should make sure that the patient is not reacting to hypoxemia. If the animal is hypoxemic, O_2 should be administered at once.

ANESTHETIC WASTE GASES AND PERSONAL SAFETY

Following the introduction of inhalant anesthetics, a survey of 303 Russian anesthesiologists in 1967 revealed a high incidence of headache, fatigue, irritability, nausea and pruritus. Since then, many medical reports have revealed that chronic exposure to trace amounts of anesthetic gases may be related to several diseases of operating room personnel.

Diseases that have been reportedly associated with exposure to trace amounts of anesthetic gases include spontaneous abortion and congenital abnormalities of the offspring of female personnel, short-term neurologic problems (nausea, headache, depression, irritability, lethargy, ataxia) and long-term neurologic problems (myoneuropathies, muscle weakness, neuron destruction, learning disabilities).

In 1977, the National Institute for Occupational Safety and Health (NIOSH) recommended that the maximal environmental concentration of halogenated anesthetics (methoxyflurane, halothane, isoflurane, enflurane) should not exceed 2 parts per million (ppm; 1 ppm = 0.001%) when used alone or 0.5 ppm when used with N_2O, and that the level of N_2O not exceed 25 ppm. Therefore, proper scavenging of gases is necessary to reduce waste gases in the operating room. Preventing leaks from anesthetic equipment and alteration of anesthetic techniques are also important.

Gas-Scavenging Systems

The most effective gas-scavenging system includes 3 major components: the *gas-capturing system,* the *interface,* and the *disposal system.*

Waste gases escape from the breathing circuit through the "pop-off" valve and enter the disposal system. The interface connects the gas-capturing system and the disposal system (Fig 6a) and serves to relieve the positive pressure caused by occlusion of the scavenging system. It is also designed to prevent the negative pressure produced by the disposal system from reaching the breathing circuit when a central vacuum is used for removal of waste gases.

Currently available disposal systems include: the noncirculating portion of the ventilation system, a central vacuum, a passive through-the-wall system, and use of a charcoal absorber. Use of the noncirculating portion of the ventilation system allows waste gases to be removed from the general air circulation. A central vacuum system combined with surgical suction has been used to eliminate waste gases, but a dedicated suction system or independent vacuum designed specifically for eliminating the waste gases is preferred. Activated charcoal absorbers (Fig 6b) can eliminate halogenated anesthetic gases from exhaled gases but do not eliminate N_2O.

Anesthetic Leaks

There are 2 major sources of anesthetic gas leaks: the *anesthetic machine* and the *breathing circuit.* An effective scavenging system in combination with a leak-free anesthetic equipment circuit is the most effective system for decreasing operating room pollution.

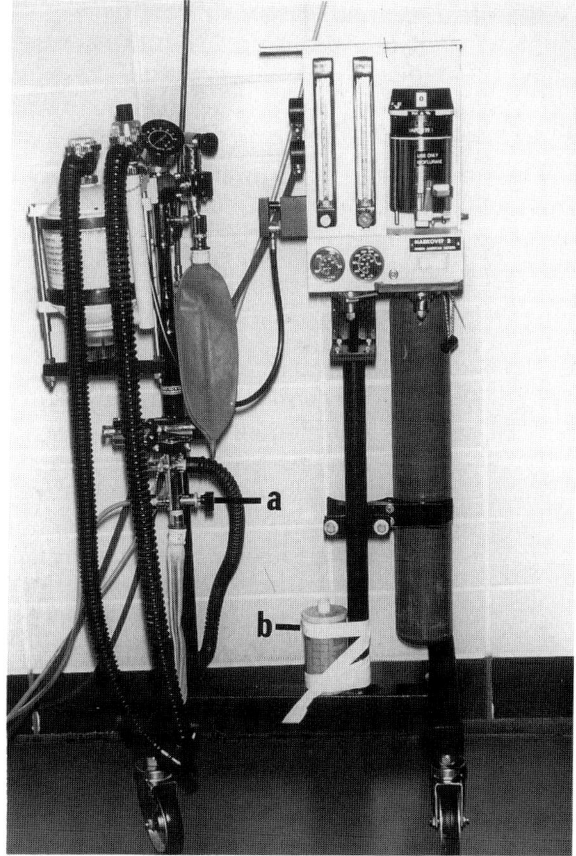

Figure 6. a. Interface connecting the gas-capturing system and the disposal system. b. Charcoal absorbers.

Thus, regular periodic maintenance of anesthesia equipment is important in decreasing operating room pollution.

Anesthesia machines should be serviced every 6 months by the manufacturer's representative, with daily routine maintenance by the technician. Service by the manufacturer should include vaporizer calibration and inspection of pressure line connectors, flow meters, CO_2 absorbers, the ventilator and the scavenging system.

The most common sources of leaks from the breathing circuit occur at the unidirectional valves, the CO_2 absorber canister, around the endotracheal tube, and from holes in the rebreathing bags and inspiratory and expiratory hoses. Leaks in the breathing circuit can be detected by occluding the Y-piece and squeezing the rebreathing bag with the "pop-off" valve closed. A loss of pressure or emptying of the rebreathing bag indicates a massive leak. A more precise method is to fill the breathing circuit and rebreathing bag with O_2. Then adjust the O_2 flow to maintain a circuit pressure of 40 cm H_2O for 30 seconds. The maximal acceptable O_2 flow rate to maintain a circuit pressure of 40 cm H_2O is 200 ml/minute. If a higher flow rate is required, the leak is excessive and the machine should be repaired before it is used.

Preferred Anesthetic Techniques

Operating room contamination can be avoided or minimized if the technician adopts the following anesthetic techniques.

- Make sure the disposal system is attached and functional.
- Avoid spilling liquid anesthetic when filling the vaporizer.
- Do not turn on the vaporizer or N_2O flow until the animal is connected to the breathing circuit.
- Use the proper size of endotracheal tube and inspect the seal between the endotracheal tube cuff and tracheal mucosa to ensure proper cuff inflation.
- Disconnect the breathing circuit from the patient as infrequently as possible during anesthesia.
- Empty the rebreathing bag into the scavenging system and fill the bag with O_2 at the end of anesthesia.
- Scavenge all nonrebreathing systems.
- Use chamber or mask induction only when necessary and make sure the mask fits tightly.
- Recap the bottle of liquid anesthetic after filling the vaporizer, even if the bottle is empty.

Though it is not possible to eliminate all trace amounts of anesthetic gases, every person in the operating room should make an effort to minimize the amount that escapes so as to provide maximal protection.

Recommended Reading

Muir WW and Hubbell JAE: *Handbook of Veterinary Anesthesia.* Mosby, St. Louis, 1989.

Paddleford RR: *Manual of Small Animal Anesthesia.* Churchill Livingstone, New York, 1988.

Short CE: *Principles and Practice of Veterinary Anesthesia.* Williams & Wilkins, Baltimore, 1987.

Warren RG: *Small Animal Anesthesia.* Mosby, St. Louis, 1983.

Notes

Notes

9

Surgical Nursing

T.P. Colville

Surgery is one of the most important activities in any veterinary practice. With most surgical procedures, the patient's future well being, if not its life, is in the hands of the surgical team. If all aspects of the surgical procedure are carried out with skill, care and accuracy, the results can be very beneficial. If, however, close attention is not paid to the many important activities of the presurgical, surgical and postsurgical periods, the consequences can be unfortunate for the patient.

The roles of veterinary technicians in surgical procedures can be many and varied. During the presurgical period, veterinary technicians are usually responsible for preparation of the patient, the surgical instruments and equipment, and the surgical environment. During surgery, the veterinary technician may be responsible for anesthesia of the patient, and will probably assist the surgeon, either directly by actually scrubbing in, or indirectly by properly opening surgical packs, suture materials, etc, and knowing how to function in a sterile surgical environment without causing contamination. In the postsurgical period, the veterinary technician is frequently responsible for postoperative patient care and monitoring, instructing clients on proper patient care during the recovery period, and removing sutures.

Definition of Surgery

Surgery is the "branch of medicine dealing with manual and operative procedures for correction of deformities and defects, repair of injuries, and diagnosis and cure of certain diseases" (*Tabor's Cyclopedic Medical Dictionary*). Commonly, surgery is thought of as procedures involving incision of the skin or other epithelial surface, manipulation of internal organs and/or tissues, and closure of the surgical wound with sutures.

Purposes of Surgery

- *Restore an animal to a normal or functional state of health.* Many surgical procedures are capable of returning an animal to a normal state of health. Such surgeries as internal fracture fixation, cystotomy for removal of urinary calculi, and surgical repair of a ruptured cranial cruciate ligament are all intended to restore normal structure and function to an animal, after healing from the surgery is complete.

  In other cases, the animal's condition dictates that normal anatomy and physiology cannot be restored, but surgery can allow the animal to return to a *functional* state of health. Such procedures as limb amputation, eye removal and mastectomy permanently alter the animal's body, but they can allow an animal to function with a reasonable quality of life.
- *Alter the anatomy and / or behavior of an animal to make it less dangerous or socially more desirable.* Surgery is sometimes performed to allow people and animals to more safely and desirably coexist. Often what are normal behavioral traits and physical characteristics in the animal world become dangerous or unpleasant when the animals are in close proximity to people. Such surgical procedures as neutering (castration, ovariohysterectomy), dehorning of cattle, and declawing of cats are intended to allow more peaceful or pleasant human-animal coexistence.
- *Alter the appearance of an animal.* Cosmetic surgery is performed to alter the appearance of an animal by modifying its normal anatomy. Included in this category are cropping the ears, docking the tail and removing the dewclaws of dogs for appearance purposes. There is ongoing debate about ethical issues surrounding cosmetic surgery in animals.
- *Prevent health problems.* Prophylactic surgery is performed to help prevent future health problems. Docking the tail of sheep helps prevent soiling and resulting infestation with fly larvae (fly strike). Removing the dewclaws from hunting dogs helps prevent trauma from catching on sticks, rocks and other objects out in the field.

- *Establish a diagnosis.* When noninvasive diagnostic procedures fail to reveal the source of an animal's problem, exploratory surgery is sometimes performed to directly visualize the affected area and establish a definitive diagnosis. For example, an exploratory laparotomy might be performed if the identity or characteristics of an abdominal mass could not be otherwise determined.

Knowledge Applied in Surgical Nursing

To function effectively as a part of the surgical team, a veterinary technician must be familiar with the various routines of surgical procedures, from preoperative preparation to postoperative care, and also needs a good working knowledge of anatomy, physiology, pathology and microbiology.

Knowledge of *anatomy* is important in understanding what parts of the body will be affected, both beneficially and adversely, by a surgical procedure. This impacts proper preoperative patient preparation and positioning, assistance during the procedure, and provision of appropriate postoperative care.

Familiarity with animal *physiology* goes hand-in-hand with knowledge of anatomy. The regenerative capacity of various parts of the body, as well as the impact surgery might have on their function(s), can be more accurately predicted with a good background in physiology.

The processes of inflammation and wound healing are included under the general subject of *pathology.* Because every surgical procedure damages normal tissue, knowledge of how the body will respond to that damage is helpful in providing care to the surgical patient.

The purpose of aseptic surgical technique is to minimize the number of microorganisms that enter the surgical wound. Proper preparation of the surgical environment, instruments, equipment and the patient are aided by knowledge of basic *microbiology* principles.

Basic Types of Surgery

Surgical procedures can usually be classified into 1 of 2 main groups – elective procedures and emergency procedures, though the division may not always be distinct.

Elective Surgery

As its name implies, elective surgery is done by choice, and, therefore, does not have to be performed immediately. It can and should be performed when conditions are most favorable and convenient. Castration, most tumor removals, and cosmetic procedures are examples of surgical procedures that are usually elective in nature.

Emergency Surgery

Emergency surgery must be performed immediately to prevent death or serious damage, even if conditions are not optimal. Conditions requiring emergency surgery might include a severely hemorrhaging ruptured organ (*eg,* the spleen), a profusely hemorrhaging external wound, or a proptosed eye.

Influence of Patient Characteristics on Surgical Procedures

Surgery can be easy, fast, simple and inexpensive, or it can be difficult, time consuming, sophisticated and very expensive. The ease and cost of surgery depend largely on the procedure performed and the extent of the precautions taken to produce an optimal outcome. The value the owner places on the animal is often the most important factor in determining what surgical procedures are to be performed and under what conditions, though other factors may enter into the decision.

An appreciation for the range of surgical options can be gained by examining 3 groups of animals and the characteristics of surgical procedures commonly performed on these animals.

Companion Animal Surgery

The human/companion animal bond often plays a significant role in determining the value an owner places on a dog, cat, bird, horse or other companion animal. The animal often becomes a member of the family, so owners are often willing to spend relatively large amounts of money on its care. This can allow relatively elaborate and expensive surgical techniques and equipment to be used, and the surgical environment can be made close to optimal.

Large Animal Surgery

Sentiment usually plays little role in the value of livestock and performance animals. Their value is usually determined by objective measures, such as market value, production or performance. The conditions under which surgery is performed is usually determined, in large measure, by the animal's economic value.

An injured race horse valued at $3,000,000 will likely receive the best-quality medical and surgical care under the best conditions. Complicated joint surgery might cost the owners many thousands of dollars, but that amount is miniscule as compared with the value of the animal and the potential monetary benefit from the procedure.

An opposite extreme would be an old stock cow, worth a few hundred dollars market value, that requires a cesarean section. The owner cannot afford to spend large sums of money to have the surgery performed under optimal circumstances, so the surgery will likely be performed, if at all, under less than ideal conditions. (Basic surgical principles should still apply to whatever extent possible, however.)

Research Animal Surgery

The conditions under which experimental surgery is performed is usually dictated by the purpose(s) of the research, the species and numbers of animals involved, and the project budget.

A toxicology research project studying the effects of substance "X" on the liver of rats might involve relatively simple, unsophisticated surgical procedures. After the rats have been exposed to various concentrations of substance "X" for varying periods, they might be anesthetized, have their liver removed for analysis and then be euthanized. The surgery would not have to be elaborate, as asepsis would not be important, so the surgery could be done very quickly and easily with a minimum of instruments and preparation.

An opposite extreme would be a research project developing a new type of artificial heart. New models of the artificial heart might be implanted in calves. The long-term survival and good health of the calves would be of paramount importance to the study of the instruments' performance, so the implantation surgery would be performed under carefully controlled conditions using elaborate and sophisticated techniques and equipment.

Basic Surgical Terminology

The language of surgery, like that of other branches of medicine, can seem cryptic until its basic principles are understood. The names of surgical instruments, supplies and equipment are discussed elsewhere in this chapter. This section discusses surgical word structure, common incision names, and common surgical procedure names.

Combining Forms

Six suffixes are commonly combined with anatomic terms to produce words describing surgical procedures.

-ectomy = to remove (to excise). For example, a splen*ectomy* is a surgical procedure to remove the spleen.

-otomy = to cut into. For example, a cysto*tomy* (incision into the urinary bladder) is often performed to remove urinary calculi (bladder stones).

-ostomy = surgical creation of an artificial opening. For example, a perineal urethro*stomy* is a surgical procedure often performed on male cats for relief of urethral obstruction. It involves excision of the penis (pen*ectomy*) and creation of a widened new urethral opening.

-rrhaphy = surgical repair by suturing. For example, abdominal hernio*rrhaphy* is the surgical repair of an abdominal hernia by suturing the defect in the abdominal musculature.

-pexy = surgical fixation. For example, gastro*pexy* (suturing of the stomach to the abdominal wall to fix it in place) is often performed in cases of gastric torsion.

-plasty = surgical alteration of shape or form. For example, pyloro*plasty* enlarges the pyloric orifice of the stomach to facilitate gastric emptying.

Abdominal Incisions

Abdominal surgery is commonly performed in animal species. Entry into the abdomen is usually gained by any of 4 common abdominal incisions. Named according to its location, each incision offers different advantages and a different exposure of the abdomen.

A *ventral midline incision* is located on the ventral midline of the animal. It offers excellent exposure of the entire abdominal cavity. Because the abdominal cavity is entered through the linea alba, where the abdominal muscles on each side are joined, the abdominal wall can be closed with a single layer of sutures in the linea alba. Closure of a ventral midline incision must be very secure, as the weight of the abdominal organs exerts tension on the incision when the animal stands. Also, any exertion by the animal can create tension on the suture line.

A *paramedian incision* is located lateral and parallel to the ventral midline of the animal. It is usually used when exposure of only one side of the abdomen is needed, such as for removal of a cryptorchid (retained) testis. The muscles of the abdominal wall are individually incised, so closure of the abdominal wall usually requires multiple layers of sutures.

A *flank incision* is generally performed either on a standing animal or one in lateral recumbency. It is oriented perpendicular to the long axis of the body, caudal to the last rib. A flank incision provides good exposure of the organ(s) immediately deep to (beneath) the incision but does not allow exploration of much of the remainder of the abdomen. It is, therefore, useful for such procedures as rumenotomy and nephrectomy, in which the organ in question lies directly beneath the incision. The muscles of the abdominal wall usually require a multiple-layer closure. In contrast to tension exerted on a ventral midline incision, the weight of the abdominal organs generally tends to keep a flank incision closed rather than pulling it apart.

A *paracostal incision* is oriented parallel to the last rib, and offers good exposure of the stomach and spleen in monogastric animals. The muscles of the abdominal wall are usually closed in multiple layers.

Any of the above incisions can be combined to increase exposure of the abdominal cavity. Because surgical incisions heal "side to side" rather than "end to end," the length of any incision, including a combined abdominal incision, has little or no effect on the overall healing time, regardless of whether the incision is 2 inches or 2 feet long, assuming adequate closure and normal tissue healing.

Common Surgical Procedures

Soft Tissue Procedures:

Ovariohysterectomy, commonly referred to as a "spay," involves removal of the ovaries and uterus.

Cesarean section is a method of delivering newborn animals in cases of dystocia (difficult labor). It consists of an abdominal incision (flank or ventral midline) and then an incision into the uterus through which the newborn(s) is (are) delivered.

Orchiectomy (castration) is the surgical removal of the testes.

Lateral ear resection is often performed in animals with chronic external ear infection. It involves removal of the lateral wall of the vertical portion of the external ear canal to allow improved ventilation and to establish drainage for exudates.

Laparotomy is an incision into the abdominal cavity, often through the flank. *Celiotomy* is another term for laparotomy.

Cystotomy is an incision into the urinary bladder, frequently for removal of urinary calculi (bladder stones).

Gastrotomy is an incision into a simple stomach, while a *rumenotomy* is an incision into a rumen.

Gastropexy involves suturing of the stomach to the abdominal wall to fix it in place. This procedure is frequently done in cases of gastric torsion.

Splenectomy is the removal of the spleen.

Thoracotomy is an incision into the thoracic cavity (chest).

Herniorrhaphy is the surgical repair of a hernia by suturing the abnormal opening(s) closed.

Enterotomy is an incision into the intestine, often for removal of a foreign body.

Intestinal resection and anastomosis involves removal of a portion of the intestine (resection) and suturing the cut ends together to restore the continuity of the intestinal tube (anastomosis).

Urethrostomy involves incision into the urethra suturing of the splayed urethral edges to the skin to create a larger urethral orifice. This procedure is frequently performed on male cats with recurrent urethral obstruction.

Mastectomy involves removal of part or all of one or more mammary glands.

Orthopedic (Bone) Procedures:

Onychectomy is the surgical removal of a claw, commonly called declawing.

Intervertebral disk fenestration is done to remove prolapsed intervertebral disk material causing pressure on the spinal cord.

Intramedullary bone pinning involves insertion of a metal rod (bone pin) into the medullary cavity of a long bone to fix fracture fragments in place.

Cranial cruciate ligament repair is performed when that stifle joint ligament has ruptured. Lack of an intact cranial cruciate ligament creates instability in the stifle, causing abnormal movement. This can damage the joint surfaces of the distal femur and proximal tibia.

Femoral head ostectomy involves amputation of the head of the femur. It is usually performed in animals with severe damage to the femoral head or neck, or a damaged acetabulum.

Wound Healing

Every surgical procedure disrupts normal tissue. In addition, surgery is often indicated to enhance healing of extensive traumatic wounds. In either case, the basic mechanisms of wound healing are the same. The primary differences are in the extent and duration of each stage of the process.

Phases of Wound Healing

The phases of wound healing include inflammation, repair and remodeling.

Inflammatory Phase: Inflammation is the body's initial vascular and cellular response to injury. It helps protect against foreign materials and invaders, removes dead tissues, and sets the stage for tissue repair. The inflammatory processes are initiated by release of chemicals from damaged cells and tissues.

For a few minutes after an acute injury. the blood vessels in the area constrict to limit hemorrhage. This transient period of vasoconstriction is quickly followed by dilation of the blood vessels in the area. Vasodilation allows blood to flow into the wound and clot. The surface of blood clots exposed externally often dehydrates to form a scab, which serves as an initial protective covering over the wound.

Blood in the dilated vessels carries antibodies, nutrients and white blood cells into the damaged area. The antibodies help provide a first line of defense against microorganisms. The nutrients are needed to "fuel" the cleanup and repair processes. The white blood cells, principally neutrophils and monocytes, begin the cleanup process by breaking down and removing foreign material, dead cells, bacteria and tissue debris.

Repair Phase: The processes of repair, which consist of capillary infiltration, fibroblast proliferation and epithelial regeneration, begin almost immediately after injury, and proceed as rapidly as the inflammatory mechanisms clean up the wound. In uncomplicated wounds, the repair phase is usually in full swing by about 3-5 days after the initial injury.

Capillaries begin growing into the damaged area initially as blind-ended "buds" off the healthy, undamaged vessels surrounding the wound. The buds join together to form intact capillaries. The developing capillary network further increases the blood supply to the healing area.

With the enhanced blood supply to the wound, fibroblasts proliferate and begin producing collagen fibers. These fibers make up the scar tissue that begins giving the wound some strength.

The soft, bright red tissue formed by the proliferating fibroblasts and capillaries is termed *granulation tissue.* A "bed" of granulation tissue must form in a skin wound before epithelium can regenerate to cover the surface of the wound.

Remodeling Phase: The remodeling phase is the final stage of wound healing. It primarily involves rearrangement of the collagen fibers in the scar to increase the strength of the healed wound. This phase begins about 4 weeks after the initial injury in an uncomplicated wound, when all of the collagen fibers have been formed, and may continue for years. There is little or no change in the outward appearance of a wound during this phase.

Types of Wound Healing

First-Intention Healing: In a wound undergoing first-intention healing, there is minimal tissue damage and minimal microbial contamination, and the skin edges are apposed (held together), usually by sutures. Healing generally proceeds smoothly, with minimal scar tissue formation. Most surgical wounds heal by first intention.

Second-Intention Healing: A wound that is healing by second-intention usually has had significant tissue damage and loss. Contamination may be extensive and the wound is left to heal open. In addition to the wound healing mechanisms described above, wound contraction helps reduce the size of an open wound as it heals. Once a granulation tissue bed forms, the wound usually begins to contract by movement of the whole thickness of the surrounding skin toward the center of the wound. This greatly decreases the amount of time necessary for the wound to close, though in some cases it may cause deformity or restrict movement if the skin is tightly adherent to the underlying structures or the wound is over a joint.

Third-Intention Healing: A wound that is healing by third intention is allowed to heal open until a granulation tissue bed forms, and then it is sutured closed.

Basic Wound Management Principles

Wound Assessment

The overall condition of the patient, as well as the characteristics and location of the wound, must be assessed before treatment decisions are made. The significance of the wound must be viewed in the context of the animal's overall status. In some injured animals, such life-threatening conditions as shock must be treated before wound therapy is begun. In other animals, such as a cat with an eyelid laceration and proptosed eye, the extent of damage to the skin and underlying tissues and the location of the wound may dictate the need for immediate attention.

Wound Lavage

Wound lavage involves copious flushing of a wound with a sterile isotonic solution. Effective lavage flushes away debris and detached tissue fragments, and decreases the number of bacteria in the wound, thus helping to speed healing. Antiseptics and antibacterials are sometimes added to wound lavage solutions, but some of these additives can damage the delicate exposed tissues of an open wound.

Wound Debridement

Removal of necrotic (dead) tissue from a wound is termed *debridement.* The process can be natural, as a part of inflammation, or surgical, when dead tissue is trimmed from a wound with scalpel or scissors. The process of inflammation debrides a wound by liquefying and carrying away dead tissue. If a wound contains large amounts of necrotic tissue, however, this process of natural debridement can slow the healing process. Physically trimming the dead tissue from a wound can significantly speed healing. Care must be exercised when debriding to avoid damaging healthy tissue.

Wound Closure or Covering

In general, wounds heal more rapidly if they are sutured closed or, if that is not feasible, if they are covered for protection. Various suture patterns and bandaging techniques can be used, depending on the characteristics and location of the wound.

Factors Affecting Wound Healing

Nutrition

Wound healing is significantly affected by a patient's nutritional status. A good-quality, balanced diet enhances wound healing by supplying the nutrients, particularly protein, needed for tissue repair. Poor nutrition deprives a healing wound of the raw materials needed for tissue repair. While many other factors affect wound healing, good nutrition should not be overlooked as an important aid to the process.

Obesity

Wounds tend to heal more slowly in obese animals because of such factors as their generally poor nutritional status, poor peripheral circulation, and increased susceptibility to infection.

Immune System Function

Any impairment of an animal's immune function can retard wound healing by direct effects on wound healing and indirect effects that allow contaminating microorganisms to proliferate and infect the wound. For example, such immunosuppressive drugs as corticosteroids and anti-cancer agents can retard wound healing and predispose to infection.

Blood Supply

Good arterial perfusion (blood supply) and venous drainage are necessary for normal healing. Improperly secured appliances, such as splints and bandages that impede circulation, can significantly delay wound healing. Wounds involving poorly perfused tissue, such as ligaments or tendons, tend to heal more slowly than wounds in very vascular areas, such as the tongue.

Age

Older animals generally have a diminished capacity for wound healing. With good care and nutrition, wounds on elderly patients heal well, but it may take longer.

Infection

While virtually all wounds have some microbial contamination, wounds are not considered infected until microorganisms actively multiply and cause tissue damage. Microorganisms in an infected wound directly delay wound healing by damaging healing tissues. This prolongs the inflammatory phase of the healing process. Microorganisms also promote extensive exudate formation and may produce toxins that further impede healing.

Movement

Movement of wound edges disturbs healing by mechanically disrupting the repair process. Healing can be enhanced by immobilizing the wound edges with sutures, bandages, and, in some cases, splints and casts.

Surgical Instruments

Surgical instruments are relatively expensive, often very delicate, and intended for specific functions. When used for the purposes for which they were intended, surgical instruments are extremely useful, and usually very long lasting. When misused, however, many surgical instruments may not last long. Scissors should not be used to cut wire. Needle holders should not be used to extract bone pins. When possible, use surgical instruments only for the function(s) for which they were intended.

Hundreds of instruments are available for use in veterinary surgery. Most practices, however, use standard sets of selected instruments organized into "packs." For example, there might be a major surgical pack, a minor pack and a suture pack. Table 1 lists examples of instrument sets in some standard surgical packs.

Common General Surgical Instruments

Scalpel: A scalpel is a surgical knife. It is the surgeon's foremost cutting instrument, and is used to make skin incisions as well as to cut and divide a variety of other organs and tissues. The original scalpels were 1-piece knives that had to be sharpened. Modern scalpels consist of handles with detachable disposable blades. The

#3 and #4 handles are most commonly used in veterinary surgery. Disposable blades are available in various sizes and shapes to fit the handles (Fig 1). The blades are packaged individually in sterile packs, so their sharpness and sterility are assured.

Scissors: Various types of scissors are used in surgery. In general they are classified according to their shape (straight or curved, Fig 2), the configuration of their points (sharp-sharp, blunt-blunt or sharp-blunt, Fig 3), and the material they are used to cut (tissue, bandages, sutures, wire, Fig 4).

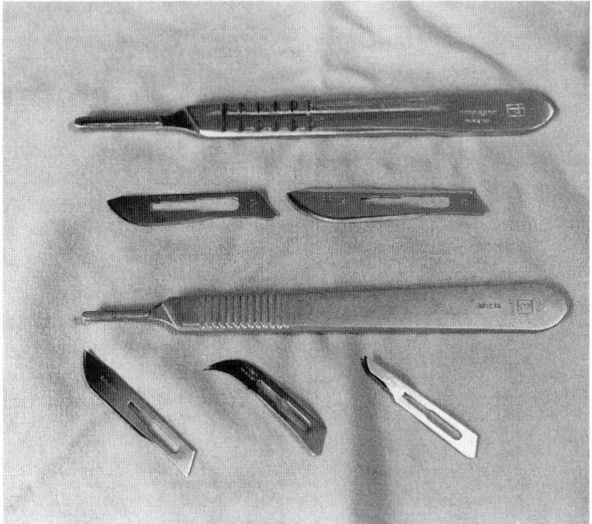

Figure 1. Scalpel handles and blades. From top to bottom: #4 scalpel handle, #20 (left) and #21 (right) blades that fit the #4 handle, #3 scalpel handle, and #10 (left), #12 (center) and #15 (right) blades that fit the #3 handle.

Figure 2. Scissor blade shapes: curved (top) and straight (bottom).

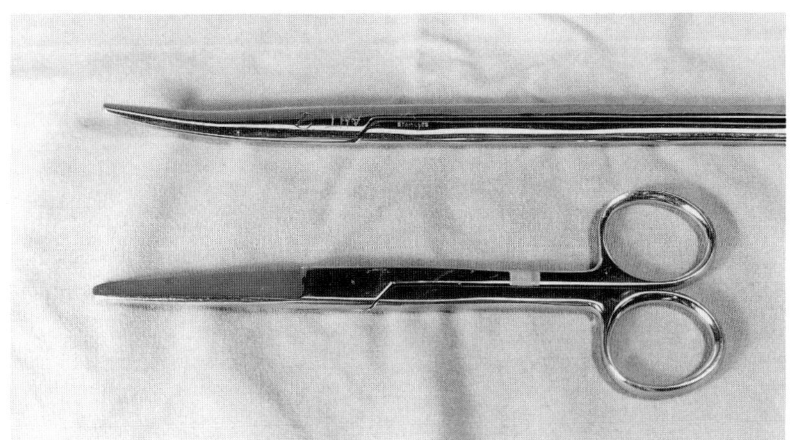

To maintain their sharpness, scissors must be used appropriately. Tissue scissors should not be used to cut sutures, and suture scissors should not be used to cut wire.

Forceps: The general term "forceps" refers to instruments that are used to grasp, manipulate or extract. Like most other surgical instruments, forceps have specific uses. Some must be held closed

Figure 3. Scissor points: sharp-sharp (left), sharp-blunt (center) and blunt-blunt (right).

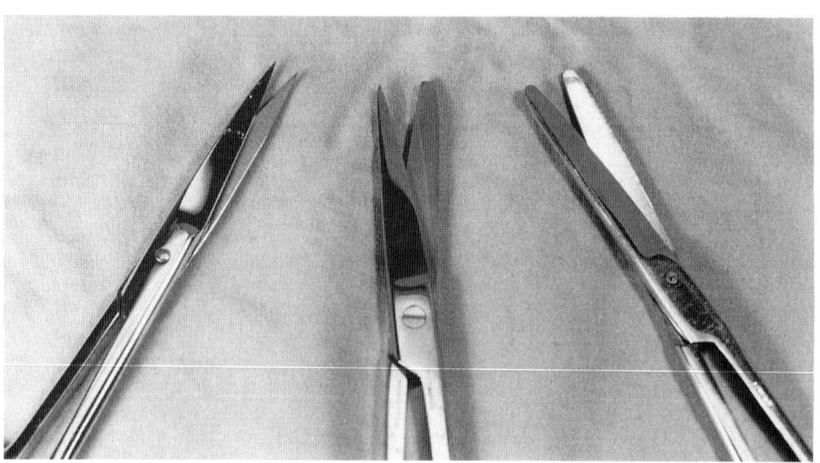

Figure 4. Scissor types: tissue scissors (top), wire scissors (center) and suture scissors (bottom).

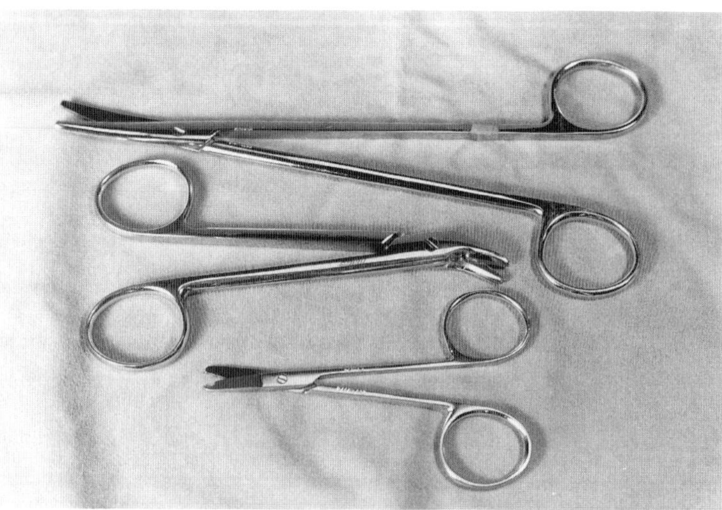

with the thumb and fingers (thumb forceps) and others have ratchet mechanisms that hold their jaws closed.

Needle holders, as their name implies, are used to grasp suture needles as they are passed through tissue during suturing. The Mayo-Hegar and Olson-Hegar scissors/needle holder are commonly used (Figs 5, 6).

Dressing and tissue forceps are similar instruments with very different uses. Thumb dressing and tissue forceps resemble "tweezers" but have different kinds of jaws (Fig 7). Dressing forceps have flat jaws with transverse grooves on their inside surfaces. They are

Figure 5. Mayo-Hegar (top) and Olson-Hegar (bottom) needle holders.

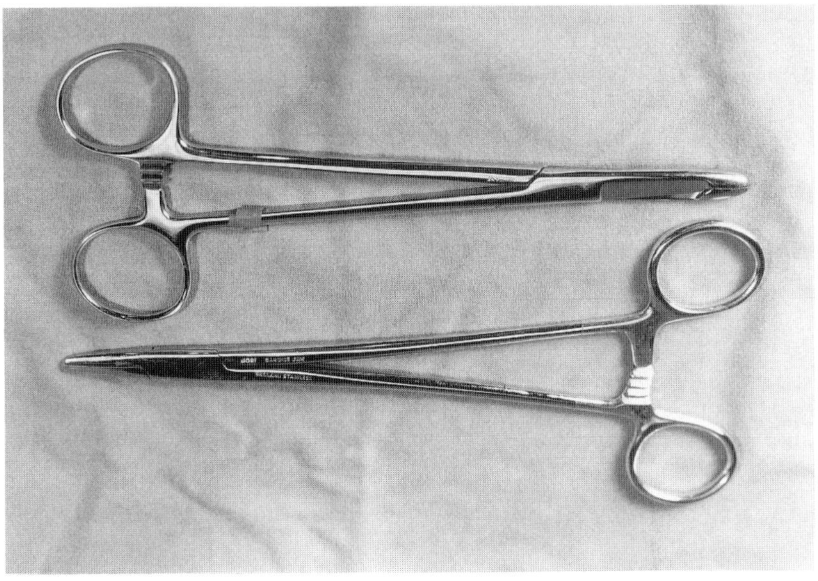

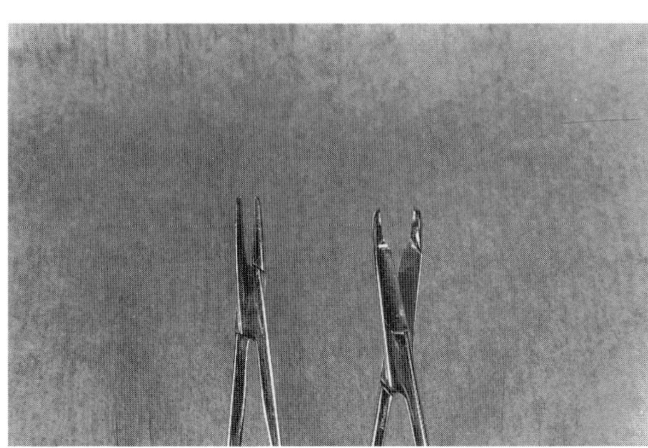

Figure 6. Closeup of Mayo-Hegar (left) and Olson-Hegar (bottom) needle holders.

designed to apply and remove dressings, and should not be used to handle tissues, as they tend to crush tissues. The tips of thumb tissue forceps have teeth that tend to separate rather than crush tissue. They are often used to grasp tissues that are being sutured. Allis tissue forceps have multiple teeth in their jaws, and a ratchet mechanism to hold them closed. They are used to grasp and manipulate organs and tissues.

Hemostats, as their name implies, are used to stop or prevent hemorrhage (hemostasis). They are usually used to clamp off blood vessels and small tissue pedicles containing blood vessels. They are available in a variety of sizes with straight or curved jaws. Mosquito forceps are relatively small hemostats used to clamp fine blood vessels (Fig 8). Kelly and Crile forceps are medium sized and differ only in how much of the inside of the jaw is covered with transverse grooves (Fig 9). The jaw of the Crile forceps is completely covered with grooves, whereas only the distal half of the Kelly forceps is grooved. Rochester-Carmalt forceps have longer, broader jaws with longitudinal grooves crossed by transverse grooves at the tips (Fig 10).

Towel forceps or towel clamps have sharp tips that curve together to a point (Fig 11). They are available in different sizes and are used to secure surgical drapes to the skin of the patient.

Sponge forceps are used to grasp surgical sponges, making them easier to manipulate in deep incisions (Fig 12).

Retractors: Retractors are used to facilitate exposure of the surgical field by holding organs and tissues out of the way, or hooking them and bringing them up into view. They may be hand held or self-retaining.

Figure 7. Thumb dressing (top) and tissue (bottom) forceps.

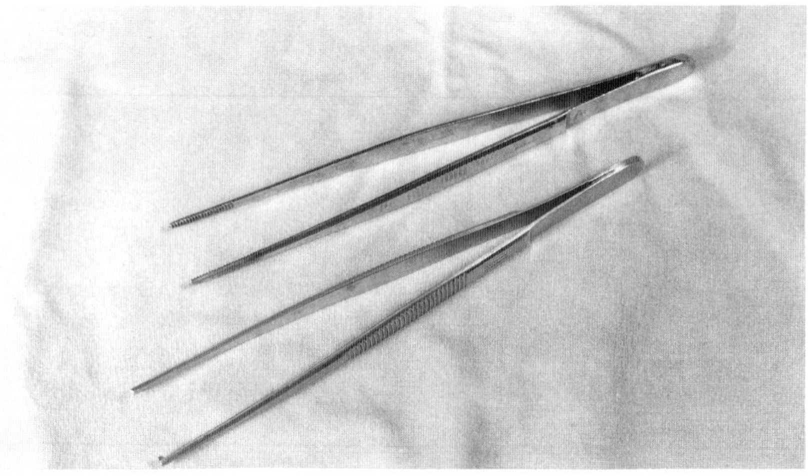

Hand-held retractors usually require an assistant to properly position and use them. U.S. Army retractors have differently sized flat blades at each end (Fig 13). A Senn retractor has a flat blade on one end and curved, fork-like tines on the other (Fig 14). A Snook's ovariohysterectomy hook has a blunt hook on one end, and is used to hook the uterus and bring it up into the incision during spay surgery (Fig 15). A grooved director is used to help shield underlying

Figure 8. Halsted (top) and Hartman (bottom) mosquito forceps.

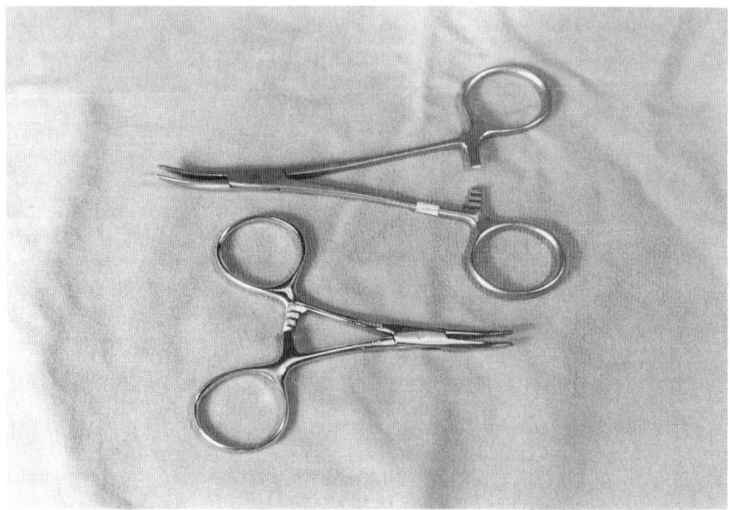

Figure 9. Kelly (top) and Crile (bottom) forceps.

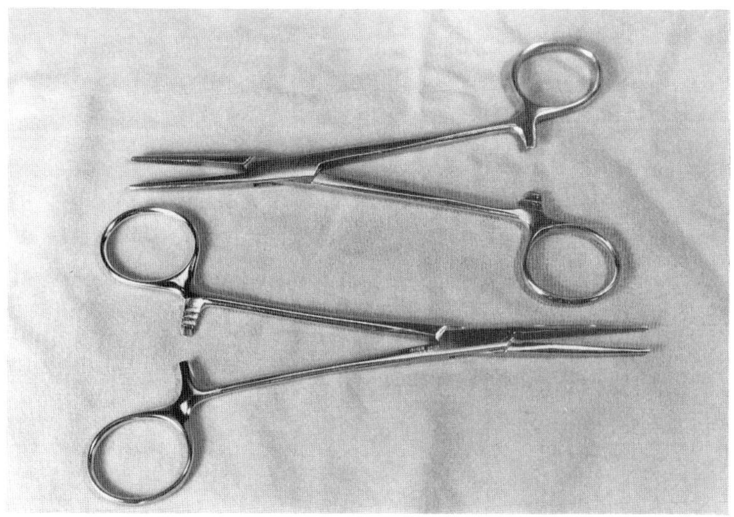

tissue when making incisions, particularly into the abdominal cavity (Fig 16).

Self-retaining retractors are held open by a ratchet locking mechanism. They can be placed and opened by one unassisted person. The Gelpi retractor has curved, sharply pointed ends directed

Figure 10. Rochester-Carmalt forceps.

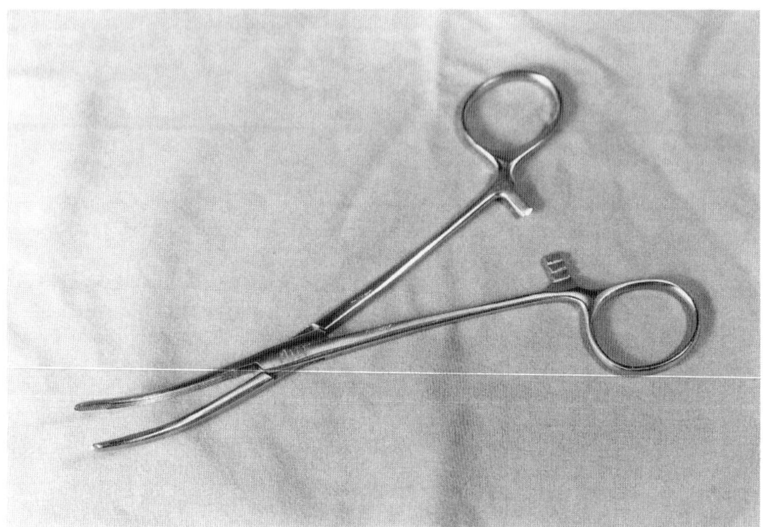

Figure 11. Backhaus towel clamps.

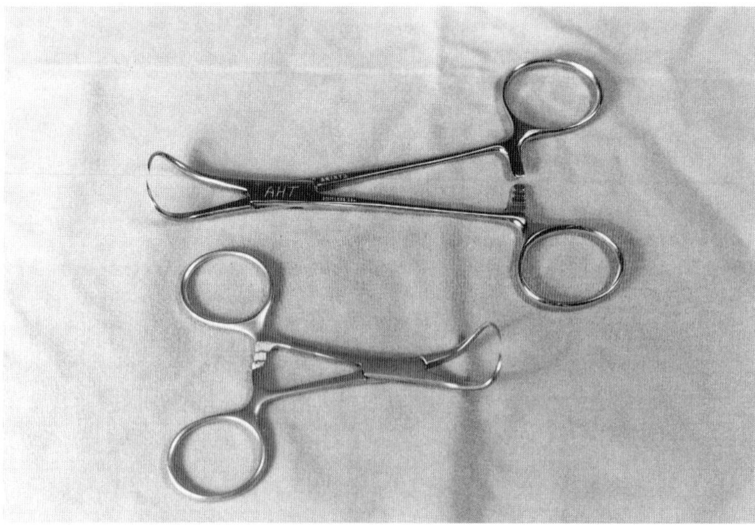

out to the sides (Fig 17). The Weitlaner retractor is similar, but has blunt, flat, fork-like tines on the ends (Fig 18).

Common Orthopedic Instruments

Orthopedic instruments are used to manipulate tough, dense tissues, such as cartilage and bone. They are generally stronger and heavier than general surgical instruments.

Rongeurs: Rongeurs are used to "chew out" small pieces of bone or cartilage (Fig 19). Their jaws are sharp and cup-shaped, and they have relatively long handles for good leverage.

Figure 12. Sponge forceps.

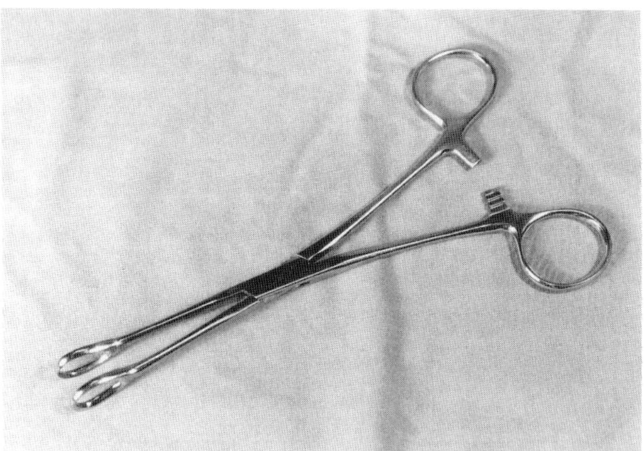

Figure 13. US Army retractor.

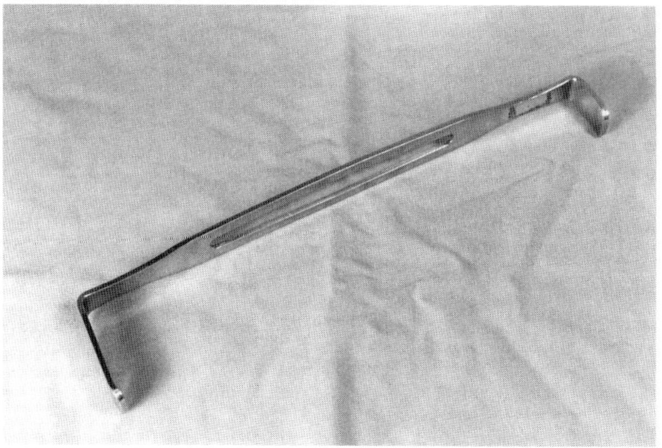

Figure 14. Senn retractor.

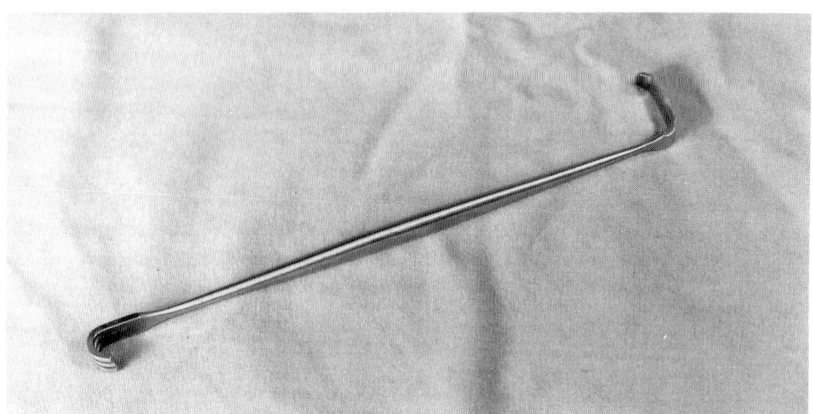

Figure 15. Snook's ovariohysterectomy hook.

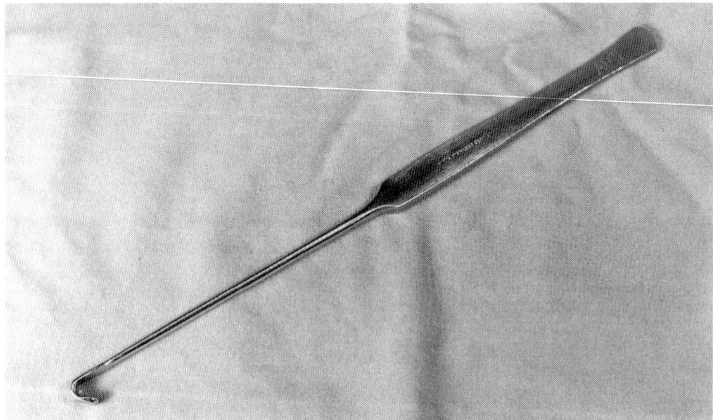

Figure 16. Grooved director.

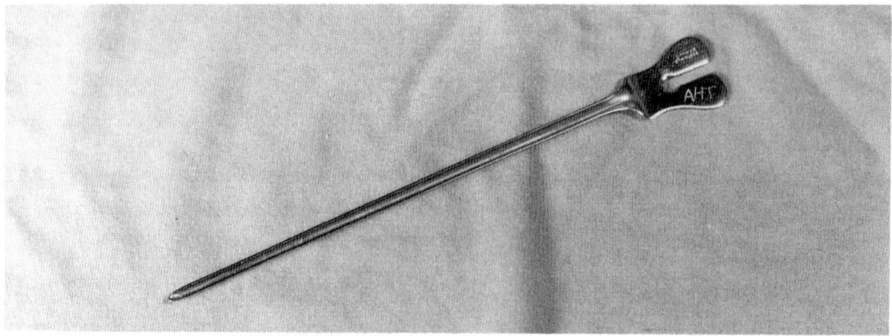

Bone-Cutting Instruments: Bone-cutting forceps have heavy, chisel-like jaws and long handles (Fig 20). They are used to cut relatively larger pieces of bone than rongeurs.

An *osteotome* is usually used with a mallet to cut through relatively thick, heavy bone (Fig 21).

Bone saws are used when relatively large areas of bone must be cut. The Gigli wire saw consists of a heavy-gauge wire with sharp ridges along its length (Fig 22). When handles are attached to each end of the wire, the wire can be drawn back and forth to saw through the bone. Care must be taken to avoid damage to surrounding soft tissues.

Trephines: A trephine is used to drill a cylinder of bone for biopsy, grafting or entry into a cavity (Fig 23). It is "T" shaped and has a cylindric saw-like cutting blade at its tip.

Figure 17. Gelpi retractor.

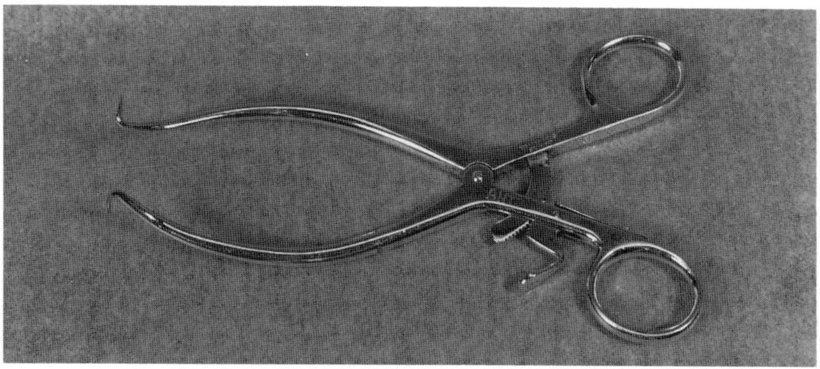

Figure 18. Weitlaner retractor.

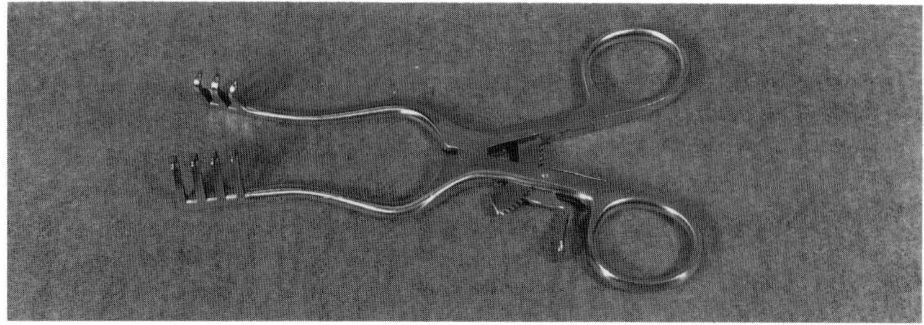

Bone-Holding Instruments: Bone forceps and clamps are used to grasp and manipulate bones and bone fragments during orthopedic procedures (Fig 24). They are fairly heavy-duty instruments, but

Figure 19. Rongeurs.

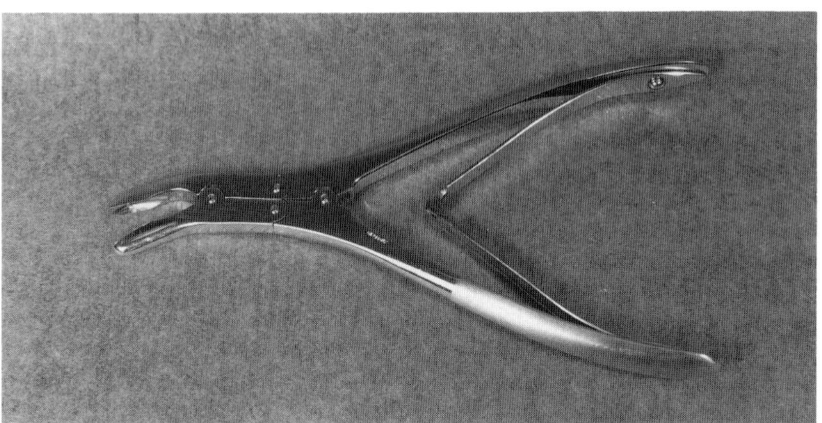

Figure 20. Bone-cutting forceps.

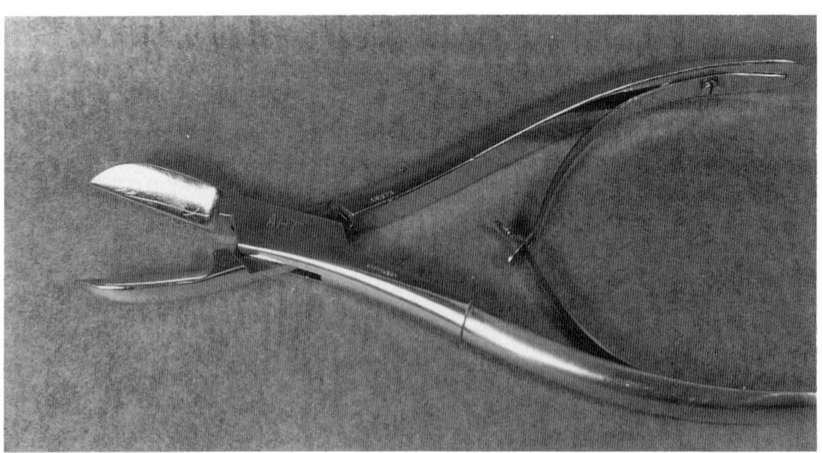

must be used and handled carefully to avoid damaging bones and surrounding soft tissues.

Periosteal Elevators: Periosteal elevators are used to elevate periosteum and other soft tissues from the surface of bones (Fig 25). The blade-like end is worked under the periosteum to elevate it from the bone's surface.

Intramedullary Pinning Instruments: Intramedullary pins are stainless-steel rods that are inserted into the medullary cavity of fractured long bones to stabilize the fracture fragments (Fig 26). Their insertion requires an intramedullary pin chuck with which to grasp them (Fig 26), and a pin cutter (Fig 27) to cut them to the proper length.

Figure 21. Osteotome (top) and mallet.

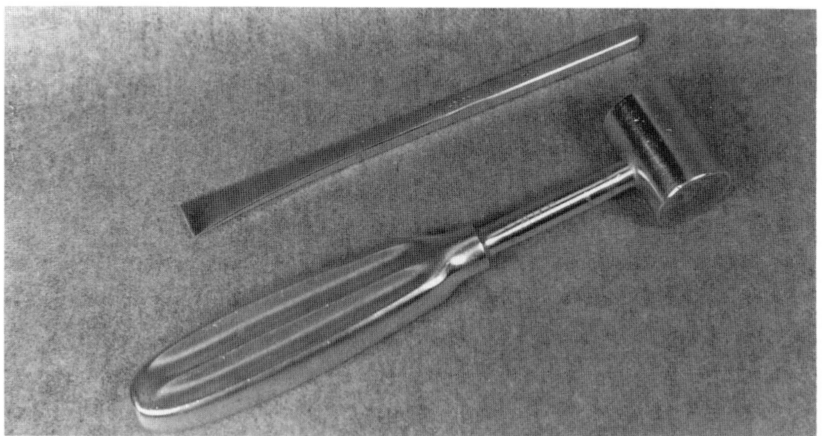

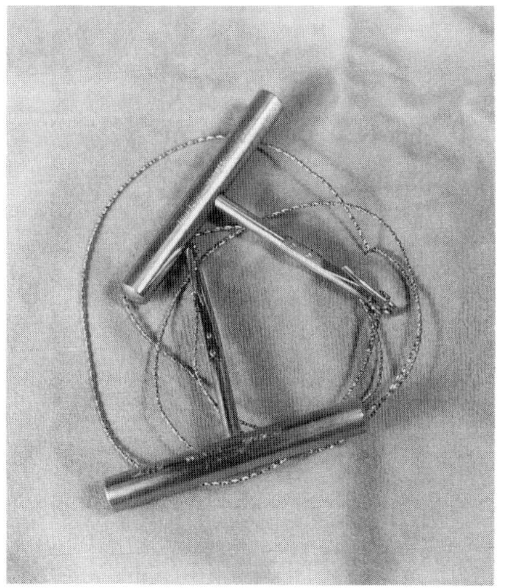

Figure 22. Gigli wire saw with handles.

Orthopedic Wire: Bone fragments are often stabilized with monofilament stainless-steel wire placed through or around the fragments (Fig 28). The wire is usually secured in place by use of a wire twister.

Bone-Plating Instruments: Stainless-steel bone plates are used to secure fracture fragments in place by insertion of screws through the plates into the bone. Their use is fairly sophisticated

Figure 23. Michel trephine.

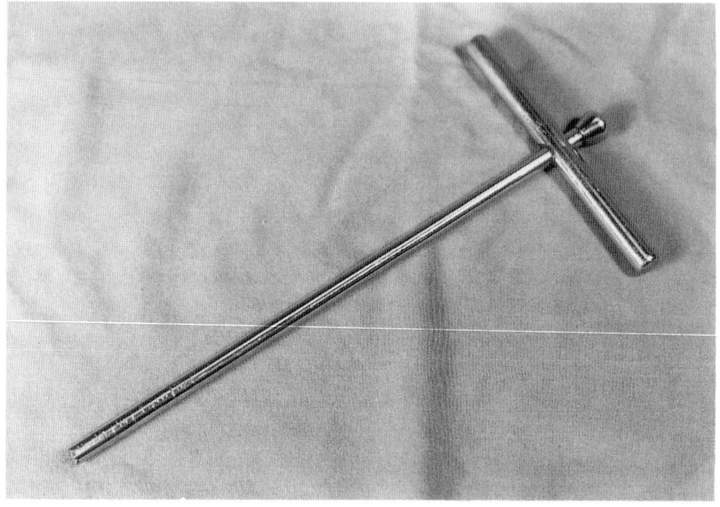

Figure 24. Loman bone-holding clamp (top) and Kern bone-holding forceps (bottom).

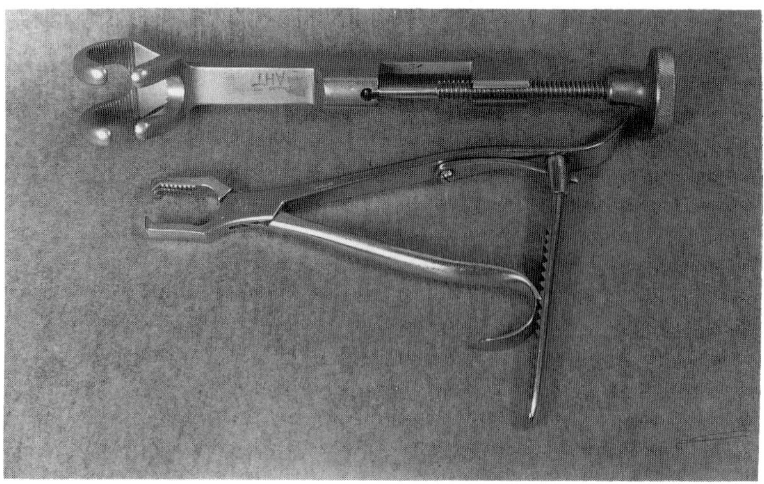

and requires a number of specialized instruments, including drills, drill guides, depth gauges, hole taps, screws and screwdrivers, in addition to the bone plates themselves.

Common Large Animal Surgery Instruments

Dehorning Instruments: Various instruments, including gouges and saws, are used to remove the horns from cattle (Fig 29). The smaller instruments are used on calves. The saws are generally used to remove the horns of adult cattle.

Castrating Instruments: Emasculators are used during open castrations to crush and sever the spermatic cord (Fig 30).

Figure 25. Periosteal elevator.

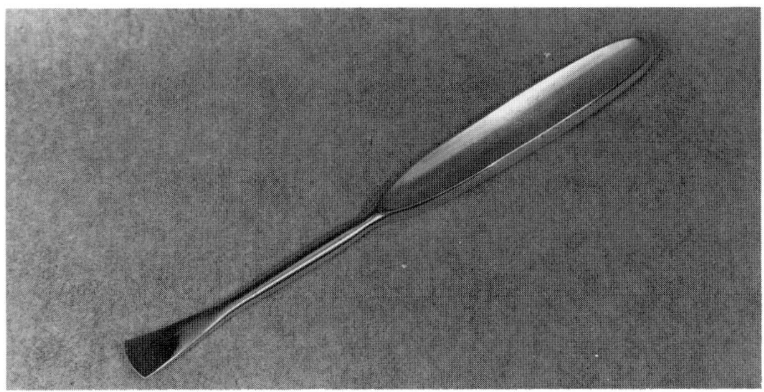

Figure 26. Intramedullary pins with a pin chuck.

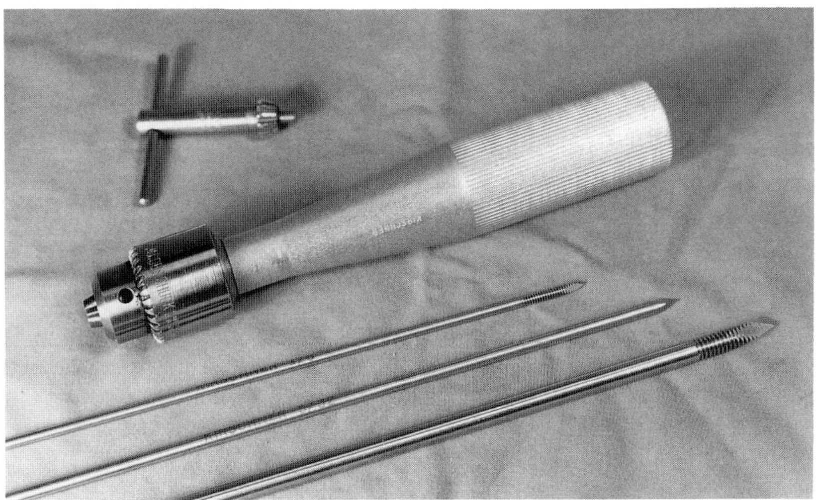

Emasculatomes are used to accomplish the same thing through the intact skin during closed castrations, particularly when fly infestation is likely to be a problem (Fig 30).

Table 1 lists instruments commonly included in standard surgical packs.

Care of Surgical Instruments

Most surgical instruments are made of what is commonly referred to as stainless steel. Actually the term "stainless" is somewhat of a misnomer. Though this type of steel does resist rust, even stainless steel is susceptible to spotting, staining and corrosion

Figure 27. Intramedullary pin cutter.

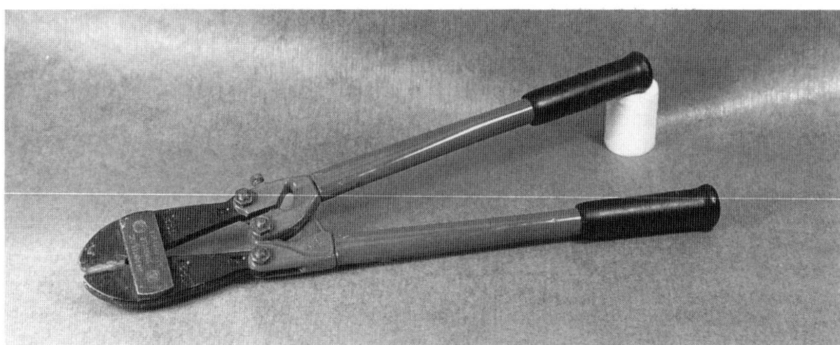

Figure 28. Stainless-steel wire in a wire twister.

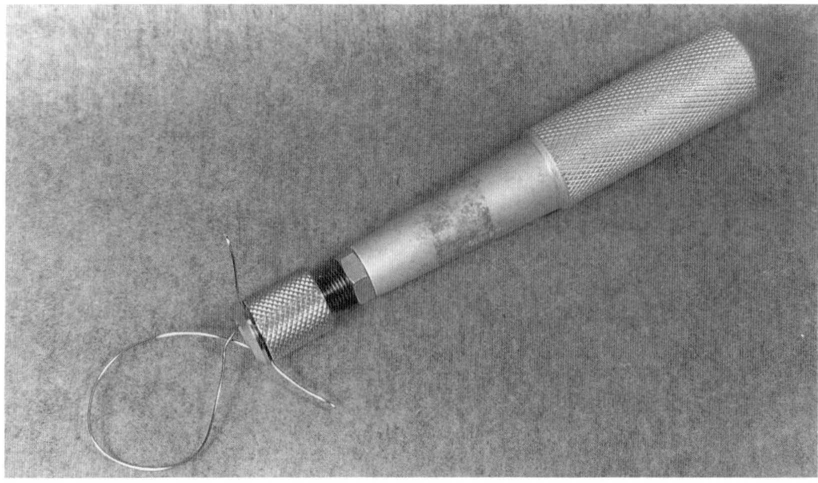

Table 1. Instruments commonly included in surgical packs.

Major Pack

1 #3 scapel handle

1 curved Metzenbaum scissors

1 straight sharp-blunt operating scissors

1 thumb tissue forceps

1 thumb dressing forceps

3 curved Rochester-Carmalt forceps

8 curved Halsted mosquito foceps

1 Mayo-Hegar needle holder

1 sponge forceps

1 Snook's ovariohysterectomy hook

2 Allis tissue forceps

2 curved Crile or Kelly forceps

6 Backhaus towel forceps

1 grooved director

assorted needles in rack

50 3 x 3 gauze sponges

1 sterilization indicator

Minor Pack

1 #3 scapel handle

1 curved Metzenbaum scissors

1 straight sharp-blunt operating scissors

1 thumb tissue forceps

1 curved Rochester-Carmalt forceps

6 curved Halsted mosquito forceps

1 Mayo-Hegar needle holder

1 Snook's ovariohysterectomy hook

6 Backhaus towel forceps

1 grooved director

assorted needles in rack

30 3 x 3 gauze sponges

1 sterilization indicator

Suture Pack

1 #3 scapel handle

1 curved Metzenbaum scissors

1 straight sharp-blunt operating scissors

1 thumb tissue forceps

1 Olson-Hegar scissors/needle holder

2 curved Halsted mosquito forceps

2 Backhaus towel forceps

assorted needles in rack

15 3 x 3 gauze sponges

1 sterilization indicator

under certain conditions. Proper care and handling of surgical instruments can significantly extend their useful life.

Cleaning

Instruments should be cleaned as soon as possible after surgery. Allowing instruments to remain soiled with blood, wound exudates and tissue fluid increases the risk of damage to the surface of the instruments. Also, if sterilization is to be effective, instruments must be extremely clean. Because blood and other organic material can inadvertently contaminate instruments not actually used dur-

Figure 29. Dehorning instruments: dehorning saw (top), Barnes dehorner (bottom left), horn gouge (bottom right).

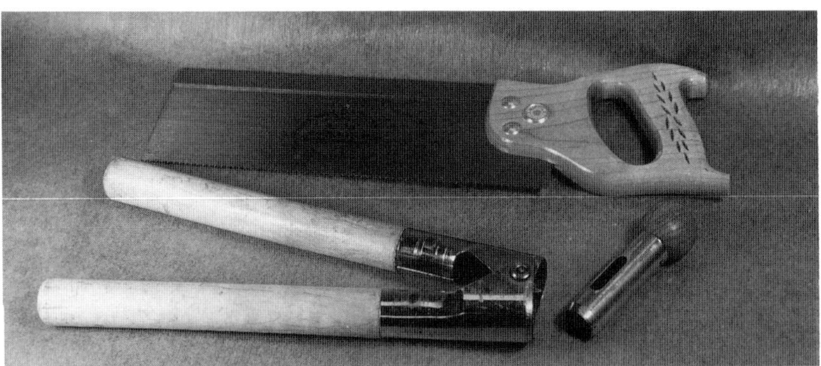

Figure 30. Emasculatome (bottom left) and emasculator (top right).

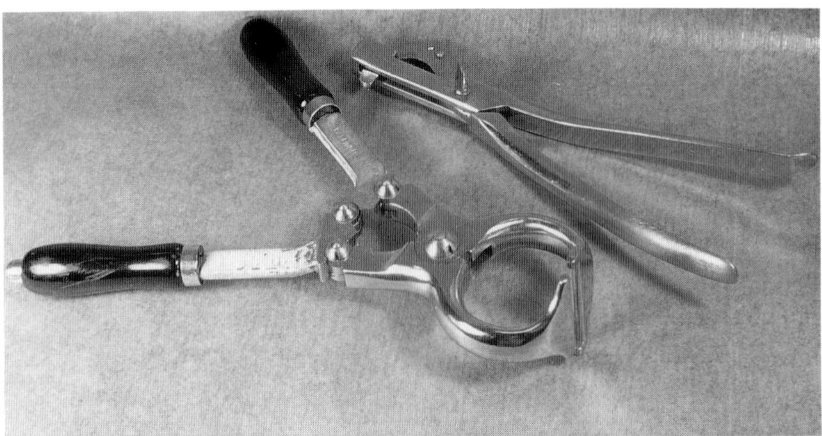

ing surgery, but sitting nearby on a tray, all instruments in the pack should be cleaned, whether or not they were used.

For manual cleaning, hinged instruments with jaws should be opened and the instruments initially soaked in a mild detergent solution. Very alkaline detergents should be avoided because of possible damage to the surface of the instruments. A scrub brush can be used to remove debris from crevices and grooves, but abrasive pads or cleansers should not be used. After cleaning, the instruments should be thoroughly rinsed, lubricated and allowed to air dry. Manual instrument cleaning is relatively inefficient at removing material from the recesses of surgical instruments.

Ultrasonic instrument cleaners are much more efficient than manual cleaning methods (Fig 31). High-frequency sound waves cause microscopic bubbles to form on all surfaces of the instruments. As rapidly as they form, the bubbles implode, creating tiny vacuum pockets that draw dirt out of the tiniest crevices and recesses. Only detergents intended for ultrasonic use should be added to the solution used to clean instruments in this manner. As with manual cleaning, hinged instruments with jaws should be open during the ultrasonic cleaning process. After ultrasonic cleaning, the instruments should be thoroughly rinsed, lubricated and allowed to air dry.

Lubricating

Without lubrication, hinged instruments can become stiff and difficult to use. Oil should not be used for lubrication, as it shields microorganisms from the sterilizing action of steam and other agents. Only water-soluble lubricants specifically designed for use

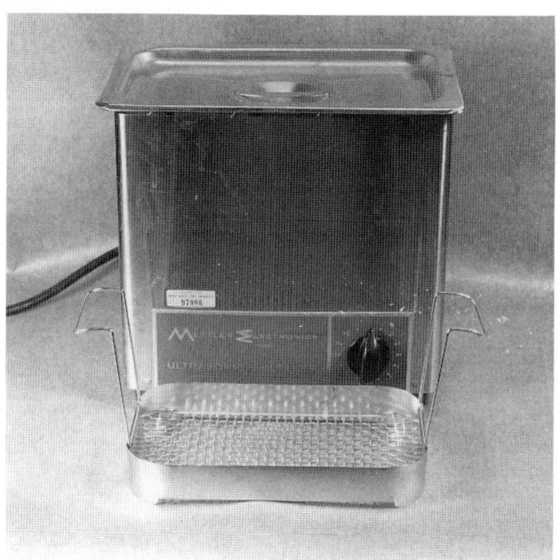

Figure 31. Ultrasonic instrument cleaner, with instrument tray removed.

on surgical instruments should be used. These lubricants penetrate into hinges and other inaccessible areas, and help prevent corrosion of instrument surfaces.

Immediately after cleaning and rinsing, instruments should be dipped into the properly diluted lubricating bath for 30 seconds. *After removal, the instruments should not be wiped or rinsed.* After the excess lubricant has been allowed to drain off, the instruments should be allowed to air dry.

Inspecting

After cleaning and drying, each instrument should be inspected before it is prepared for the next surgery. It is important that instruments be clean and free of problems to ensure proper sterilization and effective use. Things to check for include:

Hinged Instruments: Stiffness, alignment of jaws and teeth.

Sharp Instruments: Dull spots, burrs, nicks.

Instruments with Pins and Screws: Intactness and tightness of pins and screws.

Testing

Combined with a visual inspection, a few simple tests can quickly evaluate the condition of instruments:

Forceps: Close the jaws lightly. There should be no overlap and the *tips* of the jaws should come into contact first.

Test each ratchet by clamping it on the first tooth, holding the instrument by the hinge and tapping the ratchet portion lightly against a solid object. If the instrument springs open, the ratchet mechanism is faulty.

Clamp a needle in the jaws of needle holders and lock the ratchet on the second tooth. If the needle can be easily rotated by hand, the instrument is faulty.

Scissors: Scissors should easily cut 4 layers of gauze at their tip, and should cut smoothly along the entire length of the blades.

Preoperative and Postoperative Considerations

Preoperative Evaluation

Anesthesia and surgery are very stressful events that put an animal's life at risk. The role of a proper preoperative evaluation is to gather enough pertinent information to minimize that risk. That information can be gathered through a patient history, a physical examination and appropriate laboratory tests.

General Type of Surgical Procedure: Surgical procedures can be divided into 3 main categories: routine elective surgery; surgery necessary because of some disease or pathologic process; and emergency surgery.

Elective surgery consists of routine procedures, such as castrations and ovariohysterectomies. The danger with these surgeries is to confuse "routine" with "normal." Some patients undergoing routine surgery are not normal, and the preoperative evaluation must identify these abnormalities so appropriate measures can be taken to minimize risks.

An animal undergoing *surgery related to disease,* such as ovariohysterectomy for treatment of pyometra, is known to be abnormal. The preoperative evaluation should detect any changes in the animal's status and its response to any treatments that have been instituted before surgery.

With *emergency surgery,* time is of the essence. The most important preoperative considerations are monitoring the patient's condition, providing supportive care before surgery, and making appropriate preparations for the surgery. The goal is to have the prepared animal, the necessary instruments and equipment, and the veterinarian arrive at the surgery table at one time.

Patient History: An accurate patient history gives a picture of the animal's past and present health status, as related by the owner. Examples of the kind of information that should be gathered through the history include:

- Breed, gender (intact or neutered), and age
- Usual attitude and behavior
- Usual diet and appetite
- Usual elimination habits
- Current medical treatments, if any
- Past history of diseases and treatments, if any
- Past response to anesthesia and surgery, if any
- Observations on the functioning of various body systems

Physical Examination: A thorough physical examination provides important information about a patient's current health status. It should be a complete systematic evaluation of the animal, with emphasis on the cardiovascular and respiratory systems. Though not always possible in emergencies, a complete physical examination should include the following:

- Vital signs (temperature, pulse and respiratory rates)
- General appearance (conformation, attitude, etc)
- Body weight (obese, normal, emaciated)

- Skin and haircoat (lesions, general appearance)
- Lymph nodes (enlargements, asymmetry)
- Eyes (internal or external abnormalities)
- Ears (otitis, parasites)
- Nose (discharges, occlusion)
- Mouth and throat (dental disease, oropharyngeal inflammation)
- Neck and back (conformation)
- Thorax (auscultation of the heart and lungs)
- Abdomen (distension, pain or palpation)
- Genitalia (preputial/vulvar discharge, retained testes)
- Extremities (pain, swellings)
- Neurologic status (attitude, paresis)

Laboratory Evaluation: Laboratory tests can provide valuable information about the preoperative status of patients. Higher-risk animals, such as older or diseased animals, should be more thoroughly evaluated than younger animals presented for routine elective procedures. Laboratory tests useful in preoperative evaluation of patients include:

- Complete blood count
- Total plasma protein
- Parasitic examinations (fecal, heartworm test)
- Urinalysis
- Blood chemistry profile (electrolytes, enzymes, acid-base, etc)
- Specific organ function tests (kidney, liver, thyroid, etc)

Postoperative Evaluation

After a flawlessly executed surgical procedure, a patient receiving poor postoperative care can suffer devastating consequences. The postoperative period should be considered critical for all patients. Because of the possibility of unforeseen complications, it is essential that patients be continually monitored after any type of surgery.

Body Temperature: After surgery, every patient should have its rectal temperature measured at least once a day, and preferably 2-3 times a day. A 1 or 2 degree increase in rectal temperature for the first few postoperative days is a normal physiologic response to the trauma of major surgery. A higher or more prolonged temperature increase may indicate infection.

Body Weight: Daily monitoring of a surgical patient's body weight gives a measure of the animal's nutritional status and general body condition. One of the most frequently neglected aspects of postoperative patient care is provision of adequate nutrition. The healing process after surgery increases an animal's nutritional needs, particularly for protein. Those needs must be met so that healing can proceed without delay.

Attitude: An animal's behavior during the immediate postoperative period can give important information about the amount of pain it is enduring and possible complications that might be developing. If a patient is very depressed, the reasons for that state must be determined and appropriate treatment instituted quickly.

Appetite and Thirst: Surgical patients must receive adequate nutrition and fluid intake. Animals should begin eating and drinking as soon as possible after surgery. Lack of interest in food and/or water indicates problems that should be investigated without delay.

Urination and Defecation: Elimination patterns give important information about kidney and GI tract function in patients recovering from surgery. Assuming adequate fluid and food intake, urination and defecation should proceed normally.

Appearance of the Surgical Wound: The surgical incision should be examined at least daily during the immediate postoperative period. It should be evaluated by visual inspection as well as gentle palpation. Such abnormalities as fluid accumulation, inflammation and impending dehiscence (opening) of the surgical wound can be detected and corrected early if the incision is carefully evaluated.

Postoperative Complications

Hemorrhage: If not quickly corrected, postoperative hemorrhage can lead to serious consequences for an animal, even death from shock. External hemorrhage is usually relatively easy to evaluate and control because it is easily visible. Internal hemorrhage is not readily apparent and, therefore, often more serious. An animal can bleed to death through hemorrhage into the abdominal cavity or thoracic cavity. The status of an animal's cardiovascular system should be frequently monitored during the immediate postoperative period for signs that might indicate hemorrhage. Pulse rate, capillary refill time, temperature of the extremities, and color of the mucous membranes can give valuable information on cardiovascular function.

Seroma: Seromas (accumulations of serum) and hematomas (accumulations of blood) beneath the surgical incision are usually caused by "dead space" left in the incision that the body naturally fills with fluid. Though unsightly, smaller seromas and hematomas are usually of cosmetic importance only, unless the skin sutures tear out. Treatment usually involves drainage of the fluid via needle and syringe and application of a pressure bandage, or resuturing of the incision to eliminate the dead space. Seromas and hematomas can be prevented with adequate suturing.

Infection: A persistently or drastically elevated rectal temperature, depressed attitude, poor appetite, or a swollen, inflamed incision are all signs of possible postoperative infection.

Postoperative infections can be superficial, subcutaneous, within a body cavity, or spread throughout the body. Superficial infection often results in a draining wound that does not heal well. Subcutaneous infections frequently progress to abscess formation. Infection in the abdominal cavity (peritonitis) or thoracic cavity (pleuritis) often results from a penetrating injury or damage to organs in that body cavity. Septicemia is a generalized infection that spreads via the bloodstream. Fortunately, septicemia is not common after surgery.

When the danger of postoperative infection is high, as with long or potentially contaminated procedures, administration of a broad-spectrum antibacterial should be started 24 hours before surgery to achieve an effective blood level. Drug use should be continued for at least 5 consecutive days after surgery.

Wound Dehiscence: Wound dehiscence (disruption of the surgical wound) is one of the most serious postoperative complications that can occur. Possible causes of wound dehiscence include:

- Suture failure (loosening, untying, breakage)
- Infection
- Tissue weakness (old or debilitated animals, hyperadrenocorticism, prolonged corticosteroid use)
- Mechanical stress (stormy anesthetic recovery, chronic vomiting, chronic cough, excessive activity)
- Poor nutrition

Early signs of surgical wound dehiscence are frequently seen within the first 3 or 4 days after surgery. They may include a serosanguineous discharge from the incision, firm or fluctuant swelling deep to (under) the suture line, and palpation of a hernial ring or loop of bowel beneath the skin.

If only the muscle layer of an abdominal incision breaks down and the skin sutures remain intact, a doughy swelling can be palpated under the skin. This is a serious situation but is not an acute emergency. A bandage should be applied for support, and the suture line should be repaired as soon as possible.

If both the muscle layer and the skin sutures of an abdominal incision break down, the animal can eviscerate (abdominal organs protrude through suture line). If evisceration occurs, the involved organs can become bruised and grossly contaminated, and may even by mutilated by the animal itself. This is an acute emergency that must be attended to immediately. Carefully gather the exteriorized viscera in a moist towel and hold them in place near the incision while others are preparing the animal and operating room for the repair.

Aseptic Technique

Aseptic technique is the term used to describe all of the precautions taken to prevent contamination, and ultimately infection, of a surgical wound. Its purpose is to minimize contamination so that postoperative healing is not delayed.

Contamination vs Infection

Contamination of an object or a wound implies the *presence* of microorganisms within or on it. Contamination of a wound can, but does not necessarily, lead to infection.

With *infection,* microorganisms in the body or a wound *multiply and cause harmful effects.* Four main factors determine if infection occurs:

- *Number of microorganisms:* There must be sufficient microorganisms to overcome the defenses of the animal.
- *Virulence of the microorganisms:* Their ability to cause disease.
- *Susceptibility of the animal:* Some individuals have a greater natural resistance to infection than others.
- *Route of exposure to the microorganisms:* Some routes of exposure are more likely to result in infection than others.

We have no influence over the virulence of microorganisms in the environment or the susceptibility of the patient. The route of exposure to microorganisms during surgery is determined by the surgical procedure. The only factor we can significantly influence is the *number of microorganisms that enter the surgical wound.* We do that through application of strict aseptic technique before and during surgery.

Aseptic Technique

Aseptic technique in the operating room can be summarized by 6 basic rules, 4 that apply to surgical instruments and equipment and 2 that apply to surgical personnel.

Surgical Instruments and Equipment:

- *Only sterile items should touch patient tissues.*
- *Only sterile items should touch other sterile items.*

- *Any sterile item touching a nonsterile item becomes nonsterile.*
- *If the sterility of an item is in doubt, consider it nonsterile.*

Surgical Personnel:
- *Only scrubbed personnel should touch sterile items.*
- *Nonscrubbed personnel should touch only nonsterile items.*

During surgery, aseptic technique protects the exposed tissues of the patient from 4 main sources of potential contamination: the operative personnel, the surgical instruments and equipment, the patient itself, and the surgical environment.

Preparation of Operative Personnel

Normal Microbial Flora

All normal animals, including people, harbor a resident population of microorganisms living on most epithelial surfaces, especially the skin. That population is referred to as the *resident* or *normal microbial flora.* The microorganisms of the normal flora usually cause no problem on the skin surface but may cause infection if introduced into a surgical wound.

To protect surgical patients from their normal microbial flora, operative personnel must be almost completely covered to form a barrier to contamination. The hands, which will come in direct physical contact with the tissues of the patient, are of particular importance. They must be scrubbed to reduce the microbial population, and then covered with a sterile barrier in the form of latex surgical gloves.

Scrub Suit

Scrub suits are available in a variety of designs. They usually consist of trousers and a loose-fitting short-sleeved top (Fig 32). The top should be tucked into the trousers to prevent possible contamination during the surgical scrub procedure. The scrub suit should be clean and preferably not worn outside the surgical area before a surgical procedure.

The shoes worn in the operating room should be clean and also preferably not worn outside the surgical area. Shoe covers are available, however, for street shoes.

Surgical Cap

The purpose of the surgical cap is to prevent contamination from dislodged human hair. While the cap does not have to be sterile, the cap must be clean and must form an intact barrier over all of the hair (Fig 33). Surgical caps are made from a variety of materials in a variety of styles. For individuals with relatively short hair, a standard surgical cap is sufficient (Fig 33). For those with a beard, long sideburns or a very full head of hair, a hooded head cover is usually necessary (Fig 34). A bouffant-style cap can be used to contain long hair (Fig 35).

Surgical Mask

The surgical mask is worn to decrease contamination from the respiratory tract of surgical personnel by filtering the air expired

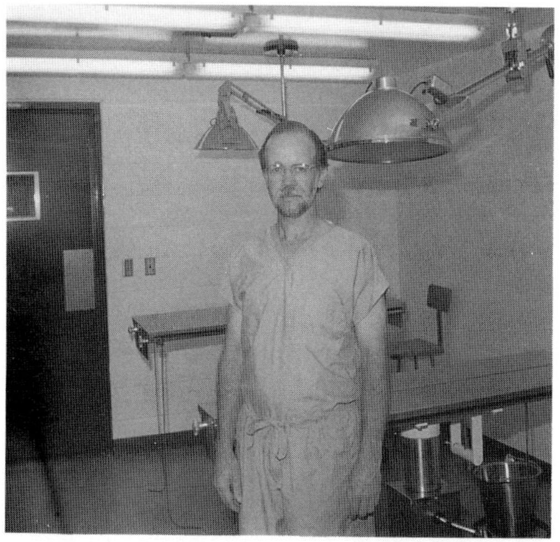

Figure 32. Scrub suit.

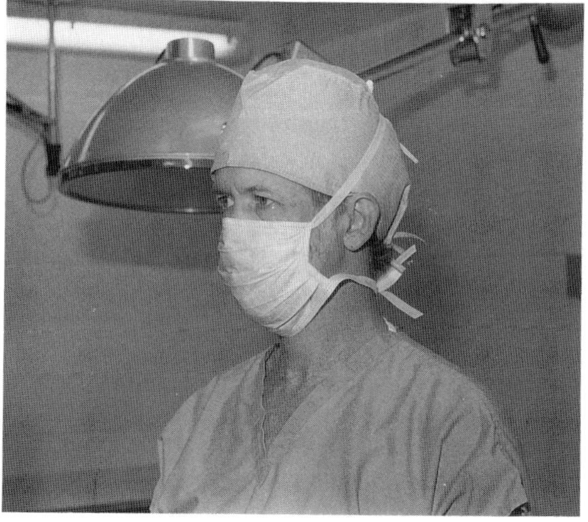

Figure 33. Standard surgical cap. Note that the beard/ sideburns are not adequately covered with this cap and mask combination.

from the nose and mouth. Available in a variety of types, styles and materials, the surgical mask should be snug fitting (Figs 34, 35). While it does not have to be sterile, the mask should be clean for each surgical procedure. With use, a mask becomes increasingly contaminated with bacteria. As it becomes moistened from the humidity in the breath, it becomes less effective as a filter.

Surgical Scrub Procedure

The purpose of the surgical scrub is to diminish the population of microorganisms on the hands and arms of surgical personnel. While it is impossible to sterilize the skin surfaces, the number of

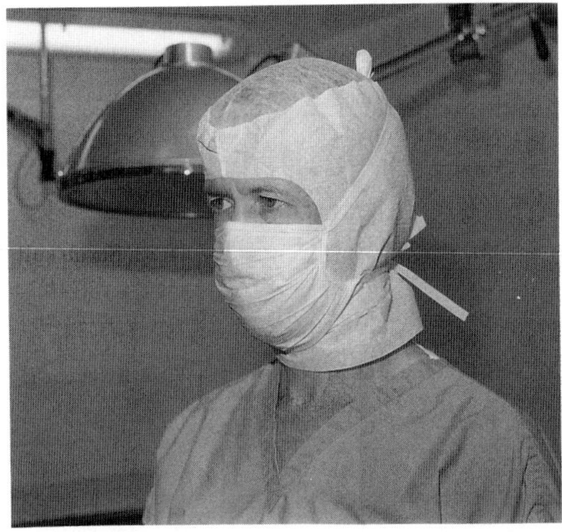

Figure 34. Surgical hood. Note that the beard/sideburns are completely covered.

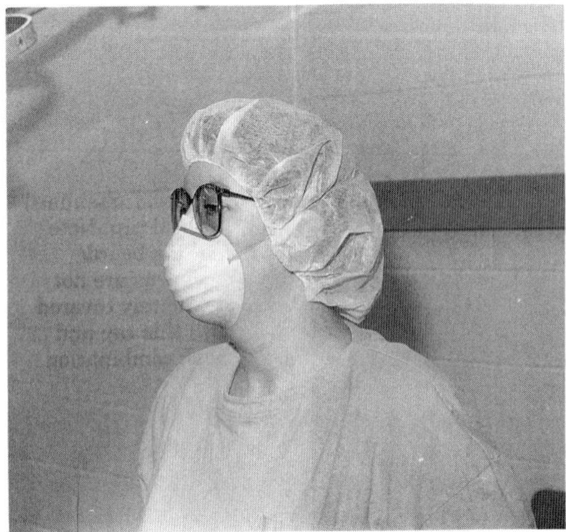

Figure 35. Bouffant surgical cap.

microorganisms can be significantly decreased before donning the surgical gown and gloves. The possibility of a defect in a latex glove or a puncture through a latex glove during surgery makes the presurgical scrub very important.

The scrub area is usually located adjacent to the operating room. It should have a deep sink to help prevent contamination from splashing water, and a water supply that can be operated without using the hands. The water supply at most surgical scrub sinks is knee controlled, though foot or elbow controls are sometimes used. A sterile scrub brush is needed. Unless the brush is disposable and already contains the surgical scrub soap, a foot-controlled scrub soap dispenser is also needed. Various surgical scrub soaps are available, but providone-iodine and chlorhexidine preparations are commonly used.

Before starting the scrub, the mask and cap should be donned and all jewelry removed from the hands. The fingernails should be short and clean and have no polish on them. During the scrub, the hands should always be held higher than the elbows so that water runs down the arms and drips off the elbows. If the hands were held lower than the elbows, water could run down from the arms and contaminate the hands. Once the scrubbing process has begun, the hands and arms should not touch anything that is nonsterile.

All surfaces of the hands and arms must receive adequate covering during scrubbing. It is convenient to think of each digit, hand and arm as having 4 surfaces that must be scrubbed: front, back and the 2 sides. The 4 surfaces of the digits, as well as their tips, are scrubbed first, then the hand and finally the arm up to the elbow. It is easiest to scrub the arm in thirds, starting with the 4 surfaces near the wrist first, then the middle third and finally the proximal third.

After a thorough general washing of the hands and arms with surgical scrub soap, the sterile scrub brush is picked up, and the scrub is carried out using the brush-stroke method or the timed method.

The *brush-stroke method* uses counted (10-20) brush strokes on all surfaces of each digit, hand and arm. The hands and arms are then rinsed and the scrub is repeated.

With the *timed method,* the hands and arms are scrubbed twice, with a rinse in between, for a total of 5-10 minutes.

At the completion of the surgical scrub, the hands and arms must be dried with a sterile towel. The towel should be grasped by bending the knees to lower the whole body rather than reaching down with the hand, so that water does not run down from the upper arm and contaminate the hand. After the hands have been carefully dried, the towel is folded or wadded up, and the first arm is dried, starting at the wrist area and working up to the elbow.

The towel is then transferred to the other hand, being careful not to grasp the surface that was just used to dry the first arm, and the other arm is dried.

Surgical Gown

After the hands are dried, the surgical gown can be donned (Fig 36). Surgical gowns are folded and wrapped for sterilization inside-out, with the arm hole/shoulder area on top when the gown pack is opened. The gown should be picked up off its sterile wrap by the arm hole/shoulder area, and allowed to unfold by gravity, with minimal shaking. The arm holes should be located and the arms slid down into the sleeves as far as the cuffs. An assistant can then fasten the ties on the back of the gown.

Once the gown has been tied in place, the front of the gown from the waist to the neck, including the arms, is considered sterile and can safely contact other sterile surfaces. The remainder of the gown surfaces is considered nonsterile and must not be allowed to come into contact with anything sterile.

Surgical Gloves

Modern latex surgical gloves act as a very thin physical barrier between the hands of the surgeon and the tissues of the patient. To preserve the sterility of the surgical field, latex gloves must have no holes or cracks. After a surgical scrub, the hands are very clean but still harbor bacteria that could contaminate a surgical wound. If a glove is accidentally punctured during surgery, it should be changed immediately or another glove applied on top of the first.

Surgical gloves should be donned in a careful manner, allowing the hands to touch only the *inside* of the gloves so as to avoid con-

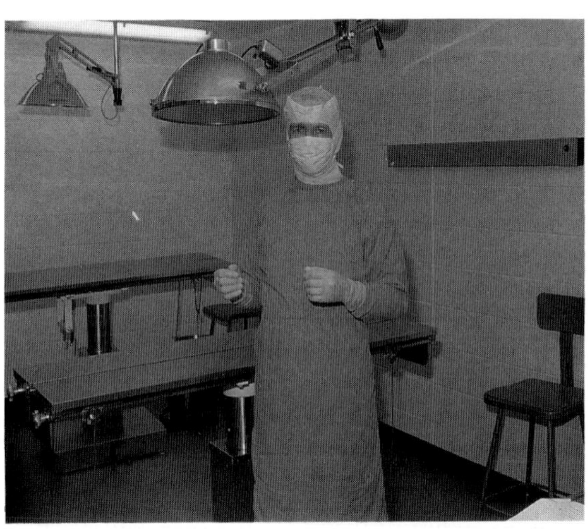

Figure 36. Surgical gown.

tamination of the outside glove surfaces. Two gloving techniques, closed and open, are commonly used.

With the *closed gloving technique,* the bare skin of the hands is never visible during the process of donning the gloves. For this technique, the hands are inserted down into, but not out through, the cuffs of the gown. The gloves are then manipulated through the gown cuff, and the hands are inserted through the gown cuffs directly into the gloves. There is less chance of accidental contamination of the outside glove surfaces with closed gloving than with the open gloving technique, but it is not always possible to use the closed gloving technique. Replacement of a damaged glove during surgery would generally require the open gloving technique, so it is important to be able to don gloves by the open method even if the closed method is generally used.

The *open gloving technique* poses more opportunities to contaminate the outside of a glove than the closed technique, but it can be very effective if done carefully. While donning gloves with this technique, it must be kept in mind that *the only thing that should touch the outside of a glove is the outside of the other glove.* The bare hands should touch only the inside of the gloves. One glove is picked up by the cuff and the other hand is slid into it, with the glove cuff left down over the hand. The gloved fingers are then placed under the cuff of the other glove and the other hand is slid into the glove. The cuff of the glove is then pulled up over the cuff of the gown all the way around. The fingers of the now completely gloved second hand are slipped under the cuff of the first glove and the cuff of the glove is pulled up over the cuff of the gown all the way around.

Surgery gloves are lubricated with a fine cornstarch type of powder to make them easier to slip on. If there is a visible layer of powder on the outside of the gloves, it should be removed with sterile moistened sponges before beginning surgery. The cornstarch granules can cause foreign-body inflammatory responses in a surgical wound.

Preparation of Surgical Equipment and Instruments

Sterilization

Sterilization is the process of destroying all microorganisms on an object. It is an "all or nothing" process. A sterile object has *no* living organisms on it. There is no such thing as "almost sterile."

Active, multiplying vegetative bacterial forms are most easily destroyed by common sterilization methods. Inactive, dormant bacterial spores are more resistant.

Ethylene Oxide Sterilization

Ethylene oxide sterilization is also referred to as "gas sterilization." Materials sterilized by this method are exposed to toxic ethylene oxide gas in adequate concentration at an appropriate temperature and humidity for a sufficient time.

While it can be used for sterilizing nearly anything, ethylene oxide gas is usually reserved for items that would be damaged by other methods of sterilization. Such items as rubber catheters, electric drills and plastic devices are commonly sterilized by this method. Ethylene oxide is not usually used for routine sterilization because of its expense and its physical and biological properties.

Ethylene oxide gas is very flammable and very irritating to body tissues. It should only be used under controlled conditions in well-ventilated areas away from sources of spark or flame. Items sterilized by this method should be allowed to "air out" for at least 24 hours before use so as to allow the toxic gas to dissipate.

Two general types of ethylene oxide sterilization units are available. The relatively expensive units resemble tabletop autoclaves. They are attached to tanks of ethylene oxide gas and operate in carefully controlled cycles using elevated processing temperatures to decrease the time required for sterilization. The less expensive units are cannisters of various shapes, sizes and materials into which plastic bags containing the items to be sterilized and ampules of ethylene oxide are placed. Scavenging systems remove the gas from the cannister and pipe it out of the area. The less expensive units operate at room temperature, and require longer exposure times, often overnight.

Chemical indicators are available to demonstrate that the exposure to ethylene oxide gas was sufficient for sterilization. One of these sterilization indicators should be placed at the center of each pack or item sterilized by this method.

Liquid Chemical Disinfection

Liquid chemical disinfection is commonly called "cold sterilization" because it involves immersion of instruments in a chemical solution that is usually at room temperature. Because most of these chemicals are effective mainly against vegetative bacterial forms, with variable efficacy against spores, their use is more appropriately termed "disinfection" rather than "sterilization."

Various liquid chemicals are used for instrument disinfection. Commonly used agents include alcohols, iodophors, phenolic compounds, and quaternary ammonium compounds. Each has different characteristics and spectrums of action, so a chemical disinfection agent should be chosen according to the criteria that are most important for a particular application. Once chosen, the solution must be carefully prepared, maintained and replaced according to the manufacturer's directions.

Because liquid chemical solutions do not dull the sharp edges of instruments as does steam in an autoclave, this method is often used to disinfect sharp-edged instruments, such as scissors and needles. The instruments must be completely clean, as the solution must contact all surfaces to be effective. The instruments must remain immersed for a sufficient time, usually ranging from a few minutes to several hours, depending on the solution used. The disinfection process can often be accelerated by warming the solution.

Use of liquid chemicals to disinfect surgical instruments has some dangers and limitations, including limited spectrum of antimicrobial action, inactivation by organic matter, and toxicity. Most commonly used solutions are effective against vegetative bacterial forms but may not kill spores, viruses and other resistant microorganisms. Many liquid chemical disinfectants are inactivated by organic matter, so instruments must be scrupulously cleaned of any blood, serum and organic debris before immersion. Finally, most chemical disinfectants are irritating to patient tissues, so they should be aseptically wiped off instruments before use.

Autoclave Sterilization

Autoclave sterilization involves exposure of instruments and equipment to high-temperature, pressurized steam in the chamber of an instrument called an autoclave (Fig 37). For autoclave sterilization to be effective, all parts of a surgical pack must be exposed to steam at the proper temperature for a sufficient length of time. In veterinary medicine, the most commonly used exposure temper-

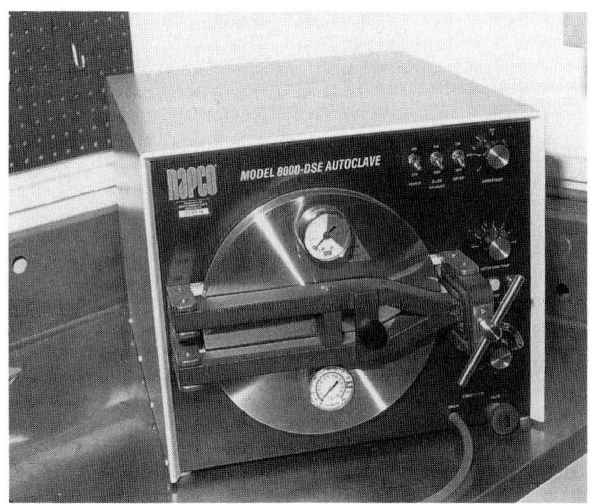

Figure 37. Autoclave.

ature/time for steam sterilization is 121 C for a minimum of 15 minutes. That means that *all* parts of the pack must receive that exposure. The time required for the steam to penetrate through the wrappings, etc, must be added to the 15-minute minimum exposure period.

Autoclave sterilization is very commonly used to sterilize surgical instruments and equipment used for routine surgery. It should be used only to sterilize instruments that are not damaged by high-temperature steam. Because steam dulls sharp edges, sharp-edged instruments (scissors, needles) are often not sterilized by this method. Also, heat-sensitive materials are usually not sterilized in an autoclave.

To achieve maximum effectiveness, the steam in the autoclave chamber must be able to circulate in and around the materials being sterilized. Sufficient space must be left for circulation of steam around the packs. Surgical packs should not be jammed tightly into the chamber. Since the steam generally flows from top to bottom in the chamber, packs should be positioned on edge rather than flat, so that steam flow is not impeded. Any bowls in a pack should also be positioned on edge so that moisture does not collect in them.

Different types of indicators have been used to confirm that the conditions for sterilization have been met in an autoclave. Some provide complete, accurate information, while others provide incomplete information. Indicators used include autoclave tape, melting pellets, culture tests and chemical autoclave indicators.

Autoclave tape resembles paper masking tape with colorless diagonal stripes that turn brown on exposure to steam (Figs 38, 39). The color change confirms exposure to steam but gives no information on the temperature of the steam or the length of the exposure.

Figure 38. Autoclave tape (top), melting pellet indicator (center) and chemical autoclave indicator (bottom) before use.

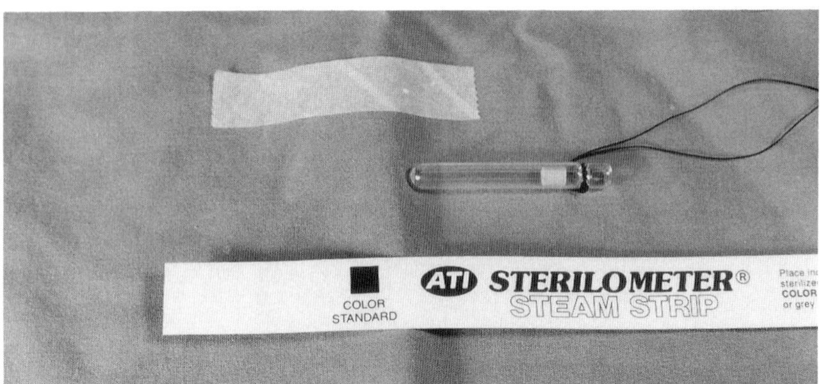

Autoclave tape is also usually applied only to the outside of the pack, so it gives no information on the conditions that prevailed inside the pack during autoclaving. Autoclave tape is useful to fasten surgical packs closed and indicates that they have been exposed to steam, but it should not be relied on to confirm the sterility of the pack contents.

The *melting pellet autoclave indicator* is an outdated and inaccurate means of determining if sterilization conditions have been met (Figs 38, 39). The indicator consists of a small sealed glass tube containing a pink pellet. The tube is placed at the center of a surgical pack and examined when the pack is opened. If the pellet has turned red and fused into place in the tube, an appropriately high temperature was reached in the pack (Fig 39). No information is provided, however, on the presence or absence of steam, or the duration of the exposure.

Commonly used *culture tests* consist of nonpathogenic bacterial spores impregnated on strips of paper. One strip is placed into a surgical pack and another is kept outside the autoclave as a control. After the pack has been autoclaved and opened for use, the spore strip is removed. The autoclaved and control strips are then (separately) placed into appropriate bacterial culture media. If autoclave sterilization was effective, the autoclaved strip should show no bacterial growth and the control strip should show growth. It may take several days to learn the results of the culture, however. While effective for periodic quality control checks, culture tests cannot be relied on as routine sterilization indicators.

Chemical autoclave indicators consist of chemical spots on paper strips or cards that change color on exposure to steam at an appropriate temperature for adequate length of time. These are often the most reliable indicators that the conditions for autoclave steriliza-

Figure 39. Autoclave tape (top), melting pellet indicator (center) and chemical autoclave indicator (bottom) after use.

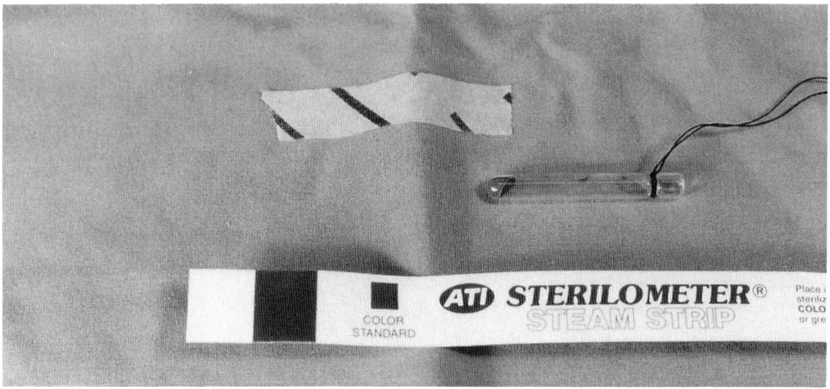

tion were met inside a surgical pack. They should be placed at the center of each autoclaved pack.

Wrapping Instrument Packs for Sterilization

Instrument packs, gowns and other items are usually wrapped in cloth or paper wraps. Individual instruments are often sealed in plastic/paper pouches for sterilization (Fig 40). The advantage of the pouches is that the instrument can be clearly seen through the transparent plastic.

Instrument packs are often double wrapped, using the same technique for each layer. Instruments and materials are placed on the open wrap in a diagonal, corner-to-corner position (Fig 41). The bottom corner is folded up over the pack, with the corner turned outward (Fig 42). The 2 side corners are folded similarly (Fig 43).

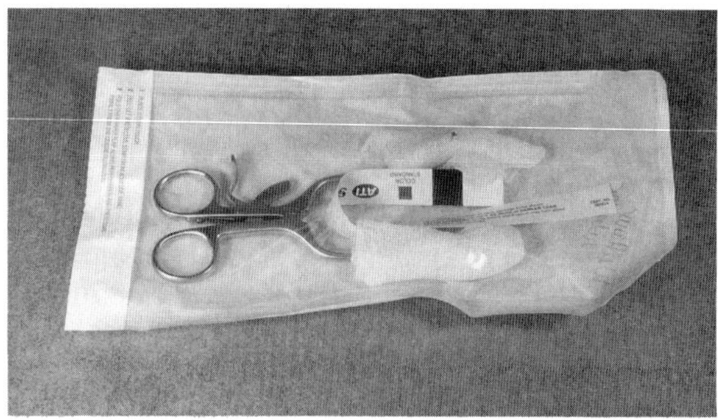

Figure 40. Surgical instrument in paper/ plastic pouch.

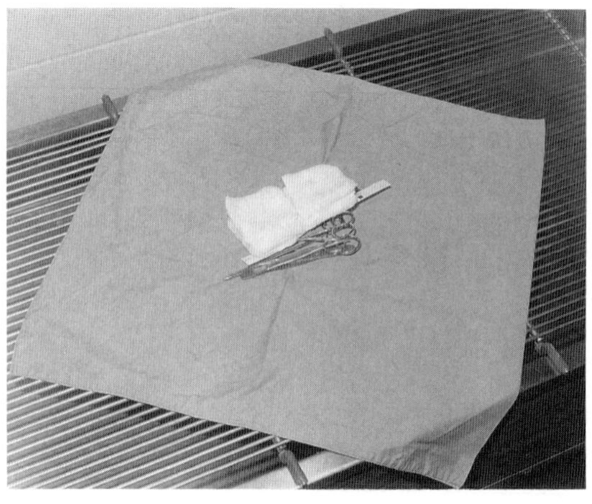

Figure 41. Wrapping a pack. The instruments are positioned on the wrap.

The last corner is folded over the pack, with the resultant flap folded inward (Figs 44, 45). The completed pack is then secured with autoclave tape (Fig 46). The tape is labeled with the contents, date, and name or initials of the person who prepared the pack.

Preparation of the Surgical Patient

The skin and haircoat of surgical patients have a normal microbial flora from which the surgical wound must be protected. On the skin surface, the normal resident microorganisms cause little or no problem for the animal. If, however, these microorganisms are in-

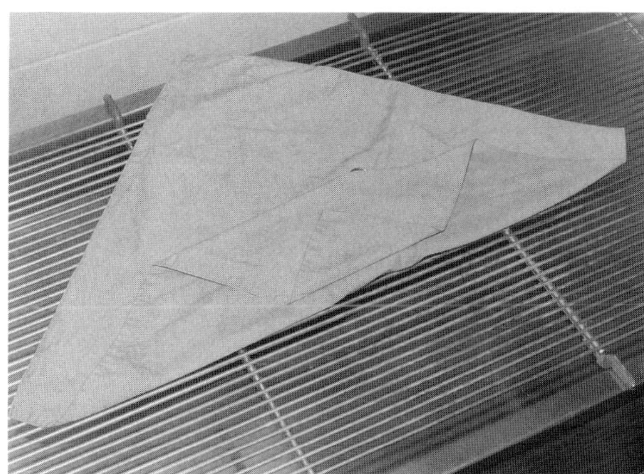

Figure 42. Wrapping a pack. The first corner is folded.

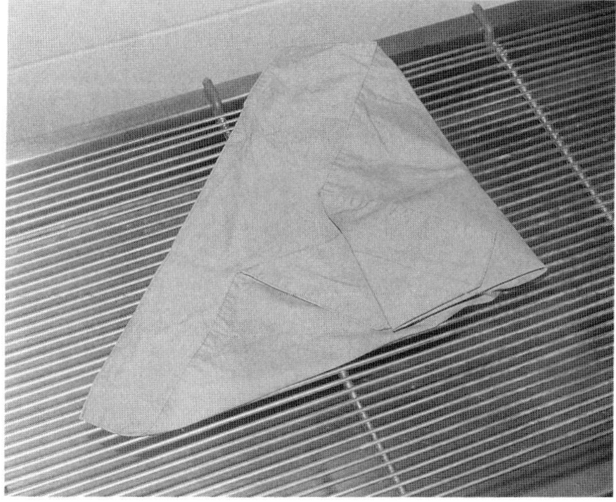

Figure 43. Wrapping a pack. The second corner is folded.

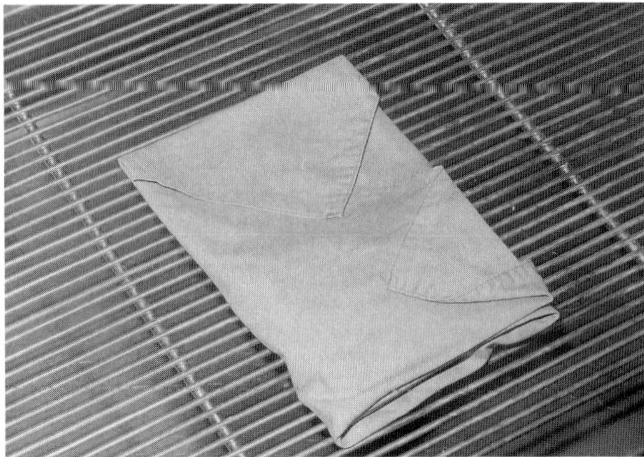

Figure 44. Wrapping a pack. The last corner is folded once.

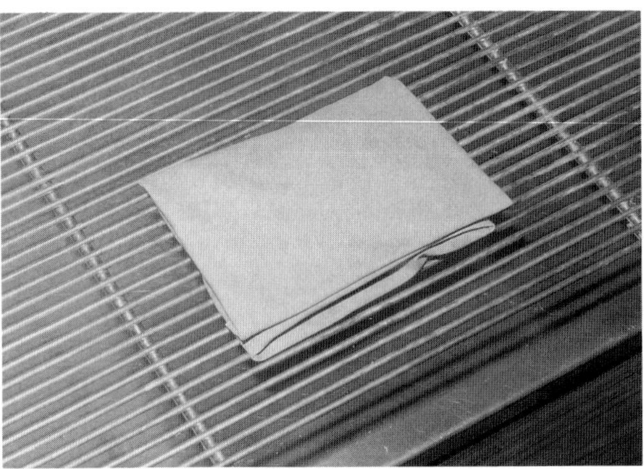

Figure 45. Wrapping a pack. The folded last corner is folded again over the pack.

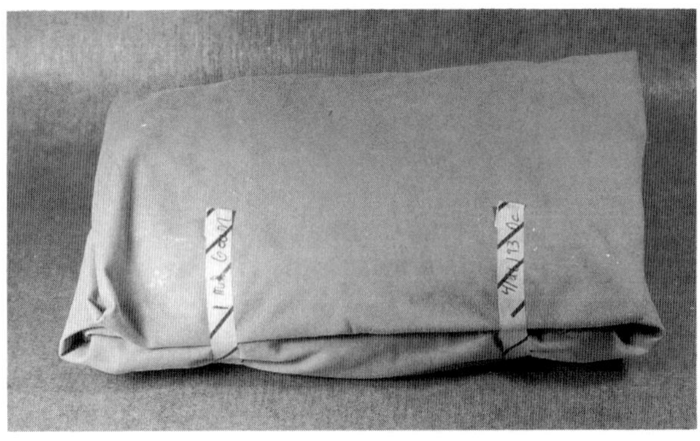

Figure 46. Surgical pack secured with autoclave tape. The dark stripes on the tape indicate that this pack has been autoclaved.

troduced beneath the skin surface into a surgical wound, they could cause infection.

To protect the internal tissues of the patient from these surface microorganisms, the hair must be removed from the surgical site, the numbers of microorganisms on the skin surface must be reduced with a preoperative surgical scrub, and sterile surgical drapes must be placed around the incision for surgery. The first 2 procedures are often conducted in a "prep" room adjacent to the surgery room, though they may be performed in the surgery room itself.

Hair Removal

Hair can be removed from the surgical site by any of several means. The most common method is by use of an electric clipper with a #40 (surgical) blade. Clipping against the grain of the hair is most effective, though clipping with the grain first may be necessary if the animal has a thick haircoat. It is useful to keep 3 principles in mind when clipping the hair: be neat (owners judge the quality of the surgery by external appearances), be gentle (avoid clipper burns and irritation), and be thorough (all of the hair must be removed at the skin surface to minimize the risk of contamination).

Another method of hair removal is with a razor. This can result in a very "close shave," but care must be exercised to avoid "presurgical incisions." The irregular contours of many areas of animal bodies can make use of a razor difficult.

Depilatories are a third method of surgical site hair removal. They are not often used in veterinary medicine, however, as long hair must first be clipped short so the depilatory cream can reach the skin surface. Skin irritation is another problem with depilatory use.

Regardless of the technique used, hair must be removed not only from the surgical site itself, but also from the area around it. This is necessary to prevent contamination from surrounding hair. Also, it prevents delays if, during surgery, the incision must be extended beyond the anticipated boundaries. The amount of hair to be removed depends on the location of the surgical site and the preferences of the surgeon. In general, the hair should be clipped at least 4 inches beyond the surgical site in all directions.

Preoperative Scrub

After the hair is removed from the surgical site, numbers of microorganisms on the patient's skin surface can be reduced with a surgical scrub very similar to that used on the hands and arms of operative personnel. Scrub soaps used are similar to those used for hand scrubbing. Povidone-iodine and chlorhexidine preparations are most commonly used. One difference from the operative personnel scrub is that a scrub brush is not used, as this would be too harsh and irritating to the patient's skin. Cotton or gauze sponges that have been sterilized or soaked in disinfectant solution or scrub soap are usually used.

The first step in the scrubbing process is usually a general wash of the clipped area with surgical scrub soap to remove any gross dirt or debris. This is followed by at least 3 surgical scrubs of the clipped area. Starting in the center of the clipped area, the incision site is thoroughly scrubbed. The scrub is then worked outward (peripherally) from the incision site in a spiral pattern, never going back over an area once it has been scrubbed. At the completion of each scrub, the scrub soap is removed from the skin with running water or sterile cotton or gauze sponges, starting over the incision site and working peripherally, and the scrub is repeated. After the last scrub, antiseptics, such as alcohol and/or povidone-iodine solution, may be sprayed or swabbed on the site.

If the patient has been prepared in another room, the patient must be very carefully transported into the surgery room, with care taken not to contaminate the freshly prepared surgery site. If the surgical site becomes contaminated, the scrubs must be repeated.

Draping

The purpose of surgical drapes is to protect exposed tissues from contamination from the surrounding skin during the surgical procedure. An attempt is generally made to cover as much of the patient as possible, leaving only the surgical site exposed.

Drapes can be made from a variety of materials, such as cloth, paper, plastic and a paper-plastic combination. They can be folded, wrapped and autoclaved, or they can be purchased prewrapped and presterilized. Drapes can be intact, in which case an aperture must be cut in the drape to expose the surgical site, or they may be "fenestrated," with built-in apertures of various sizes and shapes.

During surgery, the drapes must be protected from contact with anything that is nonsterile. With cloth and paper drapes, "strike-through" can be a potential source of contamination. If the underside of a drape (side adjacent to the patient), in contact with a contaminated area, becomes wet with saline, blood or other fluids, capillary action can draw microorganisms to the outer sterile surface, resulting in contamination. With single-layer cloth and paper drapes, a wet drape is considered contaminated. This strike-through effect can be combatted through use of multiple layers of drapes and/or use of plastic or paper-plastic combination drapes that are impervious to moisture.

Preparation of the Surgical Environment

The beneficial effects of careful preparation of the patient and operative personnel, instruments and equipment can be negated by a contaminated surgical environment. This is more likely to be the case with large animal surgery performed in the field, but poorly maintained hospital facilities can also be a significant source of contamination.

Surgery in the Field

While there is less control over the surgical environment with surgery performed in the field, it is still usually possible to take steps to minimize the risk of contamination. If possible, choose an area that is clean, and free of dust, wind and insects. Outdoors on a warm, sunny day without wind or insects is best. If surgery is to be performed in a barn, have any necessary clean bedding spread in the area as far in advance as possible to give dust a chance to settle. If there are lofts above the surgery area, people should be kept out of them so that dust and debris are not stirred up. In general, do the best job you can in preparing the surgical environment under the prevailing conditions.

Surgery in the Operating Room

To be an appropriate surgical environment, the surgery room/area in a veterinary hospital must be properly cared for. The room should be kept neat, spotlessly clean, and free of any unneeded equipment that could collect dust and increase the risk of contamination. Traffic through the surgery room should be kept to a minimum, even when surgery is not in progress. The room should be cleaned daily and weekly.

Daily cleaning should include the floors and all operating room equipment. The floor should be cleaned and disinfected with a *clean* mop or wet vacuum. Tables, lights, counters and other operating room equipment should be cleaned and wiped with disinfectant solution.

In addition to the normal daily cleaning, the operating room should receive a more thorough cleaning weekly. All interior surfaces, including the ceiling, walls, cabinets and ventilator grills, should be cleaned and disinfected.

Disinfectants used in the operating room should meet several criteria. They should be effective against a wide spectrum of microorganisms, relatively nontoxic, noncorrosive to stainless steel, plastic, etc, and reasonably economical. Disinfectant concentrates must be properly diluted, stored and used to ensure their effectiveness.

Surgery Room Conduct

Microorganisms are present everywhere in the surgery room, except on items that have been sterilized. Unfortunately, sterile instruments and equipment do not look any different from items that are nonsterile. The only way to be sure that sterile areas do not become contaminated is to observe strict rules of behavior and activity in the surgery room.

There are 2 basic "zones" or work areas within the surgery room: the "sterile zone" and the "dirty zone."

Sterile Zone

The *sterile zone* is the work area for scrubbed personnel. It includes the surgery site itself, the front of gloved and gowned personnel from the waist to the shoulders, all sterile fields, and the air spaces above the sterile fields. Sterile fields are surfaces covered by sterile drapes, wraps or covers. For example, the draped area of the patient is a sterile field, as is the instrument table covered by the sterile wrap of the instrument pack. The air spaces above the sterile fields are particularly easy for nonscrubbed personnel to violate if they are careless. The risk of contamination from microorganisms falling onto sterile surfaces by gravity is quite high, so it is important that nonscrubbed personnel stay well back from the sterile zone.

Dirty Zone

The *dirty zone* surrounds the sterile zone and is the work area for the nonscrubbed personnel. Everything in this zone is dirty (nonsterile), including anesthesia machines, intravenous fluid administration equipment, and unopened surgical and suture material packs. Items in this zone should be touched only by nonscrubbed personnel.

Rules for Scrubbed Personnel

- *Know what is sterile and what is not.* This is fundamental to maintaining an uncontaminated surgical field.
- *Keep movement and conversation to a minimum.* Movement in the surgery room increases the risk of contamination through accidentally touching something outside the sterile zone. It also sets up air currents that can carry microorganisms onto sterile fields. Excessive conversation, in addition to being

distracting, can accelerate moistening of the surgical mask, which decreases its filtering capacity.

- *Always face toward sterile fields.* It is important to always know where one is with respect to sterile fields. The front of the gown is sterile, but the back is not. If you turn your back on a sterile field, the nonsterile back of the gown could accidentally touch some part of a sterile field.
- *Do not touch anything that is not sterile with your gloved hands or any sterile part of your gown.*
- *Keep your hands elevated between waist and shoulder level.* Raising your hands up above your shoulders or lowering them below waist level increases the risk of inadvertent contamination by contact with a nonsterile item, such as a surgery light or nonsterile part of your gown. To decrease the risk of your gloved hands accidentally contacting something that is contaminated, clasp your hands in front of your body at chest level when not otherwise occupied (Fig 47).
- *Keep surgical instruments at or above the level of the surgery table.* The risk of instrument contamination increases greatly if instruments are allowed to fall below table level.
- *Pass others back to back.* The sterile fronts of scrubbed personnel must be protected from contamination when passing others in the close confines of the surgery room. If incidental contact is made between the backs of people passing each other, no harm is done, as the backs of both scrubbed and nonscrubbed personnel are nonsterile.

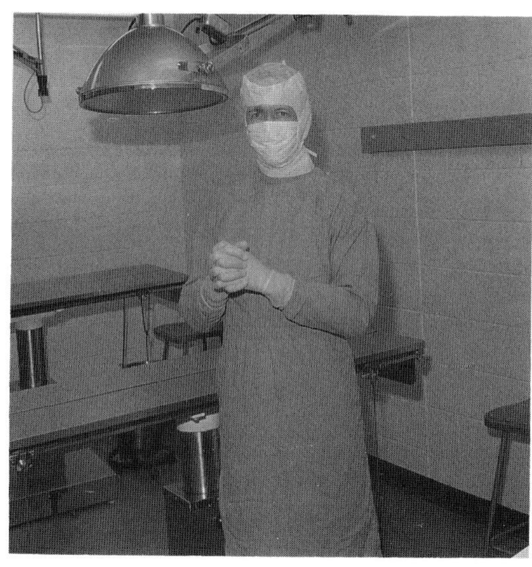

Figure 47. Gowned person with the hands clasped in front of the body and held between the waist and shoulders.

Rules for Nonscrubbed Personnel

- *Know what is sterile and what is not.*
- *Keep movement and conversation to a minimum.*
- *Always face toward sterile fields.* Both scrubbed and nonscrubbed personnel must always know where they are with respect to sterile fields. By always facing towards them, the chance of a nonscrubbed person accidentally contaminating a sterile field is considerably reduced.
- *Do not touch anything that is sterile.*
- *Always yield the right-of-way to scrubbed personnel.* Scrubbed personnel have less freedom of movement than nonscrubbed personnel, as they must protect their gloves and the sterile parts of their gown. They are also usually concentrating on the surgical procedure and may not be aware of the positions of others around them. Nonscrubbed personnel must, therefore, constantly be alert to movements of scrubbed personnel so as to stay out of their way and avoid contact.
- *Never pass between scrubbed personnel and the patient.* For this to happen, a nonscrubbed person would have entered the sterile zone or a scrubbed person would have left it. In either case, the risk of contamination is high.
- *Do not reach or lean over sterile fields.* This would violate the sterile fields and greatly increase the risk of contamination.
- *Open sterile packs aseptically.* Surgical packs should be opened by touching only the outside of the wrap and the corners, and by reaching around, rather than over, the pack as it is opened.

Suturing and Suture Materials

Suturing is the most commonly used method of surgical wound closure. It involves passage of thread-like suture material through the tissues of the patient using a suture needle. The suture material is then used to pull the wound edges together, and a knot is tied to hold everything in place. The characteristics of the animal and the surgery, the tissues being manipulated, and the surgeon's preference determine the type of suture material, suture needle, suture pattern and knot-tying technique used.

Desirable Suture Characteristics

Uniform in Size with High Tensile Strength: In the same sense that a chain is only as strong as its weakest link, suture material is only as strong as its narrowest, weakest segment. If it is uniform in size, its strength is also uniform.

Tensile strength is the resistance to tension applied linearly or lengthwise. Because most of the tension on suture material holding surgical wounds closed is linear tension, high tensile strength allows smaller-diameter suture material sizes to be used.

No Capillary Action: Suture materials that conduct fluids by capillary action can "wick" fluids, and whatever they contain, from one area/level of a surgical wound to another. More important, such porous suture materials can conduct bacterial, along with the fluid, from one level of a healing wound to another, setting up new areas of infection.

Capillary action is particularly significant when part of each suture is in contact with an area that is contaminated. For example, a porous skin suture that extends from the skin surface, with its resident population of microorganisms, could conduct bacteria from the skin surface down into the subcutaneous area.

Completely Absorbable or Inert: Ideally, once a suture material has done its job and the wound has gained sufficient strength to stay closed on its own, the suture material should be completely absorbed by the body, leaving no foreign material in the wound to promote a continued inflammatory response and slow healing.

If the suture material is not absorbed, the next best thing is for it to be completely inert and nonreactive in the body. That is, the body does not react to it and "ignores" it. The suture material should not greatly irritate the body tissues, provoking a massive foreign body inflammatory response.

Easy to Handle: The suture material should be pliable and easy to handle and tie in knots. This is particularly important with the slight loss of tactile sensation caused by surgical gloves.

Excellent Knot-Holding Characteristics: When knots are tied with suture material, there should be sufficient friction for the knot to hold securely. Without this characteristic, knots can untie and potentially cause surgical wound dehiscence.

Unfortunately, no single suture material has all of these desirable characteristics. Each has advantages and disadvantages that must be considered in determining the most appropriate suture material to use for a particular application.

Suture Sizes

Suture size refers to the diameter of the material. With the exception of wire, suture diameter is expressed in numeric units that are unique to sutures. Smaller suture sizes are expressed in "0" sizes. The more 0s (or the larger the number in front of the 0) the smaller the suture material. For example, 2-0 is larger than 6-0 material. The same size of suture material might be written as 00, or 2-0 or 2/0. Suture sizes greater than size 0 are expressed as numbers. The larger the number, the larger the diameter of the suture material. For example, #4 is larger than #2 material (Table 2).

Table 2. Except for surgical wire, suture material sizes are expressed in numeric units.

		← smaller					larger →		
. . .	0000	000	00	0	1	2	3	4	. . .

The unit of measure for the size of wire sutures is *gauge* (abbreviated as ga). In a similar fashion to the gauge sizes of hypodermic needles, the sizes are inversely proportional to the gauge. That is, the higher the number, the thinner the wire. For example, 25-ga wire is smaller than 20-ga wire (Table 3).

Table 3. The diameter of surgical wire is expressed as gauge.

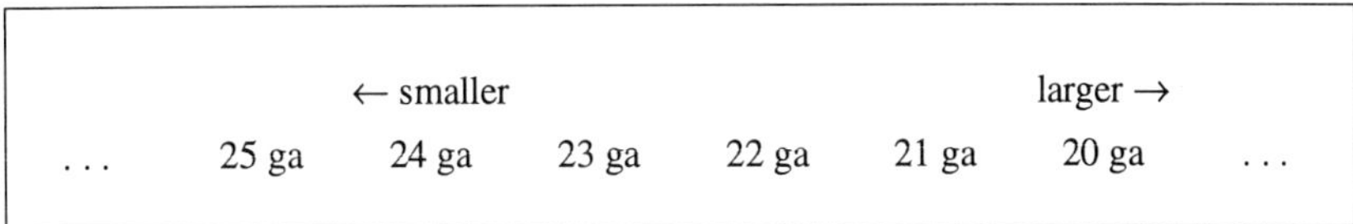

		← smaller				larger →	
. . .	25 ga	24 ga	23 ga	22 ga	21 ga	20 ga	. . .

Suture Terminology

An *absorbable suture* is one that is "digested" or broken down and absorbed by the body. As it is being broken down, it loses tensile strength. Generally, absorbable sutures should be used in tissues that heal rapidly. Surgical gut is an absorbable suture.

A *nonabsorbable suture,* as its name implies, is not broken down by the body. Unless removed, nonabsorbable sutures remain in the body and retain their tensile strength. They are often used in tissues that heal slowly. Nylon and stainless steel are nonabsorbable.

Braided suture is made up of many small filaments that are braided or twisted together. Most braided sutures conduct fluid, and potentially bacteria, by capillary action. They generally should not be used when part of the suture is exposed to contamination, as in the skin.

Monofilament suture is composed of a single fiber, similar to fishing line. Their very smooth surface allows monofilament sutures to pass through tissues easily, but also results in poor knot-holding characteristics. Several throws are often necessary to secure knots tied in monofilament suture material.

A *natural suture* is one that is derived from a natural source. Cotton, silk and surgical gut are all natural fiber sutures.

A *synthetic suture* is man-made. Synthetic sutures are often similar to, and derived from, natural fibers. Polyglactic is a synthetic suture.

Absorbable Sutures

The only commonly used absorbable suture that is from a natural source is *surgical gut.* Sometimes referred to as *catgut,* surgical gut is derived from the submucosa of sheep intestines. It is, therefore, made up largely of collagen. Two common forms of surgical gut are *plain gut,* which dissolves fairly quickly (approximately 10 days), and *chromic gut,* which, because of its treatment with chromic acid, dissolves more slowly (20-40 days). Surgical gut is inexpensive, but is not very uniform in diameter or strength, causes an inflammatory reaction, is capillary and supports bacterial growth.

Newer synthetic absorbable sutures are more expensive than surgical gut but are more uniform in diameter and strength, cause less of an inflammatory reaction, and are absorbed more slowly. Braided forms are capillary, and some very smooth sutures have poor knot-holding characteristics. Examples include polyglycolic acid (Dexon: Davis & Geck), polyglyconate (Maxon: Davis & Geck), and polyglactin (Vicryl: Ethicon).

Nonabsorbable Sutures

Nonabsorbable sutures can be divided into 3 general categories: metal sutures, natural fibers and synthetic fibers.

The only commonly used metal suture is *stainless steel,* which is available in monofilament (wire) or braided form. Stainless steel is inert and has a very high tensile strength. It is somewhat stiff and difficult to handle, however, and it takes practice to tie good square knots with it. The sharp cut ends of the suture can be irritating to the surrounding tissues. Stainless steel is becoming more commonly used in the form of surgical clips and staples.

The most common nonabsorbable natural fibers are *silk* and *cotton.* Silk is relatively inexpensive and easy to handle, and has a high tensile strength. It is, however, capillary, can cause a severe inflammatory response, and can support bacterial growth. Cotton suture is similar to silk, but its tensile strength increases when it becomes wet.

Various synthetic nonabsorbable sutures are used in surgery. Monofilament sutures, such as *polypropylene* (Prolene: Ethicon), are inert, strong and noncapillary, but they can be difficult to handle and tie because of their tendency to kink, and their very smooth surface. Braided *polyester fibers* are inert and strong, but they are expensive and some have poor knot-holding characteristics. Polyester fiber sutures can be uncoated (Mersilene: Ethicon), or may have a smooth coating of material, such as Teflon (Polydek: Deknatel). *Polymerized caprolactam* (Vetafil: Braun) is a braided synthetic fiber covered with a smooth plastic like coating. Because of its tendency to act as a nidus for infection if it becomes contaminated, it is rarely "buried" in deep tissues. It is used mainly for skin closure.

Criteria for Suture Material Selection

Because there is no such thing as a "perfect" suture material that has all of the desirable characteristics listed earlier, suture material must be selected on the basis of the requirements of each unique surgical procedure and patient. Four main criteria can be used in the selection process:

Healing Potential of the Tissue Being Sutured: Slow-healing tissues should be sutured with nonabsorbable suture material so strength is maintained during healing. If the tissue is expected to heal rapidly, absorbable sutures can probably be safely used.

Presence of Contamination or Infection: If contamination or infection is suspected, potentially capillary suture materials should be avoided. Monofilament sutures are a much safer choice.

Importance of Cosmetic Results: If the appearance of the healed skin incision is an important consideration, small-diameter, inert suture material should be used to close the skin so as to minimize scarring.

Strength Requirements: The suture material should be able to withstand the stresses encountered in the area being sutured during the healing process. The size and strength of the suture material must be appropriate for the animal, the tissue(s) being sutured, and the location of the incision.

Suture Needles

Desirable Characteristics

- *Should pass through tissues easily.*
- *Should create a hole approximately the same size as the attached suture material.*

Ideally, the "tunnel" made through tissues by the needle should be the same size and shape as the attached suture material. An overly large tunnel causes excessive tissue trauma and inflammation, and creates the opportunity for increased seepage of fluids, which can increase the risk of contamination.

Attachment of Suture Material

Eyed needles have various kinds of "eyes" through which suture material can be threaded for attachment. They can be cleaned, resterilized and reused if they have not been broken or dulled. Generally, suture material should be threaded through the eye of a suture needle only once so as to minimize the size of the tissue defect created when the needle is passed through the tissue, rather than taking several loops of material through the needle's eye.

Swaged needles have the suture material permanently attached and are intended for single use only (Fig 48). The suture material is attached at the factory by crimping the hollow end of the needle around the suture strand, which has been inserted into it. Swaged needles are very atraumatic to tissues because there is no "lump" or loop of attached suture material that must be pulled through the tunnel.

Shape

Suture needles come in a variety of shapes, but the 3 most frequently used in veterinary practice are straight, half-curved and curved (Fig 48).

Figure 48. Types of suture needles and points.

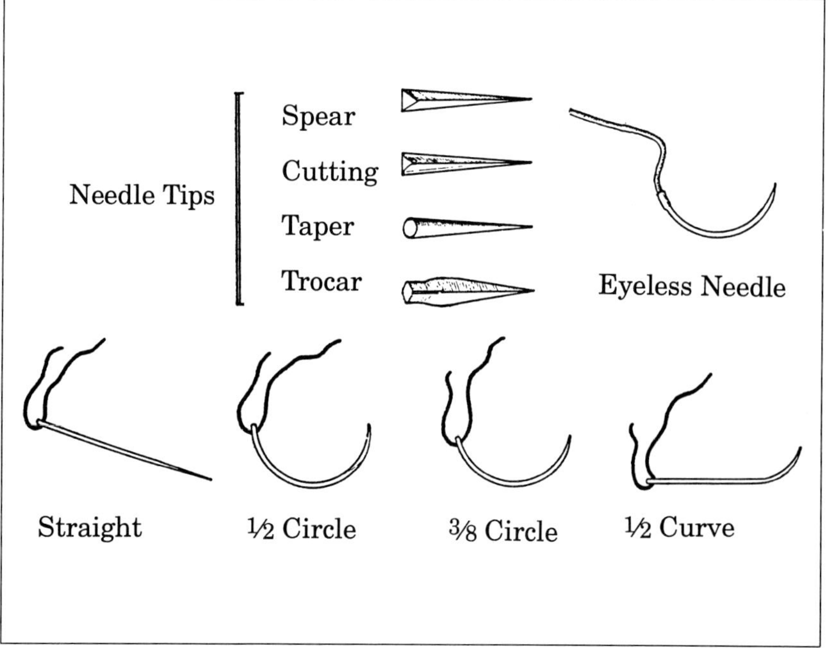

Straight needles resemble straight sewing needles (Fig 48). They are generally used when the attached suture material must be passed straight through a structure from one side to the other.

Half-curved needles are sometimes referred to as "ski" needles because their tip is curved up like a ski tip (Fig 48). They are not very commonly used.

Curved needles are most commonly used for suturing (Fig 48). They are named according to the portion of a circle they represent. Superficial wounds are often sutured with 3/8-circle needles. Deeper suturing usually requires 1/2- or 5/8-circle needles.

Point

Despite the variety of suture needle points available, most surgeons use needles with a tapered point or a cutting point.

A *tapered point* is rounded like that of a standard sewing needle (Fig 48). Taper-point needles are used for relatively soft tissues that are easily penetrated, such as abdominal organs, fat and muscle.

A *cutting* needle has a triangular tip with sharp edges (Fig 49). As its name implies, this type of needle *cuts* a hole through the tissues. Cutting needles are used for relatively tough tissues. The tip of a curved needle with a *standard cutting point* is triangular, with the triangle's apex forming the cutting edge along the concave surface of the needle (Fig 49). Standard cutting-point needles are commonly used to suture the skin. The tip of a curved *reverse cutting*

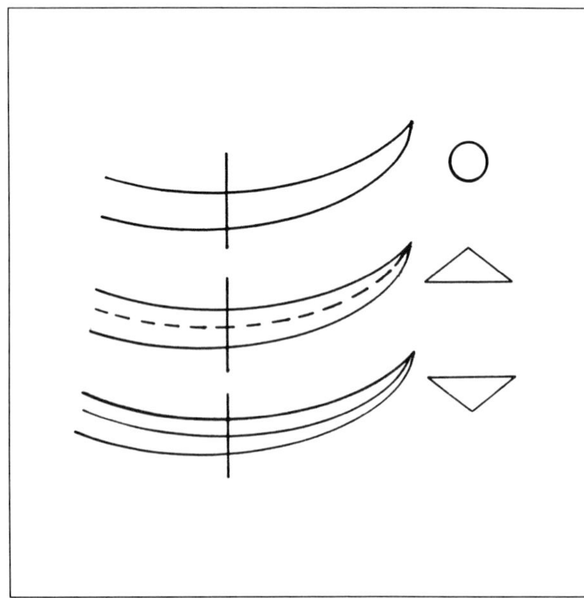

Figure 49. Types of suture needle points: tapered (top), standard cutting (center) and reverse cutting (bottom), with their respective cross sections shown at the right. (Adapted from Bellenger CR, in *Compend Cont Ed* 4:587, 1982. Courtesy of Veterinary Learning Systems)

needle is also shaped like a triangle, but the triangle's apex forms the cutting edge along the convex surface of the needle (Fig 49). Reverse cutting needles are commonly used to suture tendons and ligaments.

Surgical Knot Tying

Knots tied in suture material must be secure. Sutures are often all that holds surgical wounds together during the initial healing process. Untying of suture knots can lead to wound dehiscence.

Sutures should not, however, be tied very tightly. Excessively tight sutures can interfere with the blood supply to healing wound edges, and may even cut through tissue edges (Fig 51). Generally, knots should be tied only tight enough to bring the wound edges together.

With very few exceptions square knots should be used to tie sutures (Fig 50). Square knots have much less tendency to slip and untie than do other types of knots, such as granny knots (Fig 50). Suture knots are usually tied by hand or with the aid of a needle holder.

Numerous techniques are used for tying knots by hand. Most feel somewhat clumsy when first learned, but, with practice, knots can be tied very rapidly by hand. One disadvantage of hand ties is

Figure 50. Suture knots: 1. first tie. 2. square knot. 3. surgeon's knot. 4. triple surgeon's knot. 5. granny knot. 6. half hitch.

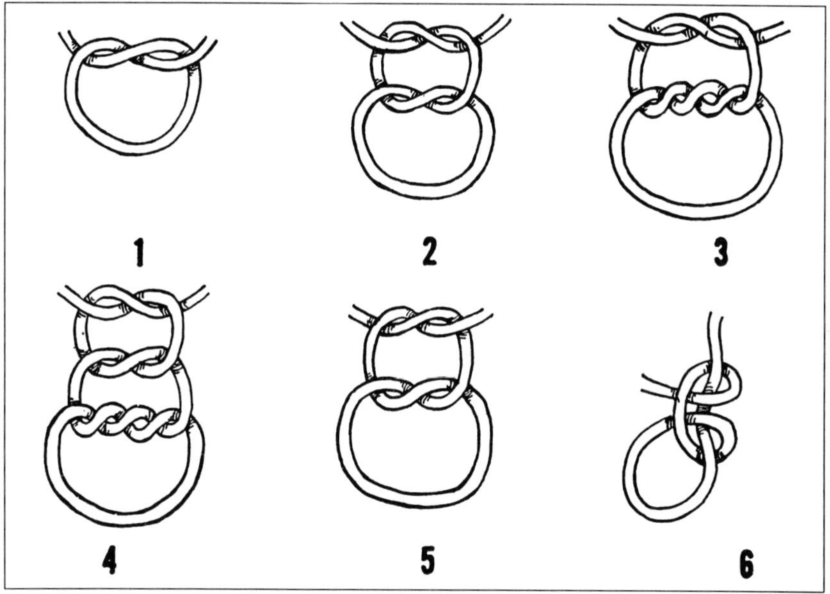

the relatively large amount of suture material that is cut off and discarded when the knot is completed.

The instrument tie usually uses a needle holder to help tie the knot. Once the needle has been passed through the tissue and the suture material has been pulled through, leaving a short strand, the long strand of the suture material (the strand with the needle attached) is looped around the needle holder, and the other, short strand, of the suture is grasped with the needle holder and pulled through. The second throw of the knot is done in a similar manner. A square knot is created if the needle holder starts either between the 2 strands or outside the 2 strands for both throws. An undesirable granny knot will result if the needle holder starts between the strands for one throw and outside the strands for the other (Fig 50).

With very smooth suture materials, such as monofilament nylon, more than 2 throws may be necessary to produce a secure knot (Figs 50, 51).

Suture Patterns

Suture patterns are the specific types "stitches" used to hold the edges of a wound together. Numerous suture patterns may be used. Which one to use in a particular situation is usually determined by

Figure 51. A. Overly tight sutures can cut through incision edges. B. With very smooth suture material, failure to tie at least 3 square knots may result in suture untying. C. If the knot holding a continuous suture becomes untied, the entire suture line may open. D. If a knot in an interrupted pattern becomes untied, only that knot is affected.

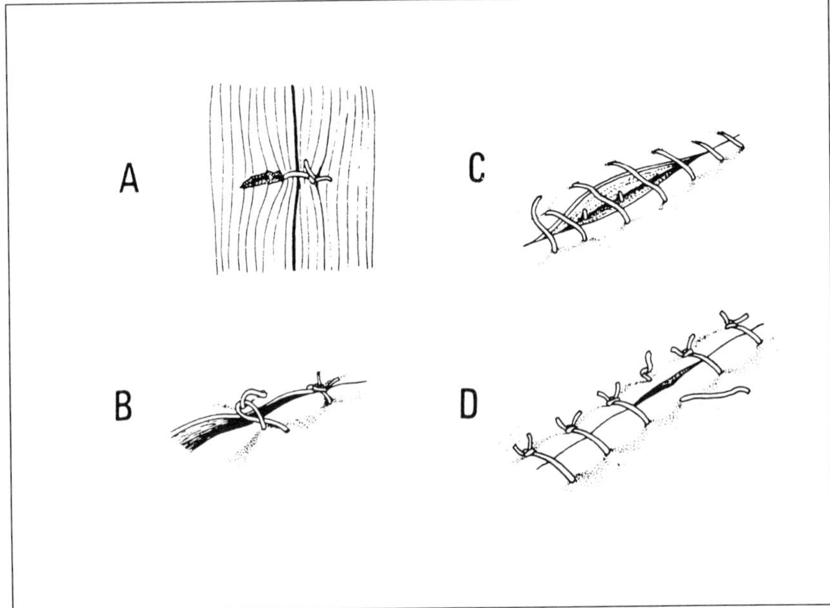

the characteristics of the organ or tissue being sutured, and the amount of tension pulling the wound apart.

Suture patterns may be placed in either a continuous or interrupted fashion. *Continuous suture patterns* are "running" stitches. The suture is tied only at the 2 ends. If either of the knots should come untied, the whole suture line will come apart. *Interrupted suture patterns* involve tying each suture individually as it is placed. Interrupted patterns are more time consuming to place, but provide more security because multiple knots are holding the wound closed.

In general, suture patterns may *appose* the wound edges (bring them together so they touch), *evert* the wound edges (turn them outward) or *invert* the wound edges (turn them inward) (Fig 52).

Appositional Suture Patterns

The *simple* suture pattern, which brings the wound edges into apposition, is very commonly used in a variety of tissues and situations. It is used internally to suture muscle and connective tissue,

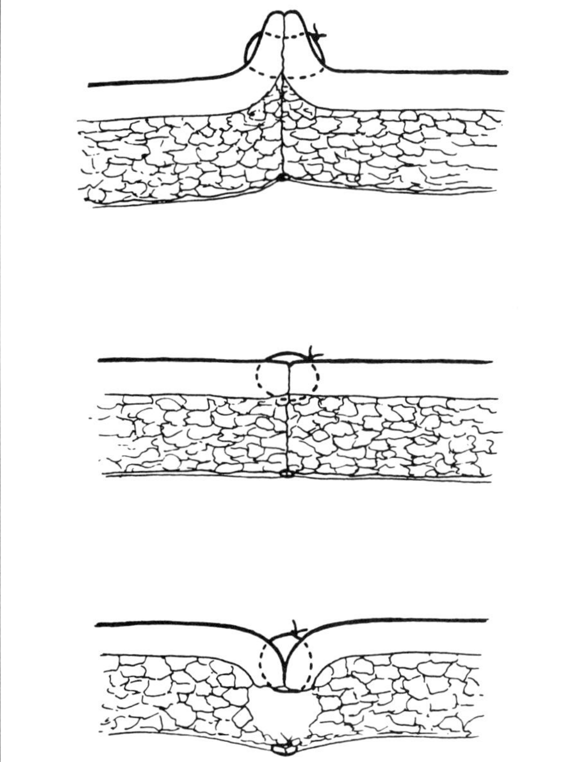

Figure 52. Everting sutures (top) are often used where tension tends to pull the wound edges apart. Appositional sutures (center) bring the wound edges precisely together. Inverting sutures (bottom) are used to close internal organs and should not be used in the skin, as they create dead space, result in excessive exudation and delay healing.

and is used externally to suture the skin. Though skin sutures are often placed as a simple interrupted pattern (Fig 53), a simple continuous pattern (Fig 54) is also used on occasion.

The simple pattern is placed by passing the suture needle into the tissue on one side of the wound, crossing the wound beneath the surface, and coming back out on the other side of the wound. This is referred to as taking a "bite" across the wound.

Everting Suture Patterns

Everting suture patterns are usually used only in the skin when excessive tension is pulling the wound edges apart. If pulled too

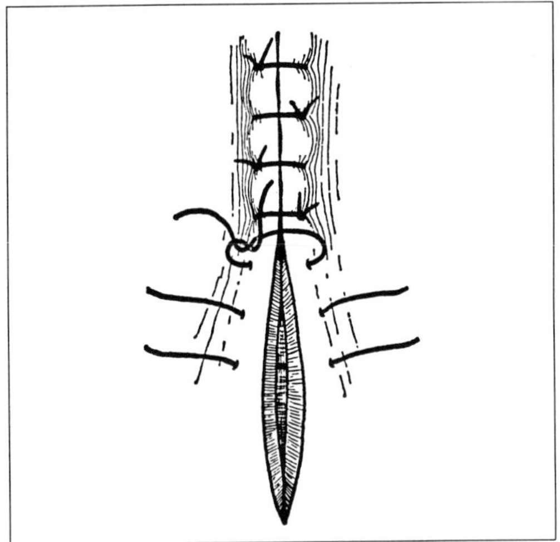

Figure 53. Simple interrupted suture pattern.

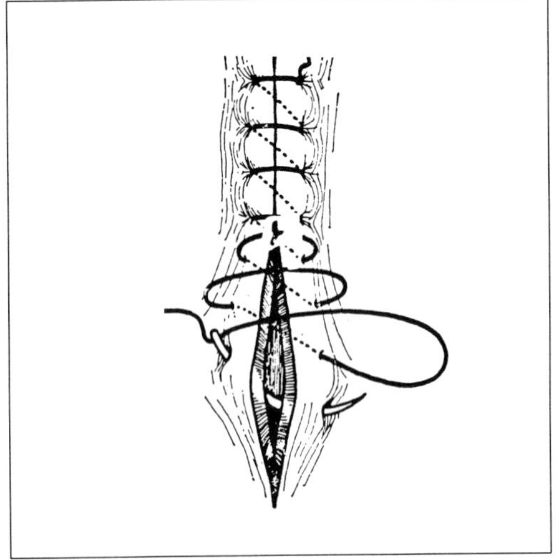

Figure 54. Simple continuous suture pattern.

tight, everting suture patterns cause the wound edges to evert. They are usually pulled just tight enough to bring the edges together (Fig 52).

The 2 most commonly used everting suture patterns are both "mattress" patterns. The *vertical mattress* pattern (Fig 55) is started by taking a large, deep bite with the needle across the wound. The needle is then reversed and a smaller, more shallow bite is taken inside the first. The *horizontal mattress* pattern (Fig 56) is similar except the 2 bites are side by side. After the first bite is taken across the incision, the needle is reversed and a second bite is taken beside the first.

Inverting Suture Patterns

Inverting patterns are used internally to close and seal wounds in hollow internal organs, such as the stomach, uterus or urinary

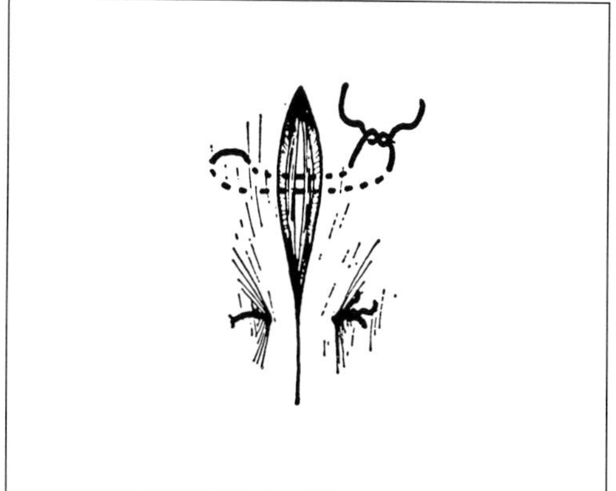

Figure 55. Vertical mattress suture pattern.

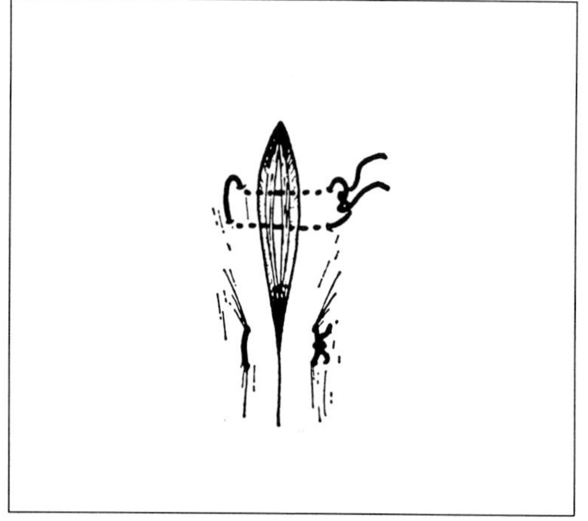

Figure 56. Horizontal mattress suture pattern.

bladder. As they are pulled tight, they invert the wound edges, forming a tight seal that helps prevent leakage. The most commonly used inverting suture patterns are the Lembert, Cushing and Connell patterns.

The *Lembert* suture pattern (Fig 57) is begun by taking a bite on one side of the wound that is perpendicular to the wound edge. The needle is then passed over the wound and a second bite is taken on the other side of the wound in line with the first bite. When the suture is tied, the wound edges invert.

The *Cushing* (Fig 58) and *Connell* (Fig 59) patterns are identical, except for the depth of each bite. The Cushing pattern passes down only to the depth of the submucosal layer of the organ. The Connell pattern passes completely into the lumen of the organ. They are otherwise placed in an identical manner. The first bite is taken on one side of the wound parallel to the wound edge. The needle is then passed over the wound, reversed, and a second bite is taken parallel to the first, in a reverse direction. When the suture is tied, the wound edges invert.

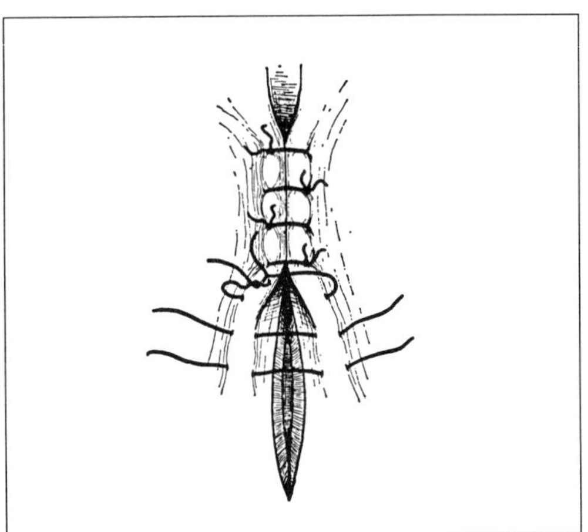

Figure 57. Lembert sutures are used to invert the edges of a wound.

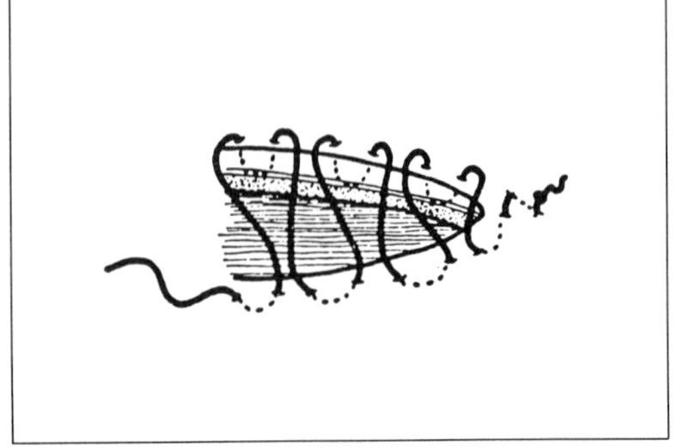

Figure 58. The Cushing suture passes only to the depth of the submucosa of a hollow organ.

Removing Skin Sutures

Skin incisions are usually closed with nonabsorbable suture material in an effort to make the outside of the incision as secure and, in some cases, esthetically appealing as possible. Because they do not dissolve on their own, these nonabsorbable sutures must be removed after an appropriate healing period (usually 7-10 days).

Proper skin suture removal is begun by grasping one or both of the ends of the suture, which were deliberately left long for that purpose, and pulling the knot away from the skin (Fig 60). Using suture removal scissors, 1 of the 2 strands of the suture beneath the knot is cut in an area that was previously beneath the skin surface, and the suture is pulled out. It is important that only one of the strands is cut so as to avoid leaving some of the suture material buried beneath the skin, where it could act as a foreign-body irritant.

Hemostasis

Hemorrhage is the escape of blood from damaged blood vessels. Its significance can range from annoying to life-threatening.

Hemostasis is the stopping of hemorrhage. The body has natural mechanisms for controlling hemorrhage, but artificial means of hemostasis often must be employed during surgical procedures.

Significance of Hemorrhage

Profuse hemorrhage can cause shock, a complex syndrome resulting from inadequate blood flow to body tissues. The inadequate blood supply can lead to generalized hypoxia and cell death, and ultimately to death of the animal.

Even hemorrhage that is not severe enough to cause shock can cause problems during and after surgery. Moderate hemorrhage can cause tissue/organ hypoxia severe enough to stress the animal and diminish normal body functions. Marginal hypoxia can also impede normal wound healing, as can hemorrhage into a wound

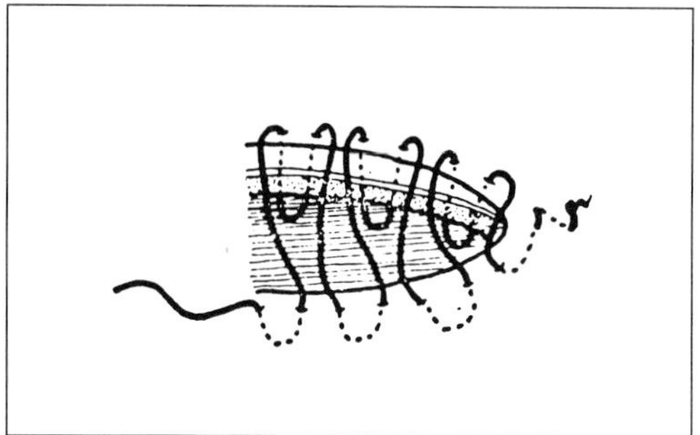

Figure 59. The Connell suture is the same as the Cushing suture, but it penetrates into the lumen of the hollow organ.

space that prevents wound edges from being brought together. Blood can obscure the surgical field and make instruments and gloves sticky. It can also wet the surgical drapes, increasing the chance of contamination. Blood is also an excellent growth medium for bacteria, which can result in problems with infection during the postoperative period.

Sources of Hemorrhage

Arteries: Blood from arterial hemorrhage is bright, cherry red and spurts rhythmically under considerable pressure. Hemorrhage from even a small to moderate-sized artery can result in considerable blood loss in a relatively short time.

Veins: Blood from venous hemorrhage is dark red and flows freely without spurts and without much pressure. Large amounts of blood can also be lost fairly quickly with venous hemorrhage.

Capillaries: Blood capillary hemorrhage oozes under very low pressure. Unless extensive, capillary hemorrhage is rarely life threatening.

Natural Hemostasis

Natural hemostasis is accomplished in the body by the initial vasospasm that occurs after an injury, and the blood clotting process.

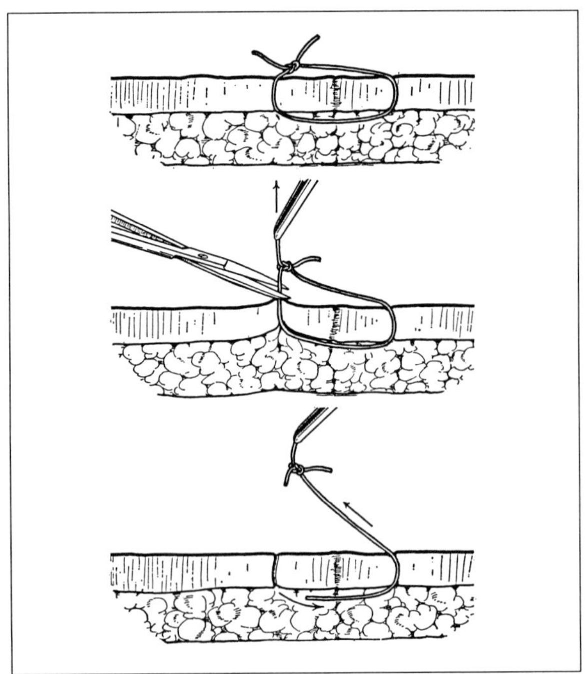

Figure 60. Proper method of removing a skin suture.

As long as blood vessel damage is not too severe or widespread, these natural hemostatic mechanisms are usually sufficient to avoid serious consequences.

When hemorrhage is severe and/or widespread, however, artificial means of hemostasis must be employed.

Methods of Hemostasis

Pressure: Pressure is a simple and often very effective method of hemostasis. It may take the form of direct digital pressure, material packed into a cavity, or a pressure bandage. Pressure is effective for relatively minor hemorrhage, and as a temporary measure for controlling more serious hemorrhage.

Crushing: Crushing with hemostatic forceps can be effective in stopping hemorrhage from relatively small, noncritical blood vessels. The vessel should be crushed using the tip of the hemostat, including as little surrounding tissue as possible.

Ligation: Ligation involves tying off the end of a hemorrhaging blood vessel with suture material, or applying a metal clip. Frequently a hemostat is applied to the end of the vessel, the vessel is ligated proximal to the instrument, and the instrument is then removed. Ligation can be effective for blood vessels of nearly any size.

Twisting: Hemostasis by twisting is accomplished by grasping a blood vessel with the tip of a hemostat and twisting the vessel before releasing the forceps. Twisting is usually effective for small blood vessels only.

Suturing: Defects in large blood vessels can sometimes be directly sutured. Suturing of tissue defects can produce hemostasis by bringing wound edges together.

Tourniquet: Tourniquets are useful to help control hemorrhage from extremities for short periods. For arterial hemorrhage, the tourniquet should be placed proximal to the site of the hemorrhage. If the hemorrhage is primarily venous in origin, the tourniquet is only effective if placed distal to the site of the bleeding.

Electrocautery: Electrocautery is accomplished using a high-frequency electric current to coagulate blood. The process causes some minor burning, which can delay healing. If proper techniques are used, however, the benefit of effective hemostasis outweighs the disadvantage of minor burning.

Topical Coagulants: Topical hemostatic substances, such as silver nitrate and alum, can be used to help stop minor superficial hemorrhage. They are irritating, so their use is confined to temporary application to surface areas of the body only.

Absorbable Coagulants: Absorbable hemostatic substances are used internally. They provide a porous surface on which a clot can form, and are then gradually absorbed by the body. Examples include gelatin sponge (Gelfoam: Upjohn) and cellulose products (Surgicel: Johnson & Johnson).

Recommended Reading

Bojrab MJ: Pre- and post-operative evaluation of the surgical patient. *Proc 15th Sem Vet Tech,* 1986.

Colville TP: Surgical sutures and needles. *Proc 15th Sem Vet Tech,* 1986.

Colville TP: The veterinary technician's guide to surgery room conduct. *Vet Technician* 7:392-396, 1986.

Heath MM: Scrubbing procedures and surgical attire. *Vet Technician* 13:345-350, 1988.

Johnston DE, in: *Nursing Care in Veterinary Practice.* Veterinary Learning Systems, Trenton, NJ, 1993.

Kagan KG: Aseptic technique. *Vet Technician* 13:205-211, 1992.

Kagan KG: Care and sterilization of surgical equipment. *Vet Technician* 13:65-80, 1992.

Knecht CD *et al: Fundamental Techniques in Veterinary Surgery.* 3rd ed. Saunders, Philadelphia, 1987.

McCurnin DM: *Clinical Textbook for Veterinary Technicians.* 2nd ed. Saunders, Philadelphia, 1990.

McCurnin DM: Surgical hemostasis. *Proc 15th Sem Vet Tech,* 1986.

Stoeberl T: Preparing the small animal patient for surgery. Anim Hlth Technician 4:271-277, 1983.

The Care and Handling of Surgical Instruments. Codman & Shurtleff, Randolph, MA, 1977.

Tracy DL and Warren RG: *Small Animal Surgical Nursing.* Mosby, St. Louis, 1983.

Notes

10

Theriogenology

S.D. Van Camp and A.R. Abdullahi

Theriogenology is the official term for veterinary obstetrics and gynecology. This name was derived from 2 Greek terms: *therio*, which means animal or beast, and *gen*, which means coming into being. The suffix *-ology*, which means the study of, was then added. Thus, theriogenology encompasses the body of knowledge that can influence *the number of animals that come into being*.

To understand theriogenology, one must understand reproductive physiology and how it is affected by management, environment, nutrition and drugs.

NORMAL REPRODUCTIVE PHYSIOLOGY

Nonpregnant Animals

Unlike women and other female primates that have *menstrual cycles*, with variable levels of sexual receptivity, the mammals that we deal with commonly in veterinary medicine have an *estrous cycle*, in which the period of sexual receptivity, *estrus*, is concentrated during a short period lasting one to several days. During the rest of the estrous cycle, the female does not accept the male's advances nor allow mating.

The *estrous cycle* is made up of 4 or 5 stages, depending on the species and whether the animal is *polyestrous* (cycles repeatedly) or *monestrous* (cycles only once during the breeding season). These estrous cycle states are:

Anestrus

This is the period of ovarian inactivity, with no behavioral signs of heat or estrus.

Proestrus

Under the influence of gonadotropin-releasing hormone (GnRH) from the hypothalamus, follicle-stimulating hormone (FSH) from the pituitary causes initial follicle development on the ovary. These growing follicles produce estrogen, which causes the genital and behavioral changes that attract the male and prepare the female's reproductive tract for mating. The proestrous female dog does not allow mating.

Estrus

This is the period of true heat, during which the female allows mating. Serum estrogen levels peak early in estrus and cause the pituitary to release luteinizing hormone (LH), which causes maturation of follicles and results in release of the egg(s) at ovulation.

Metestrus

This is a short stage during which the female may still attract males but no longer allows mating. During this stage, ovulated follicles metamorphose into corpora lutea (CLs), which begin to secrete progesterone. Metestrus is so short in some species that it is not even discussed as a separate stage and is included in diestrus.

Diestrus

This is a stage of ovarian activity without signs of heat. The CLs develop fully and produce maximum levels of progesterone to ready the uterus for the conceptus and to maintain pregnancy.

If pregnancy does not occur, prostaglandins released from the uterus destroy the CLs and stop progesterone production. The female then either enters anestrus (if it is a monestrous species such as the bitch) or reenters proestrus (if it is a polyestrous species, such as the cow).

When reading about the days of the cycle, it is important to know what is meant by "day 1." In a woman's menstrual cycle, day 1 is the first day of menstrual bleeding. However, in the estrous cycle of animals, bleeding may or may not occur and occurs at a different stage of the cycle for species that show bleeding. Therefore, when reading about the estrous cycle or interpreting graphs, one must be sure to determine if the author is defining day 1 as the first day of standing heat, as the day of or after ovulation, as the first day after heat, or as the first day of a bloody vulvar discharge, in the case of the bitch.

Pregnant Animals

If the female conceives, the embryo signals its presence to the uterus in some manner, which prevents release of prostaglandins from the uterus. Thus, the CL remains active and continues to secrete progesterone throughout pregnancy or until the placenta takes over production of progesterone. The CL is necessary throughout pregnancy in the cow, goat and bitch. To maintain pregnancy, the ewe needs it for the first 55 days of pregnancy and the queen needs it for about 45 days. The mare only needs the CL's progesterone for 100 days of its 330-day gestation. The embryologic signal of pregnancy may be estrone sulfate or a pregnancy-specific protein. As we shall see later, estrone sulfate detection may aid early pregnancy diagnosis in some animals.

Mares have an additional hormone present during part of their pregnancy. Equine chorionic gonadotropin (ECG), previously called pregnant mare serum gonadotropin (PMSG), is present from about 35 to 120 days of gestation. It acts on the ovaries to stimulate formation of secondary CLs, which fortify progesterone levels. ECG is useful in veterinary medicine because it is the basis of some blood tests for pregnancy diagnosis in mares.

Figure 1 shows development of follicles and metamorphosis of a follicle into a corpus hemorrhagicum (CH), a functional corpus luteum (CL) and, finally, into a regressed corpus albicans (CA). It also shows the temporal relationships of changes in the hormones during the estrous cycle of the mare. Figure 2 shows the hormonal relationships of pregnancy in the mare.

Progesterone is the predominant hormone necessary for maintenance of pregnancy. With the exception of ECG (PMSG), which is only found in mares, these hormonal relationships are representative for most of the animals discussed in this chapter. Several of these hormones are valuable aids for pregnancy diagnosis in the various species, but the days when applicable vary with the species.

Reproductive Physiologic Patterns

With the previous generalized review of the estrous cycle in mind, we will now discuss the specifics for various species. This information is summarized in Table 1.

Figure 1. Ovarian structures and hormones during the mare's estrous cycle. The follicle grows rapidly during the last part of the cycle in response to follicle-stimulating hormone (FSH). The follicle produces estrogen, which causes behavioral estrus and softens the cervix. Luteinizing hormone (LH) causes final maturation of the follicle, leading to release of the egg at ovulation. The postovulation follicle fills with blood to become a corpus hemorrhagicum (CH). This transforms into a corpus luteum (CL) that produces progesterone. Progesterone predominates throughout most of the cycle and would maintain pregnancy if the mare became pregnant. The CL is lysed by prostaglandins (PGF2 alpha) and progesterone levels fall. The lysed CL withers and becomes a nonfunctional corpus albicans. (From McKinnon and Voss: *Equine Reproduction,* courtesy of Lea & Febiger)

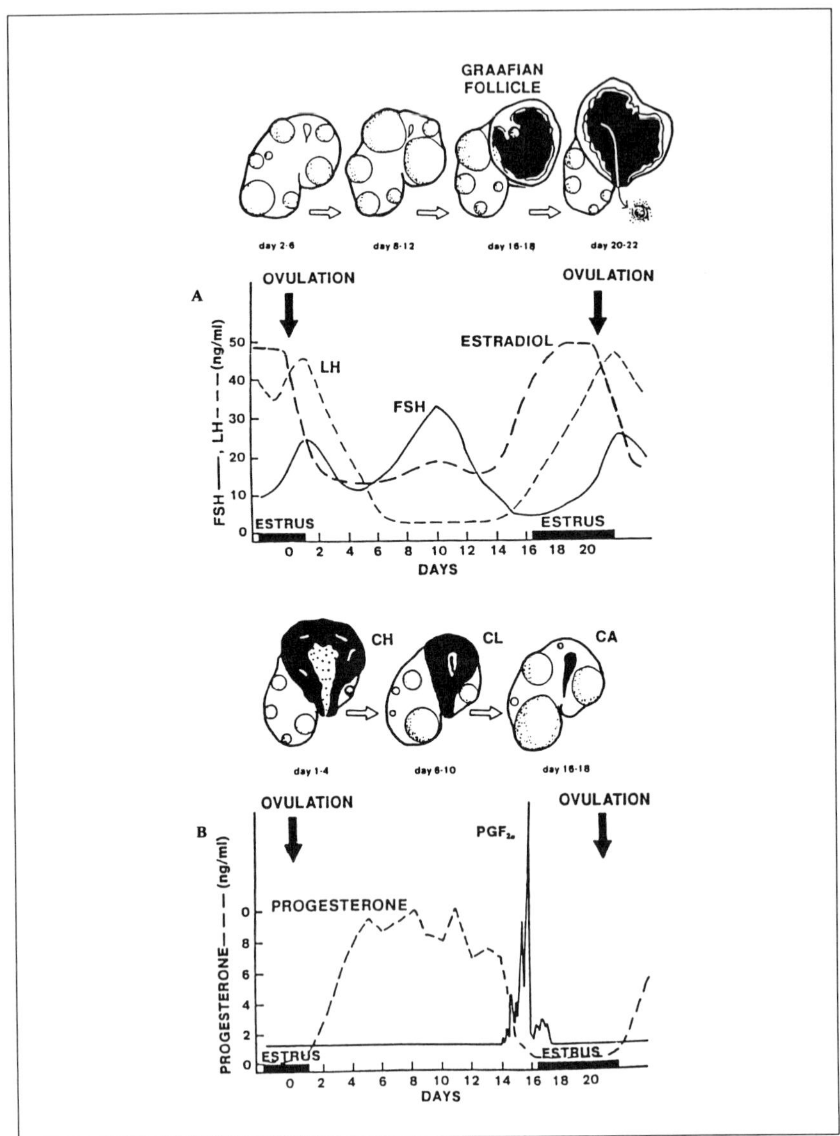

Figure 2. Hormones during pregnancy in the mare. Early pregnancy is maintained by progesterone from the corpora lutea (CL) on the ovaries. The mare develops secondary (2°) CLs in response to equine chorionic gonadotropin (ECG, previously called PMSG), which comes from the endometrial cups stimulated to form in the uterus by the fetus. The mare's placenta maintains pregnancy after 100-120 days of gestation by producing progestagens. High levels of estrogens from the fetal gonads and the placenta are present in the last part of pregnancy. Assay of ECG and estrogen levels can be used for pregnancy diagnosis in mares at the appropriate times. Progesterone is a poor hormone to use for pregnancy diagnosis. (Courtesy of Hoffman-LaRoche, Inc)

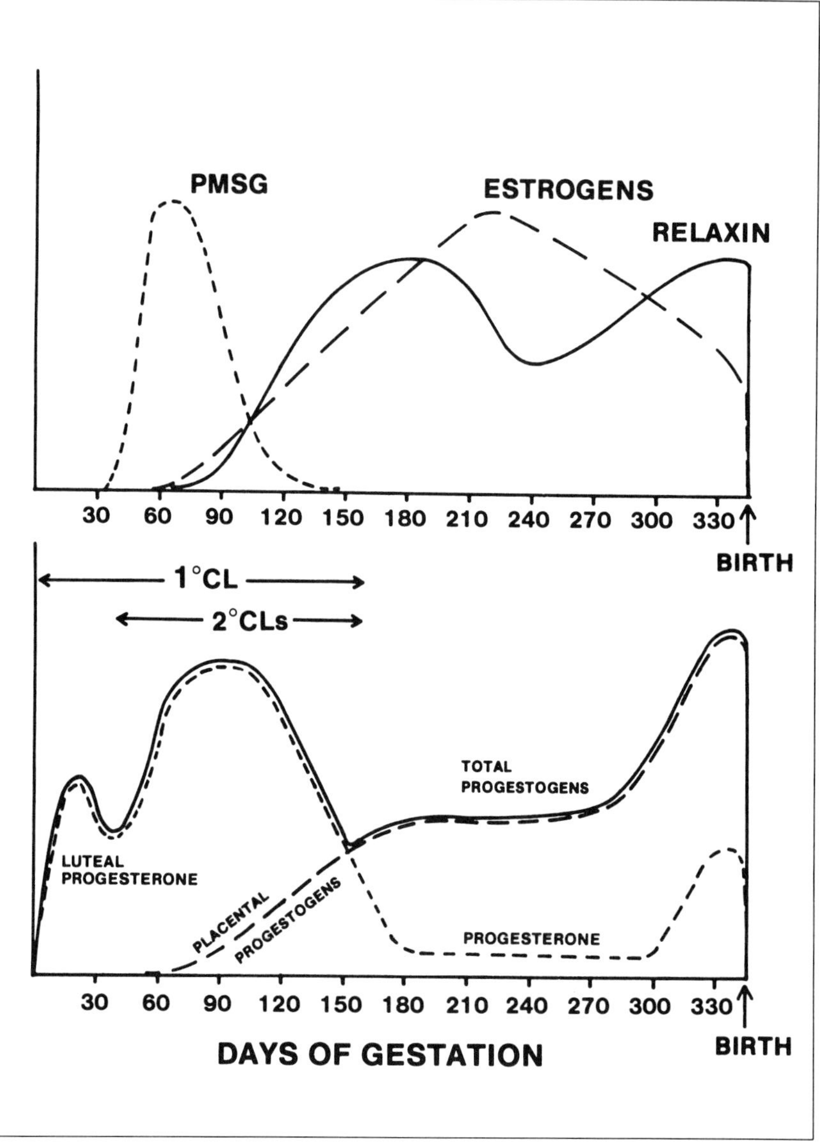

Cows

The normal cow is a polyestrous animal that cycles throughout the year, with a 1 day heat about every 21 days (range 18-23 days) unless pregnant. Heat lasts about 18 hours in cows. The signs of approaching heat in cows include nervousness, vocalization, and attempting to mount and ride other animals. A cow in "true" heat stands to be ridden by other cows. A thick, clear, tenacious string of mucus can often be seen hanging from the vulva of cows in heat. Unlike other animals, cows ovulate about 12 hours after going out of heat.

Cows that are to be bred artificially should be bred 12 hours after heat is first detected, if the herd is watched 20-30 minutes twice daily for estrous animals (Fig 3). Obviously, cows to be bred naturally must still be in standing heat. Cows often show metestrual bleeding in the mucus 1-2 days after they have ovulated. It is too late to breed cows that have evidence of metestrual blood in their mucus.

Figure 3. Signs of estrus and timing of breeding in cows. (Courtesy of *Large Animal Veterinarian*)

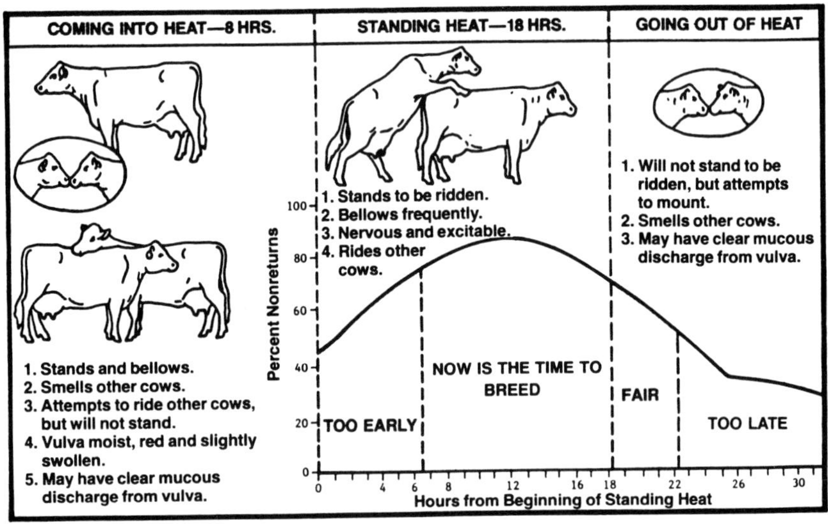

Table 1. Reproductive data for female domestic animals.

	Cycle Pattern	Cycle Length	Heat Length	Ovulation Time	Time to Breed		Gestation Length	Puberty	Age to First Breed
					Natural	Artificial Insem.			
Cow	polyestrous	21 days	18 hours	12-18 hours after heat	heat	12 hours after 1st see heat	280 days	6-16 months	14-22 months
Mare	seasonally polyestrous	21 days	5 days	24-36 hours before end of heat	day 2 and every other day of heat	same as natural	330 days (320-360 days)	18 months	2-3 years
Sow	polyestrous	21 days	2-3 days	36 hours after onset of heat	daily when in heat	same as natural	115 days	7 months	8-9 months
Bitch	seasonally polyestrous	4-7 months	7-9 days	day 2-3 of heat	days 1, 3 and 5 of heat	same as natural	63 days	6-12 months	12-18 months
Queen	seasonally polyestrous	21 days	4-10 days	induced	in heat	in heat	63 days	7-12 months	12-18 months

Mares

The mare is a seasonally polyestrous animal. Most mares stop cycling (become anestrual) during the winter; however, a few mares cycle also during the winter. The mare's natural breeding season is in the late spring and summer. Breed registration rules, however, force us to begin breeding mares in February and March. During the natural breeding season (May-August), the mare's estrous cycle is about 21 days long. They are in standing heat for about 5 days and then out of heat for 16 days.

Estrual mares (in heat) seek out the stallion. They squat and urinate frequently in the presence of the stallion, raise the tail to the side and evert (wink) the clitoris. Estrual mares stand to be mounted by the stallion. Mares that are not in heat squeal, kick, switch the tail from side to side, pin their ears back, and may attempt to bite the stallion.

Mares enter and leave the natural breeding season with very erratic cycles. They often have prolonged heats in the early spring. These early-season erratic periods result in extra labor for farm personnel and ineffective breedings. Rectal examination by a veterinarian at this time can be used to predict the optimum time for breeding. Mares usually ovulate 24-36 hours before going out of heat (Fig 1). The best time to breed a normally cycling mare is on the second day of heat and again every other day until she goes out of heat. In the early spring, when mares have prolonged heats, breeding all mares every other day may exhaust the stallion.

The veterinarian can predict ovulation, based upon changes in the follicles, as palpated rectally, and on changes in the cervix. The follicles become large and soft before ovulation. The cervix changes from a dry, firm, tight, pale organ to a very pink, edematous, soft, amorphous mass on the floor of the vagina before ovulation. Ultrasonography helps predict ovulation. The follicular wall thickens and its shape changes from round to pointed. Breeding mares based upon prediction of ovulation conserves stallion power.

After ovulation, the collapsed follicle fills with blood and becomes a corpus hemorrhagicum (CH), which is converted quickly to a corpus luteum (CL). The CL produces progesterone until it regresses if the mare has not become pregnant, and evolves to a nonfunctional corpus albicans (CA) just before the next heat.

Sows

Gilts reach puberty at about 6-7 months of age, though this varies with the breed and the time of year they are born. Pigs are nonseasonal polyestrous animals, though in a hot, humid climate they may show reduced cyclicity during the summer. Pigs are unique in that they show an early postpartum heat but do not ovulate during this heat. Then they undergo a true lactational anestrus, at which time they do not resume cyclicity until the litter is weaned.

After resumption of cycling, the sow demonstrates heat for 2-3 days every 21 (18-24) days. Heat is recognized in sows by a slightly swollen, reddened vulva. They are restless, seek out the boar, and assume a characteristic braced sawhorse stance when the boar mounts. This stance is used to detect sows and gilts in heat. A female in heat assumes this same rigid sawhorse stance if pressed on the back by a person. This is called the "riding test."

Sows ovulate in the last half of heat. They should be bred on the first day of heat and again 24 hours later for maximum conception rate and litter size.

Bitches

The bitch is a seasonally monestrous animal with a definite anestrous period between cycles. Most bitches come into season about once every 6-7 months. The heats can be at any time of the year; however, they seem to be concentrated in the spring and fall. Some may cycle only once a year, as in the Basenji. Other individual bitches may cycle every 4 months and still be considered normal.

Bitches reach puberty at 6-24 months of age, with an average of 10-12 months. Small breeds usually reach puberty earlier than large breeds.

The estrous cycle of the bitch has 5 characteristic stages. Figure 4 shows the hormonal relationships during the estrous cycle of the bitch. Vaginal smears can be used to determine the stage of the cycle (Fig 5). Owners say a bitch has come into heat when they notice attraction of males and dripping of blood from the vulva. This is actually proestrus, not estrus.

Proestrus: This stage is characterized by increased vulvar swelling, a bloody vulvar discharge, attraction to males, and courtship play, such as spinning, crouching in front, nuzzling, and even mounting the male. Proestrous females, however, do not stand to be mounted by males. A vaginal smear at this stage shows a variable amount of red blood cells (RBC) and white blood cells (WBC), and initially predominantly small, round parabasal and small intermediate vaginal epithelial cells (Fig 5). Parabasal and small intermediate cells can be recognized by their round shape and relatively large nucleus in proportion to the amount of cytoplasm.

As the bitch progresses through proestrus, the number of RBCs remains variable. The number of WBCs declines. Vaginal epithelial cells consist of large intermediate and superficial cells, both of which are thin, large and angular, with small pyknotic (dense) nuclei or no nucleus at all. The vaginal cells are becoming keratinized or cornified. The vulva is still large and edematous at this stage. Proestrus lasts an average of 9 days (range 3-17 days).

By the end of proestrus, more than 50% of the vaginal epithelial cells are anuclear (no nucleus), keratinized superficial cells (Fig 6). Serum progesterone levels begin to rise at the end of proestrus or in early estrus before ovulation. Kits are available to detect this rise and predict the time of ovulation for maximum breeding efficiency (Fig 4).

Estrus: At onset of estrus, the bitch stands to be mounted by the male. Estrus averages 9 days in the bitch but can be as short as 3 days or as long as 21 days. During estrus, the bitch lifts the tail and deflects it to the side, arches the back, and elevates the vulva.

The vulva is less turgid than in proestrus; this facilitates copulation. The estrual vulvar discharge may remain red or become straw colored. As mentioned earlier, the estrual vaginal smear consists almost entirely of superficial and large intermediate cells (Fig 5). WBCs are no longer present in the smear; RBCs may or may not be present. The presence or absence of RBCs is not a significant finding when trying to determine the stage of the cycle.

Figure 4. Hormone levels during the estrous cycle of the nonpregnant bitch. Note that progesterone levels begin to rise a few days before ovulation. This can be used to predict the best time to breed. Also note that progesterone levels remain elevated above baseline for 60 or more days even though the bitch is not pregnant; thus, progesterone assay for pregnancy is not valid in the bitch. Overt clinical pseudopregnancy occurs between 40 and 60 days as progesterone levels begin to decline. (From Kirk RW: *Current Veterinary Therapy VIII Small Animal Practice,* courtesy of W.B. Saunders)

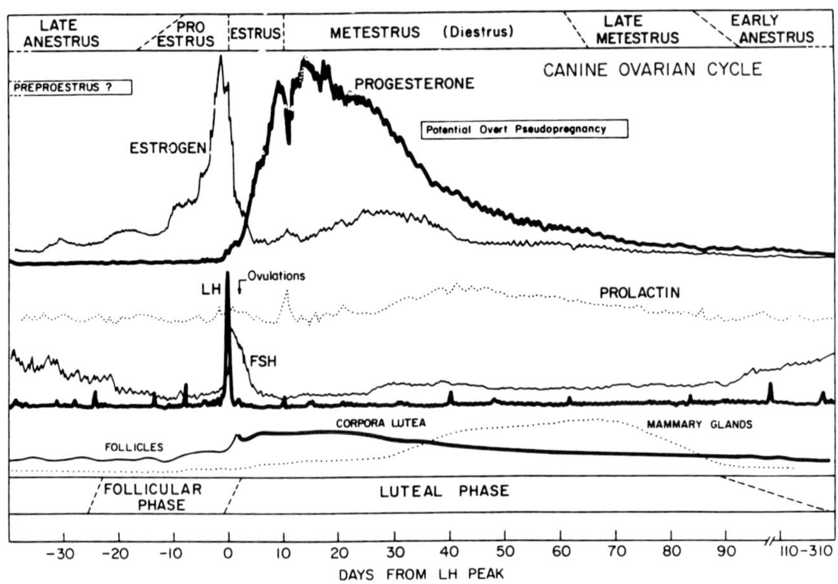

Bitches ovulate early in estrus. The best time to breed a bitch is on the first, third and fifth days of standing heat. Breeding bitches on the ninth and eleventh or eleventh and thirteenth days after the onset of vulvar bleeding is less than satisfactory because of the variable duration of proestrus and estrus. Breeding bitches on these predetermined days assumes the owner noticed the first day of vulvar discharge; however, this is often not the case. Breedings based upon the preovulatory rise in serum progesterone levels are the most effective.

During breeding, it is important to be sure that the stud has inserted the penis completely and that the bulbus glandis (enlarged caudal portion of the penis) is completely inserted into the vagina, producing the coital lock or "tie." The tie is important for stimulating contractions that help move the semen into the uterus and up the oviducts. A normal tie can last 15-30 minutes. The dogs should not be disturbed at this time. Efforts to physically separate the

Figure 5. Characteristics of vaginal cells seen on cytologic examination during various stages of the estrous cycle in the bitch.

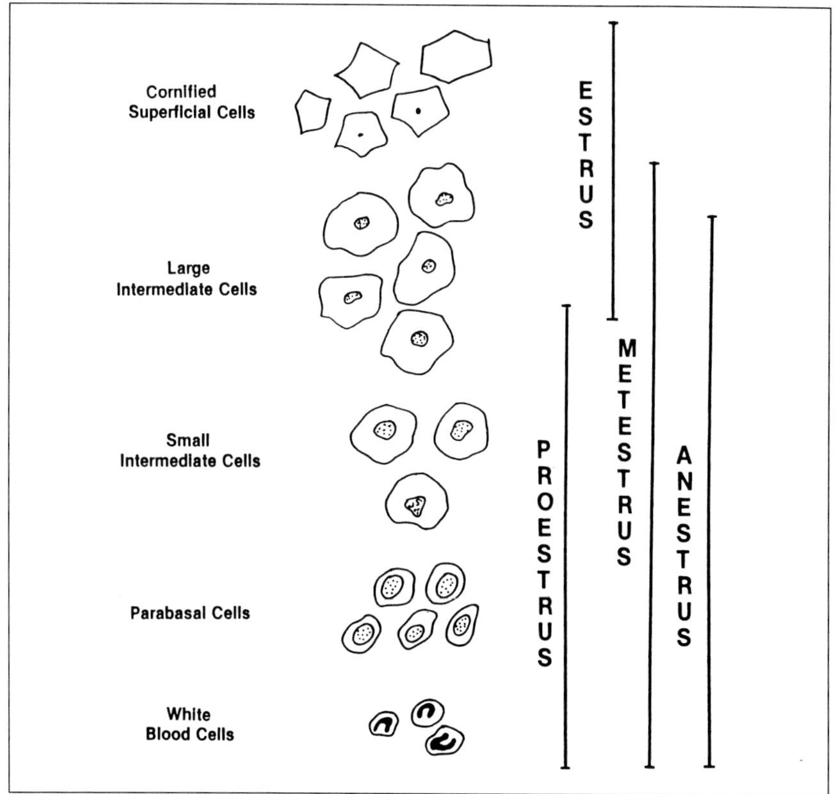

bitch and stud may injure the penis or the vagina. At the end of estrus, the bitch no longer accepts the stud dog, even though he may continue to show interest in her. The bitch then enters metestrus.

Metestrus. Metestrus is a short stage in the bitch; in fact, some authors do not even discuss it. In metestrus, the bitch refuses the male's sexual advances, and WBCs and noncornified parabasal and small intermediate cells reappear in vaginal smears. Vulvar swelling and vaginal discharge decrease rapidly during this stage. Metestrus rapidly progresses to diestrus.

Figure 6. Events during the estrous cycle in the bitch. Note that vulvar swelling and vaginal edema are greatest in proestrus and decrease during estrus. As vaginal edema subsides, wrinkling (crenulation) of the vaginal mucosa can be detected with vaginoscopy. (From Kirk RW: *Current Veterinary Therapy VIII Small Animal Practice,* courtesy of WB Saunders)

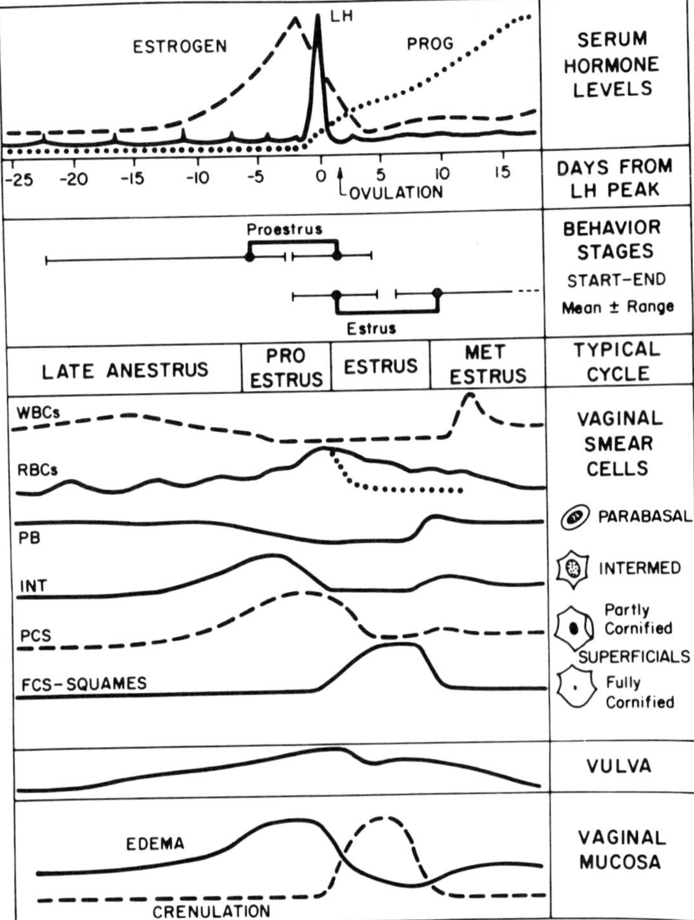

The wide range of days during which breeding can take place in the dog makes accurate prediction of whelping difficult (Fig 7). The whelping date can be predicted to occur 57 ± 1 days after the vaginal smear reverts to predominantly noncornified small intermediate and parabasal cells typical of diestrus.

Diestrus: This is the longest stage of the canine estrous cycle. It lasts about 60 days, which is nearly the same length as a normal pregnancy. There is no vulvar discharge after the first few days of diestrus. The vaginal smear contains predominantly noncornified parabasal and small intermediate cells, with a few WBCs.

Toward the end of diestrus, about the time a pregnant bitch would be ready to whelp, the nonpregnant bitch often shows *pseudopregnancy* or *false pregnancy* as serum progesterone levels decline (Fig 4). The abdomen may enlarge and the mammary glands may swell and fill with milk. The bitch may build a "nest" and even enter a false first stage of labor.

Pseudopregnant bitches often "adopt" socks, stuffed toys, or kittens as their surrogate puppies. They may have a behavior change

Figure 7. Events during the estrous cycle and pregnancy in the bitch. The wide range of days during which matings can occur makes prediction of the whelping date difficult unless based on vaginal smear changes. The final drop in progesterone levels before whelping is associated with a drop in body temperature, which is predictive of whelping. Embryo implantation (nidation) is associated with a few percentage points drop in packed cell volume (PCV). (From Kirk RW: *Current Veterinary Therapy VIII Small Practice*, courtesy of WB Saunders)

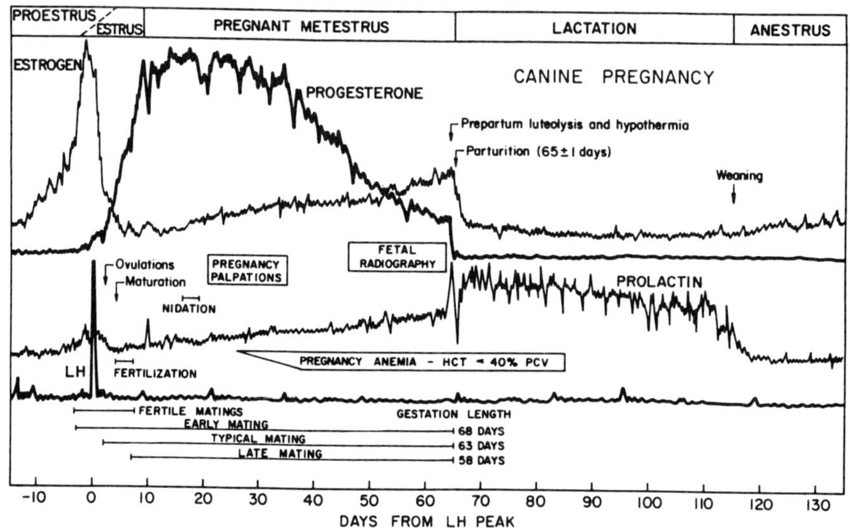

at this time and become aggressive if a person attempts to remove their "puppies." Pseudopregnant bitches have been known to raise an orphaned litter of kittens. Not all bitches show clinical signs of pseudopregnancy; however, they all undergo the same hormonal changes that could make them exhibit these signs.

Anestrus: After diestrus or pregnancy, the uterus undergoes a period of regeneration or repair during anestrus. Anestrus may last 1-11 months, depending on the breed, with 4-5 months the average. The vaginal smear at this time is mainly comprised of noncornified parabasal and small intermediate cells, with variable numbers of WBCs. At some times, WBCs can be quite numerous, making it difficult to rule out infection. Anestrous females do not attract males nor do they allow courtship or mating behavior by the stud. After anestrus, the bitch reenters proestrus and the cycle repeats itself.

Queens

Females of other domestic animals are *spontaneous ovulators.* That is, they release their eggs at a predetermined time in their cycle, after the appropriate hormonal changes. The queen, on the other hand, is an *induced ovulator,* meaning coitus is necessary to stimulate ovulation.

The queen is a seasonally polyestrous animal. If not induced to ovulate, she will have several cycles of sexual behavior before either being bred or induced to ovulate, or having the follicles regress (Fig 8). Queens have a short anestrous period between October and January, but then cycle regularly the rest of the year if they do not conceive.

Because the queen is an induced ovulator, CLs are not produced unless coitus has occurred. The cycle lasts about 14 days and is composed of 1-2 days of proestrus, 3-6 days of estrus (heat) and about 7 days of metestrus before proestrus occurs again.

Estrus: Estrus in queens is recognized by behavioral changes. They become more affectionate, vocalize, and rub up against inanimate objects and people. When petted, they arch their back, elevate the hindquarters and laterally displace the tail. Treading of the hind feet is often evident at this time.

Queens do not show the vulvar bleeding seen in bitches, but they have similar changes in the vaginal smear. Reappearance of WBCs in the smear marks the end of estrus and the beginning of metestrus. Natural breeding can be successful at any time during estrus, as the eggs are not ovulated until after breeding.

Many owners find the recurrent estrous behavior annoying. It can be stopped by inducing ovulation and pseudopregnancy after a sterile mating or false mating using a glass rod (*eg,* a sanitized rectal thermometer) to stimulate the queen's vagina. Ovulation can also be induced by injection of the appropriate luteinizing hormone. Overaggressive probing for a vaginal smear for estrus detection can also stimulate ovulation. Induced ovulation should keep a queen out of heat for 40-60 days or longer if winter is approaching.

Like dogs, cats can also show clinical signs of pseudopregnancy and experience false labor, lactation, and adoption of objects or another animal's litter.

PREGNANCY DIAGNOSIS

One of the cardinal signs of pregnancy in large animals is failure to return to heat after breeding during their breeding season. This is not true for bitches, however, because as seasonally monoestrous animals, they will not return to heat if they fail to conceive for 4-7 months. Mated but nonpregnant queens do not return to heat for several months after breeding.

Traditionally, animals have been examined for pregnancy by palpation (manual examination) of the uterus through the abdom-

Figure 8. Hormone levels during the estrous cycle and pregnancy in the queen. Psp = pseudopregnancy, Preg = pregnancy, Part = parturition. (From Kirk RW: *Current Veterinary Therapy VIII Small Animal Practice,* courtesy of WB Saunders)

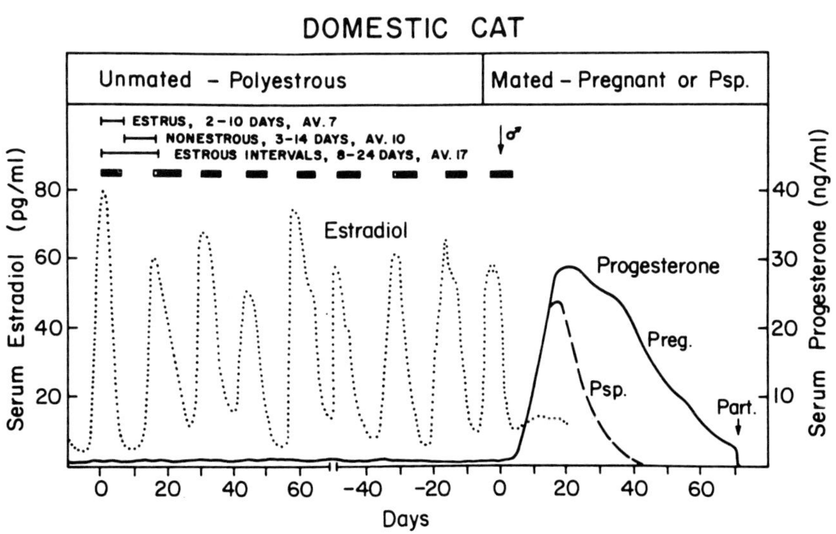

inal wall (dogs, cats, pigs, sheep, goats) or by rectal palpation (horses, cattle). Now, however, pregnancy diagnosis is becoming more technologically advanced. Various histologic, chemical, electronic, ultrasonic and radiographic techniques can be used. Figure 7 shows the hormonal relationships and events that can be used to detect pregnancy in the bitch.

Manual Examination

Bitches

Transabdominal (through the abdominal wall) palpation of the uterus can be used to diagnose pregnancy when performed during the middle and later part of gestation in bitches and queens (Fig 7). By 18-21 days postbreeding, a string of 1.3-cm swellings can be felt in the uterus. By 45-55 days, these individual swellings coalesce. The uterus feels like a long sausage, and the fetuses are difficult to palpate. By 55-63 days, the individual pups can usually be palpated again.

Queens

Fetal bulges (2-2.5 cm) in a queen can be palpated between 20 and 30 days of gestation. After 30 days, it is difficult to feel the individual fetuses, but the enlarged uterus is quite evident. Late in pregnancy, individual kittens can be palpated.

Mares

Pregnancy may be diagnosed by rectal examination as early as 19-20 days after breeding. The tone of the uterus and the chorionic or embryonic bulge can be easily identified. Later, the fetus can be palpated. Because the mare's rectum is extremely fragile, this technique should be done only by a veterinarian.

Cows

Palpation of the cow's uterus through the rectal wall reveals an amniotic vesicle at about 30-35 days. The chorioallantois can be felt as a membrane at 36-90 days. After this, the cotyledons and the fetus can be used to confirm pregnancy. Fremitus (palpable vibration) in the enlarged uterine artery is an indication of pregnancy in the middle trimester (third), when it is difficult to feel the fetus. Late in gestation, the fetus may be palpable transrectally or it may be "bumped" transabdominally (ballottement) in the ventral right flank after 6-7 months of gestation.

Sows

The sow's uterus is not usually palpated for pregnancy diagnosis; however, it is possible and can be highly accurate. Good tone in the cervix and fremitus in the uterine artery are indications of pregnancy, the latter being most evident between 60 and 110 days of gestation.

Ewes and Does

In late pregnancy, abdominal palpation can be used in a relaxed goat doe with a thin abdominal wall. This is not possible with large breeds. Many goat owners do not like abdominal ballottement as a form of pregnancy diagnosis in their does. Fasting of ewes for 12-24 hours facilitates abdominal palpation as the rumen is collapsed and the uterus is more easily identified.

Histologic Diagnosis of Pregnancy

The sow is the only animal in which this technique has been broadly applied. A vaginal biopsy 20-25 days after breeding is examined microscopically after histologic preparation. The epithelium in the biopsy specimen is only 2-4 cell layers thick if the sow is pregnant. At 20-25 days postbreeding, a nonpregnant sow that is coming back into heat typically has a very thick vaginal epithelium 10 or more layers thick. A diestrual sow also has a thin epithelium but of intermediate thickness, between that seen in estrus and pregnancy.

Chemical Diagnosis of Pregnancy

Chemical methods of pregnancy diagnosis include immunologic, endocrinologic and biologic techniques, in addition to strict chemical tests.

Progesterone Assay

Considering that blood progesterone levels remain elevated in pregnant animals, a high progesterone level in the blood at about the time of the expected subsequent estrus is an indication of pregnancy (Fig 9). The analysis is conducted between 17 and 23 days in the cow, mare and sow. Progesterone assay is not used in dogs (Fig 7) and mated cats (Fig 8) because their CLs are retained after estrus, and progesterone is secreted for the next 9-10 weeks, even if they are not pregnant.

Blood, milk or serum can be analyzed for progesterone, depending on the test kit used. The technique is very accurate for detecting nonpregnant animals, but it produces 5-15% false-positive results (incorrect diagnoses of pregnancy) because of other conditions that cause the CL to remain active and produce progesterone. Pyometra, a mummified fetus, or cystic ovaries can cause false-positive results in cows. Spontaneous prolonged diestrus can cause false-positive results in mares.

Estrogen Assay

Estrone sulfate is produced by the live fetus early in pregnancy and can be measured in blood, urine and possibly milk. Estrone sulfate assay is accurate at 18-34 days in sows, after 40 days in mares, after 70 days in cows, and after 50 days in goats. The test is probably not valid in dogs, as no estrone sulfate is present. Estrogen levels are also high in the urine of mares after 5 months of pregnancy (Fig 2). This estrogen can be detected by the *Cuboni test.* Pregnancy is indicated by dark- green fluorescence in the bottom of the test tube after urine is mixed with hydrochloric acid, sulfuric acid and benzene.

Equine Chorionic Gonadotropin Assay

Equine chorionic gonadotropin (ECG), formerly called pregnant mare serum gonadotropin (PMSG), is present in the blood of pregnant mares between 35-120+ days of gestation (Fig 2). ECG is pro-

Figure 9. Progesterone levels during postpartum cycling in cows. Note that heats occur during periods of low progesterone levels between the 1st, 2nd and 3rd cycles. Pregnant cows maintain elevated progesterone levels during pregnancy. (From Morrow DA: *Current Therapy in Theriogenology 2,* courtesy of WB Saunders)

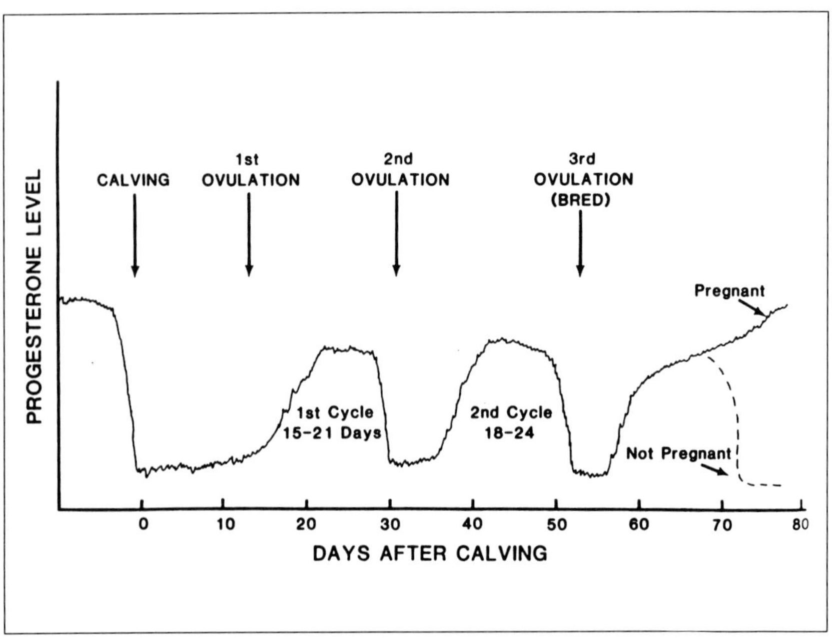

duced by endometrial cups in the uterine wall, which develop in response to the fetus. Several commercial test kits can detect this hormone.

The mare immunologic pregnancy (MIP) test is a hemagglutination-inhibition test for ECG that detects the lack of agglutination of RBCs in the pregnant mare's blood.

Biologic tests for ECG, using female rats or rabbits or male frogs, detect ovulation in females and sperm production in males after ECG-containing serum is injected into the animal.

Radioimmunoassays (RIA) and enzyme-linked immunosorbent assays (ELISA) are available for ECG detection in some laboratories. False-positive results are possible if the fetus dies after the endometrial cups are formed. The cups continue to produce detectable ECG until 120+ days of gestation, even if the fetus has been lost.

Electronic Detection of Pregnancy

Ultrasonography

The ultrasonography machine transmits high-frequency sound waves through tissues and records the echoes reflected by different tissue structures as these sound waves bounce back to the transducer. Several types of ultrasound machines are used for pregnancy detection.

The A-mode or amplitude-depth ultrasound machine bounces sound waves off of different tissue layers and records the echoes, displayed as an audible beep, a pattern of lights or a set of peaks on an oscilloscope. A-mode ultrasonography is reportedly 98% accurate at 21-90 days in sows and 18-23 days in bitches.

Doppler ultrasound detects differences in maternal and fetal pulses by reflection of the sound waves they produce. These pulses are registered as sound or as oscilloscope blips. If used properly, it is 100% accurate after 40 days of gestation in sows. It is also used in bitches after 30 days of gestation.

B-mode or brightness mode ultrasound is also known as real-time ultrasound because the image is regenerated many times per second, allowing detection of motion. It produces a visual image that can be measured, photographed or recorded on videotape or disk. Real-time ultrasound can be used to detect the embryonic vesicle in mares as early as 10-11 days after ovulation. In ewes and does it can be used transrectally between 24 and 34 days, (linear transrectal probe), and after 35 days transabdominal ultrasonography can detect pregnancy. Fetal heart beats can be detected at 25 days in mares, 20 days in cows, and 35 days in ewes and does.

Embryonic sexing can also be done using this type of ultrasound at 59-68 days in mares and 55-70 days in cows.

Electrocardiography

Fetal electrocardiograms have been used to detect the fetal heart beat in mares and cows in advanced pregnancy.

Radiography

Radiographs can be used to diagnose pregnancy in dogs and cats after 45 days of gestation, after 80 days in ewes, and after 90 days in does. At that time, the fetal skeletons and skulls are calcified and the fetuses can be counted. Radiographs are rarely used in sows because of the cost and impracticality.

PREPARTUM CARE

Some special considerations must be observed in preparing the dam for *parturition* (birth) and for nursing offspring. Nutrition is probably the most important of these.

Nutrition

The major amount of fetal growth occurs during the last third of gestation. Up until this time, dietary requirements parallel those of a nonpregnant animal, provided the dam was in good condition at the time of breeding. Nutrition is extremely important in the last trimester (third) for beef cows. The dam's nutritional status at this time affects the size and viability of the calf and also the cow's fertility by influencing the time interval until she returns to estrus after calving.

In cows, lactation is the major nutritional drain. Pregnancy is an additional stress, especially during the last third of gestation. Special attention must be paid to increased protein and caloric requirements, and calcium and phosphorus balance in the ration. To reduce some of the nutritional stress and allow dairy cows to prepare for calving, they are "dried off" (not milked) during the last 8 weeks of pregnancy. During this *dry period,* good pasture or well-cured hay and silage with a vitamin-mineral supplement are usually sufficient. An adequate dry period also improves fertility in the subsequent lactation. Cows that lose condition during lactation may require additional feed during the early dry period.

Bitches in good condition when they become pregnant and maintained on a high-quality commercial diet usually do not need special supplementation during pregnancy, except for moderate, gradual increases in total intake during the last half of pregnancy and during heavy lactation. She should be consuming 15-25% more than normal by the time she whelps. As parturition approaches, a more laxative diet is usually fed in small, frequent feedings to eliminate any digestive discomfort caused by the enlarged uterus and fetus. The well-nourished animal must be housed properly to ensure healthy neonates and a postpartum period free of complications.

Facilities

There are 3 basic requirements for an adequate area in which to give birth. It must be clean, dry and free of drafts. It must be easily observed so that assistance can be given if needed. Most important, it must be acceptable to the dam. The most "deluxe" whelping box will be abandoned by a bitch that feels more at ease in the bedroom closet.

The whelping box should be set up in a warm, draft-free, secluded place a week or so before the bitch is due to whelp, to allow her to become accustomed to it. The size varies with the size of the bitch, but it should be large enough to allow the bitch to lie down and still have plenty of room to nurse all the pups.

A queening box for female cats is similar to a whelping box. Its sides must be at least 4-6 inches high so that nursing kittens are not dragged out as the queen leaves.

Mares and cows seem to do best if allowed to give birth in a clean, well-drained pasture. Ideally it should be a spot where impending parturition can be easily observed and the dam and offspring are protected from predators. If such a pasture is not available, a well-bedded box stall at least 14 x 14 ft does nicely.

Sows are usually provided a farrowing crate, which is a narrow stall-like structure with low side rails to prevent the sow from turning around or lying down on the baby pigs. These crates usually have a heat lamp at one end to keep the baby pigs warm. The accepted practice is to house farrowing sows in a heated barn, thus eliminating the need for bedding. This also allows for easier, more thorough cleaning.

Sows should be introduced to the farrowing (delivery) area several weeks before the due date, if practical, to allow the sow to produce antibodies in her colostrum against the organisms to which the neonate will be exposed shortly after birth. Once animals are introduced to their delivery area, they must be observed regularly for signs of parturition.

Signs of Impending Parturition

As parturition approaches, several physical and behavioral signs are displayed by the dam. The mammary glands usually fill with milk one to several days before parturition, but this can occur up to several weeks before delivery in some species. At the same time, the ligaments of the tailhead relax to allow passage of the young through the birth canal.

"Waxing" of the teats occurs in mares within 24 hours of delivery; however, several false "waxes" may occur. Milk calcium levels can be monitored with dipsticks to predict foaling in mares. Many times, there is a temperature drop from the animal's norm. To check this, daily or twice-daily monitoring is usually necessary for as much as a week before the due date. The temperature decrease is a valuable tool for prediction of parturition in bitches and sows, as is the fall in serum progesterone levels. These occur 1-2 days before delivery.

About 12-24 hours before parturition, females often demonstrate anorexia and defecation and urination caused by pressure within the abdomen. The animal becomes restless and may even appear to be looking for her young, hours before they are born. Mares may have intermittent colic. Bitches, queens and sows attempt to build a nest for their young, whereas mares and cows tend to seek out an isolated area of the pasture.

Preparation for Parturition

Before parturition, steps should be taken to be sure that the perineal and mammary areas of large animals are washed and clipped. Sows are often washed completely before entering the farrowing crate. The mare's tail should be wrapped to prevent soiling and tangling with the foal and afterbirth. Mares that have had a Caslick's operation (vulvar suturing) should have their vulvar suture line reopened. This is also the time when you should gather all necessary equipment, such as obstetric chains, 7% iodine solution, towels, oxygen and other supplies you might need to assist in delivery and care of the neonate.

PARTURITION

After the preparatory changes of late pregnancy, which ready the dam and fetus for birth, parturition begins. Parturition has several common names, depending upon the species involved. *Calving* and *foaling* are self-explanatory. However, parturition in the sow or gilt is called *farrowing,* and in the bitch, it is called *whelping.* In the cat, it is called *kittening* or *queening.*

Parturition is divided into 3 stages. *Stage 1* is preliminary to expulsion of the fetus. During this stage, the uterine muscles undergo rhythmic contractions, which reposition and move the fetus caudally toward the cervix. In response to these contractions and the pressure of the fetus, the cervix relaxes fully and dilates. During first-stage labor, the dam often is anxious and restless, and shows evidence of abdominal cramps. Stage 1 ends with delivery of the fetus into the pelvic canal and rupture of the fetal membranes.

In *stage 2,* the fetus is expelled from the birth canal. Uterine contractions are stronger and accompanied by abdominal straining to help expel the fetus. The importance of abdominal straining versus uterine contractions in the birth process varies among species. Abdominal pressing is very important in foaling, but uterine contractions are relatively more important in farrowing. With successful delivery of the fetus, the dam completes stage 2 and rests during the first part of stage 3.

Stage 3 of parturition is characterized by expulsion of the placenta. Uterine contractions continue but are not as severe as those in stage 2. The uterus begins to shrink toward its nonpregnant size.

In polytocous (litter-bearing) species, the cycle of stages 1-3 repeats itself with each fetus. Actually, stages 1 and 2 may occur several times, and several fetuses may be passed before a placenta is passed in stage 3 in these species.

After delivery of the fetus, the dam rests and begins to care for the newborn. She licks it dry, which helps stimulate breathing, and licks and chews off any amniotic membrane remaining on the fetus. The bitch and queen usually chew the umbilical cord to detach the placenta. The cord usually ruptures spontaneously during delivery of a calf and during a foal's struggles to stand. The specific signs, events, and duration of the various stages of parturition vary among species (Table 2).

Calves and foals normally come out through the vulva head and feet first, in a "diving" position. Most pigs, pups and kittens are also delivered head first, but frequently 1 or both front legs are retracted alongside the body. In these small species, rear-end (breech) delivery is also common and results in normal, live offspring. Most dams deliver while lying down, but occasionally a cow or mare may deliver while standing up. This can be dangerous to the fetus.

It is often difficult to tell if a dam has finished delivering all of its offspring. Prepartum radiographs made 1 week before the due date allow one to count the number of pups or kittens in the dam. Twins in mares and cows are uncommon and can be detected by manual exploration of the vagina and uterus. However, because this is not as easily accomplished in sows, bitches and queens, you may have to rely on other signs or tests.

The bitch's abdomen may be palpated for more pups or a finger in a sterile glove may be introduced into the vagina to feel for another pup. Radiographs of the abdomen may be necessary. Some bitches and queens eat their pups, so care must be taken to differentiate ingested fetuses in the dam's stomach from those remain-

Table 2. Stages of labor in domestic species.

Stage	Cow	Mare	Sow	Bitch	Queen
I	1-4 hours (longer in heifers), restless, off feed, isolates self, allantois protudes	1-4 hours, colic, sweating, isolates self, defecation, urination, placenta ruptures	2-12 hours, 1-2 F drop in rectal temp, builds nest	6-12 hours, 1-2 F drop in rectal temp, builds nest	2-12 hours, 1-2 F drop in rectal temp, builds nest
II	½-4 hours, abdominal straining, amnion ruptures, calf delivered	5-40 minutes, forceful abdominal straining, amnion ruptures, foal delivered	1-5 hours amnion ruptures, straining, pigs delivered	3-6 hours, amnion ruptures, pups delivered	3-6 hours, amnion ruptures, kittens delivered
III	½-8 hours, uterine contractions, passes placenta	½-3 hours, rests, uterine contractions ± mild colic	⅓-4 hours, eats, drinks	½-1 hour, greenish black fluid passed	½-1 hour, brownish fluid passed
			Several fetuses often passed before placenta is passed		

ing in the dam's uterus. Sows often get up to drink and may eat after a period of rest once the last pig is delivered.

One of the most difficult situations encountered in theriogenology is to decide when parturition is not proceeding normally and that the dam is in dystocia (difficult birth) and requires assistance. Table 3 contains guidelines that have proven helpful.

MANAGEMENT OF DYSTOCIA

Dystocia (difficult birth) should be promptly corrected if the dam and offspring are to survive without permanent damage. The causes of dystocia can be classified as those due to maternal problems and those caused by fetal problems.

Some maternal causes of dystocia are uterine torsion, healed pelvic fracture restricting the birth canal, failure of the cervix to dilate, and primary uterine inertia caused by hypocalcemia (*eg,* milk fever in cows, eclampsia in bitches). Some fetal causes of dystocia are a single large pup, head enlargement from hydrocephalus (water on the brain), and positioning of a calf's forelimbs back alongside the body.

These are only a few of the many conditions that can result in dystocia. Consequently, before attempting to manage a case of dystocia, it is important to know the history of the dam. The following information should be determined: What is the due date? How long has the animal been in labor? Has the animal given birth before? If yes, when? Have any offspring already been delivered at this time? Has anyone attempted to assist the animal before you? After this information is obtained and assessed, careful examination of the dam and fetus is in order. The cause of the dystocia must be determined before attempting to deliver the offspring.

The exact procedures involved and the equipment necessary vary with the species, the cause of the dystocia, the condition of the dam and fetus, and the desires of the veterinarian involved. However, certain general principles must be kept in mind:

- *Treat life-threatening conditions to keep the dam alive until delivery is completed.* Heroic attempts to remove a fetus from a dead dam are usually unsuccessful.
- *Proper restraint is essential.* This may involve a squeeze chute or a halter and post for a cow, or general anesthesia for difficult foalings and whelpings.
- *Keep obstetric equipment in good working order, clean and disinfected.*
- *Pay strict attention to sanitation.* The vulva and perineal area should be scrubbed and rinsed thoroughly. Long-haired bitches should have the hair in this area clipped. Care

Table 3. Guidelines for intervention in dystocia.

Bitch, Queen

- intense straining that does not produce a pup or kitten in 30 minutes
- weak, intermittent straining that does not produce a pup or kitten in 2-3 hours
- an interval of over 4 hours between pups or kittens, without further labor
- illness in the dam
- a bloody, malodorous or greenish vulvar discharge
- prolonged pregnancy (overdue)
- obvious difficulty in delivering the pup or kitten (*eg,* a fetus halfway out)

Sow

- prolonged pregnancy (over 115 days)
- malodorous or bloody vulvar discharge
- expulsion of fetal feces (meconium) without expulsion of a fetus
- weak labor or cessation of labor before delivery of all fetuses
- incomplete expulsion of a fetus

Cow

- first-stage labor lasting more than 6 hours, without abdominal pressing
- second-stage labor, with abdominal pressing, lasting over 2-3 hours without progress
- rupture of the waterbag (amnion) without expulsion of the calf within 2 hours
- fetal malposition (backwards, legs retained, etc)
- fetal monstrosity (malformed fetus)

Mare

Parturition, especially stage 2, in mares is quicker and more violent than in other species. Furthermore, foals seem more susceptible to the adverse effects of dystocia than other neonates. Therefore, differentiation between a normal birth and dystocia is especially important in mares. Delivery should be assisted with:

- appearance of the red unruptured placenta at or outside the vulva at the start of second-stage labor, with evident straining
- failure of the clear amnion to appear soon after the start of second-stage labor
- failure to locate the foal's head and legs in the pelvic inlet at the beginning of second-stage labor
- rolling, repeated getting up and down and reversing of the recumbent position by the mare, without progressing through stage 2 of labor and delivering a foal
- repeated straining without delivery of a partially expelled foal
- fetal malposition (backwards, legs retained, etc) or other abnormality in delivery

should be taken to prevent feces from contaminating instruments and hands. The veterinarian should scrub his or her hands and arms thoroughly and put on a glove and sleeve before introducing the hand and/or arm into the vagina.

- *Use gentle, dexterous manipulation with plenty of lubrication.* Liberal and frequent application of lubricants facilitates manipulation and delivery. Straining during manipulation of the fetus can be suppressed by epidural anesthesia or, in the case of cattle, by passing a stomach tube into the rumen to prevent closure of the glottis.
- *After correcting the cause of the dystocia, carefully apply gentle traction to the fetus.* This may involve use of leg chains in the case of large animals or forceps for small animals. A calf-jack may also be required for large animals. Do not use a fence stretcher or hook the chains to a tractor or truck. A rule of thumb is to use no more traction than can be applied by 2 people when delivering a foal or calf. Ample lubrication greatly facilitates delivery by traction. A steady, continuous force is much more effective than short bursts of violent tugging. Constant traction allows the cervix and birth canal to expand as the fetus passes. Violent tugs often tear these tissues and can be detrimental to the fetus.
- *After delivery, examine the dam for additional fetuses and for injury that may have occurred during delivery.*

Occasionally, the fetus cannot be delivered intact through the birth canal. The veterinarian must then decide whether to perform a cesarean section or attempt to dismember the fetus (fetotomy) into parts small enough to be delivered through the vagina. The condition of the dam, uterus and fetus must be evaluated in making this decision.

A live, healthy fetus is usually delivered by cesarean section. A dead fetus can be removed by cesarean section, but many veterinarians prefer to dismember dead fetuses (fetotomy) and remove the pieces through the vagina. Fetotomy is the method of choice if the fetus is decomposing and the uterus is highly infected.

POSTPARTUM CARE

The Normal Neonate

Owners often become concerned about the condition of the neonate. Consequently, the veterinarian or veterinary staff spend a lot of time reassuring them and answering questions regarding the normality of the neonate. Table 4 contains a summary of characteristics of normal neonates.

Table 4. Characteristics of normal neonates of some domestic species.

Puppies

- can crawl and right themselves at birth
- open eyelids by 1-3 weeks
- require bitch's stimulation to urinate and defecate for about 2½ weeks
- dried umbilical cord drops off by about 2-3 days
- cannot regulate body temperature in the first few weeks (normal 94-99 F at 1-2 weeks, 97-100 F at 3-4 weeks, 100-101 F thereafter)
- can shiver by 7 days
- breathe 15-35 times/min at birth
- have a rapid pulse rate (220/min) in the first 2-3 weeks
- suckle shortly after birth
- have ear canals open by 13-17 days of age
- mostly sleep and nurse during the first week

Kittens

- can suckle and right themselves at birth
- open eyelids by 10-14 days, see well by 22-28 days
- ear canals open by 6-14 days
- require queen's stimulation to urinate and defecate for first few weeks
- double weight in first week
- sleep 90% of the time and nurse the rest of the time
- crawl by 18 days and walk by 21 days

Foals

- see, hear and shiver at birth
- breathe rapidly at first (75 breaths/min) and more slowly (35 breaths/min) by 12 hours of age
- have a pulse rate of 40-80/min, left-sided heart murmurs often present during first few days of life
- attempt to become sternally recumbent (on chest) within 2 minutes of birth
- have a suckling reflex within 5 minutes
- break the umbilical cord by about 8 minutes after birth
- stand within an hour
- nurse within 2 hours
- have a rectal temperature of 99-101 F (37.2-38.3 C)
- pass meconium within 72 hours
- urinate within 6 hours (colts) or 11 hours (fillies)

Calves

- hear, see and shiver at birth
- stand within 1-2 hours
- suckle by 2-5 hours

Piglets

- crawl toward the teats shortly after birth
- have eyes open at birth

Care of Neonates

A number of steps must be followed to ensure survival of the neonate. The most immediate concern for the newborn is a patent (clear) airway. Be sure that the fetal membranes are removed from the head and that no excess fluid is in the upper respiratory tract. In the calf, foal and pig, the nostril can be tickled with a piece of straw to stimulate a "sneezing" reflex to clear excess fluid from the airways. Often a calf is held up by the rear legs to allow fluid to drain from the nose and trachea. Pups and kittens can be held head down or gently swung.

Rubbing the neonate's back while drying it with a towel or cloth helps stimulate respiration. Licking by the dam also stimulates the neonate's respiration. Some dams, however, especially in the case of carnivores, begin to cannibalize their young. In such cases, the young must be removed and the dam restrained or tranquilized until it no longer tries to cannibalize or kill the young. This is a particular problem with inexperienced, anxious, first-time dams.

Once respiration is established, examine the newborn for congenital abnormalities. If an abnormality is found, look closer, as congenital problems often affect multiple sites. Next, the umbilical cord should be dipped in 7% iodine or some other suitable astringent disinfectant to prevent an umbilical infection, which may lead to "navel ill" and infected joints.

The next step is to ensure that the neonate locates the dam's udder or teats and nurses. This ensures adequate immunization through the dam's colostrum. Some inexperienced or poorly socialized dams may resist the neonate's attempts to nurse, and may have to be restrained or tranquilized until they become accustomed to nursing. Needle-sharp milk teeth in baby pigs may irritate and lacerate a gilt's teats. This pain can lead to cessation of nursing after a few days. Therefore, the ends of these teeth in neonatal pigs should be clipped with wire cutters at 1-2 days of age.

If the dam has little milk or the colostrum (first milk) has been lost (because of dripping before parturition), an alternative source of colostrum should be given to the neonate within 6 hours of birth before other food is ingested. Kits are available to assess the amount of antibodies absorbed from colostrum by foals and calves. Colostrum is not as essential to puppies or kittens as to other young because they acquire some of their passive immunity across the placenta. However, colostrum is still their major source of antibodies. Serum from healthy dogs can be given orally or subcutaneously to improve the natural defenses of these neonates for a short time until the first vaccinations are given.

Another item of concern is defecation and urination by the newborn. Meconium (fetal feces) impaction can cause colic in foals. Also, urinary bladder rupture is relatively common in newborn male foals. In many equine practices, an enema is routinely given to every newborn foal, along with tetanus immunization and an injection of vitamins and/or antibiotics. A better idea is to vaccinate the mare with tetanus toxoid 1 month before foaling. This allows time for production of antibodies against tetanus and their concentration in the colostrum. Thus the foal is passively immunized via the antibodies in colostrum and the mare is protected at foaling.

Feeding Orphans

If the dam rejects its young, has no milk or dies during birth, the owner must handfeed the offspring. Care must be exercised to prevent overfeeding, underfeeding or feeding the wrong type of milk.

Handfeeding the newborn is a tedious and time-consuming task. A few guidelines can be adapted to all species. Using a stomach tube reduces the time needed to feed the young that are not strong enough to have a good sucking reflex. The tube must be measured along the animal's body and marked to estimate the distance to the stomach. Care must be taken not to force passage of the tube, as this can cause irreparable damage to the esophagus.

When inserting the tube, check to see that it can be seen or felt as it moves caudally through the esophagus. If the tube is not seen or palpated, it may be in the trachea, which could cause death if milk were pumped into the lungs. Recently, esophageal feeders have been developed for use in the calf. These feeders consist of a firm tube with an enlarged end that closes the larynx when introduced into the pharynx and ensures that the fluid goes down the esophagus.

As a rule, calves and foals need 10% of their body weight in milk or milk replacer (formula) a day. Two feedings per day for most healthy calves is quite sufficient, whereas at least 4 feedings are preferred for foals.

Puppies and kittens require 25% of their body weight in milk daily. It is most desirable to feed them 6 times per day for the first 2 weeks, with 4 daily feedings thereafter until maturity. Baby pigs should be fed similarly to puppies.

There are various commercial animal milk substitutes (formulas, milk replacers) on the market. However, these may not be readily available in your area on short notice. Recipes for milk replacers are contained in Table 5. All of the formulas in Table 5 should be well blended and warmed to 35-38 C (95-100 F) before feeding. Overheating may denature the proteins in the formula.

Care of the Dam

After an uneventful parturition, the dam should be allowed to rest undisturbed so it can care for and become acquainted with its offspring. The dam should be unobtrusively observed periodically to be sure that it and the offspring are comfortable and happy. The dam should always have access to small amounts of water and feed. The udder or mammary glands should be checked for evidence of mastitis during the first few days. Dairy cows ultimately require milking and should be checked for mastitis.

The uterus should not be entered manually after an unassisted delivery, as this can unnecessarily introduce bacteria and cause a uterine infection, endangering future fertility. If a delivery has involved assistance, however, one should check the uterus and vagina, digitally or manually, for the presence of another fetus and for indications of injury to the dam. This should be done in a clean and sanitary manner. Cows that have required forced extraction of the fetus should be encouraged to stand shortly after delivery to rule out the possibility of rear-leg paralysis.

The dam should be observed to be sure all fetal membranes are passed. It is often difficult to account for all placentas with the bitch, queen and sow, as they typically eat them. Cows may eat their placenta also; however, one should attempt to prevent this, as ruminants cannot digest this material and it may cause a digestive upset or obstruction.

The bitch, queen and sow usually pass the placentas during parturition between birth of each offspring and after the last. A re-

Kittens

2⁄3 cup whole homogenized cow's milk

3 egg yolks

1 tbsp corn oil

1 dropper liquid vitamin supplement

Puppies

2⁄3 cup whole homogenized cow's milk

3 egg yolks

1 tbsp corn oil

1 dropper liquid vitamin supplement

pinch of salt

Foals

human baby formula can be used temporarily

goat milk also can be used

Baby Pigs

1 qt whole homogenized cow's milk

1 cup half and half (cream and milk)

Table 5. Recipes for milk replacers for kittens, puppies, foals and baby pigs.

tained placenta in these animals may lead to severe metritis (uterine infection); toxins from the infected uterus may be passed to the offspring in the milk and make them sick. A foul-smelling vulvar discharge several days after parturition warrants examination by a veterinarian.

Normal mares pass the placenta within 1 hour after delivery. It should be saved and filled with water so it can be examined to be sure it is all present. If the entire placenta or a piece of it is retained in the mare, a veterinarian should examine the animal. Retention of the placenta in mares may lead to laminitis (founder) if untreated.

Cows usually pass the placenta within 30 minutes to 8 hours. Those retained longer than 12 hours usually are passed within a week. Unless the cow is sick, one should not try to remove the placenta until at least 3 days after delivery. Earlier attempts may damage the cow's uterus. Manual intrusion into the uterus is not recommended.

During the first few postpartum weeks, the dam should be observed for mastitis, hypocalcemia (milk fever in the cow, eclampsia in the bitch and mare), metritis and agalactia (lack of milk).

BREEDING SOUNDNESS EVALUATION

Evaluation of Females

A reproductive examination can help assess a brood animal's chances of carrying a healthy fetus to term without endangering its health. In mares and cows, the methods and equipment used for routine examination are similar.

Rectal palpation is the most widely used method to examine the reproductive tract of large animals. With the aid of a plastic sleeve and lubricant, the veterinarian can assess the condition of the uterus, activity of the ovaries, and pregnancy status of the animal. With mares, the tail should be wrapped and tied out of the way.

After rectal examination, the vagina is usually evaluated with the aid of a speculum and light (*vaginoscopy*). The vulvar area should be cleaned thoroughly with a disinfectant scrub and dried before examination. The speculum should be lubricated with a sterile, water-soluble lubricant (*eg,* K-Y Jelly) and the labia spread to avoid contamination of the speculum as it is introduced. Once the speculum has been introduced, the vaginal walls and floor are examined for color, conformation, inflammation, and evidence of discharge. In mares, the tone and position of the cervix should be noted, as these suggest the stage of the estrous cycle.

A *uterine culture* may be performed to detect uterine infection. The best time to collect samples is during estrus. Preparation of the patient for this procedure is the same as for the vaginoscopic exam. A shielded, sterile swab is used to obtain a sample from the uterus. To avoid contamination of the swab in the vulva or vagina, it may be introduced through a speculum or by shielding with a sterile-gloved hand. After the sample is obtained, the culture swab is transferred to transport medium and sent to the laboratory for culture. Because uterine cultures are difficult to obtain in the bitch, queen and sow, one often must settle for a vaginal culture. The procedures are the same.

Uterine biopsies are an integral part of the breeding soundness examination of the mares. They are occasionally obtained to determine the cause of infertility in cows. After preparing the animal as for vaginoscopic examination, the sterilized biopsy punch is introduced with the sterile-gloved hand, through the cervix, into the uterus. The punch remains in the uterus while the hand is withdrawn and reinserted into the rectum. Once the jaws of the punch can be felt through the rectal and uterine walls, the wall of the uterus is pressed between the jaws with a finger and the jaws are closed. The closed biopsy punch is withdrawn and the biopsy sample is placed in 10% formalin or Bouin's fixative for transport to the laboratory.

In small animals, the uterus cannot be palpated per rectum but is palpated through the abdominal wall. The uterus is difficult to discern from loops of intestine. If a bitch is large enough, a finger can be inserted into the rectum. The first loop of the tissue ventral to the finger usually is the uterus.

The ovaries are not easily palpable in bitches or queens unless the animal is in heat or the ovaries are abnormally large. The uterus and ovaries can be evaluated ultrasonographically by an experienced operator. A vaginoscopic examination can be conducted with the aid of an otoscope, a nasal speculum, or a piece of small-diameter glass tubing.

In the bitch, vaginal cytology is often used to detect estrus and predict the approximate time of ovulation. A sterile cotton swab moistened with sterile saline is inserted into the cranial vagina and then rolled onto a slide. The smear is then air dried, stained with a hematologic stain, and observed microscopically. When more than 70% of the cells are cornified, the bitch is most likely in standing heat (Fig 5).

Evaluation of Males

Breeding soundness examination of males involves more than just semen evaluation. It should include a good physical examination, evaluation of the reproductive organs, and examination of the ejaculate's quantity, percentage of motile sperm, and percentage of normally shaped sperm. Procedures used in such examinations vary with the species (Table 6).

Semen can be collected by electroejaculation in the bull, ram, tom and anesthetized boar. An artificial vagina can be used in the dog, bull, tom, boar and stallion. Manual stimulation of the penis is effective in producing an ejaculate in the boar and dog. After collection of a semen sample, care must be taken to prevent the sperm from becoming cold or heat shocked, which decreases motility and produces large numbers of secondary abnormalities in the sperm.

Sperm motility is evaluated subjectively as soon after semen collection as possible, using prewarmed slides, preferably on a microscope stage warmed to about 37 C (98.6 F). The *motility score* is the percentage of individual sperm with rapid progressive motility when examined under high power. Bull sperm is evaluated for motility by examining gross motility of all the sperm in the sample under low power. Individual sperm motility is evaluated under high power after diluting the sample with saline or sodium citrate. Expensive computerized machines for assessing motility are available.

After sperm motility is evaluated, a semen smear should be stained and evaluated for *sperm morphologic characteristics*. A smear for morphologic evaluation can be made by staining the sperm with various stains, such as eosin-nigrosin, Cassarett's or fine-grain India ink (positively silhouettes sperm). The stained sample should be smeared onto a slide to produce a thin layer so that individual sperm can be seen in their entirety and counted.

Several hundred sperm should be examined and categorized as normal or affected by a primary abnormality or secondary abnormality (Fig 10). The percentage of each type of sperm should be recorded. Acceptable levels of these abnormalities for each of these species is listed in Table 6. Primary abnormalities of sperm originate in the testis, whereas secondary abnormalities are produced in the extratesticular ducts (epididymis) or are artifacts produced by careless semen handling. Primary abnormalities are predominantly abnormalities of the sperm head but also include some tail abnormalities (Fig 10).

After morphologic evaluation, the *concentration of sperm* in the sample should be evaluated in all species except the bull. In bulls, sperm production is estimated by measuring scrotal circumference. In the other species, the concentration of sperm in the sample is determined by counting sperm with a hemacytometer, Coulter counter, Spectronic 20 calibrated for sperm, or a densimeter. When using a hemacytometer, a WBC pipette or WBC Unopet chamber can be used, but care must be taken to be sure the proper dilution factors are used when calculating the concentration.

Table 6. Semen collection and evaluation in some domestic species.

	Collection Methods							Motility Evaluation		
Species	**Manual**	**Electro-ejaculator**	**Artificial Vagina (temp)**	**Volume (ml)**	**Concentration (millions/ml)**	**Sperm per Ejaculate (billion)**	**Scrotal Circumference Used**	**Gross Motility Evaluated**	**Individual Motility (minimum % acceptable)**	**Morphology (maximum % abnormal acceptable)**
Dog	yes	no	40-42 C	10 (1-25)	125 (20-540)	1.25	no	no	70%	20%
Stallion	no	no	41-50 C	70 (30-250)	120 (30-600)	8.4	yes[c]	no	70%	35%
Boar	yes	yes[a]	45-50 C	250 (125-500)	150 (25-1000)	37.5	yes[c]	no	85%	30%
Bull	yes[b]	yes	40-52 C	4 (1-15)	1200 (300-2500)	4.8	yes[d]	yes[e]	30%[e]	30%

a–must be anesthetized
b–by rectal massage of prostate and seminal vesicles
c–measured by caliper
d–measured with tape – 30 cm @ 15-18 mo; 32 cm @ 18-21 mo; 33 cm @ 21-24 mo; 34 cm @ > 24 mo old
e–general oscillation or better

Figure 10. Characteristics of normal and abnormal sperm. Primary abnormalities are of testicular origin. Secondary abnormalities occur during epididymal transport or ejaculation or after inappropriate semen handling.

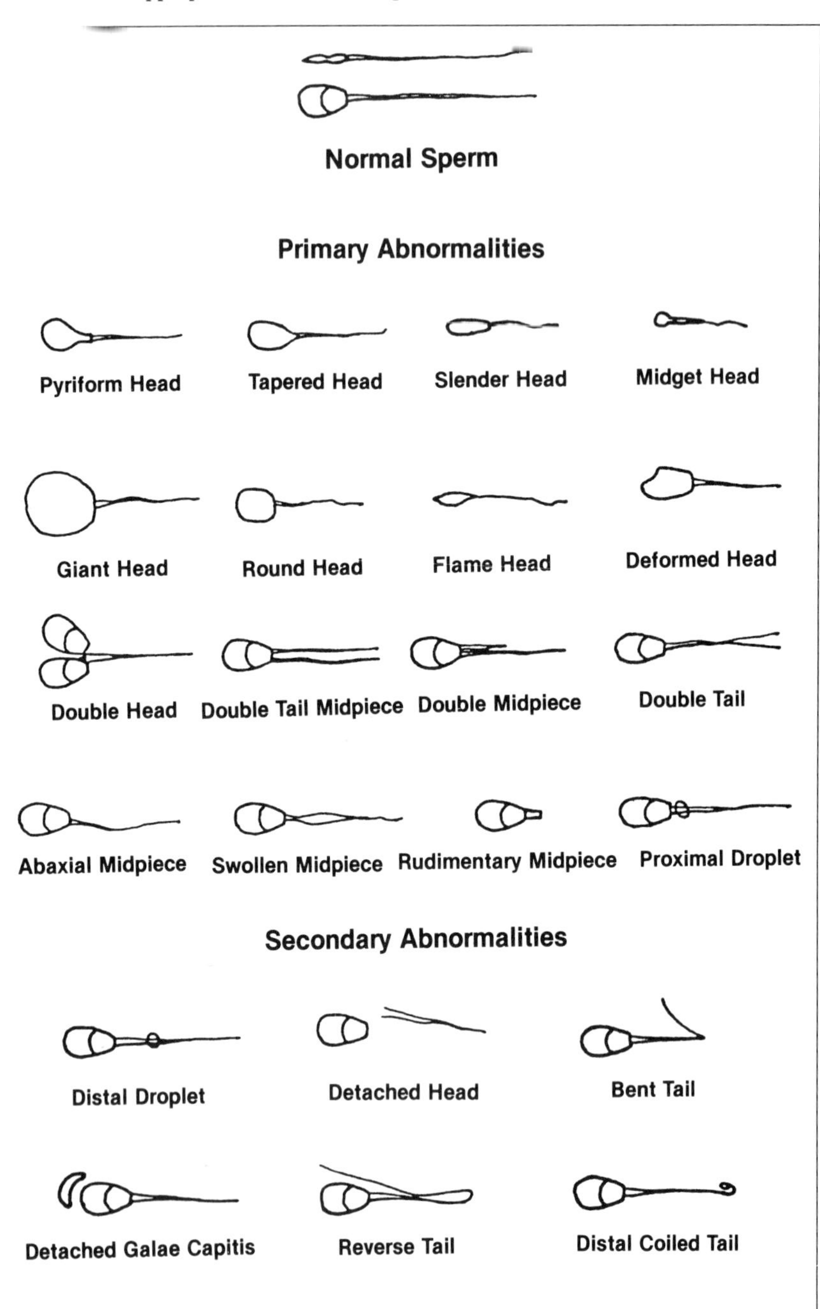

Because the volume of preejaculatory fluid can vary with the artificial means used to collect the semen, a value for the number of sperm per ejaculate is more useful than the concentration in determining the sperm output. The number of sperm per ejaculate is calculated by multiplying sperm concentration by the volume of ejaculate collected.

Any physical or behavioral abnormality of the male that prevents effective copulation is grounds for declaring that animal unsound for breeding, regardless of the semen quality. Poor semen quality may be a permanent or a temporary condition. Reevaluation in 2 months is recommended before the problem can be assumed to be permanent. The Society for Theriogenology (Hastings, NE) has male breeding soundness evaluation forms and guidelines for males of most of the common species that we deal with in veterinary medicine.

ARTIFICIAL INSEMINATION

Successful artificial insemination (AI) depends on accurate determination of the appropriate time to breed, use of high-quality semen, and careful attention to semen handling and insemination techniques.

Cows

Cows are very good about letting everyone know when they are ready to breed. However, it takes time to properly observe their behavior. It is advisable to take at least 30 minutes twice a day, early and late in the day, to observe cows for heat. Cows in heat stand to be mounted by other cows, are usually less interested in eating, act nervous, and vocalize frequently. A long strand of clear mucus is commonly seen draining from the vulva or smeared on the tail or perineum. Though standing heat is the time to breed naturally, AI requires use of the AM/PM rule. That is, cows first seen in heat in the morning (AM) should be inseminated that evening (PM) and *vice versa* (Fig 3).

Frozen semen must be handled carefully to avoid killing or damaging sperm in the straw or ampule. The thawing procedure varies and should be carried out in accordance with the recommendations of the company packaging the semen. In general, ampules are thawed in ice water for 10 minutes. Straws are thawed in warm water (90-95 F) for 45 seconds. Because thawing and refreezing kill the sperm, straws or ampules not being used should not be raised above the “frost line” in the neck of the tank of liquid nitrogen.

Once out of the storage tank, semen should be thawed and deposited in the cow within 15 minutes to ensure viability. The outer surface of the straw or ampule must be dried before loading the semen into the gun or pipette, as water kills sperm. Before inseminating the cow, make sure the vulva is wiped clean and dry.

Placing a sleeved hand just inside the rectum, apply ventral (downward) pressure to open the labia. This helps prevent contamination of the pipette and semen during passage into the vagina. Once the pipette is 3-4 inches into the vagina, extend the hand in the rectum craniad (forward) to identify and grasp the cervix, a firm cylindric structure. Encircle the cervix with the hand or hold it against the bony pelvis with the fingers. Extend the vagina to its full length to eliminate any folds in it, which could interfere with passage of the pipette through the cervix. Use your fingers as a guide to make sure the pipette is in the cervix and not in the fornix (along the thinner vaginal wall, beside the cervix).

The pipette must pass through 3-5 constrictions in the cervix. While passing through these "rings," always keep your fingers in contact with the cranial end of the pipette to guide it, as well as to protect the uterine wall from puncture as the pipette enters the uterus. When the pipette has entered the uterus about one-quarter inch, depress the plunger slowly, depositing the semen. Then withdraw the pipette and examine it for pus or blood.

Mares

Artificial insemination of mares is not as widely practiced as in cows because of breed regulations and the limited availability of frozen equine semen. However, AI may be used in addition to natural breeding to "reinforce" a service in Thoroughbreds and some other breeds. In Quarter Horses, Standardbreds and a few other breeds, AI is used when several mares must be bred at one time. A stallion's ejaculate can be diluted and still have sufficient numbers of viable sperm. Results are satisfactory when breeding is started on day 2 of heat and repeated every other day until the mare goes out of heat.

Regulations for most breeds that allow AI require that the stallion and the mare be on the same farm at the time of AI. In Hanoverians and some other breeds, freezing and shipping of semen to other locations for AI is permitted. Overnight shipping of cooled, extended semen is allowed by some breeds as long as strict record and animal identification standards are met.

Semen is collected with the aid of an artificial vagina. The temperature inside the vagina should be about 41 C (105 F) at the time of collection. A mare in heat or a "dummy" that the stallion is trained to mount is required to collect semen.

Fresh semen samples should be kept as close to 35 C (95 F) as possible to ensure sperm viability. The collection container is often equipped with a filter to help separate the gel from the remainder of the semen. Raw semen can be placed in a warm all-plastic syringe and deposited into the mare's uterus through an infusion pipette, or an extender can be added to the semen if desired.

Adding semen extender to the semen allows more mares to be inseminated and protects the sperm for a short time until deposition into the uterus. There are several acceptable commercially available semen extenders. Semen extenders often contain antibiotics to help control any bacteria that have contaminated the semen during collection or that may have been introduced into the uterus during insemination. A recipe for an acceptable semen extender is listed in Table 7. The dry portion of this extender can be mixed and prepackaged by a pharmacist and stored for up to 6 months. It must be kept in dry containers and protected from light. The liquid portions can then be added before use. The extender should be well mixed and warmed to 35 C (95 F) before adding the semen. The semen can be diluted 1:1 or 1:3 with the extender, depending on the sperm concentration in the semen. It is desirable to have 100-500 million live normal sperm per insemination dose. Extended semen can be stored or shipped for use several days later.

Sows

Sows can be inseminated with fresh or frozen semen, but AI has not been widely accepted in commercial swine production. Some reasons for reluctance of the swine industry to extensively use AI are lack of a reliable means of synchronizing heat in gilts and sows, lower conception rates and smaller litter sizes with use of AI, the limited number (6-8) of raw semen doses per ejaculate relative to the amount of time and work involved in semen collection, and the high level of management required. Also, heat detection and record keeping must be very accurate.

The best time to artificially inseminate sows depends on the heat detection techniques used. Sows checked for heat once daily

Sanalac (instant nonfat dry milk)	2.4 g
gelatin (unflavored, unsweetened)	0.4 g
glucose	4.9 g
gentamicin sulfate (50 mg/ml)	2 ml
7½ sodium bicarbonate solution (sterile)	2 ml
sterile water for injection (no preservatives)	92 ml
Total	100 ml

Table 7. Recipe for equine semen extender.

should be bred every day they stand, for at least 3 days. If heat detection is used twice daily, sows should be inseminated 12 and 24 hours after the onset of heat.

After estrus is detected, semen is collected in an artificial vagina or directly in a prewarmed vacuum-insulated container (*eg,* Thermos bottle) by manually massaging the boar's penis. Semen can be collected while the male is mounted on an estrual female or boars can be trained to mount dummies constructed for this purpose. The semen can be extended 1:4 or 1:5. One ejaculate usually contains enough sperm to inseminate 6-8 females. A minimum of 2 billion live normal sperm per semen dose is needed for adequate conception and large litter sizes. Frozen extended semen is available from at least one commercial source in the US and one in Canada.

When AI is used, relatively large volumes (50-100 ml) of semen are deposited with the aid of a spiral-tipped pipette or an infusion pipette with the most cranial inch bent at a 30-degree angle. These pipettes are actually "screwed" into the cervical rings of the sow.

Bitches

Bitches are usually artificially inseminated with fresh, undiluted semen. However, in the last few years, the American Kennel Club (AKC) has approved registration of litters produced from use of frozen dog semen when semen is collected, stored, transferred and inseminated under very strict rules. There are now 20-30 AKC-approved locations that freeze and store canine semen.

Canine semen is usually collected by manual massage of the penis. Most dogs do not require an estrual bitch present when this is done; however, some timid males may need teasing by a bitch in heat before collection. The collection should be carried out in a quiet room, with good footing for the dog and no distractions.

The dog ejaculates in 3 fractions. The first fraction is clear, contains no sperm and is discarded. The second fraction, the *sperm-rich fraction,* should be collected. The third fraction is clear; after a few drops are collected, the rest is discarded. There may be a 15- to 60-second delay between passage of fractions.

The semen is protected from cold and heat shock and transferred to a prewarmed syringe and deposited in the cranial vagina through an infusion rod. The rear of the bitch should be elevated during and for a few minutes after insemination. Some veterinarians prefer to introduce the index finger, covered with a sterile, powder-free glove, into the vagina with the infusion rod. The finger is left in the vagina for a few minutes and the dorsum of the vaginal vault is stroked gently to stimulate the coital tie between the male and female. It is thought that this induces uterine and vaginal contractions that help the sperm move into the uterus.

Canine sperm is usually not diluted because only one bitch is bred at a time. Bitches usually are artificially inseminated when the selected male cannot or will not copulate. Bitches should be inseminated on the first, third and fifth days of standing heat, or as determined by vaginal cytology and progesterone determination, if available.

Recommended Reading

Feldman EC and Nelson RW: *Canine and Feline Endocrinology and Reproduction.* Saunders, Philadelphia, 1987.

McKinnon AO and Voss JC: *Equine Reproduction.* Lea & Febiger, Philadelphia, 1993.

Morrow DA: *Current Therapy in Theriogenology 2.* Saunders, Philadelphia, 1986.

Pedersen NC: *Feline Husbandry: Diseases and Management in the Multiple-Cat Environment.* American Veterinary Publications, Goleta, CA, 1991.

Notes

Notes

Index

C, continued

D

E

F

F, continued

G

H

I

J

K

L

M

N

O

P

Q

R

S

T

T, continued

U

V

W, X, Y

Z